Annegret Kuhn · Percy Lehmann · Thomas Ruzicka (Eds.)

Cutaneous Lupus Erythematosus

Annegret Kuhn · Percy Lehmann ·
Thomas Ruzicka (Eds.)

Cutaneous Lupus
Erythematosus

With 60 Figures and 42 Tables

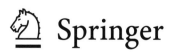
Springer

Priv.-Doz. Dr. Annegret Kuhn
Universitätsklinikum Düsseldorf
Hautklinik
Moorenstraße 5
40225 Düsseldorf, Germany

Prof. Dr. Percy Lehmann
Universitätsklinikum Witten-Herdecke
HELIOS Klinikum Wuppertal
Klinik für Dermatologie, Allergologie
und Umweltmedizin
Arrenbergerstraße 20
42117 Wuppertal, Germany

Prof. Dr. Dr. h.c. Thomas Ruzicka
Universitätsklinikum Düsseldorf
Hautklinik
Moorenstraße 5
40225 Düsseldorf, Germany

ISBN 3-540-44266-9   Springer-Verlag Berlin Heidelberg New York

Library of Congress Cataloging-in-Publication Data
Cutaneous lupus erythematosus / [edited by] Annegret Kuhn, Percy Lehmann, Thomas Ruzicka. p.; cm.
Includes bibliographical references and index.
  ISBN 3-540-44266-9 (alk. paper)
1. Lupus erythematosus. I. Kuhn, Annegret, 1967- II. Lehmann, Percy, 1953- III. Ruzicka, Thomas.
  [DNLM: 1. Lupus Erythematosus, Cutaneous–patholgoy.
2. Lupus Erythematosus, Cutaneous–therapy. WR 152 C988 2004]

Springer is a part of Springer Science+Business Media
springeronline.com

© Springer-Verlag Berlin · Heidelberg 2005

Printed in Germany

Editor: Marion Philipp
Desk Editor: Irmela Bohn
Production: PRO Edit GmbH, 69126 Heidelberg, Germany
Typesetting: SDS, Leimen, Germany
Cover design: Erich Kirchner, 69121 Heidelberg, Germany
24/3150/beu-göh – 5 4 3 2 1 0 – Printed on acid-free paper

Foreword

A comprehensive, in-depth monograph such as this focused entirely on the subject of the cutaneous manifestations of lupus erythematosus (LE) is long overdue!

LE is increasingly being recognized as a more common autoimmune disorder than was previously thought, and the cutaneous manifestations of LE are among the most common clinical features of LE at its onset and throughout its course. The most commonly recognized environmental risk factor for LE, ultraviolet light exposure from sunlight and artificial sources, necessarily transduces its disease-exacerbating effect through the skin. Cutaneous LE can be a significant contributor to psychosocial and occupational disability. In addition, the universally recognized symbols of LE – the butterfly and the wolf – relate to different cutaneous manifestations of LE.

Yet, the skin has been the least well-studied organ system that is affected by LE. This has resulted from the relative "invisibility" of the skin and skin disease to non-dermatologists who deal with patients with LE. After all, "it's only a rash." Perhaps this would be less of a problem if nondermatologist physicians were better trained in the principles and practice of recognizing and managing skin diseases during their formal medical education. Also, contributing to this is the fact that expert management of LE and rheumatic skin disease in general are at risk of being lost from the dermatologist's repertoire in some parts of the world, including the United States.

However, to a relatively small subset of academic dermatologists who subspecialize in the cutaneous manifestations of LE, the protean changes that can occur in the skin of patients with LE can be both fascinating and daunting. How a single disease process plays out so many different themes in a single organ system is truly amazing! This matrix becomes even more complex when one considers the relationships that exist between the various morphologic varieties of skin change in patients with LE and the various systemic manifestations of LE. Much is yet to be learned in this area!

We are indeed fortunate that Drs. Kuhn, Lehmann, and Ruzicka have assembled a highly experienced and expert group of individuals to address the various subjects presented in this monograph. From my perspective, this has been a wonderful, soup-to-nuts tour of our current understanding of all major aspects of LE skin disease. It is my hope that this effort will catalyze further thought and progress in this area.

Iowa City, Iowa, USA
June 2004

Richard D. Sontheimer

Preface

Lupus erythematosus (LE) is a chronic inflammatory autoimmune disease characterized by a wide spectrum of manifestations and a variable evolution. The skin is one of the most frequent sites of involvement, and thus it has long been central to the conceptual framework that physicians have used to deal with this disease. During the past few decades, the mechanisms of cutaneous LE have been under active investigation, and many clinicians and scientists around the world have spent considerable time studying the cutaneous manifestations of this disease. This research has led to the identification of subsets of LE defined by constellations of clinical and photobiological features, histologic and immunopathologic changes, and laboratory abnormalities. Besides the classic forms such as subacute cutaneous LE and discoid LE, there are uncommon variants that often lead to diagnostic difficulties. Therefore, there has long been a need for a book on the cutaneous manifestations of LE that provides not only a comprehensive description of the great variety of cutaneous abnormalities but also a synthesis of our knowledge of the relationship between cutaneous and systemic changes. Furthermore, the cutaneous manifestations of this disease are a reflection of very specific and also nonspecific immunopathologic events along with inflammatory responses, and major progress has been made in recent years in our knowledge of the skin as an immunologic organ. Many advances have also been made in understanding the induction of skin lesions of LE by ultraviolet light combined with alterations in selectins and adhesion molecules contributing to the accumulation of inflammatory cells in this disease. Animal models of LE have further provided insight into the contributing roles of various T-cell subsets. In addition, the management of cutaneous manifestations of LE is challenging, and although conventional topical and systemic therapy exists new treatment options have been introduced for patients with resistant disease.

Cutaneous Lupus Erythematosus is written by leading clinicians and scientists in a multidisciplinary effort and includes chapters on the clinical aspects, pathologic characteristics, and management of this disease. The combination of the latest clinical and scientific data supplemented with colour reproductions of the clinical and pathologic changes of the skin provides a comprehensive summary of information on cutaneous LE. This book acquaints dermatologists, rheumatologists, and general physicians with the skin manifestations of LE, and we further hope that *Cutaneous Lupus Erythematosus* will be a valuable resource for all clinicians who diagnose, treat, and manage patients with this disease. The editors would like to thank all authors for their significant contribution to accomplish this book. In addition, the editors dedicate this book to the memory of their mentor, colleague, and friend Dr. Günther

Goerz, Professor of Dermatology, University of Düsseldorf, Germany, who taught them that LE is exciting, complex, and worth spending a lifetime studying.

Düsseldorf and Wuppertal, Germany   Annegret Kuhn
June 2004   Percy Lehmann
                                                                  Thomas Ruzicka

Contents

Part III
Pathogenesis and Pathologic Features of Cutaneous Lupus Erythematosus

Part IV
Treatment and Management of Cutaneous Lupus Erythematosus

List of Contributors

ANDRADE, FELIPE, M.D., PH.D.
Instituto Nacional de Ciencias
Medicas y Nutricion "Salvador Zubiran"
Department of Immunology
and Rheumatology
Vasco de Quiroga 15
Mexico, D. F. 14000
Mexico

BACMAN, DAVID, M.D.
University of Düsseldorf
Department of Dermatology
Moorenstraße 5
40225 Düsseldorf
Germany

BEISSERT, STEFAN, M.D.
University of Münster
Department of Dermatology
Von-Esmarch-Straße 58
48149 Münster
Germany

CALLEN, JEFFREY P., M.D.
University of Louisville
School of Medicine
Department of Dermatology
310 East Broadway, Suite 200
Louisville KY 40202
USA

CASCIOLA-ROSEN, LIVIA A., PH.D.
John Hopkins University
School of Medicine
Departments of Medicine and Dermatology
5200 Eastern Avenue
Baltimore, Maryland 21224
USA

CERVERA, RICARD, M.D.
University of Barcelona
Hospital Clinic
Department of Autoimmune Diseases
Villarroel, 170
08036 Barcelona, Catalonia
Spain

CUADRADO, MARIA J., M.D., PH.D.
St. Thomas Hospital
The Rayne Institute
Lupus Research Unit
London SE1 7EH
United Kingdom

FLAIG, MICHAEL J., M.D.
Ludwig-Maximilians-University
Department of Dermatology
Frauenlobstraße 9–11
80337 München
Germany

FONT, JOSEP, M.D.
University of Barcelona
Hospital Clinic
Department of Autoimmune Diseases
Villarroel, 170
08036 Barcelona, Catalonia
Spain

FRITSCH, PETER, M.D.
University of Innsbruck
Department of Dermatology
Anichstraße 35
6020 Innsbruck
Austria

FURUKAWA, FUKUMI, M.D., PH.D
Wakayama Medical University
Department of Dermatology
811-1 Kimiidera
Wakayama 641-0012
Japan

HERNDON, THOMAS M., M.D.
Walter Reed Army Institute of Research
Department of Cellular Injury
Robert Grand Road, Building 503
Silver Spring, Maryland 20307-5100
USA

INGELMO, MIGUEL, M.D.
University of Barcelona
Hospital Clinic
Department of Autoimmune Diseases
Villarroel, 170
08036 Barcelona, Catalonia
Spain

JIMÉNEZ, SÒNIA, M.D.
University of Barcelona
Hospital Clinic
Department of Autoimmune Diseases
Villarroel, 170
08036 Barcelona, Catalonia
Spain

KARIM, YOUSUF, MRCP, MRCPATH
St. Thomas Hospital
Department of Immunology
London SE1 7EH
United Kingdom

KIND, PETER, M.D.
Hautarztpraxis
Kleiner Biergrund 31
63065 Offenbach
Germany

KUHN, ANNEGRET, M.D.
University of Düsseldorf
Department of Dermatology
Moorenstraße 5
40225 Düsseldorf
Germany

LEE, LELA A., M.D.
University of Colorado
School of Medicine
Denver Health Medical Center
Department of Dermatology
660 Bannock Street
Denver, Colorado 80204
USA

LEHMANN, PERCY, M.D.
University of Witten-Herdecke
HELIOS Klinikum Wuppertal
Department of Dermatology
Arrenberger Straße 20
42117 Wuppertal
Germany

LUGER, THOMAS A., M.D.
University of Münster
Department of Dermatology
Von-Esmarch-Straße 58
48149 Münster
Germany

MEHLING, ANNETTE, PH.D
Cognis Deutschland GmbH and Co. KG
Henkelstrasse 67
40551 Düsseldorf
Germany

MEURER, MICHAEL, M.D.
University of Dresden
Department of Dermatology
Fetscherstraße 74
01307 Dresden
Germany

MILLARD, THOMAS P., M.D.
Gloucester Royal Hospital
Department of Dermatology
Gloucester, GL1 3NN
United Kingdom

NYBERG, FILIPPA, M.D., PH.D.
Danderyds Hospital
Department of Dermatology
18288 Stockholm
Sweden

OCHSENDORF, FALK R., M.D.
University of Frankfurt
Department of Dermatology
Theodor-Stern-Kai 7
60590 Frankfurt
Germany

ORFANOS, CONSTANTIN E., M.D.
The Free University of Berlin
University Medical Center Benjamin Franklin
Department of Dermatology
Fabeckstraße 60-62
14195 Berlin
Germany

PRAMATAROV, KYRILL, M.D., PH.D.
Medical University
Department of Dermatology
1, G. Sofiiski Street
1431 Sofia
Bulgaria

PROVOST, THOMAS T., M.D.
P.O. Box 230
Milton, Delaware 19968
USA

ROSEN, ANTONY, M.D.
John Hopkins University
School of Medicine
Departments of Medicine, Cell Biology and
Anatomy
5200 Eastern Avenue
Baltimore, Maryland 21224
USA

ROSENBAUM, MICHELE L., M.D.
University of Pennsylvania
School of Medicine
Department of Dermatology
2 Rhoads Pavilion, 36th and Spruce Sts.
Philadelphia, Pennsylvania 19104
USA

RUZICKA, THOMAS, M.D.
University of Düsseldorf
Department of Dermatology
Moorenstraße 5
40225 Düsseldorf
Germany

SANDER, CHRISTIAN A., M.D.
AK St. Georg
Department of Dermatology
Lohmuehlenstrasse 4
20099 Hamburg
Germany

SCHNEIDER, MATTHIAS, M.D.
University of Düsseldorf
Department of Rheumatology
Moorenstraße 5
40225 Düsseldorf
Germany

SCHNEIDER, STEFAN W., M.D.
University of Münster
Department of Dermatology
Von-Esmarch-Straße 58
48149 Münster
Germany

SCHWARZ, THOMAS, M.D.
University of Schleswig-Holstein
Campus Kiel
Department of Dermatology
Schittenhelmstrasse 7
24105 Kiel
Germany

SHINADA, SHUNTARO, M.D.
University of Southern California Medical
Center
Los Angeles County
1200 North State Street
Los Angeles, California 90033
USA

SONTHEIMER, RICHARD D., M.D.
University of Iowa
Carver College of Medicine
Department of Dermatology
200 Hawkins Dr. 2045BT-1
Iowa City, Iowa 52242-1090
USA

SPECKER, CHRISTOF, M.D.
University of Düsseldorf
Department of Rheumatology
Moorenstraße 5
40225 Düsseldorf
Germany

STEPHANSSON, EIJA, M.D., PH.D.
Karolinska Hospital Stockholm
Department of Dermatology
17176 Stockholm
Sweden

STICHERLING, MICHAEL, M.D.
University of Leipzig
Department of Dermatology
Stephanstraße 11
04103 Leipzig
Germany

TEBBE, BEATE, M.D.
Praxis für Dermatologie und Allergologie
Hohenzollerndamm 91
14199 Berlin
Germany

TSANKOV, NIKOLAI, M.D.
Medical University
Department of Dermatology
1, G. Sofiiski Street
1431 Sofia
Bulgaria

TSOKOS, GEORGE C., M.D.
Walter Reed Army Institute of Research
Department of Cellular Injury
Robert Grand Road, Building 503
Silver Spring, Maryland 20307-5100
USA

UETRECHT, JACK, M.D., PH.D.
University of Toronto
Faculty of Pharmacy
19 Russell Street
Toronto, M4G 3L5
Canada

VON MIKECZ, ANNA, PH.D.
University of Düsseldorf
Institut für Umweltmedizinische Forschung
Auf'm Hennekamp 50
40225 Düsseldorf
Germany

WALLACE, DANIEL J., M.D.
Cedars Sinai Medical Center
UCLA School of Medicine
8737 Beverly Blvd., Suite 203
Los Angeles, California 90048
USA

WEBER, FLORIAN, M.D.
University of Innsbruck
Department of Dermatology
Anichstraße 35
6020 Innsbruck
Austria

WERTH, VICTORIA P., M.D.
University of Pennsylvania
School of Medicine
Department of Dermatology
2 Rhoads Pavilion, 36th and Spruce Sts.
Philadelphia, Pennsylvania 19104
USA

WETZEL, STEFANIE, M.D.
Ludwig-Maximilians-University
Department of Dermatology
Frauenlobstraße 9–11
80337 München
Germany

WOLLENBERG, ANDREAS, M.D.
Ludwig-Maximilians-University
Department of Dermatology
Frauenlobstraße 9–11
80337 München
Germany

YAZDI, AMIR S., M.D.
Ludwig-Maximilians-University
Department of Dermatology
Frauenlobstraße 9–11
80337 München
Germany

Abbreviations

ACA = anticardiolipin antibody
ACLE = acute cutaneous lupus erythematosus
ACR = American College of Rheumatology
ADCC = antibody-dependent cellular cytotoxicity
ANA = antinuclear antibody
APC = antigen-presenting cell
APS = antiphospholipid syndrome
ARA = American Rheumatism Association
BCR = B-cell receptor
BLE = bullous lupus erythematosus
CCLE = chronic cutaneous lupus erythematosus
cDNA = complementary DNA
CHLE = chilblain lupus erythematosus
CHS = contact hypersensitivity
CI = confidence interval
CLE = cutaneous lupus erythematosus
CR = complement receptor
CS = corticosteroids
CTLA-4 = cytotoxic T-lymphocyte activation molecule-4
DC = dendritic cell
DEJ = dermoepidermal junction
DIF = direct immunofluorescence
DLE = discoid lupus erythematosus
DM = dermatomyositis
ds-DNA = double-stranded DNA
DTH = delayed-type hypersensitivity
EADV = European Academy of Dermatology and Venereology
EBV = Epstein-Barr virus
ELISA = enzyme-linked immunosorbent assay
EM = erythema multiforme
ESR = erythrocyte sedimentation rate
FasL = Fas ligand
FITC = fluorescein isothiocyanate
G-6-PD = glucose-6-phosphate dehydrogenase
GC = glucocorticoid
GVH = graft-vs-host

HLA = human leukocyte antigen
HUVS = hypocomplementemic urticarial vasculitis
ICAM-1 = intercellular adhesion molecule-1
ICLE = intermittent cutaneous lupus erythematosus
IFN = interferon
IL = interleukin
iNOS = inducible nitric oxide synthase
IPF = immune protection factor
LAT = linker for activation of T cells
LBT = lupus band test
LE = lupus erythematosus
LEP = lupus erythematosus profundus
LET = lupus erythematosus tumidus
LFA-1 = lymphocyte function-associated antigen-1
LFT = liver function test
LP = lichen planus
MHC = major histocompatibility complex
MMF = mycophenolate mofetil
MNC = mononuclear cell
MPF = mutation protection factor
mRNA = messenger RNA
NFAT = nuclear factor of activated T cell
NKT = natural killer cell
NLE = neonatal lupus erythematosus
NZB = New Zealand Black
NZW = New Zealand White
OR = odds ratio
PABA = p-aminobenzoic acid
p-ANCAs = antineutrophil cytoplasmic antibodies with a perinuclear pattern
PCT = porphyria cutanea tarda
PDC = plasmacytoid dendritic cell
PPD = purified protein derivative
PS = phosphatidylserine
PLE = polymorphous light eruption
PNM = papular and nodular mucinosis
RAR = retinoid acid receptors
REM = reticular erythematous mucinosis
RES = reticuloendothelial system
RoRNP = Ro ribonucleoprotein
RXR = retinoid x receptors
SBC = sunburn cell
SCID = severe combined immunodeficient
SCLE = subacute cutaneous lupus erythematosus
SLAM = Systemic Lupus Activity Measure
SLE = systemic lupus erythematosus
SLEDAI = Systemic Lupus Erythematosus Disease Activity Index
snRNP = small nuclear ribonucleoprotein

SS = Sjögren's syndrome
ss-DNA = single-stranded DNA
T4N5 = T4 endonuclease V
TCR = T-cell receptor
Th1 = T helper 1
Th2 = T helper 2
TNF = tumor necrosis factor
UV = ultraviolet
VCAM-1 = vascular adhesion molecule-1
VSV = vesicular stomatitis virus

Part I
Introduction

CHAPTER 1

What is Autoimmunity: Basic Mechanisms and Concepts

Thomas M. Herndon, George C. Tsokos

In 1901, Ehrlich postulated that "organisms possess certain contrivances by means of which the immune reaction […] is prevented from acting against (its) own elements." Such "contrivances" constitute what in modern terms is designated as "tolerance" and, still in Ehrlich's words, "… are of the highest importance for the individual." Several decades later, when autoimmune diseases were described, they were interpreted as the result of a breakdown or failure of the normal tolerance to self, resulting in the development of an autoimmune response. Ehrlich's hypothesis was apparently supported by the definition of pathogenic mechanisms for different diseases considered as autoimmune in which the abnormal anti-self-immune reaction played the main role. In the 1940s, Owen, a British biologist, was involved in ontogeny studies using bovine dizygotic twins, which share the same placenta. Under these circumstances, each animal is exposed to cells expressing the genetic markers of the nonidentical twin during ontogenic development and they become tolerant to each other's antigens.

The first theory concerning tolerance, described by Burnet, Fenner, and Medawar, stated that self-tolerance is achieved by the elimination of autoreactive clones during the differentiation of the immune system. However, the development of autoimmune diseases proved that deletion of these clones was not absolute but that the remaining clones must be silenced or anergized to self-antigens, and that none of these mechanisms is foolproof for all individuals (Tsokos and Virella 2001).

Definition and General Characteristics of Tolerance

Tolerance is best defined as a state of antigen-specific immunologic unresponsiveness. This definition has several important implications: (a) When tolerance is experimentally induced it does not affect the immune response to antigens other than the one used to induce tolerance. This is a very important characteristic that differentiates tolerance from generalized immunosuppression, in which there is depression of the immune response to a wide array of different antigens. Tolerance may be transient or permanent, whereas immunosuppression is usually transient. (b) Tolerance must be established at the clonal level. In other words, if tolerance is antigen-specific it must involve the T- or a B-lymphocyte clone(s) specific for the antigen in question and not affect any other clones (von Boehmer and Kisielow 1990).

Clonal Deletion

T lymphocytes are massively produced in the thymus and, once generated, will not rearrange their receptors. Memory T cells are very long lived, and there is no clear evidence that new ones are generated after the thymus ceases to function in early adulthood. Therefore, elimination of autoreactive T cells must occur at the production site (thymus) at the time the cells are differentiating their T-cell receptor (TCR) repertoire. Once a T-cell clone has been eliminated, there is no risk of reemergence of that particular clone.

B-cell clonal deletion involves different mechanisms than T-cell clonal deletion. B cells are continuously produced by bone marrow throughout life, and they initially express low-affinity immunoglobulin (Ig) M on their membranes. In most instances, interaction of these resting B cells with circulating self-molecules neither activates them nor causes their elimination. Selection and deletion of autoreactive clones seem to take place in the peripheral lymphoid organs during onset of the immune response. At that time, activated B cells can modify the structure of their membrane immunoglobulin as a consequence of somatic mutations in their germline genes. B cells expressing self-reactive immunoglobulins of high affinity can emerge from this process, and their elimination takes place in the germinal centers of the peripheral lymphoid tissues (Blackman et al. 1990, von Boehmer 1994, Cyster et al. 1994).

Clonal Anergy

T- and B-cell clonal deletion fail to eliminate all autoreactive cells. In the case of T cells, those that recognize self-antigens not expressed in the thymus will eventually be released and will reach the peripheral lymphoid tissues. The causes of B-cell escape from clonal deletion are not as well defined, but they exist nonetheless. Thus, peripheral tolerance mechanisms must exist to ensure that autoreactive clones of T and B cells are neutralized after their migration to the peripheral lymphoid tissues. Clonal anergy is one such mechanism. Clonal anergy can be defined as the process that incapacitates or disables autoreactive clones that escape selection by clonal deletion. Anergic clones lack the ability to respond to stimulation with the corresponding antigen. The most obvious manifestation of clonal anergy is the inability to respond to proper stimulation. Anergic B cells carry IgM autoreactive antibody in their membrane but are not activated as a result of an antigenic encounter. Anergic T cells express TCR for the tolerizing antigen but fail to properly express the interleukin (IL)-2 and IL-2 receptor genes and to proliferate in response to it. Anergy results either from an internal block of the intracellular signaling pathways or from the down-regulating effects exerted by suppressor cells, and it can be experimentally induced after the ontogenic differentiation of immunocompetent cells has reached a stage in which clonal deletion is no longer possible (Singer and Abbas 1994).

There is now ample evidence suggesting that tolerance results from a combination of clonal deletion and clonal anergy. Both processes must coexist and complement each other under normal conditions so that autoreactive clones that escape deletion during embryonic development may be down-regulated and become anergic. Failure of either of these mechanisms may result in development of an autoimmune disease.

Proper stimulation of mature CD4[+] T lymphocytes requires at least two signals: one delivered by interaction of the TCR with the major histocompatibility complex (MHC) II-antigen complex and the other delivered by the accessory cell. Both signals require cell–cell contact involving a variety of surface molecules and the release of soluble cytokines. When all of these signals are properly transmitted to the T lymphocyte, a state of activation ensues. Several experiments suggest that the state of anergy develops when TCR-mediated signaling is not followed by co-stimulatory signals. If T lymphocytes are stimulated with chemically fixed accessory cells (which cannot release cytokines or up-regulate membrane molecules involved in the delivery of co-stimulatory signals) or with purified MHC-II-antigen complexes (which also cannot provide co-stimulatory signals), anergy results (Burkly et al. 1990). From the multitude of co-stimulatory pairs of molecules that have been described, the CD28/CTLA-4-B7 family is the most significant in the physiology of T-cell anergy. CD28-mediated signals are necessary for the production of IL-2, which seems to be critical for the initial proliferation of T_H0 cells and the eventual differentiation of T_H1 cells. If the interaction between CD28 and its ligand is prevented at onset of the immune response, anergy and tolerance ensue. If cytotoxic T-lymphocyte activation molecule-4 (CTLA)-4 is engaged instead of CD28, a down-regulating signal is delivered to the T-lymphocyte. Obviously, a better understanding of the regulatory mechanisms controlling the expression of alternative CD28 ligands is needed for our understanding of how a state of anergy is induced and perpetuated. It is possible that a parallel could be defined for B-cell anergy. The CD40 (B cells)-CD40 ligand (T cells) interaction is critically important for B-cell differentiation. In the absence of CD40 signaling, B cells are easy to tolerize (Rathmell et al. 1996, Thomson 1995).

It is possible to interpret the differences between high-zone and low-zone tolerance as a result of differences in the degree of co-stimulation received by T cells. In high-zone tolerance, the co-stimulatory signals are excessively strong and both T and B cells are down-regulated. Very low antigen doses fail to induce the delivery of co-stimulatory signals to T cells, and low-zone T-cell tolerance ensues (Goodnow 1992).

Down-Regulation of the Immune Response

Many different mechanisms are involved in the down-regulation of the immune response. Extreme situations of down-regulation may very well be indistinguishable from tolerance. This similarity between activation of suppressor circuits and clonal anergy is made more obvious by the fact that the experimental protocols used to induce one or the other were virtually identical. Several mechanisms have been proposed to explain the down-regulation of the immune response (Weiner et al. 1994).

Two types of mononuclear cells (MNCs) seem to be capable of suppressor activity: lymphocytes and monocytes. Recently, CD4[+] cells, which express CD25 on the surface, have been shown to act as regulators (suppressors) of the immune response in a variety of experimental conditions (Groux and Powerie 1999).

Termination of Tolerance

If tolerance depends on maintenance of a state of anergy, several possible scenarios could explain the termination of tolerance:

1. *Clonal regeneration.* Because new B lymphocytes are constantly produced from stem cells, if a tolerogenic dose of antigen is not maintained, the immune system will eventually replace aging, tolerant cells with young, nontolerant cells and recover the ability to mount an immune response.
2. *Cross-immunization.* Exposure to an antigen that cross-reacts with a tolerogen may induce activation of T-helper (Th) lymphocytes specific for the cross-reacting antigen and provide autoreactive B lymphocytes with the co-stimulatory signals necessary to initiate a response against the tolerogen.
3. *Co-stimulation of anergic clones.* It was discussed previously that anergy may be the result of incomplete stimulation of T lymphocytes. Thus, it can be postulated that proper stimulation of T lymphocytes by reestablishing the co-stimulatory pathway can terminate anergy and initiate the autoreactive process (Silverstein and Rose 2000).

Autoimmunity

Failure of the immune system to "tolerate" self-tissues may result in pathologic processes known as autoimmune diseases. At the clinical level, autoimmunity is involved in a variety of apparently unrelated diseases, such as systemic lupus erythematosus (SLE), insulin-dependent diabetes mellitus, myasthenia gravis, rheumatoid arthritis, multiple sclerosis, and hemolytic anemias. There are at least 40 diseases known or considered to be autoimmune, affecting about 5% of the general population. Their distribution by sex and age is not uniform. As a rule, autoimmune diseases predominate in females and have a bimodal age distribution. A first peak of incidence is around puberty, and the second peak is in the forties and fifties.

There are several different ways to classify autoimmune diseases. Because several autoimmune diseases are strongly linked with MHC antigens, one of the most recently proposed classifications, given in Table 1.1, groups autoimmune diseases

Table 1.1. Classification of autoimmune diseases

I. Major histocompatibility complex class II associated
A. Organ specific
(autoantibody directed against a single organ or closely related organs)
B. Systemic
(systemic lupus erythematosus – variety of autoantibodies to DNA, cytoplasmic antigens, etc)
II. Major histocompatibility complex class I associated
A. HLA-B27-related spondyloarthropathies
(ankylosing spondylitis, Reiter's syndrome, etc.)
B. Psoriasis vulgaris
(which is associated with HLA-B13, HLA-B16, and HLA-B17)

according to their association with class I or class II MHC markers. Although both sexes may be afflicted by autoimmune diseases, there is a female preponderance for the class II-associated diseases and a definite increase in the prevalence of class I-associated diseases among males.

The effector mechanisms in the development of autoimmune pathology and disease involve autoantibodies, immune complexes, and autoreactive T cells. These mechanisms are exemplified in SLE, and because LE is the study object of this book, we present them in that context in the following pages (Theofilopoulos 2002).

Systemic Lupus Erythematosus

SLE is a complex autoimmune disease involving several organs. The main effectors of disease pathology are the diverse autoantibodies, immune complexes, and autoreactive cells. Altered biology of immune cells, keratinocytes, and endothelial and possibly other cells invariably contributes to the expression of the disease. At the pathogenic level, the disease presents unprecedented complexity involving an as-yet-unspecified number of genes, immunoregulatory aberrations, and environmental and hormonal factors. Previous and current research efforts have elucidated the complex array of genetic, environmental, hormonal, and immunoregulatory factors thought to interplay in the pathogenesis of the disease.

Autoantibodies and Immune Complexes

SLE is characterized by the production of a large list of antibodies against an array of non-organ-specific self-antigens present in the nucleus, cytoplasm, cell membrane, and serum. An immune response against self is commonly part of the normal immune response and is strictly regulated. Immune cells with autoreactive potential are present in large numbers in healthy individuals, and germline genes encoding for antigen receptors of autoreactive T and B cells are part of the normal gene repertoire. Autoreactive cells are positively selected in an antigen-driven manner (Nemazee 2000, Tonegawa 1983).

IgM antibodies to DNA are frequently produced in the normal host and bind to single-stranded (ss)DNA; they have low affinity for DNA and broad cross-reactivity with a variety of other self-antigens. The production of these natural anti-DNA antibodies is tightly regulated, and they usually do not undergo isotype switching and are encoded by germline genes; affinity maturation by the process of somatic mutation does not occur. On the contrary, anti-DNA antibodies in the serum of patients with SLE have quite different features in that they have undergone isotype switching to IgG of various subclasses, and germline genes usually do not encode them because new amino acids are introduced into their variable regions to enhance affinity (somatic mutations and hypermutations). Continuous receptor editing in lupus B cells may provide an additional impetus toward production of more "pathogenic" autoantibodies. Because DNA is a highly anionic macromolecule, positively charged amino acids, particularly arginine, are introduced into the autoantibody-variable regions to enhance DNA binding. Lupus anti-DNA antibodies are thus usually charged, IgG, relatively low cross-reactive and have high affinity towards double-stranded (ds)DNA.

T cells from patients with LE, activated by nucleosomes, provide help to lupus B cells to produce anti-dsDNA of the IgG class. DNA, nucleosomes, and other intracellular autoantigens that are common targets for the lupus immune system are made accessible to immune cells during apoptosis. These autoantigens can be found in surface blebs of dying apoptotic keratinocytes after ultraviolet (UV) light exposure. It is possible that exposure of a genetically susceptible individual to environmental factors causing apoptosis may serve as the trigger to form anti-DNA and other autoantibodies. The ability of an individual to produce anti-DNA antibodies is, to some degree, genetically determined (see Chap. 15).

Several lines of evidence have led to the classification of lupus as an immune complex disease. Immune complexes have been documented in the serum of patients with LE, and both immunoglobulin and complement factors or split products have been detected in several tissues, including kidneys and skin. In addition, hypocomplementemia and increased levels of complement split factors are found in the serum and urine of patients with LE.

Cells expressing Fc and complement receptors, such as monocytes, phagocytes, and neutrophils, mediate clearance of immune complexes. Immune complex clearance is decreased in patients with LE, perhaps owing to abnormal Fc receptor function, resulting from the expression of alleles that bind IgG with lesser affinity or decreased numbers or altered allele expression of complement receptor 1.

The number of involved antigen and antibody molecules defines the lattice of an immune complex. The size and extent of lattice formation determine the rate of clearance and tissue deposition of immune complexes, and the number of Fc molecules in each immune complex defines its ability to bind to Fc receptors and trigger Fc-mediated cell functions. Large immune complexes (>Ag2Ab2) are quickly cleared by the reticuloendothelial system, and, when saturated, they deposit to tissues. Large immune complexes tend to activate complement more efficiently. Small immune complexes have a lesser tendency to deposit to tissues. The initial interaction may involve the charge of the antibody, as with deposition to kidneys, binding to an Fc or complement receptor or by specific or nonspecific binding of the F(ab')2 fragment of the involved antibody.

Immune complexes in the serum of patients with LE have distinct reasons to deposit to tissues in that those containing cationic anti-DNA antibodies facilitate binding to the kidney basement membrane. These antibodies are of IgG1, IgG2, and IgG3 subclasses and can activate complement effectively. In addition to anti-DNA antibodies, other nephrophilic antibodies can bind to the kidneys and instigate the formation of immune complexes and disease (Davidson and Diamond 2001).

Cellular and Cytokine Aberrations in Lupus Erythematosus

A great deal of literature is devoted to the description of the multiple and frequently contradictory immune cell abnormalities encountered in SLE, since aberrations of the immune cells are believed to play a major role in the pathogenesis of lupus. These studies have improved our understanding of the disease, helped us design novel treatments, and guided the search for the involved genes. Although the cellular aberrations in LE may reflect secondary effects, therapeutic modulation of the cellular abnormalities represents a plausible way to improve the management of patients with LE (Tsokos and Boumbas 2002).

Monocytes from patients with LE display a variety of abnormalities, including decreases in phagocytic activity, IL-1 production, expression of surface human leukocyte antigen (HLA)-DR, and accessory function for T-cell activation. In addition, LE monocytes fail to express the co-stimulatory B7 molecules after activation. These defects may partially explain the defective responses of lupus T cells to nominal antigens. In contrast, peripheral blood monocytes from patients with LE display increased rates of spontaneous apoptosis and can contribute to the increased levels of circulating autoantigens. Decreased phagocytic function may increase susceptibility of patients with LE to infections.

T-cell abnormalities are crucial in the pathogenesis of the disease because they regulate B-cell function, and the production of most of the pathogenic autoantibodies is T-cell dependent. T-lymphocyte abnormalities in patients with LE have been reviewed. Human studies of lupus lymphocyte biology are limited to peripheral blood lymphocytes and, in general, have established two apparently opposing (T-cell enigma) phenomena: the existence of activated T cells that provide excessive help to B cells to produce autoantibodies and yet the inability to respond in vitro to nominal antigens and produce IL-2.

The presence of activated T cells in the peripheral blood of patients with LE has been inferred from the presence of increased numbers of cells expressing DR^+ antigens and the expression of increased levels of *c-myc* messenger RNA (mRNA). Studies of *hprt* gene-mutated T cells have provided evidence for the existence of rapidly dividing T cells in the peripheral blood of patients with LE.

The existence of T cells that provide help to B cells to produce autoantibodies has been shown clearly in studies of IL-2-expanded lines and clones. Specifically, IL-2-expanded T-cell lines established from patients with lupus nephritis helped autologous B cells produce cationic anti-DNA antibodies. Most of the T-helper cell lines were $CD4^+$, whereas a small fraction were $\alpha\beta$ TCR^+ $CD4^-$ $CD8^-$ and $\gamma\delta$ TCR^+. Clones reactive with the presumptive autoantigen small nuclear ribonucleoprotein (snRNP) have been established from both patients with LE and healthy individuals who carry the HLA-DR2 or HLA-DR4 genotypes after stimulation of peripheral blood MNCs with IL-2 and snRNP and they were found to frequently use the $V\beta6$ TCR gene.

Lupus T cells have been shown to produce decreased amounts of IL-2. Both $CD4^+$ and $CD8^+$ cells are responsible for this deficiency. Decreased IL-2 secretion, in vitro, by lupus cells correlates with increased disease activity, lack of previous treatment, and increased numbers of spontaneously immunoglobulin-secreting B cells.

Peripheral blood MNCs from patients with LE produce less interferon (IFN)-γ spontaneously and after stimulation with phytohemagglutinin or IL-2 or certain viruses. Decreased IFN-γ production may contribute to a higher incidence of infections in patients with SLE. These findings contrast reports of patients with rheumatoid arthritis who developed LE after systemic administration of IFN-γ, suggesting that IFN-γ may promote autoimmunity. Lymphocytes from lupus-prone mice express increased levels of IFN-γ mRNA, and IFN-γ may promote autoimmunity by enhancing the expression of autoantigens.

The most important function of IL-6 is the promotion of immunoglobulin production by activated B cells and Epstein-Barr virus (EBV)-transformed B cells. Lupus

MNCs express high levels of mRNA for IL-6. The increased levels of IL-6 that were reported in the cerebrospinal fluid of patients with central nervous system involvement fluctuated with disease activity and may be involved in disease pathology.

Several studies have shown convincingly that IL-10 production is significantly elevated in patients with SLE and that IL-10 overproduction is implicated in the generation of anti-DNA antibodies. Up-regulated IL-10 production characterizes not only patients with LE but also healthy members of lupus multiplex families as well as affected first- and even second-degree relatives of patients with SLE. Treatment of SCID mice transplanted with human lupus MNCs with an anti-IL-10 antibody caused diminished production of anti-dsDNA antibodies.

The previously cited studies indicate that SLE is characterized by an imbalance in the ratio of type 1 (IFN-γ and IL-2)-type 2 (IL-4, IL-5, IL-6, and IL-10) cytokine-secreting MNCs. However, it is simplistic at this point to state that human lupus is a Th2 disease when there is evidence that even in NZB/NZW mice both type 2 (IL-4) and type 1 (IFN-γ and IL-12) lymphokines are needed for expression of the disease.

In contrast to the circulating T-cell pool, B cells from patients with LE are not numerically decreased but display increased proliferation rates and spontaneously secrete increased amounts of immunoglobulin, including autoantibodies. The amount of spontaneously released immunoglobulin from lupus B cells accurately correlates with disease activity. Polyclonal hypergammaglobulinemia is common in patients with SLE.

Although freshly isolated B cells and $CD4^+$ and $CD8^+$ T-lymphocyte subpopulations from patients with LE express higher levels of Fas antigen compared with normal cells, mitogenic stimulation of cell subsets causes normal Fas antigen up-regulation. The increased expression of Fas is accompanied by higher rates of spontaneous apoptosis. Activated T cells from patients with LE are relatively resistant to a TCR-mediated death stimulus, which may lead to prolonged survival of activated autoreactive cells.

The CD40-CD40 ligand (CD40L) interaction seems to be aberrant in lupus. Although the number of circulating $CD40L^+$ T cells in patients with LE is not increased compared with that in healthy individuals, its induction in lupus $CD4^+$ and $CD8^+$ T cells is both enhanced and sustained. Moreover, it was reported that lupus B cells unexpectedly express CD40L on stimulation in an equally intense manner as T cells. This abnormally regulated molecule in lupus lymphocytes is still functional because anti-CD40L monoclonal antibody inhibited the production of anti-DNA antibodies, and lupus $CD40L^+$ cells induced the expression of CD80 (B7-1) in a B-cell line. The importance of this interaction in SLE is underscored by experiments showing that administration of a single dose of anti-CD40L monoclonal antibody in mice with lupus caused significant delay in the appearance of nephritis and substantially improved the survival of such animals without compromising the nonautoimmune response.

Abnormalities in the expression of CD80 and CD86 on the cell surface of peripheral blood B cells from patients with SLE have also been reported. Levels of CD86 expression on resting and activated lupus B cells were greater than the levels of normal B cells. CD80 was also significantly overexpressed in activated but not in resting B cells from patients with LE. Therefore, overexpression of co-stimulatory molecules on circulating B cells in patients with SLE may play a role in the continuous autoreactive T-cell help to lupus B cells, leading to the production of autoantibodies.

Non-B-cell antigen-presenting cells from patients with LE fail to up-regulate in vitro surface expression of CD80 after stimulation with IFNγ in a disease-specific fashion. Replenishment of functional CD80 molecules in the culture environment significantly increased the responses of SLE T cells to tetanus toxoid and to an anti-CD3 antibody. Similarly, the decreased responses of lupus T cells to anti-CD2 antibody are reversed in the presence of CD28-mediated stimulation.

T lymphocytes may express abnormally high levels of surface molecules that facilitate attachment to endothelial or other cells. Certain pairs of molecules are involved exclusively in providing the co-stimulatory signal to T cells, whereas other pairs of molecules are involved in cell co-stimulation and adhesion/homing. Distinct sets of surface molecules participate in the cell-cell and cell-matrix adhesion process. Members of the β1-integrin family of adhesion molecules are major adhesive receptors for the extracellular matrix, and members of the β2-integrin family (VLA4 and VLA3) are involved in cell-cell and cell-extracellular matrix adhesion.

Expression of adhesion molecules is up-regulated in various disease conditions, such as atherosclerosis, inflammation, and rheumatoid arthritis. VLA4 and LFA1 are overexpressed on the surface membrane of SLE lymphocytes. Interestingly, VLA4 is overexpressed only in lymphocytes from patients with vasculitis. Lymphocytes from these patients show increased adhesion to cord vein endothelial cells (see Chap. 19).

Membrane-Mediated Signal Transduction in Lupus Immune Cells

After engagement of the antigen receptor either with a specific antigen or with an antireceptor antibody, multiple well-regulated intracellular signaling pathways are triggered in the form of biochemical cascades. A critical event in these cascades is the mobilization of Ca^{2+} from intracellular stores, followed by an influx of Ca^{2+} from the extracellular space. The Ca^{2+} response is shared by many cell types, but the presence of specialized Ca^{2+}-sensitive enzymes and transcription factors found in specific tissues dictates the transcription of cell type-specific genes.

Fresh circulating lupus T cells (whole T cells, $CD4^+$ cells, and $CD8^+$ cells) as well as lupus T-cell lines and autoantigen-specific lupus T-cell clones displayed significantly increased free intracellular Ca^{2+} responses compared with the responses of T lymphocytes, T-cell lines, or autoantigen-specific T-cell clones from healthy individuals or patients with systemic autoimmune diseases other than SLE.

The mechanism for the increased intracellular Ca^{2+} responses is not known at this point, although involvement of linker for activation of T cells (LAT) and overactivation of phospholipase C-gamma (PLC-γ) have been suggested. The possibility of defective down-regulation of the Ca^{2+} response is attractive, and one candidate for such a role is the Ca^{2+}-response down-regulator cyclic adenosine monophosphate-dependent protein kinase A type I. Activation of protein kinase A type I in T cells decreases the efflux of intracellularly stored free calcium. The Ca^{2+} pathway critically influences nuclear factor of activated T-cell (NFAT)-mediated transcription of genes such as those of CD40L and Fas ligand (FasL), and, therefore, lupus lymphocytes should express more surface membrane CD40L and FasL owing to their higher Ca^{2+} responses. Indeed, after activation, lupus T cells overexpress FasL and CD40L, which are functional.

Stimulation of lupus T cells with anti-CD3 antibodies significantly enhanced production of tyrosyl-phosphorylated cellular proteins, which reached maximal levels earlier than normal cells. The reason for this overproduction of phosphotyrosine proteins is currently unknown. The TCRζ chain (member of the zeta family of proteins) is part of the hetero-oligomeric TCR/CD3 complex. Although the TCRζ homodimer and the invariant CD3γ, δ, and ε chains do not play a role in antigen recognition, they are the signal-transducing subunits of the antigen-receptor complex. Expression of the TCRζ chain was found deficient in T cells of two thirds of the patients with LE, whereas it was always present in T cells from healthy individuals or from patients without SLE. In some patients with LE, the TCRζ mRNA was also either absent or decreased, correlating with the presence, deficiency, or absence of the ζ polypeptide. TCRζ chain deficiency was first reported in tumor-infiltrating lymphocytes in both humans and experimental models. Transcription of the ζ chain gene depends heavily on the activity of the transcription factor *elf-1*. Indeed, the levels of activated (DNA-binding) *elf-1* were found decreased in lupus T cells. TCRζ chain deficiency can explain a variety of lupus T-cell defects, such as defective CD2-mediated signaling, defective natural killer activity, and activation-induced cell death, which require an intact ζ chain.

The study of B-cell receptor (BCR)-mediated signaling of SLE B cells provides molecular insights into their disease-characterizing hyperactivity. BCR-mediated signaling abnormalities are remarkably similar to those of lupus T cells. BCR engagement produced significantly increased Ca^{2+} responses (contributed mainly by the intracellular calcium stores), increased production of inositol triphosphate, and enhanced production of tyrosyl-phosphorylated cellular proteins. It is of interest that proteins with apparent molecular size between 36 and 64 kDa were hyperphosphorylated in both B and T cells from patients with LE, whereas the baseline degree of protein tyrosyl phosphorylation did not differ between the two cell types and their normal counterparts. The signaling aberrations analyzed previously (TCR, BCR, CD2-initiated signaling, and TCRζ deficiency) are independent of disease activity, treatment status, or the presence or absence of specific SLE clinical manifestations and may thus represent intrinsic abnormalities of the lupus lymphocyte that are also disease specific, since they were not found in normal lymphocytes or in lymphocytes from patients with other systemic autoimmune rheumatic diseases. The very similar lupus T- and B-cell signaling aberrations mentioned previously could substantiate the hypothesis that a common background underlies some heterogeneous lymphocyte functional defects (Kammer and Tsokos 2000, Kammer et al. 2002, Tsokos and Liossis 1999).

Genes and Genetics

The risk for development of LE in a sibling in families with a member with LE is 20 times more than in the general population. The relatively high concordance rates for SLE in monozygotic twins (25%–57%) compared with dizygotic twins (2%–9%) supports the importance of the genetic background. It is currently believed that multiple genes confer susceptibility to SLE expression, several of which have been identified to associate with lupus. Most of these associations have been identified while investigating pathogenic mechanisms in the disease. For example, the conjecture that certain

MHC antigens should present autoantigens better than others led to unveiling of associations between the disease or individual manifestations and MHC antigens. On the other hand, the expectation that apoptosis-related genes should be associated with the expression of lupus was not fulfilled.

More recently, genome-wide searches in families with multiple affected members disclosed areas in the genome associated with lupus. Obviously, no single gene is sufficient or necessary for disease expression, and lupus diathesis is conferred by an as-yet-unidentified number of genes that differ in individual patients. Still, the fact that almost all of the rare patients with C1r/C1s and complete C4 deficiency develop lupus suggests that the number of the contributing genes may be limited in some patients. The complexity of deciphering genes involved in the expression of lupus is confounded by the number of additional environmental, hormonal, and immunoregulatory factors in a given individual or population. Finally, genetic epistasis, the interaction of different genes to produce a disease phenotype, as has been shown in animal models, may occur in patients with LE.

The long arm of human chromosome 1, which was identified in almost all of the genome-wide searches as harboring loci associated with SLE, maps several of the potential lupus loci found in these genome-wide screens as well as others implicated in lupus, such as those encoding for FcγRIIA, FcγRIIIA, TCRζ, FasL, IL-10, complement receptor 1, complement receptor 2, and C1q proteins. These molecules have been implicated in SLE by either small-scale genetic or nongenetic studies.

The impact of genetic factors is also underscored by differences in the incidence and prevalence of the disease in various races. SLE has a higher incidence and prevalence in African Americans, Afro-Caribbeans, and East Asians, and the disease may also have a more severe course and prognosis. Certain clinical (e. g., discoid skin lesions and nephritis) and serologic (e. g., anti-Sm autoantibodies) manifestations are found more frequently in the African American LE population, and the high prevalence of severe nephritis encountered therein is responsible for the severe prognosis. Detailed genetic analysis may reveal the molecular basis for such interracial differences.

In summary, multiple genetic loci or genes contribute to susceptibility for the development of SLE. Genetic analyses may increase our understanding of the disease heterogeneity and provide a molecular basis for the racial differences in disease prevalence, manifestations, severity, and prognosis. The pathogenic contribution and complex interaction of lupus-susceptibility genes needs to be clarified by additional studies, and the precise role and contribution of each of the lupus-related genes should be addressed (Gregersen 1997).

Hormones

Although lupus affects prepubertal males and females equally, during puberty it manifests a striking preference for females that is maintained throughout the reproductive years. Thus, female hormonal factors play a permissive role at least, whereas male hormonal factors play a protective one in the expression of SLE. This has been further supported by studies in murine strains in which it has been clearly shown that estrogens have deleterious effects on lupus-prone experimental animals, whereas androgens are protective.

Estrogens act on target cells after binding to their cytoplasmic estrogen receptors, which belong to the group of nuclear receptors. The estrogen-estrogen receptor complex acquires transcription factor activity, and, after entrance into the nucleus and binding to specific estrogen-response elements found in the promoters of several genes, it modulates their transcription. Estrogen receptors are located in the cytoplasm and on the cell surface membrane. In murine T cells, membrane estrogen receptors, on binding to estradiol, mediate a rise in the concentration of intracellular calcium, which is a pivotal second messenger. Estrogen response elements are found in the promoters of the proto-oncogenes *c-fos* and *c-jun* and affect their transcription and, therefore, the levels of the transcription factor AP-1, which is a *fos/jun* heterodimer. Estrogens cause a significant increase in the amounts of calcineurin transcripts and also in calcineurin phosphatase activity in SLE T cells. The latter finding may provide a molecular explanation for the role of estrogens in autoimmunity (Tsokos and Boumpas 2002).

Environmental Factors

Various environmental factors, such as UV light, heavy metals, organic solvents, and infections, influence a genetically susceptible host in triggering the expression of SLE. Exposure to UV light causes photosensitivity (more frequently in the white LE population) and is a known disease-exacerbating factor. UV light causes apoptotic cell death of keratinocytes and cell surface expression of autoantigens previously "hidden" in the cytoplasm or nucleus. Autoantigens presented on surface membrane blebs of discrete size become accessible for immune recognition and attack. The latter may result in local inflammation and the appearance in the circulation of autoantibodies. UV light irradiation of cultured human keratinocytes induced changes consistent with apoptosis, and the autoantigens were clustered in two kinds of blebs of the cell surface membrane, the smaller blebs containing endoplasmic reticulum, ribosomes, and the (auto)antigen Ro/SSA and the larger blebs containing nucleosomal DNA, Ro/SSA and La/SSB, and the small ribonucleoproteins. UV-mediated apoptotic cell death may yield increased serum concentrations of autoantigens that activate immune cells. In addition, the activated apoptotic cascade may allow further degradation of autoantigens, which may lead to the exposure of cryptic and potentially more immunogenic antigens, which would permit expansion of the autoimmune response (see Chap. 2). UV light and ionizing irradiation, along with other apoptotic stimuli, lead to the generation of new phosphoproteins, which apparently act as autoantigens since they are recognized by lupus serum. These phosphoproteins associate with U1-snRNP and may, therefore, alter splicing of various genes. In addition, it is known that cell stress induced by exposure to radiation, heavy metals, toxins, and drugs causes activation of various kinases, including p38 and the Jun N-terminus mitogen-activated protein kinases, which may also contribute to this process. These studies are important in revealing the biochemistry of the stressed cell and its repercussions in the production of new autoantigens. In addition, the altered cell biochemistry may affect gene transcription in the immune cells, which may render them autoreactive. Such candidate genes may include adhesion and co-stimulatory molecules (ICAM-1, CD40L, etc.).

Clinical experience suggests that SLE may be initiated or may relapse after an infection, but, despite repeated efforts, a lupus-causing microorganism has never been identified. It has been hypothesized that infectious agents can dispropor-tionately trigger an endogenously dysregulated immune system for the development or exacerbation of SLE. Among the common pathogens, the herpesvirus EBV has received the most attention. Antibodies against EBV have cross-reactivity with the lupus-specific autoantigen Sm. It was recently reported that newly diagnosed young patients with LE have a significantly higher percentage of seropositivity for EBV infection than controls. Other tested herpesviruses did not follow this pattern. EBV DNA was found in the lymphocytes of all 32 young patients with LE tested and two thirds of controls. Whether EBV-infected individuals become more susceptible to the development of LE or patients with LE are become more susceptible to EBV infection or whether a third factor increases susceptibility to both is currently not known.

Molecular mimicry between autoantigens and antigens expressed by viruses and other pathogens have been extensively considered in the pathogenesis of autoimmune diseases. Epitopes of the SLE-associated 60-kd Ro/SSA autoantigen share sequences with the vesicular stomatitis virus (VSV) nucleocapsid protein, which may explain the presence of anti-Ro/SSA antibodies. In addition, immunization of animals with VSV proteins causes production of anti-Ro/SSA autoantibodies and anti-VSV antibodies. Additional examples of molecular mimicry include that between the B/B′ component of the Sm antigen and the human immunodeficiency virus type 1 p24 gag protein and the D component of the Sm antigen and the EBV nuclear antigen type 1 protein of EBV.

Alternatively, viral infection can break tolerance to self-antigens, as was shown in transgenic mice expressing a VSV glycoprotein. Autoantibodies to VSV glycoprotein cannot be induced by VSV glycoprotein in adjuvant or by recombinant vaccinia virus expressing VSV glycoprotein, but they are triggered by infection with wild-type VSV. The latter is an attractive mechanism because it can explain disease flares that follow infections.

Viral proteins may interfere with the function of proteins involved in cell death and survival. For example, adenoviral proteins may activate or inhibit p53 and bcl-2. Interestingly, viral proteins may mimic chemokine receptors or ligands. These exam-ples further complicate elucidation of the pathogenic involvement of viruses and other infectious agents in the development of the autoimmune response.

The syndrome of drug-induced LE has many similarities, but also important dif-ferences, to the idiopathic SLE syndrome. Because it represents a disease entity wherein the inciting factor is known, it is a good model to study certain aspects of SLE pathogenesis. Drugs that cause the SLE-like syndrome have been reported to induce DNA hypomethylation. Lupus T-cell DNA is hypomethylated, and the activity of the methylation-inducing enzyme DNA methyltransferase is decreased. Non-T cells from patients with SLE did not share this abnormality, which affected only half of the patients tested, and, moreover, this abnormality was not disease specific. Treat-ment of T cells with DNA methylation inhibitors induces up-regulation of the adhe-sion/co-stimulatory molecule lymphocyte function-associated antigen (LFA)-1. The significance of this event is underscored by studies in animal models in which infu-sion of T cells overexpressing LFA-1 can mediate the production of anti-dsDNA autoantibodies and the appearance of glomerulonephritis. It is thus possible that drugs inducing DNA hypomethylation can initiate an autoimmune process by up-regulating the co-stimulatory molecule LFA-1 (Dighiero and Rose 1999, Tsokos and Boumpas 2002).

Conclusions

In a genetically susceptible host, exogenous and hormonal factors influence the immune system at multiple levels, leading to numerous immunoregulatory abnormalities. The latter leads to generation of effector mechanisms of autoimmune pathology, including autoantibodies, immune complexes, autoreactive cells, and byproducts of immune activation, including lymphokines. T cells interact with B cells by cognate and noncognate means to help them produce autoantibodies. Autoantigens are revealed to the immune system because stressful stimuli such as UV light irradiation of keratinocytes (from exposure to sunlight) induce surface expression of previously hidden nuclear or cytoplasmic constituents. Immune complexes formed in excess amounts are cleared in decreased rates, resulting in increased serum levels and enhanced tissue deposition (Fig. 1.1).

Recent advances in scanning the human genome are expected to identify all genes involved in expression of the disease. When this is accomplished, we may be able to provide accurate genetic counseling and identify genes whose products are involved in the pathogenesis of the disease and the expression of pathology.

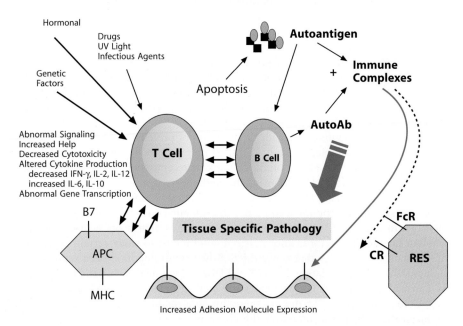

Fig. 1.1. Summary of the major cellular aberrations involved in the pathogenesis of lupus erythematosus (LE). Multiple genetic, environmental, and hormonal factors instigate a variety of cellular and cytokine abnormalities. These abnormalities lead to increased production of autoantibodies, which either directly or after forming complexes with autoantigens and activating complement deposit in tissues and initiate an inflammatory response. Immune complexes are formed in excessive amounts in patients with LE and are cleared at decreased rates because the numbers or the function of Fc and complement receptors are decreased. APC, antigen-presenting cells; autoAb, autoantibody; CR, complement receptor; FcR, Fc receptor; IFN, interferon; IL, interleukin; MHC, major histocompatibility complex; RES, reticuloendothelial system; uv, ultraviolet

Although better use of immunosuppressants and improved health care delivery have effectively decreased disease morbidity and mortality, there still is a long way to go before conquering this disease. Understanding the immunoregulatory abnormalities has helped in designing rational approaches to expand our therapeutic armamentarium. Biologic agents that can specifically reverse certain immune aberrations should further help patients with LE by improving survival and quality of life, and limiting adverse effects.

References

Blackman M, Kapler J, Marrack P (1990) The role of the T lymphocyte receptor in positive and negative selection of developing T lymphocytes. Science 248:1335–1341

Burkly LC, Lo D, Flavell RA (1990) Tolerance in transgenic mice expressing major histocompatibility molecules extrathymically on pancreatic cells. Science 248:1364–1368

Cyster JG, Hartley SB, Goodnow CC (1994) Competition for follicular niches exceeds self-reactive cells from the recirculating B-cell repertoire. Nature 371:389–395

Davidson A, Diamond B (2001) Autoimmune diseases. N Engl J Med 345:340–350

Dighiero G, Rose NR (1999) Critical self-epitopes are key to the understanding of self-tolerance and autoimmunity. Immunol Today 20:423–428

Goodnow GC (1992) Transgenic mice and analysis of B-cell tolerance. Ann Rev Immunol 10:489–518

Gregersen PK (1997) Genetic analysis of rheumatic diseases. In Kelley WN, Harris ED Jr, Ruddy S, Sledge CB (eds) Textbook of rheumatology, vol 1. W.B. Saunders, Philadelphia, pp 209–227

Groux H, Powrie F (1999) Regulatory T cells and inflammatory bowel disease. Immunol Today 20:442–445

Kammer GM, Tsokos GC (2000) Molecular aberrations in human lupus. Mol Med Today 6:418–424

Kammer GM, Perl A, Richardson BC, Tsokos GC (2002) Altered T cell signal transduction in systemic lupus erythematosus: a primary disorder. Arthritis Rheum 46:1139–1154

Nemazee D (2000) Receptor editing in B cells. Adv Immunol 74:89–126

Rathmell JC, Townsend SE, Xu JC, Flavell RA, Goodnow C (1996) Expansion or elimination of B cells in vivo: dual roles for CD40- and Fas (CD95)-ligands modulated by the B cell antigen receptor. Cell 87:319–329

Silverstein AM, Rose N (2000) There is only one immune system! The view from immunopathology. Semin Immunol 12:173–178

Singer GG, Abbas AK (1994) The fas antigen is involved in peripheral but not thymic deletion of T lymphocytes in T cell receptor transgenic mice. Immunity 365–371

Theofilopoulos AN (2002) An overview. In: Theofilopoulos AN, Bona AN (eds) The molecular pathology of autoimmune diseases. Taylor & Francis, Ann Arbor, pp 1–16

Thomson CB (1995) Distinct roles for the costimulatory ligands B7-1 and B7-2 in helper cell differentiation. Cell 81:979–982

Tsokos GC, Liossis SNC (1999) Immune cell signaling defects in human lupus: activation, anergy and death. Immunol Today 20:123–128

Tsokos GC, Virella G (2001) Tolerance and autoimmunity. In: Virella G (ed) Medical immunology. Marcel Decker, New York, pp 313–339

Tsokos GC, Boumpas DT (2002) Human systemic lupus erythematosus. In: Theofilopoulos AN, Bona AN (eds) The molecular pathology of autoimmune diseases. Taylor & Francis, Ann Arbor, pp 261–287

Tonegawa S (1983) Somatic generation of antibody diversity. Nature 302:575–581

von Boehmer H (1994) Positive selection of lymphocytes. Cell 76:219–228

von Boehmer H, Kisielow P (1990) Self-nonself discrimination by T cells. Science 248:1369–1373
Weiner HL, Friedman A, Miller A, Khoury SJ, al-Sabbagh A, Santos L, Sayegh M, Nussenblatt RB,
    Trentham DE, Hafler DA (1994) Oral tolerance: immunologic mechanisms and treatment of
    animal and human organ-specific autoimmune diseases by oral administration of auto anti-
    gens. Ann Rev Immunol 12:809–837

CHAPTER 2

Photoimmunology

Stefan Beissert, Annette Mehling, Thomas Schwarz

Among the wide-ranging environmental factors affecting human life, ultraviolet (UV) irradiation can be regarded as one of the most significant. Although UV light has an essential impact on terrestrial and aquatic ecology and is a fundamental necessity for the life of humans, animals, and plants, mid-wavelength UVB (290–320 nm) in particular can also exert hazardous effects on health. UV radiation not only plays an instrumental role in the development of skin cancer but also has profound effects on local and systemic inflammatory responses. While studying the biological effects of UVB irradiation, it has become evident that UV exposure can significantly compromise the immune system. The implications of the immunosuppressive properties of UV irradiation are manifold because UVB-induced immunosuppression not only is responsible for the inhibition of protective cell-mediated immunity but also contributes to the initiation, development, and perpetuation of several skin disorders (Fisher et al. 1997, Kochevar 1995, Kraemer 1997, Kripke 1990, Unna 1894, Urbach et al. 1974). These effects include induction of inflammation and cell death, premature skin aging, exacerbation of infectious diseases, and induction of skin cancer and photosensitive diseases such as cutaneous lupus erythematosus (LE), polymorphous light eruption, and solar urticaria. Some of these clinical effects of solar irradiation were first described more than 100 years ago (Unna 1894). Therefore, detailed knowledge about the mechanisms underlying UVB-mediated immunomodulation is of utmost importance. Extensive investigations have been performed in the field of photoimmunology in the past three decades, and it has become much clearer by which mechanisms UVB irradiation suppresses immunity (Beissert 2002, Beissert and Granstein 1996, Beissert and Schwarz 1999, DeFabo and Kripe 1979, Köck et al. 1990, Setlow 1974). Most of the experiments were performed in mice using the contact hypersensitivity (CHS) or delayed-type hypersensitivity (DTH) model to haptens as well as photocarcinogenesis experiments (Beissert 2002, Beissert and Schwarz 1999). These models have provided important information not only for photoimmunology but also for immunology per se. In the following section, the effects of UV exposure on the murine and human immune systems are briefly reviewed.

UV-Induced Local Immunosuppression

Application of hapten onto low-dose UVB-exposed human or murine skin leads to inhibition of the induction of CHS. This effect has also been termed "UV-induced local immunosuppression". The UV-induced changes in epidermal Langerhans' cell function, as well as the UV-induced release of soluble immunosuppressive factors (interleukin [IL]-10, tumor necrosis factor [TNF]-α, IL-1α, and cis-urocanic acid), which influence the local micromilieu, have been proposed to be the major players contributing to this phenomenon (Black et al. 1978, Enk et al. 1993, 1995, Grewe et al. 1993, Kock et al. 1990, Noonan et al. 1988, Toews et al. 1980, Ullrich 1995a, b).

In the early 1980s, Streilein's research group (Streilein and Bergstresser 1988) observed that low-dose UVB irradiation is capable of suppressing CHS responses to epicutaneously applied haptens in some strains of mice, and later studies revealed that genetic factors influence individual immunologic (un)responsiveness (Toews et al. 1980). Mouse strains in which immunosuppression was observed were designated UVB susceptible (e.g., C3H/HeN and C57BL/6), whereas strains resistant to the adverse effects of UV irradiation were termed "UVB resistant" (C3H/HeJ and BALB/c) (Streilein and Bergstresser 1988, Streilein et al. 1994). Further studies revealed that the genotype can be polygenically inherited and that the relevant autosomal loci controlling these traits can be found in the alleles *lps* and *tnf* (Yoshikawa and Streilein 1990). Further circumstantial evidence for the relevance of the *tnf* locus was supplied by experiments in which suppression of CHS in UVB-susceptible animals was prevented when its gene product was blocked by neutralizing anti-TNF-α antibodies (Moody-cliffe et al. 1994). In keeping with these results, a diminished capacity to mount a CHS response when hapten was applied to murine skin after injection of subinflammatory doses of TNF-α has also been demonstrated. UV irradiation also induces morphologic alterations in epidermal Langerhans' cells. This leads to their immobilization, whereby the reduction of CHS responses ensues, and similar changes can be observed after injections of TNF-α. The involvement of TNF-α in the emigration of Langerhans' cells from irradiated skin into the regional lymph nodes has also been reported by other research groups (Cumberbatch and Kimber 1992). Nonetheless, the role of TNF-α was made questionable by the report that normal Langerhans' cell migration after hapten application onto unirradiated skin was observable in TNF receptor 1 (p55)-deficient mice but that the treatment of these mice with neutralizing anti-TNF-α antibodies still had the effect of reducing Langerhans' cell migration (Cumberbatch and Kimber 1992, Kondo et al. 1995, Wang et al. 1996). This suggests that TNF receptor 1 may not be crucial for this process and indirectly implied that the TNF receptor 2 (p75) is required for Langerhans' cell migration. Because of the possible similarities between UVB- and TNF-α-mediated effects, the same group used these mouse models to study the role of the known TNF-α signaling pathways in UV-induced local suppression (Kondo et al. 1995). UVB irradiation similarly abrogated CHS responses in both mutant and wild-type mice as well as in mice deficient in TNF-α receptor 1+2, once again precluding TNF-α receptor 1 as a integral factor in the effects caused by UV in local cutaneous immunity. Taken together, the data obtained from the studies with these gene-targeted mice put the role of TNF-α signaling into a different perspective and suggest a minor role, if any, for the classic TNF-α signaling pathway in UVB-induced local immunosuppression and point to other factors as key mediators in this process.

UVB susceptibility and UVB resistance are not limited to mice but can also be found to a certain degree in humans (Yoshikawa et al. 1990). In addition, an association between the immunosuppressive effects of UVB and the development of skin cancer is evidenced by the significantly higher incidence of skin cancer in photosensitive patients. Once again, in accordance with the evidence provided by the mouse models, microsatellite markers and single nucleotide polymorphisms link these phenotypes to the TNF-α locus, suggesting that TNF-α or other genes contained in this region are plausible determinants of UVB susceptibility in humans (Niizeki et al. 2001). With the advent of human genome sequencing, a better marker(s) for UV susceptibility will be identified in the near future and will help clarify these controversial findings.

It is well documented that exposure to UVB radiation impairs Langerhans' cells in their activity to present antigens (Aberer et al. 1982, 1991, Caceres-Dittmar et al. 1995, Greene et al. 1979, Simon et al. 1990, Stingl et al. 1981, 1983, Tang and Udey 1991). Low-dose exposure of Langerhans' cells to UVB also leads to the preferential activation of CD4$^+$ cells of the T helper 2 (Th2) subset but does not result in the activation T helper 1 (Th1) cells (Simon et al. 1990). A follow-up study on this reported that UVB irradiation converts Langerhans' cells from immunogenic to tolerogenic antigen-presenting cells because of induction of specific clonal anergy in CD4$^+$ Th1 cells (Simon et al. 1991). Because hapten sensitization represents a primary syngeneic response and these studies used either allogeneic primary systems or primed syngeneic systems, an extrapolation of these findings to the in vivo situation for hapten sensitization may not be feasible, as neither of these model systems is an appropriate surrogate for suppression of a primary immune response.

UV-Induced Systemic Immunosuppression

Exposure of mice to relatively large doses of UVB radiation ($>2\,\text{kJ/m}^2$) inhibits both CHS responses after application of haptens to sites not exposed to UV and the induction of DTH responses (Beissert 2002, Beissert and Schwarz 1999, Noonan and DeFabo 1990, Toews et al. 1980, Ullrich 1995a). Because the Langerhans' cells critically involved in local immunosuppression were not altered in their number or morphology in non-UVB-exposed skin areas, this was indicative of effector mechanisms other than those involved in UV-induced local immunosuppression. Various mechanisms are considered to be involved in this so-called UV-induced systemic immunosuppression, including aberrant signaling due to damage of the photoreceptor DNA, conformational changes in the photoreceptor urocanic acid, and the release of a plethora of soluble factors with suppressive properties, such as IL-1α, TNF-α, PGE$_2$, and IL-10 (Beissert et al. 1995a, b, Black et al. 1978, Enk et al. 1995, Grewe et al. 1993, Köck et al. 1990, Niizeki and Streilein 1997, Noonan et al. 1988, Schwarz et al. 1994, Tan and Stoughton 1969, Ullrich et al. 1990, Yamawaki et al. 1998).

In particular, the role of IL-10 in UV-induced immunosuppression and regulation of cutaneous immune responses has been emphasized by several research groups (Beissert et al. 1995a, b, Enk et al. 1995, Niizeki and Streilein 1997, Ullrich 1994, Yamawaki et al. 1998). Intraperitoneal IL-10 administration was found to inhibit the elicitation phase but not the induction phase of CHS responses (Schwarz et al. 1994). On the other hand, both the induction and the elicitation of DTH immunity are suppressed by IL-10 treatment, indicating that CHS and DTH responses are related but distinct immune reactions. Increased concentrations of IL-10 were detected in the serum of UVB-exposed mice, and application of neutralizing anti-IL-10 antibodies significantly inhibited the UV-induced suppression of DTH responses to alloanti-gens, suggesting that IL-10 functions as a main mediator of UV-induced systemic immunosuppression (Beissert and Schwarz 1999, Beissert et al. 1996, Ullrich 1994). These findings are in agreement with the observation that spleen cells from UVB-treated mice are unable to present antigen to Th1 cells, whereas antigen presentation to Th2 cells was even enhanced (Ullrich 1994). Abrogation of both effects was achieved by application of neutralizing anti-IL-10 antibodies. To directly address the role of IL-10 in UV-induced systemic immunosuppression, IL-10-deficient mice were used (Beissert et al. 1996). The induction of DTH responses in IL-10-deficient mice could not be suppressed by UVB irradiation, whereas the induction of CHS responses was suppressed after UVB exposure. These data clearly demonstrate the in vivo rele-vance of IL-10 as a key mediator of UV-induced systemic immunosuppression. Fur-thermore, because IL-10 is one of the key cytokines involved in skewing the immune balance toward Th2-like immunity, such findings support the concept that UV expo-sure inhibits Th1-type immune responses.

The concept of a Th2 shift in systemic immunosuppression is further supported by the observation that immune suppression is blocked in mice treated with neutral-izing anti-IL-4 antibodies (Shreedhar et al. 1998a). Although UVB irradiation does not directly induce the release of this key Th2 cytokine, the IL-4 effects might be mediated indirectly via the UVB-induced release of prostaglandin E_2 by ker-atinocytes. Accordingly, this concept was substantiated by the observation that cyclooxygenase-2 inhibitors block IL-4 production after UV treatment. This alludes to the activation of a cytokine cascade (prostaglandin $E_2 \rightarrow$ IL-4 $\rightarrow$ IL-10) after UVB exposure that finally results in systemic immunosuppression (Shreedhar et al. 1998a). Recent observations in humans revealed that UVB irradiation stimulates the immi-gration of neutrophils into the skin, which could give rise to type 2 T-cell responses in UVB-exposed skin via secretion of IL-4 (Teunissen et al. 2002). Hence, there is sub-stantial evidence that exposure to UVB radiation generates a shift toward a Th2 immune response in vivo, thus explaining the fact that mostly Th1-mediated cellular immune reactions are impaired by UVB irradiation.

UV-Induced Antigen-Specific Immunotolerance

Another of the many consequences of UV irradiation for the immune system is that it also interferes with cell-mediated immunity to allergens by inducing anti-gen-specific tolerance (Beissert and Granstein 1996, Elmets et al. 1983, Toews et al. 1980, Ullrich 1995a, b). Mice having received an initial immunization through UVB-exposed skin do not mount an immune response after resensitization with the same antigen at a later time (Elments et al. 1983). These same mice showed no compromised immune responses when being sensitized against a different, unrelated antigen, suggesting that UVB irradiation leads to antigen-specific rather than general suppression of the immune system. Subsequent investigations revealed that the induction of antigen-specific tolerogenic suppressor/regulatory T cells was the root of the observed immunosuppression (see "UV-Induced Suppressor/Regulatory T Cells") and that this also occurred in the model of systemic immuno-suppression.

Once again, there is a correlation between mice and humans in that UVB irradiation can impair CHS responses due to antigen-specific tolerance, depending on the study, in approximately 10% of the human subjects tested (Yoshikawa et al. 1990). In accordance with the mouse models, tolerance induced in these few volunteers was antigen specific, since they reacted with pronounced CHS responses on subsequent sensitization with a nonrelated antigen. Even higher percentages of human volunteers developing tolerance when the antigen was initially applied onto skin areas exposed to erythemogenic UVB doses were reported in a further study (Cooper et al. 1992). These variations may be due to the different UV irradiation protocols used. Nevertheless, both studies demonstrate the existence of a subtype of humans who develop tolerance when the sensitizing antigen is first applied onto UVB-exposed skin.

Erythemogenic UVB doses not only cause the emigration and subsequent depletion of Langerhans' cells in the skin but also result in the infiltration of CD1a$^-$ HLA-DR$^+$ CD36$^+$ macrophages in the skin (Cooper et al. 1992). These macrophages can then activate autoreactive T cells (Cooper et al. 1985, 1986), specifically, CD4$^+$ "suppressor-inducer" cells, which in turn induce the maturation of suppressor T cells (Baadsgaard et al. 1988, 1990). In addition, these macrophages, which also express CD11b$^+$, can release the immunosuppressive cytokine IL-10 at considerable concentrations, probably representing the major source for epidermal IL-10 protein in human UV-exposed skin (Kang et al. 1994). This is of particular relevance in light of the fact that IL-10 seems to be play a major role in UVB-induced immunosuppression (see "UV-Induced Systemic Immunosuppression"). In vitro studies have shown that on UVB exposure, the macrophages infiltrating the epidermis can also induce CD4$^+$ T lymphocytes, which lack expression of the IL-2 receptor alpha chain (Stevens et al. 1995). Down-regulation of the IL-2 receptor alpha chain seems to be connected with effects caused by transforming growth factor, another immunosuppressive mediator.

UV-Induced Suppressor/Regulatory T Cells

UV-induced skin tumors from UV-suppressed mice grow progressively when transferred to mice immunocompromised by UV, yet typically regress when transplanted into immunocompetent mice (Fisher and Kripke 1978, 1982, Kripke et al. 1979). Furthermore, the transfer of T lymphocytes from UVB-irradiated mice into healthy recipients also results in the failure to reject UVB-induced tumors (Spellman and Daynes 1977, Spellmann et al. 1977). Analogous results were obtained using the hapten model of sensitization (Elmets et al. 1983, Noonan et al. 1981), in which injection of T lymphocytes from lymph nodes or spleens originating from UVB-irradiated and hapten-sensitized mice suppress CHS responses in the recipients. In correlation to the studies previously mentioned, the recipients could still generate a normal CHS response to a non-cross-reacting hapten (Elmets et al. 1983, Noonan et al. 1981). Taken together, these findings corroborate the hypothesis that UV-induced tolerance is mediated via induction of hapten-specific suppressor T cells. Yet, because of the poor characterization of the molecular mechanisms and the phenotypes of the cells generating these suppressive phenomena, the term "suppressor T cells" was almost banned and the entire concept of suppression drawn into question (Shevach 2001, 2002). However, the persistent hunt for suppressor T cells by investigators in photoimmunology and other fields finally resulted in the discovery of these regulatory T cells, thus justifying both the search for and the concept of suppressor T cells (Chatenoud et al. 2001, Shevach 2001, 2002).

Tolerance can be induced by the transfer of lymphocytes in both local and systemic suppression. However, different subsets of T cells seem to be responsible for the immunosuppressive effects. Systemic UVB-induced suppression (see "UV-Induced Systemic Immunosuppression") is mediated by antigen-specific $CD3^+$, $CD4^+$, and $CD8^-$ suppressor cells (Elmets et al. 1983, Ullrich et al. 1990). The results of a study initiated by Elmets et al. (Elmets et al. 1983) revealed that in local UV-induced immunosuppression, treatment of cells from UVB-irradiated animals with antibodies directed against Lyt-1 (CD4) completely abrogated their ability to transfer suppression, whereas treatment of cells with antibodies directed against Lyt-2 (CD8) inhibited suppression partially. Accordingly, Schwarz et al. (Schwarz et al. 1998) reported that in the UV low-dose model, suppression was prevented when the transferred T lymphocytes were depleted of $CD8^+$ cells. It is important to note that suppressor T cells in this particular experimental design influence the induction but not the elicitation of CHS, since introduction of UVB-induced suppressor T cells into previously sensitized mice does not affect the CHS response in recipients (Glass et al. 1990, Schwarz et al. 2004). This observation might indicate that effector T cells dominate suppressor T cells.

On the heels of the discovery of suppressor T cells, the field of immunosuppression and suppressor T cells has experienced a tremendous revival. Many studies have been conducted to further characterize this cell type. Both human and murine $CD4^+$ T cells subjected to chronic activation with CD3 in the presence of IL-10 induce $CD4^+$ T-cell clones with low proliferative capacity, low levels of IL-2, and no IL-4, yet are able to produce high levels of IL-10 (Shevach et al. 2001). Studies in severe combined immunodeficient (SCID) mice demonstrated that these antigen-specific T-cell clones can suppress the proliferation of $CD4^+$ T cells in response to antigen and can be used to prevent T-cell-mediated colitis (Groux et al. 1997, Sakaguchi et al. 1995). This particular subset of $CD4^+$ T cells was designated regulatory T cells. Another subset of $CD4^+$ regulatory T cells is characterized by the constitutive expression of the a chain of the IL-2 receptor (CD25) (Chatenoud et al. 2001, Sakaguchi et al. 1995, Shevach 2001). Interestingly, $CD4^+CD25^+$ regulatory T cells constitute approximately 10% of all human and murine peripheral $CD4^+$ T cells. The results of these and other studies have inspired a great deal of new research investigating the role of suppressor/regulatory T cells, currently making this area of research one of the most intensively studied subjects in general immunology. Whether the cells are termed "regulatory" or "suppressor" is more a matter of semantics, but because of this new breakthrough, the concept of suppressor T cells has been redeemed and is now "socially accepted" in the immunologic community (Chatenoud et al. 2001, Shevach et al. 2001).

The first successful cloning of regulatory T cells from UVB-irradiated mice was achieved by Shreedhar et al. (Shreedhar et al. 1998b). Mice were sensitized with fluorescein isothiocyanate after UVB treatment. The T cells cloned from these mice were phenotypically analyzed as $CD4^+$, $CD8^-$, TCR-α/β^+, MHC-restricted T cells specific for the fluorescein isothiocyanate antigen. They secreted IL-10 but not IL-4 or interferon-γ, whereas cells from nonirradiated control animals produced high amounts of interferon-γ and little IL-4 and IL-10 (Shreedhar et al. 1998b). The cytokine pattern of the UVB-induced cells was related but not identical to that of T regulatory 1 cells; thus, the authors designated these cells as T regulatory 2-type cells. In vitro experiments established that these cells can block antigen-presenting cell functions, including IL-12 production. Even more important, injection of precisely these now-characterized T cells into untreated recipients suppressed the induction of CHS against fluorescein isothiocyanate.

Although many studies previously pointed the finger at suppressor T cells of the CD8 type, the previously mentioned reports and many more provide increasing evidence that most belong to the CD4 type. In this respect, the role of CD4+CD25+ regulatory T cells in eliciting UVB-induced tolerance remains to be determined. First, clues as to the importance of CD4+ T cells in generating UVB-induced immunosuppression were recently found using major histocompatibility complex class II knockout mice (Krasteva et al. 2002). These animals are resistant to the immunosuppressive effects of UVB irradiation, indicating that UVB-induced immunosuppression is due to preferential activation of CD4+ suppressor/regulatory T cells and a result of deficient priming or expansion of effector CD8+ T cells (Krasteva et al. 2002).

T-suppressor cells also express the negative regulatory molecule cytotoxic T-lymphocyte activation molecule-4 (CTLA-4) on their surfaces. CTLA-4 is functionally relevant for immunosuppression because inhibition of CTLA-4 by a neutralizing antibody inhibits the induction of tolerance and immunosuppression after the transfer of T cells (Schwarz et al. 2000). In vitro stimulation of suppressor T cells induces the release of IL-2, interferon γ, high amounts of IL-10 but no IL-4, a cytokine secretion pattern reminiscent of that of regulatory T cells. Evidence for one possible mode of action by which CTLA-4 could exert its effects, namely, by the induction of IL-10, results from the observation that transfer of suppression was inhibited when recipients received neutralizing anti-IL-10 antibodies.

As is now fairly obvious, there is a distinct heterogeneity of suppressor cells, and this becomes even more apparent by the observation that UVB-induced natural killer T (NKT) cells are involved in the suppression of tumor immune responses (Moodycliffe et al. 2000). NKT cells express intermediate amounts of T-cell receptor molecules and co-express surface antigens usually found on natural killer cells (NK1.1, DX5, and Ly49a). Moodycliffe et al. supplied compelling data that UVB-induced suppressor T cells may actually belong to the NKT type and that these cells can suppress DTH and antitumoral immunity. It remains to be seen to what extent these cells, which have also been detected in UV-exposed humans, play a role in the etiology of tumor progression of UVB-induced skin cancers (Hersey et al. 1983).

Intracellular Mechanisms Involved in UV-Induced Immunosuppression

Several candidate molecules have been proposed as the cellular photoreceptors for UVB irradiation whereby nuclear DNA is considered the major UVB-absorbing chromophore (Applegate et al. 1989, Gordon and Haseltine 1982, Tan and Stoughton 1969). UVB irradiation has been found to primarily induce two types of photolesions in DNA, cyclobutane pyrimidine dimers and 6-4-photoproducts (Freeman et al. 1986, 1989, Ley et al. 1991, Mitchell and Nairn 1989, Yarosh et al. 1994). For many years, it has been proposed that UVB-induced DNA damage plays an essential role in UVB-induced immunosuppression, since the formation of DNA photoproducts by UV light is associated with various cellular responses, including the activation of many genes.

Data to support this hypothesis stems from the marsupial model *Monodelphis domestica* (Ley et al. 1991). In contrast to humans, UVB-induced DNA lesions in this animal are excised via a repair process called photoreactivation. As a result, DNA damage is removed more rapidly when these animals are exposed to visible light after UVB irradiation. Correspondingly, exposing these animals to visible light immediately after UVB irradiation significantly reduced the UVB-mediated inhibition of CHS responses. Because this photoreactivation removes DNA lesions, the inference was made that UVB-induced DNA damage is critically involved in signaling processes elicited by UVB-induced damage and the ensuing immunosuppression.

This hypothesis was further supported by studies using the DNA excision repair enzyme T4 endonuclease V (T4N5), which increases the rate of repair of UV-induced DNA damage in human cells (Yarosh et al. 1984). Topical application of T4N5 incorporated into a liposomal delivery system to the UVB-damaged skin prevented UV-induced impairment of the CHS response (Kripke et al. 1992). Further supporting data were provided by studies in which the release of the cytokines IL-10 and TNF-α triggered by UV irradiation of keratinocytes was considerably suppressed after treatment with T4N5 (Kibitel et al. 1991, Nishigori et al. 1996). Further evidence was made available by studies conducted in a mouse model in which essential components of the nucleotide excision repair system, the endogenous repair system, were knocked out (Boonstra et al. 2001). These animals are more susceptible to UV-induced immunosuppression, and these studies underlined that both global and transcription-coupled repair are needed to mitigate immunomodulation by UVB. The substantial role of DNA damage in the processes involved in UVB-induced immunosuppression was recently also confirmed in humans in vivo. In research conducted by Stege et al., nickel was used as a model contact sensitizer, and volunteers who were hypersensitive to nickel were treated with a placebo or the DNA repair enzyme photolyase immediately after UVB exposure (Stege et al. 2000). Nickel-specific hypersensitivity reactions were prevented after photolyase treatment, once again supporting the role of DNA damage as an essential factor involved in impaired immune responsiveness after UV irradiation.

Recent published studies documented a potential connection between DNA damage and IL-12 (Schmitt et al. 2000, Schwarz et al. 2002). IL-12 was able to reduce cyclobutane pyrimidine dimers in both mice and humans, and the reduction of UVB-induced damage seemed to depend on nucleotide excision repair, since this unique effect was not observed in knockout mice in which the nucleotide excision repair was defective. Because DNA damage is a key factor in the modulation of the immunosuppressive effects elicited by UVB radiation and IL-12 alleviates UVB-induced immunosuppression, it is tempting to speculate whether at least part of the immunoreconstitutive effects of IL-12 originate from its ability to decrease DNA damage. The observation that IL-12 inhibits UVB-induced IL-10 release, which is mediated via DNA damage, gives further support to this speculation (Nishigori et al. 1996, Schmitt et al. 2000). On the other hand, one should not forget the evidence of extranuclear cellular UVB targets involved in photoimmunology. UVB radiation effects the release of many cytokines, which can modulate immune responses and may also interfere with the biological activities of immune mediators, whether they be depletion or alteration of the functionality of antigen-presenting or T cells. For example, UVB irradiation interferes with the signal transduction pathway of interferon-γ and IL-2, both important immunomodulatory cytokines (Aragane et al. 1997, Kulms and Schwarz 2001). An alternative means by which UVB irradiation could have an effect is by inhibiting the phosphorylation of important signal transduction proteins involved in the signaling of these two cytokines.

Conclusion

Most of the published studies indicate the inhibitory effects of UV irradiation, especially on cellular immune responses. However, UV exposure is also known to induce and activate cell-mediated diseases such as systemic and certain forms of cutaneous LE. Thus, it seems that there is a paradox in the effects of UV irradiation on health. However, systemic LE, for example, is thought to represent a Th2-type disease with increased autoantibody production and B-cell activation, resulting in cutaneous inflammation, as well as internal organ involvement. For efficient B-cell activation and (auto-)antibody production, help from T cells, especially Th2 cells, is required. Because UV irradiation induces a shift toward Th2 rather than Th1 immune responses and Th2 cells have been shown to be involved in the activation of B cells, it might be possible that UV-induced/activated Th2 cells contribute to the development and/or deterioration of LE after UV light exposure. Furthermore, IL-10 represents an important growth factor for B cells. Multiple investigations have demonstrated up-regulation of IL-10 production after UV irradiation in mice and humans. Therefore, it would be possible that UV-induced IL-10 production contributes to B-cell survival under certain circumstances and thereby contributes to disease development. Together, these findings suggest how UV light exposure might be able to induce and/or exacerbate autoimmune disorders.

Acknowledgements. Due to space limitations, many studies could not be referenced or mentioned. We apologize to their authors. This work was supported by the German Research Association (DFG) project BE 1580/2–3, SFB 293, IZKF grant Lo2/065/04, and a European Community Grant QLK4-CT-2001-00115.

References

Aberer W, Schuler G, Stingl G, Hönigsmann H, Wolff K (1981) Ultraviolet light depletes surface markers of Langerhans cells. J Invest Dermatol 76:202–210

Aberer W, Stingl G, Stingl-Gazze LA, Wolff K (1982) Langerhans cells as stimulator cells in the murine primary epidermal cell-lymphocyte reaction: alteration by UV-B irradiation. J Invest Dermatol 79:129–135

Applegate LA, Ley RD, Alcalay J, Kripke ML (1989) Identification of the molecular target for the suppression of contact hypersensitivity by ultraviolet irradiation. J Exp Med 170:1117–1131

Aragane Y, Kulms D, Luger TA, Schwarz T (1997) Down-regulation of interferon gamma-activated STAT1 by UV light. Proc Natl Acad Sci USA 94:11490–11495

Baadsgaard O, Fox DA, Cooper KD (1988) Human epidermal cells from ultraviolet light-exposed skin preferentially activate autoreactive CD4$^+$2H4$^+$ suppressor-inducer lymphocytes and CD8$^+$ suppressor/cytotoxic lymphocytes. J Immunol 140:1738–1744

Baadsgaard O, Salvo B, Mannie A, Dass B, Fox DA, Cooper KD (1990) In vivo ultraviolet-exposed human epidermal cells activate T suppressor cell pathways that involve CD4$^+$CD45RA$^+$ suppressor-inducer T cells. J Immunol 145:2854–2861

Beissert S (2002) Use of mutant mice in photoimmunological and photocarcinogenic investigations. Methods 28:130–937

Beissert S, Granstein RD (1996) UV-induced cutaneous photobiology. Crit Rev Biochem Mol Biol 31:381–404

Beissert S, Schwarz T (1999) Mechanisms involved in UV-induced immunosuppression. J Invest Dermatol Symp Proc 4:61–64

Beissert S, Hosoi J, Grabbe S, Asahina A, Granstein RD (1995a) IL-10 inhibits tumor antigen presentation by epidermal antigen-presenting cells. J Immunol 154:1280–1286

Beissert S, Ullrich SE, Hosoi J, Granstein RD (1995b) Supernatants from UVB radiation-exposed keratinocytes inhibit Langerhans cell presentation of tumor-associated antigens via IL-10 content. J Leukoc Biol 58:234–240

Beissert S, Hosoi J, Kühn R, Rajewsky K, Müller W, Granstein RD (1996) Impaired immunosuppressive response to ultraviolet radiation in IL-10-deficient mice. J Invest Dermatol 107:553–557

Black AK, Greaves MW, Hensby, CN, Plummer NA (1978) Increased prostaglandins E$_2$ and F$_2$ in human skin at 6 and 24 hours after ultraviolet B irradiation (290–320 nm). Br J Clin Pharmacol 5:291–295

Boonstra A, van Oudenaren A, Baert M, van Steeg H, Leenen PJ, van der Horst GT, Hoeijmakers JH, Savelkoul HF, Garssen J (2001) Differential ultraviolet-B-induced immunomodulation in XPA, XPC, and CSB DNA repair-deficient mice. J Invest Dermatol 117:141–146

Caceres-Dittmar G, Arizumi K, Xu S, Tapia FJ, Bergstresser PR, Takashima A (1995) Hydrogen peroxide mediates UV-induced impairment of antigen presentation in a murine epidermal-derived dendritic cell line. Photochem Photobiol 62:176–183

Chatenoud L, Salomon B, Bluestone JA (2001) Suppressor T cells – they're back and critical for regulation of autoimmunity! Immunol Rev 182:149–163

Cooper KD, Fox P, Neises G, Katz SI (1985) Effects of ultraviolet radiation on human epidermal cell alloantigen presentation: initial depression of Langerhans cell-dependent function is followed by the appearance of T6-Dr$^+$ cells that enhance epidermal alloantigen presentation. J Immunol 134:129–137

Cooper KD, Neises GR, Katz SI (1986) Antigen-presenting OKM5$^+$ melanophages appear in human epidermis after ultraviolet radiation. J Invest Dermatol 86:363–370

Cooper KD, Oberhelman L, Hamilton TA, Baadsgaard O, Terhune M, LeVee G, Anderson T, Koren H (1992) UV exposure reduces immunization rates and promotes tolerance to epicutaneous antigens in humans: relationship to dose, CD1a$^-$DR$^+$epidermal macrophage induction, and Langerhans cell depletion. Proc Natl Acad Sci USA 89:8497–8501

Cumberbatch M, Kimber I (1992) Dermal tumour necrosis factor-alpha induces dendritic cell migration to draining lymph nodes, and possibly provides one stimulus for Langerhans' cell migration. Immunology 75:257–263

DeFabo EC, Kripke ML (1979) Dose-response characteristics of immunologic unresponsiveness to UV-induced tumors produced by UV-irradiation of mice. Photochem Photobiol 30:385–390

Elmets CA, Bergstresser PR, Tigelaar RE, Wood PJ, Streilein JW (1983) Analysis of the mechanism of unresponsiveness produced by haptens painted on skin exposed to low dose ultraviolet radiation. J Exp Med 158:781–794

Enk AH, Angeloni VL, Udey MC, Katz SI (1993) Inhibition of Langerhans cell antigen-presenting function by IL-10: a role for IL-10 in induction of tolerance. J Immunol 151:2390–2398

Enk CD, Sredni D, Blauvelt A, Katz SI (1995) Induction of IL-10 gene expression in human keratinocytes by UVB exposure in vivo and in vitro. J Immunol 154:4851–4856

Fisher GJ, Wang ZQ, Datta SC, Varani J, Kang S, Voorhees JJ (1997) Pathophysiology of premature skin aging by ultraviolet light. N Engl J Med 373:1419–1428

Fisher MS, Kripke ML (1978) Further studies on the tumor-specific suppressor cells induced by ultraviolet radiation. J Immunol 121:1139–1144

Fisher MS, Kripke ML (1982) Suppressor T lymphocytes control the development of primary skin cancer in ultraviolet-irradiated mice. Science 216:1133–1134

Freeman SE, Gange RW, Matzinger EA, Sutherland BM (1986) Higher pyrimidine dimer yields in the skin of normal humans with higher UVB sensitivity. J Invest Dermatol 86:34–36

Freeman SE, Hachham H, Gange RW, Maytum DJ, Sutherland JC, Sutherland BM (1989) Wavelength dependence of pyrimidine dimer formation in DNA of human skin irradiated in situ with ultraviolet light. Proc Natl Acad Sci USA 86:5605–5609

Glass MJ, Bergstresser PR, Tigelaar RE, Streilein JW (1990) UVB radiation and DNFB skin painting induce suppressor cells universally in mice. J Invest Dermatol 94:273–278

Gordon LK, Haseltine WA (1982) Quantitation of cyclobutane pyrimidine dimer formation in double and single-stranded DNA fragments of defined sequences. Radiat Res 89:99–112

Greene MI, Sy MS, Kripke ML, Benacerraf B (1979) Impairment of antigen-presenting cell function by ultraviolet radiation. Proc Natl Acad Sci 76:6591–6595

Grewe M, Trefzer U, Ballhorn A, Gyufko K, Henninger H, Krutmann J (1993) Analysis of the mechanism of ultraviolet (UV) B radiation-induced prostaglandin E_2 synthesis by human epidermoid carcinoma cells. J Invest Dermatol 101:528–531

Groux H, O'Garra A, Bigler M, Rouleau M, Antonenko S, de Vries JE, Roncarolo MG (1997) A $CD4^+$ T-cell subset inhibits antigen-specific T-cell responses and prevents colitis. Nature 389:737–742

Hersey P, Haran G, Hasic E, Edwards A (1983) Alteration of T cell subsets and induction of suppressor T cell activity in normal subjects after exposure to sunlight. J Immunol 31:171–174

Kang K, Hammerberg C, Meunier L, Cooper KD (1994) $CD11b^+$ macrophages that infiltrate human epidermis after in vivo ultraviolet exposure potently produce IL-10 and represent the major secretory source of epidermal IL-10 protein. J Immunol 153:5256–5264

Kibitel JT, Yee V, Yarosh DB (1991) Enhancement of ultraviolet-DNA repair in denV gene transfectants and T4 endonuclease V-liposome recipients. Photochem Photobiol 54:753–760

Kochevar IE (1995) Molecular and cellular effects of UV radiation relevant to chronic photoaging. In: Gilchrest BA (ed) Photodamage. Blackwell Science, Cambridge, pp 51–67

Kock A, Schwarz T, Kirnbauer R, Urbanski A, Perry P, Ansel JC, Luger TA (1990) Human keratinocytes are a source for tumor necrosis factor α: evidence for synthesis and release upon stimulation with endotoxin or ultraviolet light. J Exp Med 172:1609–1614

Kondo S, Wang B, Fujisawa H, Shvji GM, Echtenacher B, Mak TW, Sauder DN (1995) Effect of gene-targeted mutation in TNF receptor (p55) on contact hypersensitivity and ultraviolet B-induced immunosuppression. J Immunol 155:3801–3805

Kraemer KH (1997) Sunlight and skin cancer: another link revealed. Proc Natl Acad Sci USA 94:11–14

Krasteva M, Aubin F, Laventurier S, Kehren J, Assossou O, Kanitakis J, Kaiserlian D, Nicolas JF (2002) MHC class II-KO mice are resistant to the immunosuppressive effects of UV light. Eur J Dermatol 12:10–19

Kripke ML (1990) Effects of UV radiation on tumor immunity. J Natl Cancer Inst 82:1392–1396

Kripke ML, Thorn RM, Lill PH, Civin PI, Pazimono NH, Fisher MS (1979) Further characterization of immunological unresponsiveness induced in mice by ultraviolet radiation. Growth and induction of nonultraviolet-induced tumors in ultraviolet-irradiated mice. Transplantation 28:212–217

Kripke ML, Cox PA, Alas LG, Yarosh DB (1992) Pyrimidine dimers in DNA initiate systemic immunosuppression in UV-irradiated mice. Proc Natl Acad Sci USA 89:7516–7520

Kulms D, Schwarz T (2001) Ultraviolet radiation inhibits interleukin-2-induced tyrosine phosphorylation and the activation of STAT5 in T lymphocytes. J Biol Chem 276:12849–12855

Ley RD, Applegate LA, Fry RJM, Sanchez AB (1991) Photoreactivation of ultraviolet radiation-induced skin and eye tumors of Monodelphis domestica. Cancer Res 51:6539–6542

Mitchell DL, Nairn RS (1989) The biology of the (6-4) photoproduct. Photochem Photobiol 49:805–819

Moodycliffe AM, Kimber I, Norval M (1994) Role of tumor necrosis factor-alpha in ultraviolet B light-induced migration of dendritic cells and suppression of contact hypersensitivity. Immunology 81:79–84

Moodycliffe AM, Nghiem D, Clydesdale G, Ullrich SE (2000) Immune suppression and skin cancer development: regulation by NKT cells. Nat Immunol 1:521–525

Niizeki H, Streilein JW (1997) Hapten-specific tolerance induced by acute, low-dose ultraviolet B radiation of skin is mediated via interleukin-10. J Invest Dermatol 109:25–30

Niizeki H, Naruse T, Hecker KH, Taylor JR, Kurimoto I, Shimizu T, Yamasaki Y, Inoko H, Streilein JW (2001) Polymorphisms in the tumor necrosis factor (TNF) genes are associated with susceptibility to effects of ultraviolet-B radiation on induction of contact hypersensitivity. Tissue Antigens 58:369–378

Nishigori C, Yarosh DB, Ullrich SE, Vink AA, Bucana CD, Roza L, Kripke ML (1996) Evidence that DNA damage triggers interleukin 10 cytokine production in UV-irradiated murine keratinocytes. Proc Natl Acad Sci USA 93:10354–10359

Noonan FP, DeFabo EC (1990) Ultraviolet-B dose-response curves for local and systemic immunosuppression are identical. Photochem Photobiol 52:801–808

Noonan FP, DeFabo EC, Kripke ML (1981) Suppression of contact hypersensitivity by UV radiation and its relationship to UV-induced suppression of tumor immunity. Photochem Photobiol 34:683–689

Noonan FP, DeFabo EC, Morrison H (1988) Cis-urocanic acid, a product formed by ultraviolet B irradiation of the skin, initiates an antigen presentation defect in splenic dendritic cells in vivo. J Invest Dermatol 90:92–99

Sakaguchi S, Sakaguchi N, Asano M, Itoh M, Toda M (1995) Immunologic self-tolerance maintained by activated T cells expressing IL-2 receptor alpha-chains (CD25). Breakdown of a single mechanism of self-tolerance causes various autoimmune diseases. J Immunol 155:1151–1164

Schmitt DA, Walterscheid JP, Ullrich SE (2000) Reversal of ultraviolet radiation-induced immune suppression by recombinant interleukin-12: suppression of cytokine production. Immunology 101:90–96

Schwarz A, Grabbe S, Riemann H, Aragane Y, Simon M, Manon S, Andrade S, Luger TA, Zlotnik A, Schwarz T (1994) In vivo effects of interleukin-10 on contact hypersensitivity and delayed type hypersensitivity reactions. J Invest Dermatol 103:211–216

Schwarz A, Grabbe S, Mahnke K, Riemann H, Luger TA, Wysocka M, Trinchieri G, Schwarz T (1998) IL-12 breaks UV light induced immunosuppression by affecting CD8$^+$ rather than CD4$^+$ T cells. J Invest Dermatol 110:272–276

Schwarz A, Beissert S, Grosse-Heitmeyer K, Gunzer M, Bluestone JA, Grabbe S, Schwarz T (2000) Evidence for functional relevance of CTLA-4 in ultraviolet-radiation-induced tolerance. J Immunol 165:1824–1831

Schwarz A, Stander S, Berneburg M, Bohm M, Kulms D, van Steeg H, Grosse-Heitmeyer K, Krutmann J, Schwarz T (2002) Interleukin-12 suppresses ultraviolet radiation-induced apoptosis by inducing DNA repair. Nat Cell Biol 4:26–31

Schwarz A, Maeda A, Wild MK, Kernebeck K, Gross N, Aragane Y, Beissert S, Vestweber D, Schwarz T (2004) Ultraviolet radiation-induced regulatory T cells not only inhibit the induction but can suppress the effector phase of contact hypersensitivity. J Immunol 172:1036–1043

Setlow RB (1974) The wavelengths in sunlight effective in producing skin cancer: a theoretical analysis. Proc Natl Acad Sci 71:3363–3366

Shevach EM (2001) CD4$^+$CD25$^+$ regulatory T cells-certified professionals. J Exp Med 193:F41–F45

Shevach EM (2002) CD4$^+$CD25$^+$ suppressor T cells: more questions than answers. Nat Rev Immunol 2:389–400

Shevach EM, McHugh RS, Piccirillo CA, Thornton AM (2001) Control of T-cell activation by CD4$^+$CD25$^+$ suppressor T cells. Immunol Rev 182:58–67

Shreedhar V, Giese T, Sung VW, Ullrich SE (1998a) A cytokine cascade including prostaglandin E₂, IL-4, and IL-10 is responsible for UV-induced systemic immune suppression. J Immunol 160:3783–3789

Shreedhar VK, Pride MW, Sun Y, Kripke ML, Strickland FM (1998b) Origin and characteristics of ultraviolet-B-radiation-induced suppressor T lymphocytes. J Immunol 161:1327–1335

Simon JC, Cruz PD Jr, Bergstresser PR, Tigelaar RE (1990) Low dose ultraviolet B-irradiated Langerhans cells preferentially activate CD4+ cells of the T helper 2 subset. J Immunol 145:2087–2091

Simon JC, Tigelaar RE, Bergstresser PR, Edelbaum D, Cruz PD Jr (1991) Ultraviolet B radiation converts Langerhans cells from immunogenic to tolerogenic antigen-presenting cells. Induction of specific clonal anergy in CD4+ T helper 1 cells. J Immunol 146:485–489

Spellman CW, Daynes RA (1997) Modification of immunological potential by ultraviolet radiation. II. Generation of suppressor cells in short-term UV-irradiated mice. Transplantation 24:120–126

Spellman CW, Woodward JG, Daynes RA (1977) Modification of immunological potential by ultraviolet radiation. I. Immune status of short-term UV-irradiated mice. Transplantation 24:112–119

Stege H, Roza L, Vink AA, Grewe M, Ruzicka T, Grether-Beck S, Krutmann J (2000) Enzyme plus light therapy to repair DNA damage in ultraviolet-B-irradiated human skin. Proc Natl Acad Sci USA 97:1790–1795

Stevens SR, Shibaki A, Meunier L, Cooper KD (1995) Suppressor T cell-activating macrophages in ultraviolet-irradiated human skin induce a novel, TGF-beta-dependent form of T cell activation characterized by deficient IL-2r alpha expression. J Immunol 155:5601–5607

Stingl G, Gazze-Stingl LA, Aberer W, Wolff K (1981) Antigen presentation by murine epidermal langerhans cells and its alteration by ultraviolet B light. J Immunol 127:1707–1713

Stingl LA, Sauder DN, Iijima M, Wolff K, Pehamberger H, Stingl G (1983) Mechanism of UV-B induced impairment of the antigen-presenting capacity of murine epidermal cells. J Immunol 130:1586–1591

Streilein JW, Bergstresser PR (1988) Genetic basis of ultraviolet-B effects on contact hypersensitivity. Immunogenetics 27:252–258

Streilein JW, Taylor JR, Vincek V, Kurimoto I, Chimizu I, Tie T, Golomb C (1994) Immune surveillance and sunlight-induced skin cancer. Immunol Today 15:174–179

Tan EM, Stoughton RB (1969) Ultraviolet light induced damage to desoxyribonucleic acid in human skin. J Invest Dermatol 52:537–542

Tang A, Udey MD (1991) Inhibition of epidermal Langerhans cell function by low dose ultraviolet B radiation, ultraviolet B radiation selectively modulates ICAM-1 (CD54) expression by murine LC. J Immunol 146:3347–3355

Teunissen MB, Piskin G, Nuzzo S, Sylva-Steenland RM, de Rie MA, Bos JD (2002) Ultraviolet B radiation induces a transient appearance of IL-4+ neutrophils, which support the development of Th2 responses. J Immunol 168:3732–3739

Toews GB, Bergstresser PR, Streilein JW (1980) Epidermal Langerhans cell density determines whether contact hypersensitivity or unresponsiveness follows skin painting with DNFB. J Immunol 124:445–453

Ullrich SE (1994) Mechanisms involved in the systemic suppression of antigen-presenting cell function by UV irradiation. Keratinocyte-derived IL-10 modulates antigen-presenting cell function of splenic adherent cells. J Immunol 152:3410–3416

Ullrich SE (1995a) Modulation of immunity by ultraviolet radiation: key effects on antigen presentation. J Invest Dermatol 105:30S–36S

Ullrich SE (1995b) The role of epidermal cytokines in the generation of cutaneous immune reactions and ultraviolet radiation-induced immune suppression. Photochem Photobiol 62:389–401

Ullrich SE, McIntyre WB, Rivas JM (1990) Suppression of the immune response to alloantigen by factors released from ultraviolet-irradiated keratinocytes. J Immunol 145:489–498

Unna PG (1894) Die Histopathologie der Hautkrankheiten, Hirschwald, Berlin.

Urbach F, Epstein JH, Forbes PD (1974) Ultraviolet carcinogenesis: experimental, global and genetic aspects. In: Fitzpatrick TB, Pathak MA, Harber LC, Seiji M, Kukita A (eds) Sunlight and man. McGraw Hill, Tokyo, pp 258–283

Wang B, Kondo S, Shivji GM, Fujisawa H, Mak TW, Sauder DN (1996) Tumour necrosis factor receptor II (p75) signalling is required for the migration of Langerhans' cells. Immunology 88:284–288

Yamawaki M, Katiyar SK, Anderson CY, Tubesing KA, Mukhtar H, Elmets CA (1998) Genetic variation in low-dose UV-induced suppression of contact hypersensitivity and in the skin photocarcinogenesis response. J Invest Dermatol 111:706–708

Yarosh D, Bucana C, Cox P, Alas L, Kibitel J, Kripke ML (1994) Localization of liposomes containing a DNA repair enzyme in murine skin. J Invest Dermatol 103:461–468

Yoshikawa T, Streilein JW (1990) Genetic basis of the effects of ultraviolet light B on cutaneous immunity. Evidence that polymorphism at the TNF-α and Lps loci governs susceptibility. Immunogenetics 32:398–405

Yoshikawa T, Rae V, Bruins-Slot W, van den Berg JW, Taylor JR, Streilein JW (1990) Susceptibility to effects of UVB radiation on induction of contact hypersensitivity as a risk factor for skin cancer in humans. J Invest Dermatol 95:530–536

CHAPTER 3

The Epidemiology of Lupus Erythematosus 3

SÒNIA JIMÉNEZ, RICARD CERVERA, MIGUEL INGELMO, JOSEP FONT

Lupus erythematosus (LE) is an autoimmune disorder that includes a broad spectrum of clinical forms, ranging from those with lesions confined to the skin to others with more generalized involvement, then termed "systemic LE (SLE)". Although previously considered a rare disease, LE now seems to be relatively common in certain groups, probably owing to the development of several immunologic tests that identify many atypical or benign cases that otherwise might not be diagnosed. Furthermore, since the introduction in 1982 by the American College of Rheumatology (ACR) of a set of more sensitive criteria for SLE classification, more cases are now being detected. It is noteworthy that cutaneous manifestations account for 4 of the 11 revised criteria for the classification of SLE.

In the present chapter, we present the most important data regarding the incidence and prevalence of LE in the general population; the epidemiology of the main clinical and immunologic features of LE, with special emphasis on the more relevant cutaneous manifestations; overall information on the patterns of disease expression in specific subsets; and studies on mortality in LE.

Incidence and Prevalence of Lupus Erythematosus

Incidence

The incidence of LE in the general population varies according to the characteristics of the population studied, ie, predominant age or sex group, race, ethnicity, national origin, or period of time studied, and changes in diagnostic classification (Abu-Shakra et al. 1995b, Boumpas et al. 1995, Cervera et al. 1993, 2003, Drenkard et al. 1994, Fessel 1974, Font and Cervera 1993, Font et al. 1991, 1993, Fukase 1980, Ginzler et al. 1982, Gladman 1996, Gourley et al. 1997, Gudmundsson and Steisson 1990, Helve 1985, Hochberg 1987, Hochberg et al. 1995, Hopkinson et al. 1994, Iseki et al. 1994, Johnson and Nived 1990, Johnson et al. 1995, Karlson et al. 1997, Maskarinec and Katz 1995, McCarty et al. 1995, Meddings and Grennan 1980, Merrell and Shuldman 1955, Michet et al. 1985, 2001, Nived et al. 1985, Nepom and Schaller 1984, Nossent 1992, Pistiner et al. 1991, Samanta et al. 1992, Siegel and Lee 1973, Studenski et al. 1987, Swaak et al. 1989, Symmonds 1995, Tan et al. 1982, Ting and Hsieh 1992, Uramoto et al. 1999, Villar et al. 1980, Vlachoyiannopoulos et al. 1993, Wallace et al. 1981, Ward et al. 1995a, b). Furthermore, most studies only focus on SLE.

Table 3.1. Incidence of systemic lupus erythematosus in several studies in Europe

Study location (reference)	Study year	Incidence[a]
Sweden (Nived et al. 1985)	1985	4.8
England (Nottingham) (Hopkinson et al. 1994)	1994	3.7
Iceland (Gudmundsson and Steisson 1990)	1990	3.3
England (Birmingham) (Johnson et al. 1995)	1995	3.8

[a] Per 100,000 persons per year (males and females).

Table 3.2. Incidence of systemic lupus erythematosus in several studies in the United States

Study location (reference)	Study year	Incidence[a]
New York (Siegel and Lee 1973)	1965	2.0
San Francisco (Fessel 1974)	1973	7.6
Baltimore (Hochberg et al. 1995)	1977	4.6
Rochester (Michet et al. 1985)	1979	2.2
Pittsburg (McCarty et al. 1995)	1990	2.4
Rochester (Uramoto et al. 1999)	1992	5.8

[a] Per 100,000 persons per year (males and females).

In Europe, the annual incidence of SLE ranges from 3.3 cases per 100,000 persons in Iceland (Gudmunsson and Steisson 1990) to 4.8 cases per 100,000 persons in Sweden (Nived et al. 1985) (Table 3.1). In the United States, the annual incidence of SLE has been estimated in several studies, with rates ranging from 2.0 to 7.6 cases per 100,000 persons (Fessel 1974, Hochberg et al. 1995, McCarty et al. 1995, Michet et al. 1985, Siegel and Lee 1973, Uramoto et al. 1999) (Table 3.2). According to Rochester data, the rates increased by a factor of 2.5 between 1950–1954 (Michet et al. 1985) and 1975–1979 (Uramoto et al. 1999). Information from other continents is more scarce. In Okinawa, Japan, Iseki et al. (Iseki et al. 1994) identified 566 newly diagnosed cases of SLE between 1971 and 1991, corresponding to an average annual incidence of 3.0 cases per 100,000 persons. On the Island of Curacao, the annual incidence between 1980 and 1989 was 4.6 cases per 100,000 persons (Nossent 1992).

Prevalence

The studies on prevalence in the general population also show marked differences. This variability may result from differences in methods of case ascertain and socio-economic causes. However, geographic differences cannot be excluded and may result from differences in genetic or environmental factors.

In Europe, the study by Hochberg (Hochberg 1987) in England and Wales reported a prevalence in 1987 of 12.5 cases per 100,000 women of all ages, which was increased to 17.7 in women aged 15–64 years. A more recent study by Hopkinson et al. (Hopkinson et al. 1994) indicates a prevalence of 24.6 cases per 100,000 persons in Nottingham. Johnson et al. (Johnson et al. 1995) reported a prevalence of 27.7 cases per 100,000 persons. The greater prevalence in Europe has been described in Sweden,

Table 3.3. Prevalence of systemic lupus erythematosus in several studies in Europe

Study location (reference)	Study year	Prevalence[a]
Finland (Helve 1985)	1978	28.0
England-Wales (Hochberg 1987)	1982	12.5[b]
Sweden (Nived et al. 1985)	1982	39.0
England (Leicester) (Samanta et al. 1992)	1989	26.1
Iceland (Gudmundsson and Steisson 1990)	1990	36.0
England (Nottingham) (Hopkinson et al. 1994)	1990	24.6
England (Birmingham) (Johnson et al. 1995)	1991	27.7
Ireland (Gourley et al. 1997)	1993	25.4

[a] Per 100,000 persons (males and females).
[b] Females only.

Table 3.4. Prevalence of systemic lupus erythematosus in several studies in the United States

Study location (reference)	Study year	Prevalence[a]
New York (Siegel and Lee 1973)	1965	14.6
San Francisco (Fessel 1974)	1973	50.8
Rochester (Michet at el. 1985)	1980	40.0
Hawaii (Maskarinec and Katz 1995)	1989	41.8

[a] Per 100,000 persons (males and females).

where there were 39 registered cases per 100,000 persons (Nived et al. 1985) (Table 3.3). The overall prevalence in the United States has been reported to range from 14.6 to 50.8 cases per 100,000 persons (including white and black people) (Maskarinec and Katz 1995, Michet et al. 1985, Nived et al. 1985, Siegel and Lee 1973) (Table 3.4). In New Zealand, Australia, and Japan, SLE prevalence rates of 15, 52, and 21 cases per 100,000 persons, respectively, have been observed (Anstey et al. 1993, Fukase 1980, Meddings and Grennan 1980).

Epidemiology of the Main Clinical and Immunologic Features of Lupus Erythematosus

Tables 3.5 and 3.6 describe the frequencies of the different clinical and immunologic features from a series of 1,000 patients with SLE derived from seven European countries ("Euro-Lupus cohort") (Cervera et al. 1993). Cutaneous and articular features are the most frequent organic manifestations, and they appear in most patients. Also, several potentially serious features, such as renal, serositic, neurologic, and hematologic manifestations, are relatively frequent. Malaise is the most frequent systemic feature, and it is present in nearly all patients. Antinuclear antibodies and antidoubled-stranded DNA antibodies were the most common immunologic features. Similar prevalences have been described in other series from different European and American countries (Abu-Shakra et al. 1995a, Estes and Christian 1971, Font et al. 1991, Fries et al. 1974, Ginzler et al. 1982, Gripenberg and Helve 1991, Johnson and Nived 1990, Kellum and Haserike 1964, Nepom and Schaller 1984, Reveille et al. 1990, Rubin et al. 1985, Seleznick and Fries 1991, Ting and Hsieh 1992, Urowitz et al. 1976).

Table 3.5. Clinical manifestations in a series of 1,000 European patients with systemic lupus erythematosus (Cervera et al. 1993)

Clinical Manifestation	Prevalence (%)
Arthritis	84
Malar rash	58
Fever	52
Photosensitivity	45
Nephropathy	39
Serositis	36
Raynaud's phenomenon	34
Neurologic involvement	27
Oral ulcers	24
Thrombocytopenia	22
Sicca syndrome	16
Livedo reticularis	14
Thrombosis	14
Lymphadenopathy	12
Discoid lesions	10
Myositis	9
Hemolytic anemia	8
Lung involvement	7
Subacute cutaneous lesions	6
Chorea	2

Table 3.6. Immunologic features in a series of 1,000 European patients with systemic lupus erythematosus (Cervera et al. 1993)

Serologic Feature	Prevalence (%)
Antinuclear antibodies	96
Anti-DNA antibodies	78
Anti-Ro/SSA antibodies	25
Anti-La/SSB antibodies	19
Anti-RNP antibodies	13
Anti-Sm antibodies	10
Rheumatoid factor	18
IgG anticardiolipin antibodies	24
IgM anticardiolipin antibodies	13
Lupus anticoagulant	15

Epidemiology of the Cutaneous Manifestations of Lupus Erythematosus

The cutaneous manifestations of LE have been classified by Gilliam and Sontheimer (Gilliam and Sontheimer 1981) into chronic cutaneous LE (CCLE), subacute cutaneous LE (SCLE), and acute cutaneous LE (ACLE). Any of these forms can appear in patients with LE confined to the skin or in patients with SLE. Overall, cutaneous manifestations appear in 72%–85% of patients with SLE (Dubois and Tuffanelli 1964). They can occur at any stage of the disease, but they are the first manifestations of SLE in 23%–28% of patients (Table 3.7).

CCLE includes classic localized discoid LE (DLE), generalized DLE, hypertrophic/verrucous DLE, lupus panniculitis (lupus profundus), and chilblain LE. DLE is characterized by inflammatory plaques with scaling, follicular, plugging, atrophic scarring, central hypopigmentation, and peripheral hyperpigmentation. Approximately 5% of patients with isolated localized DLE subsequently develop SLE. It has been postulated that SLE is seven-fold more common than DLE. Chronic discoid lesions may be the initial manifestation of SLE in approximately 10% of patients, and they can occur during the course of the disease in 15%–30% of patients. It has been suggested that patients with SLE and discoid lesions may have a more benign clinical course, with less severe renal disease, than unselected patients with SLE (Callen 1985). In another study that included 136 patients with DLE (Le Bozec et al. 1994), the authors described the development of SLE in 11 of them. Interestingly, most of these patients developed SLE within 5 years of the onset of the cutaneous lesions, and 4 of the 11 had a poor prognosis, with renal or neurologic involvement.

SCLE occurs in 10%–15% of patients with SLE and includes the papulosquamosus (psoriasiform) and annular-polycyclic variants. These lesions are usually widespread, symmetrical, and nonscarring. They occur in a characteristic, photoexposed distribution, with an LE-specific histopathology. A few patients may have a combination of psoriasiform and annular lesions, although most predominantly have either one or other subtype (Sontheimer 1989). Approximately, 50% of patients with isolated SCLE subsequently develop SLE. Patients in this subset of LE frequently have anti-Ro antibodies (Sontheimer et al. 1982) and are HLA-B8-DR3/2 positive (Johansson-Stephansson et al. 1989). SCLE may be associated with other systemic autoimmune diseases, and photoactive medications may induce lesions of SCLE.

ACLE appears in 30%–60% of patients with SLE. It includes localized (malar) erythema, widespread (face, scalp, neck, upper chest, shoulders, extensor arms, and back of hands) erythema, and bullous (toxic epidermal necrolysis-like) LE. Additionally, nonspecific but disease-related cutaneous manifestations can appear in patients with LE, including photosensitivity, alopecia, urticaria, livedo reticularis, dermal vasculitis, and Raynaud's phenomenon (Yell et al. 1996).

The prevalence of photosensitivity ranges from 28% to 71%. It is one of the major diagnostic criteria for SLE. Photosensitivity precedes the clinical onset of internal manifestations of SLE in about one third of patients. Some patients may not notice erythema after prolonged UV exposure, but hours or days later they may note increased arthralgia, malaise, or fever.

Table 3.7. Prevalence of cutaneous manifestations in systemic lupus erythematosus in several series

Cutaneous Manifestation	Dubois and Tuffanelli 1964 (n=520)	Estes and Christian 1972 (n=150)	Lee et al. 1977 (n=110)	Grigor et al. 1978 (n=375)	Weinstein et al. 1987b (n=84)	Worral et al. 1990 (n=100)	Pistiner et al. 1991 (n=464)	Yell et al. 1996 (n=73)
All types of skin lesions (%)	72	81	NA	NA	82	90	55	100
Raynaud's phenomenon (%)	18.4	21	46	32	NA	NA	25	60
Photosensitivity (%)	32.7	NA	50	28	NA	48	37	63
Mucous membrane (%)	9.1	7	NA	34	34.5	36	19	55
Malar rash (%)	20.9	NA	NA	NA	21	NA	34	45
Urticaria (%)	6.9	13	5	NA	NA	NA	4	44
Alopecia (%)	21.3	37	38	64	NA	NA	NA	40
Chronic discoid lesions (%)	28.6	14	28	22	11	NA	23	25
Butterfly blush (%)	36.7	39	36	68	NA	NA	NA	14
Vasculitis (%)	NA	21	NA	70	18	NA	NA	11
Bullae (%)	0.4	2	NA	NA	NA	NA	NA	8
Psoriasiform rash (%)	NA	2	NA	NA	NA	NA	NA	7

NA, not applicable.

Hair loss is a common and characteristic finding in patients with SLE. The variability in recording alopecia resulted in its exclusion from the ACR criteria. It may be scarring, if preceded by DLE, or nonscarring.

Urticaria, angioedema, and Raynaud's phenomenon are common cutaneous vascular reaction patterns. Some patients with SLE described lesions suggestive of urticarial vasculitis, with prevalences ranging from 7% (Provost et al. 1980) to 22% (O'Loughlin et al. 1978). Dermal vasculitis has been reported in 18% to 70% of patients with SLE. Livedo reticularis may be associated with the antiphospholipd syndrome and has been reported as an initial manifestation of SLE in many patients (Weinstein et al. 1987a). Other skin disorders have been occasionally reported in patients with SLE, such as sclerodactyly, erythromelalgia, erythema multiforme, chronic ulcers, splinter hemorrhages, rheumatoid nodules, and acanthosis nigricans.

Mucous membrane involvement was thought to be relatively uncommon in SLE. Dubois and Tuffanelli (Dubois and Tuffanelli 1964) found only a 9% incidence. However, on careful inspection, more than 50% of patients with SLE may have mucosal lesions, mainly oral ulcers (Jonsson et al. 1984).

Patterns of Disease Expression in Specific Lupus Erythematosus Subsets

Effects of Age

LE can appear in people of any age. However, in most patients, the LE symptoms appear between ages 15 and 40 years, with a mean age of 29–32 years (Cervera et al. 1993). Conversely, LE can appear before 15 years of age in 8%–15% of patients and in a similar percentage of older patients (>55 years) (Cervera et al. 1993, Font et al. 1991, Nepom and Schaller 1984, Ting and Hsieh 1992). In some studies carried out recently (Gudmundsson and Steisson 1990, Hochberg et al. 1995, Ting and Hsieh 1992), the mean age of appearance of symptoms has increased to 41–47 years.

It is interesting to note that, in several studies, patient age at the beginning of symptoms can modify the clinical and immunologic characteristics of LE. Thus, in the Euro-Lupus project (Cervera et al. 1993), patients whose disease appeared during childhood had a greater incidence of renal disease and a lower incidence of rheumatoid factor. Conversely, patients whose disease appeared at an elderly age presented a lower incidence of malar rash, arthritis, and renal disease as initial manifestations, thus making difficult their diagnosis.

Effects of Sex

Clinical studies have consistently demonstrated a female predominance. Thus, in the greater European series (Cervera et al. 1993), which included 1000 patients, 91% were females, and in the greater American series (Ginzler et al. 1982), which included 1103 patients, 88% were females. In general, this percentage ranges from 78% to 96% in most studies, with a female-male ratio of approximately 10:1. This excess of females is especially noteworthy in the 15- to 64-year-old age group, where ratios of age- and sex-specific incidence rates show a 6- to 10-fold female excess. No such excess was noted in patients 14 years and younger and in those 65 years and older. These age-related differences in the female-male ratios have been considered to be related to hormonal changes.

Effects of Ethnic and Social Factors

A greater incidence and prevalence of LE has consistently been found in blacks than in whites (Siegel and Lee 1973). A study in Birmingham, England, found higher age-adjusted incidence and prevalence rates in Afro-Caribbean people than in whites (Johnson et al. 1995). Incidence rates (age adjusted) were 25.8 and 4.3 cases per 100,000 persons per year in Afro-Caribbean people and whites, respectively, and prevalence rates were 112 and 21 cases per 100,000 persons. In this study, the age distribution of incidence cases differed significantly, with a younger median age in Afro-Caribbean females of 34.5 years compared with 41 years in white females. Some data also exist regarding an excess prevalence of LE in Asians compared with whites. In Birmingham (Johnson et al. 1995), the age-adjusted annual incidence and prevalence rates of LE in Asians were 20.7 and 46.7 cases per 100,000 persons, respectively, compared with 4.3 and 20.7 cases per 100,000 persons in whites, respectively.

The cases described in Africa until the past decade were very scarce. Although there are no good epidemiologic studies, currently it is considered that these differences could be attributed to the associated socioeconomic conditions that favor or hinder diagnosis and correct treatment. For example, since this disease affects fundamentally young women, with an age at onset of 15–40 years, it is possible that the incidence will be greater in countries with rapid population growth. Also, in countries and social groups with worse socioeconomic conditions, a more severe clinical presentation could be more frequent (Symmonds 1995).

Effects of Familial or Hereditary Factors

Studies in relatives of patients with SLE, particularly in homozygous twins, reveal a higher-than-expected incidence of the disease, thus suggesting the influence of hereditary factors. Nevertheless, the frequency in relatives is relatively low and ranges according to the series from 3% to 18%. Recent studies indicate that there are no notorious differences between the patients with SLE who have other affected relatives (familial SLE) and those who do not (sporadic SLE) (Michel et al. 2001).

Mortality Studies

Survival of patients with LE has increased significantly in the past 40 years. Studies performed in 1955 (Merrell and Shuldman 1955) showed a survival rate lower than 50% at 5 years, whereas recent studies (Abu-Shakra et al. 1995a, Gripenberg and Helve 1991, Pistinier et al. 1991, Seleznick and Fries 1991) indicate that approximately 93% of patients with LE survive more than 5 years, and 85% survive more than 10 years. In the Euro-Lupus project (Cervera et al. 2003), 92% survival was found after 10 years from the time of entry into the study, slightly higher than that found in the American studies. This is probably because of a more homogeneous care system in Europe and better management of patients with LE in the present decade (earlier diagnosis, more appropriately used anti-LE therapies, and advances in medical therapy in general).

The improved survival of patients with LE has been associated with an alteration in the patterns of mortality. In 1976, Urowitz et al. (Urowitz et al. 1976) described a bimodal pattern of mortality, emphasizing inflammatory activity as the principal cause of death in patients with a recent diagnosis of SLE, whereas cardiovascular events were the most important cause of death in those with long evolution. Recently, epidemiologic studies observed that although one third of the deaths can be attributed to SLE activity, the complications of the therapy and other noninflammatory manifestations are important causes of death in these patients. This is the case with antiphospholipid antibody-related thrombotic events ("antiphospholipid syndrome"), which were responsible for 26.7% of the deaths in the Euro-Lupus cohort.

Prognosis studies and investigation of variables affecting mortality in LE have identified a wide range of significant factors (Cervera et al. 2003, Fries et al. 1974, Ginzler et al. 1982, Pistiner et al. 1991, Reveille et al. 1990, Seleznick and Fries 1991, Studenski et al. 1987, Wallace et al. 1981). In the Euro-Lupus project, only nephropathy at the beginning of the study was found to have prognostic significance for lower survival probability. However, 88% of patients with nephropathy at the beginning of the study survived after a 10-year follow-up period. Other studies performed in the United States (Reveille et al. 1990) observed that black patients (who more frequently have renal disease) and those with worse socioeconomic conditions or a lower cultural level have the most aggressive course and greater mortality.

References

Abu-Shakra M, Urowitz MB, Gladman DD, Gough J (1995a) Mortality studies in systemic lupus erythematosus. Results from a single center. I. Causes of death. J Rheumatol 22:1259–1264

Abu-Shakra M, Urowitz MB, Gladman DD, Gough J (1995b) Mortality studies in systemic lupus erythematosus. Results for a single center. II. Predictor variables for mortality. J Rheumatol 22:1265–1270

Anstey A, Bastian I, Dunckley H, Currie BJ (1993) Systemic lupus erythematosus in Australian aberigines: high prevalence, morbidity and mortality. Aust N Z J Med 23:646–651

Boumpas DT, Fessler BJ, Austin HA III, Balow JE, Kippel JH, Lockshin MD (1995) Systemic lupus erythematosus: emerging concepts. Part 2: Dermatologic and joint diaseas, the antiphospholipis syndrome, pregnancy and hormonal therapy, morbidity and mortality, and pathogenesis. Ann Intern Med 123:42–53

Callen JP (1985) Systemic lupus erythematosus in patients with chronic cutaneous (discoid) lupus erythematosus. Clinical and laboratory findings in seventeen patients. J Am Acad Dermatol 12:278–288

Cervera R, Khamashta MA, Font J, Sebastiani GD, Gil A, Lavilla P, Domenech I, Aydintug AO, Jedryka-Goral A, de Ramon E, Galeazzi M, Haga HJ, Mathieu A, Houssiau F, Ingelmo M, Hughes GRV, and the European Working Party on Systemic Lupus Erythematosus (1993) Systemic lupus erythematosus: clinical and imunological patterns of disease in a cohort of 1000 patients. Medicine (Baltimore) 72:113–124

Cervera R, Khamashta MA, Font J, Sebastiani GD, Gil A, Lavilla P, Mejia JC, Aydintug AO, Chwalinska-Sadowska H, de Ramon E, Fernandez-Nebro A, Galeazzi M, Valen M, Mathieu A,

Houssiau F, Caro N, Alba P, Ramos-Casals M, Ingelmo M, Hughes GR (2003) Morbidity and mortality in systemic lupus erythematosus during a 10-year period. A comparison of early and late manifestations in a cohort of 1000 patients. Medicine (Baltimore) 82:299–308

Drenkard C, Villa AR, Alarcón-Segovia D, Pérez-Vazquez ME (1994) Influence of the antiphospholipid syndrome in the survival of patients with systemic lupus erythematosus. J Rheumatol 21:1067–1072

Dubois EL, Tuffanelli DL (1964) Clinical manifestations of SLE. Computer analysis of 520 cases. J Am Med Assoc 190:104–111

Estes D, Christian C (1971) The natural history of systemic lupus erythematosus by prospective analysis. Medicine (Baltimore) 50:85–95

Fessel WJ (1974) Systemic lupus erythematosus in the community: incidence, prevalence, outcome and first symptoms; the high prevalence in black women. Arch Intern Med 134:1027–1035

Font J, Cervera R (1993) 1982 revised criteria for classification of systemic lupus erythematosus-Ten years later. Lupus 2:339–341

Font J, Pallarés L, Cervera R, Lopez-Soto A, Navarro M, Bosch X, Ingelmo M (1991) Systemic lupus erythematosus in the elderly: clinical and immunological characteristics. Ann Rheum Dis 50:702–705

Font J, Pallarés L, Cervera R, Vivancos J, Lopez-Soto A, Herrero C, Darnell A, Torras A, Mirapeix E, del Olmo JA et al (1993) Lupus eritematoso sistémico: estudio clínico e inmunológico de 300 pacientes. Med Clin (BARC) 100:601–605

Fries JF, Weyl S, Hellman HR (1974) Estimating prognosis in diasease activity. Am J Med 57:561–566

Fukase M (1980) The epidemiology of systemic lupus erythematosus in Japan. In: Fukase M (ed) Systemic lupus erythematosus. University Park Press, Baltimore S 3–10

Gilliam JN, Sontheiner RD (1981) Distinctive cutaneous subsets in the spectrum of lupus erythematosus. J Am Acad Dermatol 4:471–475

Ginzler EM, Diamond HS, Weiner M, Schlesinger M, Fries JF, Wasner C, Medsger TA Jr, Ziegler G, Klippel JH, Hadler NM, Albert DA, Hess EV, Spencer Green G, Grayzel A, Worth D, Hahn BH, Barnett EV (1982) A multicenter study of outcomes in systemic lupus erythematosus. I. Entry variables as predictors of prognosis. Arthritis Rheum 25:601–611

Gladman DD (1996) Prognosis and treatment of systemic lupus erythematosus. Curr Op Rheumatol 8:430–437

Gourley IS, Patterson CC, Bell AL (1997) The prevalence of systemic lupus erythematosus in Nothern Ireland. Lupus 6:399–403

Grigor R, Edmons J, Lewkonia R, Bresnihan B, Hughes GR (1978) Systemic lupus erythematosus. A prospective analysis. Ann Rheum Dis 37:121–128

Gripenberg M, Helve T (1991) Outcome of systemic lupus erythematosus. A study of 66 patients over 7 years with special reference to the predictive value of anti-DNA antibody detrminations. Scand J Rheumatol 20:104–109

Gudmundsson S, Steisson K (1990) Systemic lupus erythematosus in Iceland 1975 though 1984. A nationwide epidemiological study in an unselected population. J Rheumatol 17:1162–1167

Helve T (1985) Prevalence and mortality rates of systemic lupus erythematosus and causes of death in SLE patients in Finland. Scand J Rheumatol 14:43–46

Hochberg MC (1987) Prevalence of systemic lupus erythematosus in England and Wales, 1981–2. Ann Rheum Dis 46:664–666

Hochberg MC, Perlmutter SL, Medsger TA, Steen V, Weisman MH, White B, Wigley FM (1995) Prevalence of self-reported physician-diagnosed systemic lupus erythematosus in the USA. Lupus 4:454–456

Hopkinson ND, Doherty M, Powell RJ (1994) Clinical features and race-specific incidence/prevalence rates of systemic lupus erythematosus in geographically complete cohort of patients. Ann Rheum Dis 53:675–680

Iseki K, Miyasato F, Oura T, Uehara H, Nishime K, Fukiyama K (1994) An epidemiologic analysis of end-stage lupus nephritis. Am J Kidney Dis 23:547–554

Johnson H, Nived O (1990) Estimating the incidence of systemic lupus erythematosus in a defined population using multiple sources of retrieval. Br J Rheumatol 29:185–188

Johnson AE, Gordon C, Palmer RG, Bacon PA (1995) The prevalence and incidence of systemic lupus erythematosus in Birmingham, England. Arthritis Rheum 38:551–558

Jonsson R, Heyden G, Westberg NG (1984) Oral mucosal lesions in systemic lupus erythematosus. A clinical, histopathological and immunopathological study. J Rheumatol 11:38–42

Johansson-Stephansson E, Koskimies S, Partanen J, Kariniemi AL (1989) Subacute cutaneous lupus erythematosus. Genetic markers and clinical and immunological findings in patients. Arch Dermatol 125:791–796

Karlson EW, Daltroy LH, Lew RA, Wright EA, Patridge AJ, Fossel AH, Roberts WN, Stern SH, Straaton KV, Wacholtz MC, Kavanaugh AF, Grosflam JM, Liang MH (1997) The relation ship of socioeconomic status, race and modifiable risk factors to outcomes in patients with systemic lupus erythematosus. Arthritis Rheum 40:47–56

Kellum RE, Haserike JR (1964) Systemic lupus erythematosus, a statistical evaluation of mortality based on a consecutive series of 229 patients. Arch Intern Med 113:200–207

Le Bozec P, La Guyadec T, Crickx B (1994) Chronic lupus erythematosus in lupus disease. Retrospective study of 136 patients. Presse Med 23:1598–15602

Lee P, Urowitz MB, Boockman AA, Koehler BE, Smythe HA, Gordon DA, Ogryzlo MA (1977) Systemic lupus erythematosus. A review of 110 cases with reference to nephritis, the nervous system, infections, aseptic necrosis and prognosis. Q J Med 46:1–32

Maskarinec G, Katz AR (1995) Prevalence of systemic lupus erythematosus in Hawaii: Is there a difference between ethnic groups? Hawaii Med J 54:406–409

Meddings J, Grennan MD (1980) The prevalence of systemic lupus erythematosus (SLE) in Dunedin. N Z Med J 91:205–206

Merrell M, Shuldman LE (1955) Determination of prognosis in chronic disease, illustrated by systemic lupus erythematosus. J Chron Dis 1:12–32

McCarty DJ, Manzi S, Medsger TA, Ramsy-Goldman R, La Porte PE, Kwoh CK (1995) Incidence of systemic lupus erythematosus. Race and gender differences. Arthritis Rheum 38: 1260–1270

Michel M, Johanet C, Meyer C, Frances C, Wittke F, Michel C, Arfi S, Tournier-Lasserve E, Piette JC (2001) Familial lupus erythematosus: clinical and immunological features of 125 multiplex families. Medicine (Baltimore) 80:153–158

Michet CJ, McKenna CH, Elveback LR, Kaslow RA, Kurland LT (1985) Epidemiology of systemic lupus erythematosus and other connective tissue diseases in Rochester, Minnesota, 1950 through 1979. Mayo Clin Proc 60:105–113

Nepom BS, Schaller JG (1984) Chilhood systemic lupus erythematosus. Prog Clin Rheumatol 1:33–69

Nived O, Sturfelt G, Wolheim F (1985) Systemic lupus erythematosus in an adult population in southern Sweden: Incidence/prevalence and validity of ARA revised criteria. Br J Rheumatol 24:147–154

Nossent JC (1992) Systemic lupus erythematosus on the Caribbean island of Curacao: An epidemiological investigation. Ann Rheum Dis 51:1197–1201

O'Loughlin S, Schoeter AL, Jordan RE (1978) Chronic urticaria-like lesions in systemic lupus erythematosus. Arch Dermatol 114:879–883

Pistiner M, Wallace DJ, Nessim S, Metzger AL, Klinenberg JR (1991) Lupus erythematosus in the 1980s: a survey of 570 patients. Semin Arthritis Rheum 21:55–64

Provost TT, Zone JJ, Synowski D (1980) Unusual cutaneous manifestations of systemic lupus erythematosus: I. Urticaria-like lesions. Correlations with clinical and serological abnormalities. J Invest Dermatol 75:495–499

Reveille JD, Bartolucci A, Alarcón GS (1990) Prognosis in systemic lupus erythematosus. Negative impact of increasing age at onset, black race, and thrombocytopenia, as well as causes of death. Arthritis Rheum 33:37–48

Rubin LA, Urowitz MB, Gladman DD (1985) Mortality in systemic lupus erythematosus: the bimodal pattern revisited. Q J Med 55:87–98

Samanta A, Roy S, Feehally J, Symmons D (1992) The prevalence of diagnosed systemic lupus erythematosus in whites and Indian Asian immigrants in Leicester City, UK. Lupus 1(suppl):123

Seleznick MJ, Fries JF (1991) Variables associated with decreased survival in systemic lupus erythematosus. Semin Arthritis Rheum 21:73–80

Siegel M, Lee SL (1973) The epidemiology of systemic lupus erythematosus. Semin Arthritis Rheum 3:1–54

Sontheimer RD, Maddison PJ, Reichlin M (1982) Serologic and HLA associations in subacute cutaneous lupus erythematosus, a clinical subset of lupus erythematosus. Ann Intern Med 97:664–671

Sontheimer RD (1989) Subacute cutaneous lupus erythematosus: a decade's perspective. Med Clin North Am 73:1073–1090

Studenski S, Allen NB, Caldwell DS, Rice JR, Polisson RP (1987) Survival in systemic lupus erythematosus: A multivariate analysis of demographic factors. Arthritis Rheum 30:1326–1332

Swaak AJ, Nossent J, Bronsveld W, Van Rooyen A, Nieuwenhuys EJ, Theuns L, Smeenk RJ (1989) Systemic lupus erythematosus: I. Outcome and survival: Dutch experience with 110 patients studied prospectively. Ann Rheum Dis 48:447–454

Symmonds DPM (1995) Frequency of lupus in people of African origin. Lupus 4:176–178

Tan EM, Cohen AS, Fries JF, Masi AT, McShane DJ, Rothfield HF, Schaller JG, Talal N, Winchester RJ (1982) The 1982 revised criteria for classification of SLE. Arthritis Rheum 25:1271–1272

Ting CK, Hsieh KH (1992) A long term immunological study of childhood onset systemic lupus erythematosus. Ann Rheum Dis 51:45–51

Uramoto KM, Michet CJ, Thumboo J, Sunku J, O'Fallon WM, Gabriel SE (1999) Trends in the incidence and mortality of systemic lupus erythematosus 1992. Arthritis Rheum 42:46–50

Urowitz MB, Bookman AAM, Koeler BE, Gordon DA, Smythe HA, Ogryzlo MA (1976) The bimodal mortality pattern of systemic lupus erythematosus. Am J Med 60:221–225

Villar J, Sánchez de Cos J, Pachón J, Maestre J, Pastor L, Martin M, Carneado J, Salgado V (1980) Lupus erythematosus disseminatus. Evaluation of the clinical and biological manifestations in 54 cases. Rev Clin Esp 159:21–26

Vlachoyiannopoulos PG, Karassa FB, Karakostas KX, Drosos AA, Moutsopoulos HM (1993) Systemic lupus erythematosus in Greece. Clinical features, evolution and outcome: a descriptive analysis of 292 patients. Lupus 2:303–313

Wallace DJ, Podell T, Weiner J, Klinenberg JR, Forouzesh S, Dubois EL (1981) Systemic lupus erythematosus: Experience with 609 patients. JAMA 245:934–938

Ward MM, Pyun E, Studenski S (1995a) Long-term survival in systemic lupus erythematosus. Patients characterisctics associated with poorer outcomes. Arthritis Rheum 38:274–283

Ward MM, Pyun E, Studenski S (1995b) Causes of death in systemic lupus erythematosus. Long-term follow-up of an inception cohort. Arthritis Rheum 38:1492–1499

Weinstein C, Miller MH, Axtens R, Buchanan R, Littlejohn GO (1987a) Livedo reticularis associated with increased titres of anticardiolipin antibodies in systemic lupus erythematosus. Arch Dermatol 123:596–600

Weinstein C, Miller MH, Axtens R, Littlejohn GO, Dorevitch AP, Buchanan R (1987b) Lupus and non-lupus cutaneous manifestations in systemic lupus erythematosus. Aust NZ J Med 17:501–506

Worral JG, Snaith ML, Batchelor JR, Isenberg DA (1990) SLE: a rheumatological view. Analysis of the clinical features, serology and immunogenetics of 100 SLE patients during long-term follow-up. Q J Med 74:319–330

Yell JA, Mbuagbaw J, Burge SM (1996) Cutaneous manifestations of systemic lupus erythematosus. Br J Dermatol 135:355–362

CHAPTER 4

Historical Background of Cutaneous Lupus Erythematosus

PERCY LEHMANN

The term *lupus érythémateaux* was used for the first time by Cazénave (Cazénave 1851) in 1851 to distinguish the noninfectious forms of lupus from cutaneous tuberculosis (lupus vulgaris). Cazénave referred in his original paper to Biett's earlier report on this disease, which was termed *erytheme centrifuge,* as being a very good description of what nowadays would be called *discoid lupus erythematosus* (DLE). Also, in 1845, Hebra (Hebra 1845) precisely described systemic manifestations of LE that occurred in patients who had the classic "butterfly erythema," which he named "seborrhea congestive". Since the earlier descriptions had always discussed LE in the context of cutaneous tuberculosis, it is very much Cazénave's achievement to have clearly separated LE from an infectious disease, thus clearing the way for further studies on this complex disease following other hypotheses and directions.

Based on Hebra's work, further clinical and histopathologic studies on the relation of cutaneous lesions and systemic manifestations of LE were performed. Kaposi (Kaposi 1869, 1872, 1880) recognized the relationship of DLE and systemic LE (SLE) and extensively described the butterfly erythema as a facial cutaneous sign of SLE. Accordingly, through his continuous efforts, which are reflected in several publications between 1869 and 1880, Kaposi is nowadays recognized as the first describer of SLE. In 1872, Kaposi described SLE as an acute febrile eruption with pronounced painful joint involvement and a characteristic facial erythema that he termed "erysipelas perstans faciei" (Fig. 4.1).

The most extensive description on the systemic manifestations of LE at that time must be referred to Osler in 1895 (Osler 1895) in his work titled "On the visceral complications of erythema exsudativum multiforme". Although he had not adopted the term "lupus erythematosus" from his European colleagues, he based his studies on their work, and, thus, the investigations dealing with this fascinating and complex disease reached the New World by the end of the 19th century.

In an article published by the *Journal of the American Medical Association* in 1923, Goeckerman (Goeckerman 1923) pointed again in depth to the systemic nature of LE ("lupus erythematosus as a systemic disease"). In Europe, Hutchinson (Hutchinson 1888) emphasized at the end of the 19th century the multisystem nature of LE and the different expressions and variations of the disease with respect to cutaneous and systemic manifestations in different patients.

In summary, the complex disease LE was first recognized and evaluated by its visible cutaneous manifestations before the analysis and study of its systemic manifestations established the multisystem nature of LE.

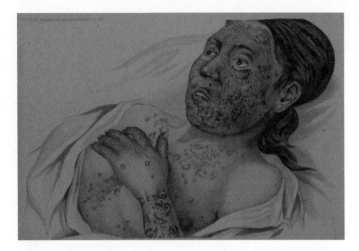

Fig. 4.1. Historical drawing of cutaneous lupus erythematosus (from Kaposi's *Handatlas der Hautkrankheiten* [Kaposi 1898])

Clinical and Histologic Classifications of Lupus Erythematosus

On establishing the unifying concept that LE comprised a common disease with heterogenous expressions, attempts were undertaken to develop a clinical classification of the different forms of LE.

In 1921, Brocq (Brocq 1921) subdivided LE into three different forms: DLE, disseminated DLE, and SLE. In 1934, O'Leary (O'Leary 1934) further developed the classification, trying to connect the cutaneous manifestations to certain systemic involvements. He stressed that disseminated DLE represented the transition from a localized cutaneous disease to a multisystem systemic illness, namely, SLE. At that time, no serologic markers had been identified, which later helped better characterize the different subsets in the LE spectrum. The concept of a disease spectrum was, finally, emphasized by Dubois and Tuffanelli (Dubois and Tuffanelli 1964). They extensively described 520 consecutive patients with SLE, with precise characterization of the various cutaneous and systemic disease expressions, therefore demonstrating the disease continuum from the relatively benign forms of limited skin disease such as localized DLE to the potentially fatal fully expressed SLE. Between these two poles a spectrum of characteristic disease manifestations was recognized in which clinical, histopathologic, serologic, immunologic, and photobiologic features composed the fundamentals for the specific diagnosis of an LE subset with a well-established prognostic value.

The modern and generally accepted classification of LE is based mostly on the work of Gilliam, Sontheimer, and their coworkers (Gilliam and Sontheimer 1981a, b, 1982, 1983). Based on the spectrum concept of Dubois, they concentrated on the relationships that exist between the various cutaneous and systemic manifestations of LE. Clinical, histopathologic, photobiologic, immunologic, and genetic studies led

Gilliam and Sontheimer to the extensive in-depth description of the immunogenetically homogeneous LE subset, namely, subacute cutaneous LE (SCLE). This work led to the modern classification of LE and has been widely agreed on. This progress had been made possible by the rapid developments in biochemistry, immunology, and molecular biology that were integrated into clinical science and helped investigate the various phenomenologic expressions of LE. Examples include the discovery of the LE cell factor by Hargraves et al. (Hargraves et al. 1948) in 1948 and the development of the antinuclear antibody assay in 1957 by Friou (Friou 1957). These laboratory investigations prompted the era of intense research on clinical-serologic correlations.

The discovery and characterization of numerous antibodies led to a better understanding of the various expressions of LE sometimes assuming a marker function for the disease.

Photobiology

Of the different external factors that have detrimental effects on disease activity, the sun's radiation has been best studied. Already in Cazénave's original description (Cazénave 1881) it was mentioned that outdoor workers were predisposed to the disorder and that exacerbations of the disease were related to environmental factors. Hutchinson (Hutchinson 1888) reported in his Harveian Lectures on Lupus, published in 1888, that patients with LE did not tolerate exposure to the sun. In 1915, Pusey (Pusey 1915) described a young lady with LE that first appeared after some days of extensive golfing in the summertime. The lesions disappeared after strict avoidance of the sun, only to reexacerbate the next summer after a golf tournament. Freund (Freund 1929) evaluated in a study from 1920 to 1927 the admission of patients with LE to the Department of Dermatology in Berlin. He demonstrated an increased prevalence of new LE cases in May and June and concluded that climatic factors were responsible for this climax in the number of new patients with LE.

Shortly after these observations it became clear that artificial light sources were also able to induce LE. Jesionek (Jesionek 1916), a German pioneer of phototherapy, warned clinicians in 1916 not to apply phototherapy in patients with LE. He described two cases in which phototherapy had caused dramatic exacerbation of the disease with induction of systemic multiorgan involvement for previously limited DLE. In 1929, Fuhs (Fuhs 1929) reported a patient with exacerbated "lupus erythematosus subacutus" after irradiation with an artificial light source. Possibly, this is the first description of the exquisite light sensitivity of the SCLE subset. The author unsuccessfully tried to determine the action spectra and dosages that led to disease induction.

Epstein (Epstein et al. 1965) was the first investigator to introduce the repeated exposure technique, which enabled him and his coworkers to induce LE lesions in 5 of 25 patients. Baer and Harber (Baer and Harber 1965) also tested a limited number of patients, and Freeman et al. (Freeman et al. 1969) as well as Cripps and Rankin (Cripps and Rankin 1973) performed for the first time studies with monochromatic radiation, because of these studies, the action spectrum of LE was ascribed to the ultraviolet (UV) B range. In 1990, our group (Lehmann et al. 1990) demonstrated that the action spectrum of LE reaches into the long-wave UVA region. In the original study, 128 patients with LE had been tested using a standardized phototest protocol.

This study was extended, and over the ensuing 15 years 405 patients with LE were phototested (Kuhn et al. 2001). Other groups confirmed the published results (Leenutaphon and Boonchai 1999, Nived et al. 1993, Walchner et al. 1997, Wolska et al. 1989). During these studies, a rare subset of cutaneous LE, namely LE tumidus (LET), turned out to be even more photosensitive than SCLE (Kuhn et al. 2001). LET was first mentioned by Gougerot and Burnier (Gourgerot and Burnier 1930) in 1930, but since then LET has been documented rarely in the literature.

In 1981, Provost and coworkers (Provost 1983, Provost and Reichlin 1981, Provost et al. 1983, 1985) described the anti-Ro/SSA autoantibody as a serologic marker for neonatal LE and the association of these autoantibodies with a group of patients with LE and exquisite photosensitivity. Subsequently, Norris and colleagues demonstrated that UV irradiation modulates the expression of Ro/SSA antigens by epidermal keratinocytes (LeFeber et al. 1984, Norris and Lee 1985). For the first time, a molecular explanation for photosensitivity of patients with LE was presented. Ten years later, in 1994, Casciola-Rosen et al. (Casciola-Rosen et al. 1994) studied UV-induced apoptosis of keratinocytes of patients with LE. They demonstrated the compartmentalization of specific nucleosome constituents to the cytoplasmatic cell surface blebs of apoptotic keratinocytes. This was hypothesized to be a possible first step in the cascade that finally leads to an autoimmune disease.

References

O'Leary PA (1934) Disseminated lupus erythematosus. Minn Med 17:637–644

Baer RL, Harber LC (1965) Photobiology of lupus erythematosus. Arch Dermatol 92:124–128

Brocq L (1921) Précis-atlas de pratique dermatologique. G Doin, Paris, pp 468–477

Casciola-Rosen LA, Anhalt G, Rosen A (1994) Autoantigens targeted in systemic lupus erythematosus are clustered in two populations of surface structures on apoptotic keratinocytes. J Exp Med 179:1317–1330

Cazénave PLA (1851) Lupus érythémateux (érythéme centrifuge). Ann Mal Peau Syph 3:297–299

Cripps DJ, Rankin J (1973) Action spectra of lupus erythematosus and experimental immunoflourescence. Arch Dermatol 107:563–567

Dubois EL, Tuffanelli DL (1964) Clinical manifestations of systemic lupus erythematosus. JAMA 190:104–111

Epstein JH, Tuffanelli DL, Dubois EL (1965) Light sensitivity and lupus erythematosus. Arch Dermatol 91:483–485

Freeman RG, Knox JM, Owens DW (1969) Cutaneous lesions of lupus erythematosus induced by monochromatic light. Arch Dermatol 100:677–682

Freund H (1929) Inwieweit ist der Lupus erythematodes von allgemeinen Faktoren abhängig? Dermatol Wochenschr 89:1939–1946

Friou GJ (1957) Clinical application of lupus serum: nucleoprotein reaction using fluorescent antibody technique. J Clin Invest 36:890

Fuhs E (1929) Lupus erythematosus subacutus mit ausgesprochener Überempfindlichkeit gegen Quarzlicht. Z Hautkr 30:308–309

Gilliam JN, Sontheimer RD (1981a) Distinctive cutaneous subsets in the spectrum of lupus erythematosus. J Am Acad Dermatol 4:471–475

Gilliam JN, Sontheimer RD (1981b) Skin manifestations of SLE. Clin Rheum Dis 8:207–218

Gilliam JN, Sontheimer RD (1982) Subacute cutaneous lupus erythematosus. Clin Rheum Dis 8:343–352

Gilliam JN, Sontheimer RD (1983) Clinically and immunologically defined subsets of lupus erythematosus. Dermatol Clin 2:147–165

Goeckerman WH (1923) Lupus erythematosus as a systemic disease. JAMA 80:542–547

Gourgerot H, Burnier R (1930) Lupus érythémateux tumidus. Bull Soc Fr Dermatol Syphil 37:1291–1292

Hargraves MM, Richmond H, Morton R (1948) Presentation of two bone marrow elements: The "tart" cell and the "LE" cell. Mayo Clin Proc 23:25–28

Hebra F (1845) Bericht über die Leistungen in der Dermatologie. In: Jahresbericht über die Fortschritte der gesamten Medizin in allen Ländern. Enke Verlag, Erlangen, pp 226–227

Hutchinson J (1888) Harveian lectures on lupus. Lecture III. On the various forms of lupus vulgaris and erythematosus. Br Med J 1:113–118

Jesionek A (1916) Richtlinien der modernen Lichttherapie. Strahlentherapie 7:41–65

Kaposi M (1869) Zum Wesen und zur Therapie des Lupus erythematodes. Arch Dermatol Syph 1:18–41

Kaposi M (1872) Neue Beiträge zur Kenntnis des Lupus erythematodes. Arch Dermatol Syph 1:36–78

Kaposi M (1880) Pathologie und Therapie der Hautkrankheiten. In: Vorlesungen für praktische Ärzte und Studierende (2nd ed). Urban & Schwarzenberg, Vienna, pp 608–615

Kaposi, M (1898–1900) Handatlas der Hautkrankheiten fur Studierende und Ärzte. Wilheld Braumüller, Vienna

Kuhn A, Richter-Hintz D, Oslislo C, Ruzicka T, Megahed M, Lehmann P (2000) Lupus erythematosus tumidus, a neglected subset of cutaneous lupus erythematosus: report of 40 cases. Arch Dermatol 136:1033–1040

Kuhn A, Sonntag M, Richter-Hintz D, Oslislo C, Megahed M, Ruzicka T, Lehmann P (2001) Phototesting in lupus erythematosus: a 15-year experience. J Am Acad Dermatol 45:86–95

Leenutaphong V, Boonchai W (1999) Phototesting in oriental patients with lupus erythematosus. Photodermatol Photoimmunol Photomed 15:7–12

LeFeber WP, Norris DA, Ran SR, Lee LA, Huff JC, Kubo M, Boyce ST, Kotzin BL, Weston WL (1984) Ultraviolet light induces binding of antibodies to selected nuclear antigens on cultures of human keratinocytes. J Clin Invest 74:1545

Lehmann P, Holzle E, Kind P, Goerz G, Plewig G (1990) Experimental reproduction of skin lesions in lupus erythematosus by UVA and UVB radiation. J Am Acad Dermatol 22:181–187

Nived O, Johansen PB, Sturfelt G (1993) Standardized ultraviolet-A exposure provokes skin reaction in systemic lupus erythematosus. Lupus 2:247–250

Norris DA, Lee LA (1985) Antibody-dependent cellular cytotoxicity and skin disease. J Invest Dermatol 85:165S–175S

Osler W (1895) On the visceral complications of erythema exsudativum multiforme. Am J Med Sci 110:629–646

Provost TT (1983) Neonatal lupus erythematosus. Arch Dermatol 119:619–622

Provost TT, Reichlin M (1981) Antinuclear antibody-negative systemic lupus erythematosus. J Am Acad Dermatol 4:84–89

Provost TT, Arnett TC, Reichlin M (1983) Homozygous C2 deficiency, lupus erythematosus, and anti-Ro(SS-A) antibodies. Arthritis Rheum 26:1279–1281

Provost TT, Herrera-Esparza R, Diaz LA (1985) Nucleoprotein autoantibodies in lupus erythematosus. J Invest Dermatol 85:133–139

Pusey WA (1915) Attacks of lupus erythematosus following exposure to sunlight or other weather factors. Arch Dermatol Syph 34:388

Walchner M, Messer G, Kind P (1997) Phototesting and photoprotection in LE. Lupus 6:167–174

Wolska H, Blaczyk M, Jablonska S (1989) Phototests in patients with various forms of lupus erythematosus. Int J Dermatol 28:98–103

Part II
Classification
and Clincial Aspects
of Cutaneous Lupus
Erythematosus

CHAPTER 5

Classification of Cutaneous Lupus Erythematosus

ANNEGRET KUHN, THOMAS RUZICKA

The clinical expression of skin involvement in patients with lupus erythematosus (LE) is very common and shows great variation. Therefore, it has been difficult to develop a unifying concept of the cutaneous manifestations of this disease, and much attention has been paid to the issue of classifying LE from the dermatologic perspective in the past. However, the only universally accepted criteria for the classification of LE are those of the American Rheumatism Association (ARA), now known as the American College of Rheumatology (ACR), which were established in 1971 (Cohen et al. 1971) and revised in 1982 (Tan et al. 1982) and 1997 (Hochberg 1997). This classification system includes 11 clinical and laboratory criteria for the classification of systemic LE (SLE) primarily for the purpose of providing some degree of uniformity to the patient populations of clinical studies. For rheumatologists and internists, however, the ARA classification criteria for SLE might be most meaningful, whereas a histologic classification of nephritis would likely be of greater value to nephrologists, and a clinical and histopathologic classification of the cutaneous manifestations of LE would be most useful to dermatologists (Sontheimer 1997). Unfortunately, a classification criteria system for the more mildly affected patients who suffer predominantly from cutaneous LE (CLE) has not yet been established. There is still continuous debate within the dermatology community concerning classification criteria for patients having a form of CLE without systemic disease activity that would be recognized by the ARA criteria system as SLE (Sontheimer 1997).

In 1977, Gilliam (Gilliam 1977) initially proposed a nomenclature for cutaneous manifestations of LE, with several refinements soon thereafter (Gilliam and Sontheimer 1981, 1982), that was presented in the context of a new clinical-histopathologic classification system. The new nomenclature attempted to bring some order to the high level of confusion that existed in the literature resulting from the use of ambiguous and competing terms for the plethora of skin lesions that can be encountered in patients with LE. The unique and clinically relevant relationships that exist between individual skin lesions and aspects of the underlying systemic disease process should not be overlooked, and the new developments in immunology should best be integrated into the management of patients with cutaneous manifestations of LE (Sontheimer 1997). The classification system developed by Gilliam divided all skin lesions with any association to LE into those that are histologically specific for LE (LE-specific skin disease) and those that do not share this pattern of histopathologic changes (LE-nonspecific skin disease). Three broad categories of LE-specific skin lesions had been suggested: acute CLE (ACLE), subacute CLE (SCLE), and chronic CLE (CCLE) with its variants, such as discoid LE (DLE). The adjectives "acute," "subacute," and "chronic" used in these designations conform to the classic dermatologic definitions of these terms. In contrast, LE-nonspecific skin lesions, such as calcinosis cutis, sclerodactyly, cutaneous vasculitis, and rheumatoid nodules, are those that in some way are related to the under-lying LE autoimmune disease process but can also be encountered in other disease set-tings. This nomenclature by Gilliam was meant to be a more logical classification sys-tem for the extremely varied skin lesions that can be encountered in patients with LE, and the various categories within this classification system were not meant to rigidly define subsets of LE (Sontheimer 1997). In most patients, one form of LE-specific skin involvement will predominate; however, with any arbitrary subdivision of a disease continuum such as LE, overlapping features can occur. For example, patients who have predominantly SCLE lesions can also develop ACLE or scarring CCLE lesions at some point in the course of their disease. Furthermore, a small percentage of patients pre-senting with CCLE or SCLE skin lesions can subsequently die of complications of SLE. However, there are certain patterns of systemic disease activity or inactivity that can be seen to occur in conjunction with the three categories of LE-specific skin disease.

Since the initial formulation of the Gilliam nomenclature and classification system more than 2 decades ago, several attempts have been made to improve on this system or to provide altogether new approaches to the problem of classification of cutaneous manifestations of LE. In 1991, Beutner et al. (Beutner et al. 1991) first presented the results of their studies on a new criteria set developed by the European Academy of Dermatology and Venereology (EADV) for the purpose of classification of patients with CLE. The European system differs from the ARA classification criteria for SLE by using a greater number of better-defined dermatologic criteria, such as Raynaud phe-nomenon, alopecia, and urticarial vasculitis. Furthermore, the group by Beutner et al. (Beutner et al. 1992, 1993) subsequently presented additional work in this area, which includes an effort to develop a new criteria set for identifying SLE in patients with cuta-neous disease using a two-step model. However, although commendable in its goals and its systemic approach, this classification scheme has not yet gained wide accept-ance. As others have pointed out (Halmi et al. 1993), the approach advocated by Beut-ner et al. is more cumbersome to use than the ARA criteria classification system, and, as a result, it is less useful to the practicing clinician. More recently, Parodi and Rebora (Parodi and Rebora 1997) supported the value of the EADV criteria, finding them to be somewhat less sensitive but more specific than the ARA criteria for patients with CLE. This group strongly recommended that the ARA criteria should not be used in patients with CLE as they are too sensitive, poorly specific, and altogether misleading. In 1993, Halmi et al. (Halmi et al. 1993) proposed a new three-part classification scheme for LE that included a bridging category between CLE and SLE that was termed "intermediate LE". Patients with this form were defined as those with skin lesions showing histopathologic features of LE and fulfilling more than 1 but less than 4 of the 11 ARA criteria for the diagnosis of SLE. In this system, CLE was defined as having only one such criterion, namely, isolated CLE lesions, and SLE was defined as having four or more such criteria. The positive and negative aspects of this classification system were subsequently debated in a public forum by a panel of experienced clinicians (Rothfield et al. 1994). Although attractive in some aspects, the mere counting up of classification criteria can at times be misleading, especially when attempting to use such criteria for diagnosis rather than classification. An identical classification system to that described by Halmi et al. was used by Watanabe and Tsuchida in 1995 (Watanabe and Tsuchida

1995) in their elegantly executed efforts to better document the relationships that exist between the cutaneous and systemic manifestations of LE in Japanese patients.

Further efforts have been made to simplify the classification of LE by developing classification trees through the methods of recursive partitioning (Edworthy et al. 1988). In addition, much work has been expanded to subclassify the cutaneous manifestations of this disease into more uniform patient groups (Costner et al. 2003, Sontheimer and Provost 1996), and a variety of subclassification criteria have been used: clinical features, laboratory findings, histopathologic and immunohistologic patterns, genetic associations, and, more recently, phototesting results. Provocative phototesting has been crucial in further characterizing a highly photosensitive form of CLE, namely, LE tumidus (LET) (Kuhn et al. 2000). Although LET was first mentioned by Hoffmann in 1909 (Hoffmann 1909), and some years later by Gougerot and Bournier (Gougerot and Burnier 1930), this subtype had since been somewhat "forgotten" or rarely described in the literature. In 1990, Goerz et al. (Goerz et al. 1990) emphasized for the first time the extreme photosensitivity as a major characteristic of LET, and additional studies showed that these patients were more photosensitive than those with other forms of CLE (Kuhn et al. 2001a). Furthermore, in our experience the prognosis in patients with LET is generally more favorable than in those with other forms of CLE and, interestingly, LET lesions can disappear spontaneously within days or weeks, even if the disease recurs chronically in these patients. Nevertheless, characteristic LET lesions can also occur in patients with SLE (Jolly et al. 2004). Recent studies of more than 60 patients with LET further confirmed that this subtype of CLE has so many characteristic features that it should be considered as a separate entity and differentiated from ACLE, SCLE, and CCLE (Kuhn et al. 2000, 2001b, 2002a, b, 2003). Meanwhile, there is no doubt about LET being a separate entity, and further case reports of this disease followed from groups other than our own (Alexiades-Armenakas et al. 2003, Hsu et al. 2002, Pacheco et al. 2002). Therefore, based on the recent published data on LET we developed a modified classification system including LET as an intermittent subtype of CLE (ICLE) (Kuhn 2003). In addition, bullous skin lesions associated with different forms of LE (BLE) have also been added to the new

Table 5.1. Düsseldorf Classification of Cutaneous Lupus Erythematosus 2003

Acute cutaneous lupus erythematosus (ACLE)
Subacute cutaneous lupus erythematosus (SCLE)

Chronic cutaneous lupus erythematosus (CCLE)
   Discoid lupus erythematosus (DLE)
     Hypertrophic/verrucous variant
     Teleangiectoid variant
   Lupus erythematosus profundus (LEP)
   Chilblain lupus erythematosus (CHLE)

Intermittent cutaneous lupus erythematosus (ICLE)   Lupus erythematosus tumidus (LET)

Bullous lesions in lupus erythematosus (BLE)
   LE-specific bullous skin lesions
   LE-nonspecific bullous skin lesions
   Primarily bullous skin disorders associated with LE

"Düsseldorf classification of CLE 2003" (Table 5.1). The various types of vesicular and bullous skin lesions that can occur in patients with LE have been divided into those that show or do not show LE-specific histopathology (Sontheimer 1997, Yell and Wojnarowska 1997). Furthermore, a number of primarily blistering diseases, such as bullous pemphigoid, dermatitis herpetiformis, and pemphigus vulgaris, has been reported in relationship to LE. Whether these bullous skin disorders are the result of the LE autoimmune disease process or develop as a mere chance occurence in patients who also have LE is not clear.

References

Alexiades-Armenakas MR, Baldassano M, Bince B, Werth V, Bystryn JC, Kamino H, Soter NA, Franks AG (2003) Tumid lupus erythematosus: criteria for classification with immunohistochemical analysis. Arthritis Rheum 15:494–500
Beutner EH, Blaszczyk M, Jablonska S, Chorzelski TP, Vijay K, Wolska H (1991) Studies on criteria of the European Academy of Dermatology and Venereology for the classification of cutaneous lupus erythematosus. Int J Dermatol 30:411–417
Beutner EH, Jablonska S, White DB, Blaszczyk M, Chorzelski TP, Cunningham RK, Davis BM (1992) Dermatologic criteria for classifying the major forms of cutaneous lupus erythematosus: methods for systematic discriminant analysis and questions on the interpretation of findings. Clin Dermatol 10:443–456
Beutner EH, Blaszczyk M, Jablonska S, Chorzelski TP, White D, Wolska H, Davis B (1993) Preliminary, dermatologic first step criteria for lupus erythematosus and second step criteria for systemic lupus erythematosus. Int J Dermatol 32:645–651
Cohen AS, Reynolds WE, Franklin EC, Kulka JP, Ropes MW, Shulman LE, Wallace SL (1971) Preliminary criteria for the classification of systemic lupus erythematosus. Bull Rheum Dis 21:643–648
Costner MI, Sontheimer RD, Provost TT (2003) Lupus erythematosus. In: Sontheimer RD, Provost TT (eds) Cutaneous manifestations of rheumatic diseases. Williams & Wilkins, Philadelphia, pp 15–64
Edworthy SM, Zatarain E, McShane DJ, Bloch DA (1988) Analysis of the 1982 ARA lupus criteria data set by recursive partitioning methodology: new insights into the relative merit of individual criteria. J Rheumatol 15:1493–1498
Gilliam JN (1977) The cutaneous signs of lupus erythematosus. Cont Educ Fam Phys 6:34–70
Gilliam JN, Sontheimer RD (1981) Distinctive cutaneous subsets in the spectrum of lupus erythematosus. J Am Acad Dermatol 4:471–475
Gilliam JN, Sontheimer RD (1982) Skin manifestations of SLE. Clin Rheum Dis 8:207–218
Goerz G, Lehmann P, Schuppe HC, Lakomek HJ, Kind P (1990) Lupus erythematosus. Z Hautkr 65:226–234
Gougerot H, Burnier R (1930) Lupus érythémateux tumidus. Bull Soc Franc Dermatol Syphil 37:1219–1292
Halmi BH, Dileonardo M, Jacoby RA (1993) Classification of lupus erythematosus. Int J Dermatol 32:642–644
Hochberg MC (1997) Updating the American College of Rheumatology revised criteria for the classification of systemic lupus erythematosus. Arthritis Rheum 40:1725
Hoffmann E (1909) Demonstrationen: Lupus erythematodes tumidus. Derm Zeitschr 16:159–160
Hsu S, Hwang LY, Ruiz H (2002) Tumid lupus erythematosus. Cutis 69:227–230
Jolly M, Laumann AE, Shea CR, Utset TO (2004) Lupus erythematosus tumidus in systemic lupus erythematosus: novel association and possible role of early treatment in prevention of discoid lupus erythematosus. Lupus 13:64–69

Kuhn A (2003) Neue klinische, photobiologische und immunhistologische Erkenntnisse zur Pathophysiologie des kutanen Lupus erythematodes. In: Hautklinik. Düsseldorf: Heinrich-Heine University, Habilitationsschrift

Kuhn A, Richter-Hintz D, Oslislo C, Ruzicka T, Megahed M, Lehmann P (2000) Lupus erythematosus tumidus – a neglected subset of cutaneous lupus erythematosus: report of 40 cases. Arch Dermatol 136:1033–1041

Kuhn A, Sonntag M, Richter-Hintz D, Oslislo C, Megahed M, Ruzicka T, Lehmann P (2001a) Phototesting in lupus erythematosus: a 15-year experience. J Am Acad Dermatol 45:86–95

Kuhn A, Sonntag M, Richter-Hintz D, Oslislo C, Megahed M, Ruzicka T, Lehmann P (2001b) Phototesting in lupus erythematosus tumidus – review of 60 patients. Photochem Photobiol 73:532–536

Kuhn A, Sonntag M, Lehmann P, Megahed M, Vestweber D, Ruzicka T (2002a) Characterization of the inflammatory infiltrate and expression of endothelial cell adhesion molecules in lupus erythematosus tumidus. Arch Dermatol Res 294:6–13

Kuhn A, Sonntag M, Sunderkotter C, Lehmann P, Vestweber D, Ruzicka T (2002b) Upregulation of epidermal surface molecule expression in primary and ultraviolet-induced lesions of lupus erythematosus tumidus. Br J Dermatol 146:801–809

Kuhn A, Sonntag M, Ruzicka T, Lehmann P, Megahed M (2003) Histopathologic findings in lupus erythematosus tumidus: review of 80 patients. J Am Acad Dermatol 48:901–908

Pacheco TR, Spates ST, Lee LA (2002) Unilateral tumid lupus erythematosus. Lupus 11:388–391

Parodi A, Rebora A (1997) ARA and EADV criteria for classification of systemic lupus erythematosus in patients with cutaneous lupus erythematosus. Dermatology 194:217–220

Rothfield NF, Braverman IM, Moschella S, Sontheimer RD, Provost TT, Fitzpatrick TB, Tuffanelli DL (1994) Classification of lupus erythematosus: an open forum. Fitzpatrick's J Clin Dermatol 1:912

Sontheimer RD, Provost TT (1996) Lupus erythematosus. In: Sontheimer RD and Provost TT (eds) Cutaneous manifestatons of rheumatic diseases. Williams & Wilkins, Baltimore, pp 1–71

Sontheimer RD (1997) The lexicon of cutaneous lupus erythematosus – a review and personal perspective on the nomenclature and classification of the cutaneous manifestations of lupus erythematosus. Lupus 6:84–95

Tan EM, Cohen AS, Fries JF, Masi AT, McShane DJ, Rothfield NF, Schaller JG, Talal N, Winchester RJ (1982) The 1982 revised criteria for the classification of systemic lupus erythematosus. Arthritis Rheum 25:1271–1277

Watanabe T, Tsuchida T (1995) Classification of lupus erythematosus based upon cutaneous manifestations. Dermatological, systemic and laboratory findings in 191 patients. Dermatology 190:277–283

Yell JA, Wojnarowska F (1997) Bullous skin disease in lupus erythematosus. Lupus 6:112–121

CHAPTER 6

Clinical Manifestations of Cutaneous Lupus Erythematosus

ANNEGRET KUHN, RICHARD SONTHEIMER, THOMAS RUZICKA

The clinical manifestations of cutaneous lupus erythematosus (CLE) include the subtypes acute CLE (ACLE); subacute CLE (SCLE); chronic CLE (CCLE), with its variants discoid LE (DLE), chilblain LE (CHLE), and LE profundus (LEP); and LE tumidus (LET), as well as bullous skin lesions associated with LE (BLE) (see Chap. 5).

Acute Cutaneous Lupus Erythematosus

The typical clinical manifestations of ACLE are characterized by a localized erythema known as the "malar rash" or "butterfly rash" on the central portion of the face or by a generalized, more widespread form (Fabbri et al. 2003, Sontheimer and Provost 2003). Localized ACLE may only affect the skin transiently, and the lesions may last for only several days up to a few weeks. Therefore, at the onset of disease, the patients may mistake this rash for sunburn and may seek medical advice only after the lesions have persisted for a longer period. Generalized ACLE, also known as "photosensitve lupus rash", is a less common variety and may be located anywhere on the body; however, it has a predilection for sun-exposed areas of the face, extensor aspects of the arms and forearms, and the dorsal aspects of the hands. It generally presents as a maculopapular or exanthematous eruption with a pruritic component. In most of the patients, systemic manifestation is strongly associated with ACLE, preceding by weeks or months the onset of a multisystem disease along with the confirmatory serologic findings (Watanabe and Tsuchida 1995, Wysenbeek et al. 1992, Yung and Oakley 2000). Since dermatologists are not usually the primary managers of such patients, few data concerning this form are available in the dermatologic literature.

ACLE has been reported in 20%–60% of large lupus patient cohorts, and it is more common in women than in men (Cervera et al. 1993, Pistiner et al. 1991, Wysenbeek et al. 1992). In one study, women were found to be six times more often affected than men, and the patients were on average in their second or third decade of life (Ng et al. 2000). Ultraviolet (UV) exposure is a common exogenous factor to be capable of precipitating ACLE (Kuhn et al. 2001a, Wysenbeek et al. 1989), and photosensitive patients sometimes report an exacerbation of their systemic symptoms after sun exposure. Furthermore, infections, especially with subtle types of viruses, or certain drugs, e.g., hydralazine, isoniazide, and procainamide, have also been found to induce or aggravate this disease (Pramatarov 1998, Rubin 1999). A possible association with HLA-DR2 and -DR3 has been suspected, and familial associations or concordance in twins suggest a genetic component.

Fig. 6.1. Localized acute cutaneous lupus erythematous (ACLE). Classic butterfly rash characterized by symmetrical erythema on the malar areas of the face

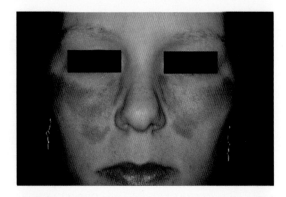

Fig. 6.2. Localized acute cutaneous lupus erythematous (ACLE). Erythematous lesions on the face of a patient that became confluent and hyperkeratotic

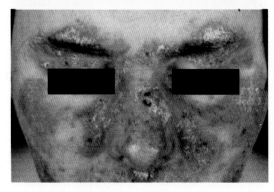

The localized form of ACLE usually begins with small, discrete erythematous macules and papules, occasionally associated with fine scales involving both the malar areas and the bridge of the nose while sparing the nasolabial folds (Fig. 6.1). This classic "malar rash" or" butterfly rash" can disappear without scarring and pigmentation or gradually becomes confluent and hyperkeratotic (Fig. 6.2), and facial swelling may be severe in some patients with this disease (Norden et al. 1993, Yell et al. 1996). Similar lesions have also been found to occur on the forehead, the V-area of the neck, the upper limbs, and the trunk. Furthermore, patients with ACLE may have diffuse thinning or a receding frontal hairline with broken hairs (lupus hair), telangiectasias and erythema of the proximal nail fold, and cuticular abnormalities (Patel and Werth 2002). Superficial ulcerations of the oral and/or nasal mucosa are frequently accompanied with ACLE and may cause extreme discomfort in some patients. The posterior areas of the hard palate are most commonly affected; however, the gingival, buccal, and lingual mucosa may also be involved. In general, ACLE lesions are nonscarring, and the simultaneous occurrence of ACLE and other variants of CLE, such as DLE, is uncommon.

Some patients experience an extremely acute, generalized form of ACLE that presents as a maculopapular rash and can develop a more prolonged disease activity (Fabbri et al. 2003, Sontheimer 1997). In the few existing reports in the literature, this form is characterized by a generalized eruption of symmetrically distributed small,

Fig. 6.3. Generalized acute cutaneous lupus erythematous (ACLE). Erythematous plaques over the dorsal aspects of the hands in a patient with severe SLE

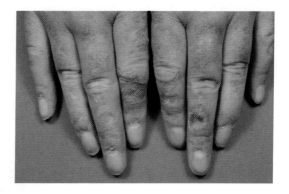

confluent erythematous macules and papules with a pruritic component. The color of the lesions is usually red or, less frequently, dull red or livid, and there have been reports of patients presenting with severe involvement of the oral mucosa or the palms and phalanges (Fig. 6.3) (Braverman 1981, McCauliffe 2001). In contrast to the classic malar erythema of ACLE, the generalized form is a rather uncommon cutaneous manifestation that may be located anywhere on the body, although the preferred sites are above the waistline (Sontheimer and Provost 2003, Yell et al. 1996). It may resemble a drug eruption or can simulate toxic epidermal necrolysis, and it frequently occurs after sun exposure. As with "malar rash" or "butterfly rash", the onset of the generalized form usually coincides with exacerbation of systemic disease. Its incidence is estimated to be approximately 5%–10% of patients with SLE (Cardinali et al. 2000, Tan et al. 1982), but the sporadic observations published in the dermatologic literature probably underestimate the real prevalence of this from.

Subacute Cutaneous Lupus Erythematosus

SCLE, a subset with specific clinical and serologic features occurring preferentially in white females, was first discussed as a distinct entity by Gilliam in 1977 (Gilliam 1977), with expanded descriptions in 1979 (Sontheimer et al. 1979), 1981 (Gilliam and Sontheimer 1981), and 1982 (Gilliam and Sontheimer 1982). This subtype shows a significant coincidence with HLA-DR2 or -DR3, and patients with overlapping manifestations of Sjögren's syndrome or high levels of anti-Ro/SSA antibodies are more likely to have HLA-B8, -DR3, -DRw6, -DRw52, and -DQ2 (Sontheimer et al. 1981). Certain drugs, especially hydrochlorothiazide, angiotensin-converting enzyme inhibitors, and calcium channel blockers have been associated with the onset and/or exacerbation of this disease (Reed et al. 1985, Srivastava et al. 2003). In recent years, terbinafine has also been reported to induce SCLE with high titers of antinuclear antibodies (ANAs) and antihistone antibodies in genetically susceptible persons (Bonsmann et al. 2001, Callen et al. 2001). Furthermore, most patients with this subtype are sensitive to sunlight and exposure to UV irradiation can precipitate or aggravate SCLE lesions (Kuhn et al. 2001a). Patients with SCLE typically have prominent cutaneous and musculoskeletal complaints but generally do not develop a severe

Fig. 6.4. Papulosquamous subacute cutaneous lupus erythematosus (SCLE). Psoriasiform lesions with superficial scale and the tendency for individual lesions to merge into a vetiform pattern

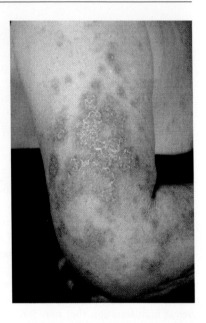

systemic disease, and only half of them have four or more of the American Rheumatism Association (ARA) criteria for the diagnosis of systemic lupus erythematosus (SLE) (Cohen and Crosby 1994, Crowson and Magro 2001, Tan et al. 1982). Therefore, SCLE can be considered a relatively benign illness that is intermediate in severity between ACLE and CCLE (Sontheimer 1989).

Initially, SCLE lesions present with erythematous macules and papules that evolve into scaly papulosquamous or annular/polycyclic plaques (Sontheimer et al. 1981). Approximately 50% of patients have predominantly papulosquamous or psoriasiform lesions (Fig. 6.4), and the other half have the annular/polycyclic type (Fig. 6.5); a few patients may develop both forms of lesions (Sontheimer 1985a, Sontheimer et al. 1979). However, some groups have observed a predominance of the papulosquamous lesions, whereas others have noted an abundance of the annular/polycyclic type (Callen and Klein 1988, Chlebus et al. 1998, Cohen and Crosby 1994, David-Bajar 1993, Fabbri et al. 1990, Herrero et al. 1988, Molad et al. 1987). One recent study found that 42% of the patients with SCLE studied exhibit the annular/polycyclic form, 39% had the papulosquamous form, and 16% showed both manifestations (Parodi et al. 2000). Generally, lesions of this subtype heal without scarring but can leave long-lasting and permanent vitiligo-like pigmentary changes as a "clue" for the clinical diagnosis (Fig. 6.6) (Milde and Goerz 1994). SCLE has a characteristic distribution of lesions in sun-exposed areas, in particular the upper chest and back, the deltoid aspect of the shoulders, the extensor surface of the arms, and less commonly the face or scalp. In the study by Parodi et al. (Parodi et al. 2000), the neck was affected in 83% of patients, with 66% exhibiting lesions on the face, 39% on the extensor arms, 21% on the dorsal hands, 16% on the lower limbs, and 12% on the scalp. Interestingly, 27%–100% of patients with SCLE have been reported to be abnormally photosensitive, and experimental studies showed positive phototest results in 63% after UVA or

Fig. 6.5. Annular subacute cutaneous lupus erythematosus (SCLE). Polycyclic lesions with central hypopigmentation and inflamed erythematous borders on the extensor aspects of the arm

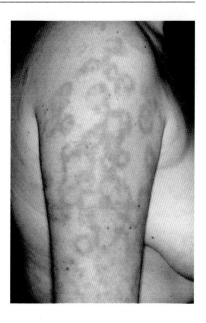

UVB irradiation (Kuhn et al. 2001a). However, some ethnic groups, such as Japanese and Chinese, seem to be less photosensitive (Nishikawa and Provost 1991, Shou-yi et al. 1987). A prevalence of polymorphous light eruption of 60%–70% has also been demonstrated in patients with SCLE, as well as phototoxic reactions when photosensitizing medications were prescribed (Millard et al. 2000).

Several other skin lesions that are not specific for LE have been described in patients with SCLE (Parodi et al. 2000, Sontheimer 1989). The most frequently encountered of these include nonscarring alopecia, painless mucous membrane lesions, livedo reticularis, periungual telangiectasias, and Raynaud's phenomenon (Callen et al. 1986, Callen and Klein 1988, David et al. 1984, Herrero et al. 1988, Molad et al. 1987, Sanchez-Perez et al. 1993, Sontheimer 1985a). Cutaneous vasculitis of the lower extremities is a frequent finding in anti-Ro/SSA antibody-positive patients with SCLE also described under the rubric of Sjögren's syndrome/LE overlap syndrome (Provost et al. 1988). Furthermore, cutaneous calcinosis may be seen rarely in patients with SCLE, and HPV-11-associated squamous cell carcinomas of the skin were noted in one patient with SCLE (Cohen et al. 1992). In one additional case, annular/polycyclic SCLE lesions were reported over time to progress to plaques of morphea (Rao et al. 1990).

Patients with SCLE may also develop localized facial ACLE, which has been seen in 7%–100% of patients (David et al. 1984, Fabbri et al. 2003, Molad et al. 1987, Shouyi et al. 1987, Sontheimer 1985a). However, ACLE skin lesions tend to be more transient, to heal less often with pigmentary changes, and to be more edematous and less scaly than SCLE lesions. ACLE more commonly affects the malar areas of the face; in general, SCLE involves the face much less often. Several reports have also noted that up to 29% of patients with SCLE manifest DLE lesions during their clinical course and, interestingly, 19% of the original cohort of patients with SCLE had classical DLE

Fig. 6.6. Hypopigmentation in subacute cutaneous lupus erythematosus (SCLE). Permanent vitiligo-like depigmentation in the face of a patient with SCLE

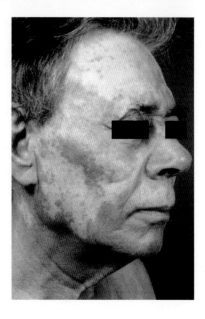

(Callen and Klein 1988, David et al. 1984, Molad et al. 1987, Shou-yi et al. 1987, Sontheimer 1985a, Sontheimer et al. 1979). These lesions can predate the onset of SCLE lesions; however, DLE lesions are generally associated with a greater degree of pigmentary changes, may display atrophic dermal scarring, and are more characteristically associated with follicular plugging and adherent scaling than SCLE lesions. Furthermore, DLE lesions are characteristically indurated, whereas SCLE lesions are not (David-Bajar et al. 1992).

In addition to the common forms of SCLE, several unusual varieties of this subtype have been reported. Infrequently, SCLE lesions present initially with an appearance of erythema multiforme, which can simulate Rowell's syndrome (erythema multiforme-like lesions occurring in patients with SLE in the presence of anti-La/SSB autoantibodies) (Rowell et al. 1963, Sontheimer 1985b). Lyon et al. (Lyon et al. 1998) reported two cases of delayed diagnosis of SCLE because of the clinical and histologic similarities between SCLE and erythema multiforme. Furthermore, lesions similar to erythema annulare centrifugum can be seen in some patients, and, as a result of hyperacute basal cell layer injury, on rare occasions, the active edge of annular SCLE lesions undergoes a vesicular change that breaks down to produce a striking crusted appearance (Grant 1981, Wechsler and Stavrides 1982). On at least one occasion such lesions have progressed to mimic toxic epidermal necrolysis (Bielsa et al. 1987), and in a study by Herrero et al. (Herrero et al. 1988), vesiculobullous changes were present in 38% of the SCLE population, which coincided histologically with focal areas of necrosis. In 1988, one patient with SCLE was reported to initially present exfoliative erythroderma (DeSpain and Clark 1988) and this was also noted more recently by Mutasim (Mutasim 2003). Other patients presented with a curious acral distribution of annular lesions (Scheinman 1994) or a form of SCLE with widespread plaques (Tsutsui et al. 1996). Pityriasisform (Caproni et al. 2001, Hymes et al. 1986) and exanthematous (Sontheimer 1985b) variants of SCLE have been mentioned anecdotally on rare occasions. In addition, follicular erythematous lesions are occasionally seen in patients with SCLE, and it has been reported to be associated with generalized poikiloderma (Pramatarov et al. 2000).

Chronic Cutaneous Lupus Erythematosus

Several different entities can be allocated to the group of CCLE, such as DLE, with its "hypertrophic/verrucous" and "telangiectoid" variants; and the more rare subtypes LEP and CHLE.

Discoid Lupus Erythematosus

The most common form of all chronic cutaneous variants is DLE, which can be localized or generalized, both with and without systemic manifestations of LE. Typical DLE lesions may be present at the onset of SLE in about 5%–10% of patients, and approximately 30% of patients may develop DLE lesions, usually of the generalized type, during the course of SLE (Cervera et al. 1993, Hymes and Jordon 1989, Tebbe et al. 1997). The localized form presents with sharply demarcated, erythematokeratotic, atrophic or scarring lesions, and it is often seen on the face and scalp, whereas the generalized form also involves the regions below the neck (Fabbri et al. 2003, McCauliffe 2001, Patel and Werth 2002). DLE occurs mostly in the third to fourth decade of life; however, in two recent studies, more than 40 children with DLE ranging in age from 2 to 16 years have been described in the literature (Cherif et al. 2003, Moises-Alfaro et al. 2003). Earlier reports indicated that DLE may be more prevalent in whites than in blacks, but epidemiologic studies showed that it can affect any race (Findlay and Lups 1967, Ng et al. 2000, Tebbe and Orfanos 1997). Besides the genetic predisposition, the clinical manifestations may often be provoked or aggravated by exogenous factors, such as UV irradiation, cold, mechanical trauma, and, in rare cases, infections or drugs (Djawari 1978, Kuhn et al. 2001a, Lodin 1963). Association with HLA-B7, -B8, -Cw7, -DR2, -DR3, and -DQw1 has been described in the literature (Fischer et al. 1994, Knop et al. 1990).

Most commonly, DLE begins unilaterally or bilaterally, with flat or slightly elevated, sharply demarcated, erythematous macules or papules with a scaly surface. Early lesions most commonly evolve into larger, coin-shaped ("discoid"), confluent, disfiguring plaques of varying size (from a few millimeters to approximately 15 cm) owing to peripheral growth demonstrating a prominent adherent scale formation (Fig. 6.7) (Crowson and Magro 2001). When the adherent scale is peeled back from more advanced lesions, follicle-sized keratotic spikes similar in appearance to carpet tacks can be seen to project from the undersurface of the scale ("the carpet tack sign"). Telangiectasia and hyperpigmentation can replace the active inflammation, and the patches may give a poikilodermatous appearance. Pigmentary changes are common, especially in dark-skinned people, with white hypopigmentation in the central area and a hyperpigmented zone at the active border. Furthermore, in some ethnic groups, such as Indians from the Asian subcontinent, DLE can also present as isolated areas of macular hyperpigmentation (George et al. 1992). The skin lesions are

Fig. 6.7. Classic discoid lupus erythematosus (DLE). Slightly infiltrated, erythematous plaques with scarring atrophy in a patient with therapeutically refractory facial DLE

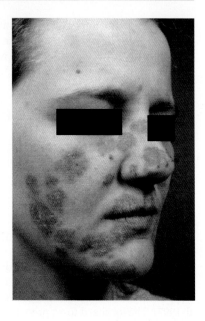

generally progressive, and resolution of the lesions leaves more or less evident atrophy and scarring, depending on the duration and severity of the lesions during the active phase. This may result in considerable mutilations, particularly when present in acral regions on the face, such as the tip of the nose and the ears, or in irreversible scarring alopecia on the scalp. A characteristic pitted, acneiform scarring is also a common feature of the perioral area (Fig. 6.8).

Cutaneous lesions of DLE predominantly occur in light-exposed areas, such as the face, particularly the cheeks and ears, but the forehead, eyebrows, eyelids, nose, and lips can also be included (Fabbri et al. 2003, McCauliffe 2001, Patel and Werth 2002). Symmetrical, butterfly-shaped DLE plaques will occasionally be found over the malar areas and the bridge of the nose. Such lesions are not to be confused with the more transient, edematous erythema reactions that occur over the same distribution in patients with ACLE. As with ACLE, DLE usually spares the nasolabial folds. However, DLE lesions may further affect sun-protected areas, such as inguinal folds and palmoplantar skin, and involvement of the scalp can be found in approximately 60% of patients with this subtype (Sontheimer and Provost 2003). At the latter location, DLE may even be the only cutaneous manifestation in 10% of cases and thus presents a classical differential diagnosis of scarring alopecia (Fig. 6.9) (Prystowsky and Gilliam 1975). In one series, irreversible scarring alopecia resulting from permanent follicular destruction occurred in more than 30% of patients (Wilson et al. 1992); in some patients, DLE on the scalp progresses to the point of total, irreversible scarring alopecia and may be accompanied by secondary bacterial superinfection (Fig. 6.10). The irreversible scarring alopecia that is the result of persistent DLE activity in localized areas differs from the more widespread, reversible, nonscarring alopecia that patients with SLE often develop during periods of systemic disease activity. There is also an increased incidence of alopecia areata in patients with DLE (Werth et al. 1992). Fur-

Fig. 6.8. Perioral pitted scarring in discoid lupus erythematosus (DLE). Perioral DLE lesions often resolve with a striking acneiform pattern of pitted scarring

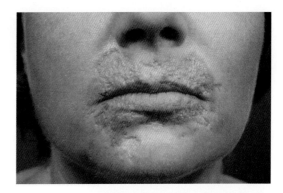

Fig. 6.9. Discoid lupus erythematosus (DLE) of the scalp. Irreversible scarring alopecia as a result of persistent activity in localized areas

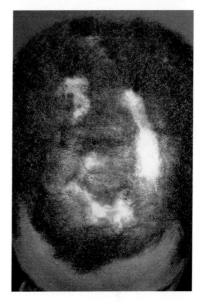

thermore, DLE lesions occurring below the neck are most commonly found on the extensor aspects of the arms and the V-area of the neck. However, in the generalized form, such lesions can occur at virtually any site on the body, although the presence of DLE lesions solely below the neck is extremely uncommon. Painful erosive palmar-plantar DLE involvement can predominate in some cases, producing significant disability and presenting an especially difficult management problem (Ashinoff et al. 1988, Parrish et al. 1967). Small, follicularly oriented erythematous papules of less than 1 cm in diameter present as follicular DLE at the elbows but may occur at any other part of the body as well. These lesions may also be more common in Chinese and other Asian patients (Wong 1969).

Mucous membrane involvement can be found in 25% of patients with DLE and other forms of CCLE (Andreasen and Poulsen 1964, Botella et al. 1999, Burge et al. 1989). It does not necessarily reflect systemic manifestation or high disease activity; however, it is included in the list of the 11 diagnostic ARA criteria for the diagnosis

Fig. 6.10. Total irreversible alopecia in discoid lupus erythematosus (DLE). In this patient, the disease process has progressed to the point of total irreversible scarring alopecia with secondary bacterial superinfection

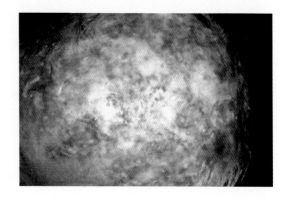

of SLE (Tan et al. 1982). Urman et al. (Urman et al. 1978) extensively studied oral ulcerations in 47 (26%) of 182 patients with SLE and noted no significant correlation between the oral ulcerations and cutaneous manifestations. Interestingly, an increased frequency of these mucosal lesions was associated with increased overall clinical activity, but no detectable correlation was found between oral ulcerations and serologic parameters. Oral, mainly buccal, manifestations are most common, with the palate, alveolar processes, and tongue less frequently involved, but nasal, conjunctival, and anogenital mucous membranes may also be affected at times. Individual lesions begin as painful, erythematous patches, later maturing to a chronic plaque that has a sharply marginated, irregularly scalloped white border with radiating white striae and telangiectasia (Fig. 6.11). The surface of these plaques overlying the palatal mucosa often have a well-defined meshwork of raised hyperkeratotic white strands that encircle zones of punctate erythema (Burge et al. 1989). The centers of older lesions cause atrophy and may become depressed and, occasionally, undergo painful ulceration. Sometimes mucosal DLE resembles lichen planus, with a honeycomb appearance, and squamous cell carcinoma as a long-term complication should be suspected and excluded in any case of chronic asymmetrical induration of either mucosal or cutaneous lesions (Miyagawa et al. 1996, Reichart 2003, Sherman et al. 1993, Voigtlander and Boonen 1990). Well-defined DLE plaques also can appear on the vermillion border of the lips or can present as a diffuse cheilitis, especially on the more sun-exposed lower lip, causing considerable discomfort and disfiguration (Fig. 6.12). Mucosal lesions of the nose may result in nasal septum perforation, especially in association with generalized DLE or SLE (Bach 1980, Rahman et al. 1999). Similarly, ocular affections that are mainly located at the palpebral conjunctiva and the lower margin of the eyelids can cause permanent loss of eye lashes, ectropion, and corneal stromal keratitis (Afshari et al. 2001, Raizman and Baum 1989). Conjunctival DLE lesions begin most commonly as small areas of nondescript inflammation producing considerable disability, and as the early lesions progress, scarring becomes more evident (Frith et al. 1990, Heiligenhaus et al. 1996, Meiusi et al. 1991).

The nails can be involved as a very uncommon site of occurrence; however, periungual telangiectasias and erythema of the proximal nail fold are significant cutaneous features that can occur in patients with DLE prone to developing systemic disease. Furthermore, focal lesions of DLE occurring over the nail fold can produce nail

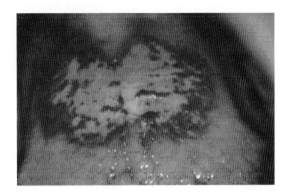

Fig. 6.11. Mucosal discoid lupus erythematosus (DLE). Typical appearance of a buccal lesion on the hard palate with a honeycomb appearance

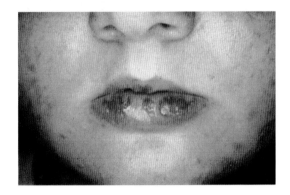

Fig. 6.12. Cheilitis in discoid lupus erythematosus (DLE). Diffuse small lesions on the vermillion border of the upper lip causing considerable discomfort

plate dystrophy (Kanwar et al. 1993). The nail unit can also be impacted by other forms of CLE as well as SLE, producing red lunulae, clubbing, paronychia, pitting, leukonychia striata, and onycholysis (Costner et al. 2003).

The appearance of DLE lesions or other forms of CLE in unusual locations and on completely sun-protected areas may be evidence that these lesions can follow in the wake of any form of trauma to the skin (Koebner's phenomenon or isomorphic response) (Ueki 1994). Rowell and Goodfield (Rowell and Goodfield 1992) stated that in their series, DLE lesions were initiated by trauma in 11% of patients, sunburn in 5%, infection in 3%, and exposure to cold in 2%. Furthermore, DLE lesions have been noted to occur following exposure to x-ray, diathermy, and chemical burns and have arisen in scars associated with herpes zoster. DLE lesions have also been reported to occur in the scars of smallpox vaccination (Lupton 1987). It has long been observed that DLE lesions develop mainly during the summer and can be precipitated by sun exposure; however, this occurs less frequently than with ACLE, SCLE, or LET (Lehmann 1996). Photosensitivity in DLE can manifest in several ways: discoid lesions may themselves be specifically induced and exacerbated by UV radiation, but the development of polymorphous light eruption (PLE) can also be seen. A prevalence of PLE has been reported in 50% of patients with DLE by Millard et al. (Millard et al. 2000). However, in contrast to PLE, it is predominantly UVB that aggravates DLE lesions, although longer UVA lengths can also be deleterious in some patients

(Lehmann et al. 1990, Nived et al. 1993, Walchner et al. 1997, Wolska et al. 1989). In experimental studies, characteristic skin lesions have been induced by UV irradiation in 42% of patients with DLE. Approximately 50% of these patients reacted to both UVB and UVA irradiation, 33% to UVB only, and 14% to UVA only (Kuhn et al. 2001a). Interestingly, in more than 50% of patients, sun exposure does not seem to be related to the cause of their disease, and DLE lesions in the hair-bearing scalp, external auditory canal, or perineal areas are examples where this form of CCLE is not related to light exposure.

Hypertrophic/Verrucous Variant of Discoid Lupus Erythematosus

Hypertrophic/verrucous lesions in association with CLE were first described by Bechet in 1940 (Bechet 1940); in this very rare variant, the hyperkeratosis that is usually present in DLE lesions is greatly exaggerated. Classic DLE lesions are often present elsewhere on the body, aiding in diagnosis (Callen 1985, Santa Cruz et al. 1983) and, recently, a patient with SLE and hypertrophic lesions has also been reported (Cardinali et al. 2004). However, only approximately 2% of patients with DLE show a hyperkeratotic type of lesion (Mascaro et al. 1997, Sontheimer and Provost 2003).

Clinically, hypertrophic DLE consists of dull, red, and indurated lesions that can appear as unique or multiple papulonodular elements covered by keratotic scale, as larger plaques covered by an adherent multilayered ostraceous horny white or yellowish material, or as regionally diffuse hyperkeratosis that looks like a chalky dust applied over the skin (Fig. 6.13) (Daldon et al. 2003). The entity "lupus erythematosus hypertrophicus et profundus" seems to represent a further very rare variant affecting the face, associated with the additional features of violaceus or dull red, indurated, rolled borders, and striking central, crateriform atrophy (Dammert 1971, Otani 1977, Winkelmann 1983). Nevertheless, the name of this entity is somewhat ambiguous because its pathology does not include a significant degree of LEP.

The verrucous, indurated, hyperkeratotic plaques can occur at any site where classical DLE lesions develop, although the extensor aspects of the arms and limbs, the upper back, and the face are the most frequently areas affected (Daldon et al. 2003, Mascaro et al. 1997). Recently, conjunctival hypertrophic lesions have been reported in a patient with a history of chronic blepharoconjunctivitis (Uy et al. 1999). When the palms and soles are involved, hypertrophic DLE produces localized or partially diffuse keratoderma, up to 1- to 3-mm thick, that makes finger mobility more difficult (Rothfield 1993).

Differential diagnosis must take into consideration verrucous psoriasis, hyperkeratotic lichen planus, prurigo nodularis, keratoacanthoma, and squamous cell carcinoma (Daldon et al. 2003, Perniciaro et al. 1995, Romero et al. 1977, Vinciullo 1986). Squamous cell carcinoma needs special consideration because it is well known that it can develop on chronic lesions of DLE, and until date, more than 100 cases of squamous cell carcinoma arising on scars of CCLE have been reported in white and African American patients (Caruso et al. 1987, De Berker et al. 1992, Sherman et al. 1993). In most cases, a male predominance, long evolution of previous CCLE lesions (mean time for development of squamous cell carcinoma over CCLE is 30.8 years), and high metastatic tendency (40%), especially when in labial location, was found (Millard and Barker 1978).

Fig. 6.13. Hypertrophic/verrucous variant of discoid lupus erythematosus (DLE). Skin lesions on the elbow are entirely covered by a thickened shield of hyperkeratosis

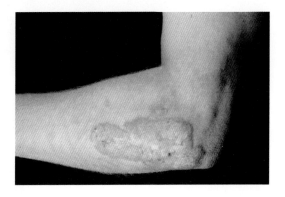

Patients with hypertrophic DLE rarely develop systemic disease; however, the clinical course is characterized by chronicity and resistance to treatment (Daldon et al. 2003, Spann et al. 1988). The lesions may respond, in some cases, to local cryotherapy (with carbon dioxide or liquid nitrogen), topical glucocorticosteroid application, and systemic antimalarial drug therapy. Topical tretinoin and systemic isotretinoin therapy have also been found to be effective (Green and Piette 1987, Seiger et al. 1991).

Telangiectoid Variant of Discoid Lupus Erythematosus

The telangiectoid variant of DLE is extremely rare, consisting of purplish plaques or blotchy reticulate telangiectasia that may develop on the face, neck, ears, dorsal aspects of the hands, breast, front of the knees, and back of the heels or sides of feet (Fig. 6.14) (Bechet and Elizabeth 1948, Mascaro et al. 1997). The lesions are mostly associated with further CCLE lesions or can replace active inflammation in patients with DLE developing a poikilodermatous appearance and prominent atrophic scarring. Efficient management of telangiectoid lesions can be difficult; however, argon laser treatment has been reported to yield an excellent cosmetic result without any short-term side effects (Kuhn et al. 2000d).

Chilblain Lupus Erythematosus

CHLE, a rare manifestation of CCLE distinguished by Hutchinson in 1888 (Hutchinson 1888), is strongly influenced by environmental factors (Breathnach and Wells 1979, Doutre et al. 1992, Helm and Jones 2002, Rowell 1987, Uter et al. 1988). This subtype seems to be more frequent in women and, interestingly, very uncommon in the United States, as Tuffanelli and Dubois (Tuffanelli and Dubois 1964) failed to detect such lesions among 520 patients; however, these patients were collected for the most part from the warm Southern California area. In contrast, Millard and Rowell (Millard and Rowell 1978) detected 17 cases with this subtype in a review of 150 patients with CLE (11.3%). Four of these patients demonstrated erythema multiforme-like lesions, and 3 of these 17 patients subsequently developed features of SLE. One further reported case of CHLE was induced by pregnancy and disappeared after delivery (Stainforth et al. 1993). The pathogenesis is unknown, but microvascular injury secondary to exposure to cold, damp weather or a drop in temperature and possible

Fig. 6.14. Telangiectoid variant of discoid lupus erythematosus (DLE). Multiple erythematous plaques and reticulate telangiectasia on the face that produce large areas of disfigurement on confluence

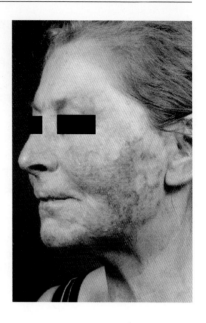

hyperviscosity from immunologic abnormalities may play a role (Mascaro et al. 1997, Yell et al. 1996). In most reported cases, patients with CHLE present a polyclonal hypergammaglobulinemia, increased serum immunoglobulin levels, and a positive rheumatoid factor. In addition, anti-double-stranded DNA or anti-Ro/SSA antibodies have often been detected, but laboratory examinations usually fail to reveal evidence of cryoglobulins, cryofibrinogens, or cold agglutinins (Su et al. 1994). In a few patients, CHLE has been described in association with antiphospholipid syndrome (Allegue et al. 1988, De Argila Fernandez-Auran et al. 1996). The evolution of lesions in patients with CHLE is usually chronic, and sometimes these lesions precede other manifestations of SLE (Doutre et al. 1992). The risk of developing SLE is estimated to be approximately 20%, but in this rare form of CCLE, only a few studies have been reported; nevertheless, long-term follow-up of these patients is warranted (Viguier et al. 2001). Most patients progressing to SLE have arthralgia, manic depressive psychoses, or a reduced creatinine clearance, presumably from renal involvement. Furthermore, most patients with CHLE have or have had typical DLE lesions on the face; however, the evolution of both types of lesions is different, and chilblain manifestations usually persist when classic DLE disappears.

Clinically, CHLE is characterized by symmetrically distributed, circumscribed, sometimes infiltrated, pruriginous or painful areas of livid and purple plaques that appear and exacerbate during cold, damp weather periods (Fig. 6.15). There is only a slight tendency to central regression, and the lesions, in their evolution, may ulcerate or present firmly adherent hyperkeratosis (Kuhn et al. 2000c, Sontheimer and Provost 2003). The lesions of CHLE involve mostly the dorsal and lateral parts of the hands and feet, the ears, the nose, the elbows, the knees, or the calves (Helm and Jones 2002, Su et al. 1994). On toes and fingers, the lesions develop on the back or on the pads (Doutre et al. 1992, Fisher and Everett 1996), and fissuring of the knuckles as well as

Fig. 6.15. Chilblain lupus erythematosus (CHLE). Red-purple patches on the finger end joints that are precipitated by cold, damp climates

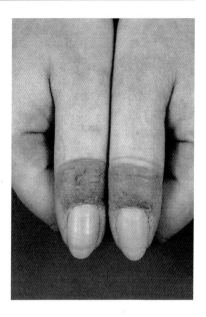

accompanying hyperhidrosis are common, producing a great deal of discomfort (Costner et al. 2003). Ulceration is frequent in digital pulp lesions, and they easily become necrotic on the soles (Mascaro et al. 1997). When located in the periungual zone, the nail plate may develop mild to severe dystrophy.

Because CHLE lesions are highly reminiscent of simple chilblains or pernio lesions (Viguier et al. 2001), one could question whether such patients have simple pernio that in the predisposed individual produces a Koebner's phenomenon resulting in DLE. The terms "chilblain lupus" and "perniotic lupus" have been used to describe such lesions. Unfortunately, the term "lupus pernio" has also been used for such lesions, although this term is more properly used to designate a form of cutaneous sarcoidosis (James 1992). For a positive diagnosis of CHLE, it has been proposed to establish two groups of major and minor criteria (Su et al. 1994). Major criteria include (a) cold-induced or cold-aggravated lesions in acral locations and (b) evidence of LE on histopathology or direct immunofluorescence. Minor criteria include (a) the coexistence of SLE or other manifestations of CLE, (b) positive response to LE therapy, and (c) negative results of cryoglobulin and cold agglutinin studies. The diagnosis of CHLE may be affirmed if the patient fulfills both major criteria and at least one of the minor criteria. A chronic form of CHLE occurs especially in older persons who have underlying vascular abnormalities, such as acrocyanosis, Raynaud's phenomenon, atherosclerosis, or erythrocyanosis. In such patients, this subtype of CCLE can last for several months and tends to recur annually, sometimes with hemorrhagic blisters, erosions, or ulcers.

Lupus Erythematosus Profundus

LEP, historically referred to as "Kaposi-Irgang disease" or also known as "lupus panniculitis", is a rare variant of CCLE in which pathologic changes occur primarily in the lower dermis and subcutaneous tissue. In 1883, subcutaneous nodules associated with LE were first described by Kaposi (Kaposi 1883), but the term "lupus profundus" was coined by Irgang (Irgang 1940) in 1940. Subsequently, different authors reported new cases and contributed to define the clinical and histopathologic characteristics of this disease (Arnold 1956, Sanchez et al. 1981, Tuffanelli 1971, Winkelmann 1970). Middle-aged women are predominantly affected; however, in a recent study it has been shown that LEP in Asian patients is more frequent in a younger age group compared with the Caucasian population (Ng et al. 2002). The course of this subtype of CCLE is usually chronic and characterized by periods of remission and exacerbation. The major morbidity is usually disfigurement and disability related to pain, and the lesions finally resolve, leaving deep atrophic scars (Kuhn et al. 2000c, Mascaro et al. 1997). LEP can be found in approximately 2%–10% of patients with SLE and other autoimmune diseases; however, patients with LEP present more commonly without further or only mild signs of systemic manifestations. In some extensive cases, association of LEP with serious systemic disease or a lethal outcome has been reported, although there is a relatively low incidence of renal involvement (Grossberg et al. 2001). Serologically, ANAs may be found to be low in titer or nonexistent, and hypergammaglobulinemia has been reported in some cases of LEP along with low total complement and C4 levels (Martens et al. 1999). Approximately 70% of patients with LEP also have other lesions of CLE, particularly discoid or hypertrophic lesions, often overlying the panniculitis lesions (Balabanova et al. 1992, Suss et al. 1994). When LEP exists in the absence of other LE-specific lesions, the diagnosis has been questioned. Therefore, it is important to obtain biopsy specimens to confirm the diagnosis because a number of cases of subcutaneous lymphoma have given a clinical appearance of lupus profundus (Magro et al. 1997, Ng et al. 2002). Physical factors, such as trauma, may often be directly related to the lesions of LEP (Tuffanelli 1971); however, the relevance of photosensitivity in this rare subtype of CCLE is unknown (Fabbri et al. 2003).

Single or multiple sharply defined, persistent, asymptomatic or sometimes painful subcutaneous plaques or nodules of varying sizes are the typical lesions of LEP (Costner et al. 2003, Peters and Su 1989). The overlying skin ultimately becomes attached to the firm lesions, producing a deep depression into the subcutis with a normal or erythematous, inflammatory surface (Fig. 6.16). Dystrophic calcifications or ulcerations within older lesions of LEP, leaving atrophic scars or sometimes resembling lipatrophy, may occur and at times can be a prominent clinical feature of the disease requiring surgical excision. In addition, LEP may produce breast nodules that can mimic carcinoma, clinically and radiologically (Holland et al. 1995, Peters 2000), and linear involvement of the extremities or the scalp has also been observed (Nagai et al. 2003, Tada et al. 1991). Most lesions of LEP are usually found in areas of increased fat deposition, such as the trunk, buttocks, and proximal upper and lower extremities, but the shoulders and thighs are further sites of predominant involvement (Martens et al. 1999). LEP may also develop on the scalp clinically simulating alopecia areata (Kossard 2002) and in unusual zones on the face, such as the parotid

Fig. 6.16. Lupus erythematosus profundus (LEP). Subcutaneous nodules leaving extensive depressed, atrophic areas on the upper arm with hyperpigmented borders

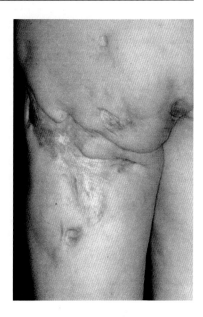

region. Interestingly, periorbital edema as an initial symptom of LEP has been described in several patients as the only clinical manifestation of the disease (Franke et al. 1999, Lodi et al. 1993, Magee et al. 1991).

Lupus Erythematosus Tumidus

In 1909, the term "lupus erythematosus tumidus" was first used by Hoffmann (Hoffmann 1909) at a meeting of the Berlin Dermatological Society, and, in 1930, five further patients were reported by Gougerot and Burnier (Gougerot and Burnier 1930, 1931, 1932) to describe a disease with erythematous, indurated, nonscarring lesions on the face with minimal or absent surface changes. However, the next case reports of LET were not mentioned until 1965 in the German and French literature (Bazex et al. 1965, Casala et al. 1971, De Graciansky et al. 1965), and in the following years, only a few further cases were reported (Dekle et al. 1999, Mosquera Vieitez et al. 1984, Ruiz and Sanchez 1999). This might be due to the fact that other authors have not considered LET as a separate entity different from other variants of CLE, and it is likely that skin lesions described under different designations, such as "urticarial plaque lupus erythematosus," represent the same disease entity (Sontheimer and Provost 1996). Because some skin conditions share a variety of similar features, a correct diagnosis demands attention to rather subtle details and appreciation of the characteristic signs as well as the course of the disease. In 2000, our group (Kuhn et al. 2000a) analyzed 40 patients with LET and defined diagnostic criteria for the classification of this disease. Meanwhile, there is no doubt about LET being a separate entity, and further reports by other groups have been published indicating that the incidence of LET seems to be higher than found in earlier studies (Alexiades-Armenakas et al. 2003, Hsu et al. 2002,

Jolly et al. 2004, Pacheco et al. 2002). Interestingly, most case reports of LET in the literature are published by European countries indicating that many more patients are seen in the Caucasian population (Sontheimer 2000).

The importance of reevaluating this form lies in the characteristic clinical and histopathologic picture, in its remarkable photosensitivity, and in the course of the disease (Kuhn 2003). In several aspects, the cutaneous manifestations of LET differ from other variants of CLE. Scarring, the hallmark of DLE, does not occur in LET, even in patients with recurrent skin lesions at the same site for many years, and epidermal atrophy has not developed in any case. Follicular plugging and adherent hyperkeratotic scaling, which are further features of DLE, also have not been seen in any of the patients with LET. Hypopigmentation, frequently evident in patients with SCLE after the active phase with erythema and scaling, has never been detected in LET (David-Bajar and Davis 1997). Because some of the patients with LET present with annular skin lesions, there might be a possibility of developing annular erythema associated with Sjögren's syndrome; however, this rare entity has only been reported for Asian patients (Kuhn et al. 2000b). Furthermore, association with systemic disease seems to be very rare in patients with LET (Alexiades-Armenakas et al. 2003, Jolly et al. 2004); however, none of our patients fulfilled four or more ARA criteria for the diagnosis of SLE (Kuhn et al. 2000, Tan et al. 1982). Although joint symptoms occurred temporarily, no signs of inflammatory joint disease or rheumatoid arthritis have been detected, and further systemic manifestations, such as renal, central nervous system, or lung involvement, have not yet been appreciated in any of the patients. Therefore, the prognosis in patients with LET is generally more favorable than in those with other forms of CLE and several patients who had been followed for more than 15 years showed no recurrence after local or systemic treatment. However, this would need to be confirmed by long-term investigations in a greater number of patients.

LET is mostly found in males, and the mean onset of the disease is nearly the same as that described for DLE; therefore, compared with SCLE or SLE, patients with LET are older when the disease begins (Bangert et al. 1984). However, even children may be affected, and, interestingly, one boy had already developed LET skin lesions when he was 9 months old (Kuhn et al. 1997). LET in childhood seems similar to the adult form of the disease, with the same clinical and histologic features, but, to date, only three children with LET have been published in the literature (two boys and one girl aged 9 months to 3 years at disease onset) (Sonntag et al. 2003). Interestingly, photoprovocation tests, which had been performed in two of the young patients, demonstrated no characteristic skin lesions after UV irradiation, although the patients had a positive history of photosensitivity, and ANAs were not detectable. During 6-year follow-up, no signs of systemic involvement had developed in any of the three children.

Clinically, LET is characterized by succulent, urticaria-like, single or multiple plaques with a bright reddish or violaceous, smooth surface on sun-exposed areas, such as the face, upper back, V-area of the neck, extensor aspects of the arms, and shoulders (Fig. 6.17); the lesions spare the knuckles, inner aspect of the arms, and axillae, and have never been detected below the waist (Kuhn et al. 2000a). The swollen appearance of the lesions and the absence of clinically visible epidermal involvement are the most important clinical features of this subtype. The borders are sharply limited, and, in some cases, there is a tendency for the lesions to coalesce in the periphery,

Fig. 6.17. Lupus erythematosus tumidus (LET). Succulent, elevated, urticaria-like erythematous plaques on the right cheek

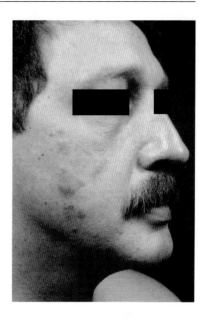

producing a gyrate configuration, or to swell in the periphery and flatten in the center (Fig. 6.18) (Mascaro et al. 1997). Some patients develop erythematous, annular lesions on the cheeks and upper extremities imitating the annular type of SCLE, and, recently, a patient with LET following the lines of Blaschko has been reported (Pacheco et al. 2002). LET lesions can also coexist with DLE lesions (Ruiz and Sanchez 1999) and have been reported to mimic alopecia areata when present on the scalp (Werth et al. 1992). However, other nonspecific LE lesions, such as hypopigmentation, mucous membrane ulcers, diffuse alopecia, livedo reticularis, and vasculitis, have never been seen in any patient.

It has long been suggested that this subset of CLE is characterized by a remarkable photosensitivity (Goerz et al. 1990). Provocative phototesting according to a standardized protocol revealed that patients with LET are more photosensitive than those with other forms of CLE. In a study by our group (Kuhn et al. 2001b), characteristic

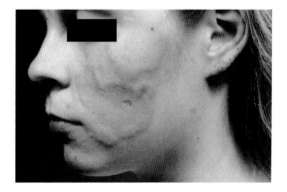

Fig. 6.18. Polycyclic/annular form of lupus erythematosus tumidus (LET). Confluent, non-scarring lesions on the face with a tendency to coalesce in the periphery and flatten in the center

skin lesions were induced by UV irradiation in 43 (72%) of the 60 patients; 30 patients (50%) reacted to UVA and 29 (48%) to UVB irradiation. Combined UVA and UVB irradiation has been used in 30 patients; 19 of these patients (63%) reacted to this testing regimen. Interestingly, 19 (32%) of the 60 patients with LET reacted to more than one wavelength of UV irradiation. However, because of the latency period in developing positive phototest reactions, it may be difficult for patients to link sun exposure to their skin lesions. In contrast to the studies by Kind et al. (Kind et al. 1993) in 1993, our data further showed a positive photoprovocation test reaction in all 10% of the ANA-positive patients, and all 15% of the patients who had moderate ANA titers also developed skin lesions after UV irradiation. In addition, our data revealed a positive correlation of anti-Ro/SSA and anti-La/SSB antibodies and positive provocative phototest reactions, as has been described for patients with SCLE and neonatal LE.

Histologic analysis of skin lesions is necessary to confirm the diagnosis of LET, and, therefore, it represents one of the major criteria of this disease (Kuhn et al. 2003). The most frequent features in biopsy specimens from LET lesions are a moderate to dense, fairly well-circumscribed lymphocytic dermal infiltrate in a perivascular and periadnexal pattern and abundant interstitial mucin deposition. Occasionally, some neutrophils are present, and, in a few cases the dermis shows edema in its upper part; however, in contrast to other forms of CLE, epidermal changes, such as atrophy and follicular plugging, as well as vacuolar degeneration of the dermoepidermal junction or basement membrane thickening are absent. Skin biopsy specimens from UV-induced lesions of LET taken after provocative phototesting present with a similar pattern compared with primary lesions, but a more dense infiltrate of lymphocytes is seen, and interstitial mucin deposition is less prominent. Direct immunfluorescence staining of lesional skin specimens of LET has mostly been negative for immunoglobulin or complement components (Kind and Goerz 1988). In our recent study (Kuhn et al. 2003), biopsy specimens from primary skin lesions demonstrated immunoglobulin deposits (IgG, IgM) along the dermoepidermal junction in 24% of patients with LET, but IgA as well as complement components were not identified in any specimen from primary or UV-induced lesions.

In the past years, immunohistologic studies helped characterize the skin lesions of patients with LET and supported the clinical findings that LET represents a distinct subset of CLE with a similar immunopathomechanism rather than a different disease (Alexiades-Armenakas et al. 2003, Kuhn et al. 2002a, b). Epidermal surface molecules, such as intercellular adhesion molecule-1 (ICAM-1), histocompatibility class II molecule (HLA-DR), and 27E10, a distinct marker for cell activation and differentiation, were equally up-regulated in primary and UV-induced lesions of patients with LET, DLE, and SCLE (Kuhn et al. 2002b). Furthermore, skin specimens from patients with LET demonstrated an inflammatory infiltrate composed of more than 75% CD4[+], CD8[+], and HLA-DR[+] cells; interestingly, CD45RO[+] cells in contrast to CD45RA[+] cells were the prevailing inflammatory cell population. Compared with skin specimens from patients with DLE and SCLE, the mean expression of CD4[+] and CD8[+] cells was higher (but not significant) in LET, and no differences were observed with the other three antibodies (Kuhn et al. 2002a). In contrast to controls, ICAM-1, vascular adhesion molecule-1, E-selectin, and P-selectin showed the same expression pattern in skin specimens from patients with DLE, SCLE, and LET.

LET bears striking similarities to PLE, Jessner's lymphocytic infiltration of the skin, reticular erythematous mucinosis (REM), and pseudolymphoma (Ruhdorfer et al. 1998). The clinical distinction between PLE and LET can be difficult; however, LET shows a much more delayed reaction after sun exposure, and healing of skin lesions takes much longer, even when sun exposure is avoided and a sun block is applied daily (Holzle et al. 1987, Lehmann et al. 1986). Furthermore, in contrast to LET, desensitization phototherapy or photochemotherapy are the most effective forms of preventive treatment in PLE (Bilsland et al. 1993, Ortel et al. 1986). Histologic investigations provide further criteria to differentiate PLE from LET, both showing a superficial and deep lymphocytic infiltration and no changes at the dermoepidermal junction (Ackerman 1997). However, in contrast to LET, a marked edema is seen in the papillary dermis and interstitial mucin deposition is not detectable, which is best accomplished by colloidal iron staining. Interestingly, in two studies determining ANAs in patients with PLE, 10%–14% also showed titers of 1:80 or higher, correlating positively in one study with a longer duration of skin lesions (Murphy and Hawk 1991, Petzelbauer et al. 1992)

Jessner's lymphocytic infiltration of the skin is a relatively uncommon disorder with asymptomatic, papulonodular, nonscarring lesions most often located on the face that has not always been considered a specific disease entity. Until today, no unanimity exists concerning its nosology (Weyers et al. 1998). Several studies demonstrated that clinical and histopathologic criteria are insufficient to distinguish Jessner's lymphocytic infiltration of the skin from different subtypes of CLE (Akasu et al. 1992, Bonczkowitz and Weyers 1996). In a more recent report (O'Toole et al. 1999), the occurrence of these two conditions in one family further supports the theory that Jessner's lymphocytic infiltration of the skin is in the same disease spectrum as CLE. In addition, Weber et al. (Weber et al. 2001) supposed by provocative phototesting that Jessner's lymphocytic infiltration of the skin might be a photosensitive variant of LET. Histologically, Jessner's lymphocytic infiltration of the skin shows a patchy perivascular and sometimes periadnexal infiltrate consisting of lymphocytes, few histiocytes, and plasma cells. The infiltrate often shows a tendency to arrange itself around cutaneous appendages and blood vessels, and it may extend into subcutaneous fat (Ashworth and Morley 1988, Bonczkowitz and Weyers 1996). However, in contrast to LET, mucin deposition seems not to be a major histologic criteria in patients with Jessner's lymphocytic infiltration of the skin and was not described in the original report by Jessner and Kanof in 1953 (Jessner and Kanof 1953).

Reticular erythematous mucinosis is a further rare disease with skin lesions ranging from erythematous, indurated papules to reticulated, macular erythema on the central chest or upper back. In contrast to LET, young to middle-aged women are mostly affected. Interestingly, some authors also consider REM to be a variant of CLE because antimalarial agents have been reported to be the most effective therapy, and patients with REM have shown aggravation of the rash on exposure to sunlight (Braddock et al. 1993, Cohen et al. 1990). However, only a few attempts have been made to quantify the light intolerance or to provoke the skin by phototesting in this disease (McFadden and Larsen 1988), and, in addition, treatment of REM with a large dose of UVB radiation has even been suggested (Yamazaki et al. 1999). Histologic analysis of REM shows no or minimal vacuolar degeneration at the dermoepidermal junction and a mild to dense perivascular and perifollicular infiltrate of lymphocytes with abundant mucin deposition in the dermis (Vanuytrecht-Henderickx et al. 1984). Furthermore, pseudolymphoma can also clinically simulate LET; however, in most cases, histologic analysis shows a top-heavy, usually wedge-shaped infiltrate of small lymphocytes as well as plasma cells and eosinophils and no interstitial mucin deposition (Ploysangam et al. 1998, Weinberg et al. 1993).

In summary, LET is a distinct subset of CLE with characteristic clinical features requiring correlation with photobiologic, serologic, histologic, and immunohistologic findings because, taken in isolation, other diagnoses can be indicated. The reported data emphasize the importance of defining LET as a separate entity with an intermittent course and demonstrate that this disease has been neglected in the literature since first mentioned in 1909.

Bullous Lesions in Lupus Erythematosus

The frequency of bullous lesions associated with LE (BLE) is low, and it has been reported that less than 5% of patients with SLE and skin changes had chronic vesiculobullous lesions (Gammon and Briggaman 1993, Yell and Wojnarowska 1997). Confusion has always existed concerning the nosology and classification of the bullous skin changes that can occur in patients with LE, and there has been no consensus in this area for a long time. In 1997, Sontheimer (Sontheimer 1997) divided the various types of vesicular and bullous skin lesions that can be encountered in patients with LE into those that have or do not have LE-specific pathology and proposed the following classification scheme:

(1) Bullae may develop in LE-specific skin lesions such as ACLE or other cutaneous forms of LE as a direct extension of the vacuolar degeneration of the epidermal basal layer. Skin cleavage occurs as a result of dissolution of the basal cell layer, resulting in subepidermal cleavage that may have the clinical appearance of toxic epidermal necrolysis. Anti-Ro/SSA antibody-positive patients seem to be at increased risk of developing this complication following UV light exposure (Gilliam et al. 1985, Kulick et al. 1983). Documentation of LE as the causal factor in this type of bullous skin change can be difficult because such patients are also frequently taking systemic medication and toxic epidermal necrolysis, therefore, also commonly develops as a result of drug hypersensitivity reaction. In patients with SCLE, vesiculobullous changes may also occur at the active advancing edge of annular lesions (Grant 1981, Sontheimer 1985b, Wechsler and Stavrides 1982), and subepidermal bullous changes have also been reported to be present in DLE lesions; however, these changes seem to be extremely rare (Nagy and Balogh 1961).

(2) On unusual occasions, bullous eruptions or vesiculobullous lesions, unassociated with LE skin lesions, occur in patients with SLE (Bacman et al. 2004, Camisa and Sharma 1983, Gammon et al. 1985, Hall et al. 1982, Olansky et al. 1982, Penneys and Wiley 1979). These lesions predominantly involve flexural or extensor skin (Fig. 6.19), the upper trunk, and the supraclavicular regions, but the face and the mucosal membranes are also predilection sites. The bullae arise on erythematous or normal skin, tend to be tense, and may approach the size of blisters in

Fig. 6.19. Bullous skin lesions associated with lupus erythematosus (BLE). Firm bullous lesions on the extensor aspect of the lower arm in a patient with SLE

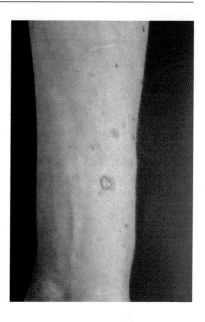

bullous pemphigoid or may resemble the vesiculobullous lesions of dermatitis herpetiformis. If the bullous lesions rupture, they leave erosions, crusts, and pigmentary changes, and when they regress, scars, milium cysts, or calcinosis cutis can remain (Eckman and Mutasim 2002). In this form of bullous skin lesions, the activity of blistering may or may not coincide with the activity of the patient's systemic disease, and occasionally, mild and serious cases associated with organ-threatening disease have been reported (Gammon and Briggaman 1993, Sontheimer 1997). An important and interesting feature of these patients is also the dramatic response to treatment with dapsone even with very small doses (Hall et al. 1982, Yung and Oakley 2000). However, the drug could not be tapered and discontinued without rapid recurrence of the lesions. In a recent study, the efficacy of methotrexate in bullous SLE has also been reported in one patient (Malcangi et al. 2003). Histologically, the subepidermal blisters demonstrate neutrophilic microabscesses in dermal papillae along with a perivascular and periadnexal infiltration consisting of lymphocytes and neutrophils (Megahed 2004). Direct immunofluorescence shows linear or granular deposits of IgG, IgA, and/or IgM and complement along the basement membrane zone, and immunoelectron microscopic studies demonstrate IgG deposits at or below the lamina densa (Gammon and Briggaman 1993, Yell and Wojnarowska 1997). Furthermore, indirect immunofluorescent studies are positive using a 1 M NaCL split skin demonstrating mostly dermal binding (Gammon et al. 1985), and Western blot analysis showed that these autoantibodies bind to the noncollagenous portion of type VII collagen (Shirahama et al. 1998). These data further demonstrated that the autoantibodies in this bullous form of LE bind to the same epitopes as described in epidermolysis bullosa (Barton et al. 1986, Lapiere et al. 1993). Prior to these studies, two other groups had performed acid elution studies on skin of patients with SLE, demonstrating autoantibodies reactive against human skin (Landry and Sams 1974, Nicholas and Gilliam 1981, 1982). It is highly likely that these investigators were dealing with autoantibodies reactive against type VII collagen. In more recent studies, Chan et al. (Chan et al. 1999) concluded that patients with bullous SLE may have autoantibodies to multiple basement membrane components, such as bullous pemphigoid antigen-1, laminin-5, and laminin-6. Furthermore, Yell and Wojnarowska (Yell and Wojnarowska 1997) demonstrated that two of seven patients also showed epidermal binding and, in one case, this was also associated with dermal binding.

In addition, a variety of primarily blistering diseases have been anecdotically reported to occur in patients with cutaneous and systemic manifestations of LE, in particular, dermatitis herpetiformis (Davies et al. 1976), bullous pemphigoid (Miller et al. 1978), pemphigus erythematosus (Chorzelski et al. 1968), pemphigus foliaceus (Blanchet et al. 1981), epidermolysis bullosa acquisita (Dotson et al. 1981), and linear IgA dermatoses (Lau et al. 1991). A non-autoimmune blistering skin disease, porphyria cutaneous tarda, has also been reported in patients with different forms of LE (Gibson and McEvoy 1998, Weatherhead and Adam 1985); however, this association could also be merely fortuitous.

References

Ackerman AB (1997) Lupus erythematosus. In: Ackerman AB (ed) Histologic diagnosis of inflammatory skin diseases. Williams & Wilkins, Baltimore, pp 525–546

Afshari NA, Afshari MA, Foster CS (2001) Inflammatory conditions of the eye associated with rheumatic diseases. Curr Rheumatol Rep 3:453–458

Akasu R, Kahn HJ, From L (1992) Lymphocyte markers on formalin-fixed tissue in Jessner's lymphocytic infiltrate and lupus erythematosus. J Cutan Pathol 19:59–67

Alexiades-Armenakas MR, Baldassano M, Bince B, Werth V, Bystryn JC, Kamino H, Soter NA, Franks AG (2003) Tumid lupus erythematosus: criteria for classification with immunohistochemical analysis. Arthritis Rheum 15:494–500

Allegue F, Alonso ML, Rocamora A, Ledo A (1988) Chilblain lupus erythematosus and antiphospholipid antibody syndrome. J Am Acad Dermatol 19:908–910

Andreasen JO, Poulsen HE (1964) Oral discoid and sytemic lupus erythematosus. Acta Odont Scand 22:389–400

Arnold HL (1956) Lupus erythematosus profundus: commentary and report of four more cases. Arch Dermatol 73:15–33

Ashinoff R, Werth VP, Franks AG (1988) Resistant discoid lupus erythematosus of palms and soles: successful treatment with azathioprine. J Am Acad Dermatol 19:961–965

Ashworth J, Morley WN (1988) Jessner and Kanof's lymphocytic infiltration of the skin: a familial variant. Dermatologica 177:120–122

Bach GL (1980) Nasal septum perforation in disseminated lupus erythematosus, case report and literature review. Z Rheumatol 39:22–27

Bacman D, Ostendorf B, Megahed M, Ruzicka T, Schneider M, Kuhn A (2004) Bullous systemic lupus erythematosus. Hautarzt 55:392–395

Balabanova MB, Mateev GS, Obreschkova EW, Wassileva ST, Pramatarov KD (1992) Lupus erythematodes hypertrophicus et profundus. Z Hautkr 67:812–815

Bangert JL, Freemann RG, Sontheimer RD, Gilliam JN (1984) Subacute cutaneous lupus erythematosus and discoid lupus erythematosus. Comparative histopathologic findings. Arch Dermatol 120:332–337

Barton DD, Fine JD, Gammon WR, Sams WMJ (1986) Bullous systemic lupus erythematosus: an unusual clinical course and detectable circulating autoantibodies to the epidermolysis bullosa acquisita antigen. J Am Acad Dermatol 16:369–373

Bazex A, Salvador R, Dupre A, Parant M, Christol B (1965) Are we justified in considering Jessner's and Kanof's lymphocytic infiltration as a nosologic entity? Hautarzt 16:250–254

Bechet PE (1940) Hypertrophic lupus erythematosus. Arch Dermatol 42:211–213

Bechet PE, Elizabeth NJ (1948) Lupus erythematosus telangiectoides. Arch Dermatol 58: 128–133

Bielsa I, Herrero C, Font J, Mascaro JM (1987) Lupus erythematosus and toxic epidermal necrolysis. J Am Acad Dermatol 16:1265–1267

Bilsland D, George SA, Gibbs NK, Aitchison T, Johnson BE, Ferguson J (1993) A comparison of narrow band phototherapy (TL-01) and photochemotherapy (PUVA) in the management of polymorphic light eruption. Br J Dermatol 129:708–712

Blanchet P, Auffret N, Fouchard J, Lesavre P, Durupt G, Civatte J (1981) Association of thymoma, superficial pemphigus, nephrotic syndrome and lupus biology. Ann Dermatol Venereol 108:471–472

Bonczkowitz M, Weyers W (1996) Abgrenzung von Lupus erythematodes und lymphozytischer Infiltration. Verch Dtsch Ges Path 80:235–240

Bonsmann G, Schiller M, Luger TA, Stander S (2001) Terbinafine-induced subacute cutaneous lupus erythematosus. J Am Acad Dermatol 44:925–931

Botella R, Alfonso R, Silvestre J, Ramon R (1999) Discoid lupus erythematosus-like lesions and stomatitis. Arch Dermatol 135:847–850

Braddock SW, Kay HD, Maennle D, McDonald TL, Pirruccello SJ, Masih A, Klassen LW, Sawka AR (1993) Clinical and immunologic studies in reticular erythematous mucinosis and Jessner's lymphocytic infiltrate of skin. J Am Acad Dermatol 28:691–695

Braverman IM (1981) Connective tissue (rheumatic) diseases. In: Braverman IM (ed) Skin signs of systemic diseases. WB Saunders, Philadelphia, pp 255–377

Breathnach SM, Wells GC (1979) Chilblain lupus erythematosus with response to chemical sympathectomy. Br J Dermatol 101:49–51

Burge SM, Frith PA, Juniper RP, Wojnarowska F (1989) Mucosal involvement in systemic and chronic cutaneous lupus erythematosus. Br J Dermatol 121:727–741

Callen JP (1985) Discoid lupus erythematosus – variants and clinical associations. Clin Dermatol 3:49–57

Callen JP, Kulick KB, Stelzer G, Fowler JF (1986) Subacute cutaneous lupus erythematosus. Clinical, serologic, and immunogenetic studies of forty-nine patients seen in a nonreferral setting. J Am Acad Dermatol 15:1227–1237

Callen JP, Klein J (1988) Subacute cutaneous lupus erythematosus. Clinical, serologic, immunogenetic, and therapeutic considerations in seventy-two patients. Arthritis Rheum 31: 1007–1013

Callen JP, Hughes AP, Kulp-Shorten C (2001) Subacute cutaneous lupus erythematosus induced or exacerbated by terbinafine: a report of 5 cases. Arch Dermatol 137:1196–1198

Camisa C, Sharma HM (1983) Vesicobullous systemic lupus erythematosus: report of two cases and a review of the literature. J Am Acad Dermatol 9:924–933

Caproni M, Cardinali C, Salvatore E, Fabbri P (2001) Subacute cutaneous lupus erythematosus with pityriasis-like cutaneous manifestations. Int J Dermatol 40:59–62

Cardinali C, Caproni M, Bernacchi E, Amato L, Fabbri P (2000) The spectrum of cutaneous manifestations in lupus erythematosus – the Italian experience. Lupus 9:417–423

Cardinali C, Giomi B, Caproni M, Fabbri P (2004) Cutaneous hypertrophic lupus erythematosus in a patient with systemic involvement. Skinmed 3:49–51

Caruso WR, Stewart ML, Nanda VK, Quismorio FPJ (1987) Squamous cell carcinoma of the skin in black patients with discoid lupus erythematosus. J Rheumatol 14:156–159

Casala AM, Bianchi C, Bianchi O, Stringa SG (1971) Lupus erythematosus tumidus (lymphocytic infiltration of the skin) and chronic lupus erythematosus associated in the same patient. Immunofluorescent study. Bull Soc Fr Dermatol Syphil 78:256–258

Cervera R, Khamashta MA, Font J, Sebastiani GD, Gil A, Lavilla P, Domenech I, Aydintug AO, Jedryka-Goral A, de Ramon E, Galezzi M, Haga HJ, Mathieu A, Houssiau F, Ingelmo M, Hughes GRV (1993) Systemic lupus erythematosus: clinical and immunologic patterns of disease expression in a cohort of 1,000 patients. The European Working Party on Systemic Lupus Erythematosus. Medicine (Baltimore) 72:113–124

Chan LS, Lapiere JC, Chen M, Traczyk T, Mancini AJ, Paller AS, Woodley DT, Marinkovich MP (1999) Bullous systemic lupus erythematosus with autoantibodies recognizing multiple skin basement membrane components, bullous pemphigoid antigen 1, laminin-5, laminin-6, and type VII collagen. Arch Dermatol 135:569–573

Cherif F, Mebazaa A, Mokni M, El Euch D, Azaiz MI, Dhahri AB (2003) Childhood discoid lupus erythematosus: a Tunisian retrospective study of 16 cases. Pediatr Dermatol 20:295–298

Chlebus E, Wolska H, Blaszczyk M, Jablonska S (1998) Subacute cutaneous lupus erythematosus versus systemic lupus erythematosus: diagnostic criteria and therapeutic implications. J Am Acad Dermatol 38:405–412

Chorzelski T, Jablonska S, Blaszczyk M (1968) Immunopathological investigations in the Senear-Usher syndrome (coexistence of pemphigus and lupus erythematosus). Br J Dermatol 80: 211–217

Cohen LM, Tyring SK, Rady P, Callen JP (1992) Human papillomavirus type 11 in multiple squamous cell carcinomas in a patient with subacute cutaneous lupus erythematosus. J Am Acad Dermatol 26:840–845

Cohen MR, Crosby D (1994) Systemic disease in subacute cutaneous lupus erythematosus: a controlled comparison with systemic lupus erythematosus. J Rheumatol 21:1665–1669

Cohen PR, Rabinowitz AD, Ruszkowski AM, DeLeo VA (1990) Reticular erythematous mucinosis syndrome: review of the world literature and report of the syndrome in a prepubertal child. Pediatr Dermatol 7:1–10

Costner MI, Sontheimer RD, Provost TT (2003) Lupus erythematosus. In: Sontheimer RD and Provost TT (eds) Cutaneous manifestations of rheumatic diseases. Williams & Wilkins, Philadelphia, pp 15–64

Crowson AN, Magro C (2001) The cutaneous pathology of lupus erythematosus: a review. J Cutan Pathol 28:1–23

Daldon PE, Macedo de Souza E, Cintra ML (2003) Hypertrophic lupus erythematosus: a clinico-pathological study of 14 cases. J Cutan Pathol 30:443–438

Dammert K (1971) Lupus erythematosus hypertrophicus et profundus. Acta Derm Venereol 52:315–316

David KM, Thornton JC, Davis B, Sontheimer RD, Gilliam JN (1984) Morbidity and mortality in patients with subacute cutaneous lupus erythematosus (SCLE). J Invest Dermatol 82:408–409

David-Bajar KM, Bennion SD, DeSpain JD, Golitz LE, Lee LA (1992) Clinical, histologic, and immunofluorescent distinctions between subacute cutaneous lupus erythematosus and discoid lupus erythematosus. J Invest Dermatol 99:251–257

David-Bajar KM (1993) What's new in cutaneous lupus syndromes: subacute cutaneous lupus erythematosus. J Invest Dermatol 100:2S–8S

David-Bajar KM, Davis BM (1997) Pathology, immunopathology, and immunohistochemistry in cutaneous lupus erythematosus. Lupus 6:145–157

Davies MG, Marks R, Waddington E (1976) Simultaneous systemic lupus erythematosus and dermatitis herpetiformis. Arch Dermatol 112:1292–1294

de Argila Fernandez-Auran D, Revenga Arranz F, Iglesias Diez L (1996) Perniosis and lupus anticoagulant. Rev Clin Esp 196:24–27

de Berker D, Dissaneyeka M, Burge S (1992) The sequelae of chronic cutaneous lupus erythematosus. Lupus 1:181–186

de Graciansky P, Grupper C, Sirkis L (1965) Dermatomycosis caused by Tricophyton rubrum simulating lupus erythematosus tumidus. Bull Soc Fr Dermatol Syphil 72:809–811

Dekle CL, Mannes KD, Davis LS, Sangueza OP (1999) Lupus tumidus. J Am Acad Dermatol 41:250–253

DeSpain JD, Clark DP (1988) Subacute cutaneous lupus erythematosus presenting as erythroderma. J Am Acad Dermatol 19:388–392

Djawari D (1978) Drug-induced lupus erythematosus. Z Hautkr 53:180–188

Dotson AD, Raimer SS, Pursley TV, Tschen J (1981) Systemic lupus erythematosus occurring in a patient with epidermolysis bullosa acquisita. Arch Dermatol 117:422–426

Doutre MS, Beylot C, Beylot J, Pompougnac E, Royer P (1992) Chilblain lupus erythematosus: report of 15 cases. Dermatology 184:26–28

Eckman JA, Mutasim DF (2002) Bullous systemic lupus erythematosus with milia and calcinosis. Cutis 70:31–34

Fabbri P, Bernacchi E, Neri R (1990) Subacute cutaneous lupus erythematosus. Review of the literature and immunological studies of 11 patients. G Ital Dermatol Venereol 125:329–336

Fabbri P, Cardinali C, Giomi B, Caproni M (2003) Cutaneous lupus erythematosus: diagnosis and management. Am J Clin Dermatol 4:449–465

Findlay GH, Lups JG (1967) The incidence and pathogenesis of chronic discoid lupus erythematosus. An analysis of 191 consecutive cases from the Transvaal. S Afr Med J 41:694–698

Fischer GF, Pickl WF, Fae I, Anegg B, Milota S, Volc-Platzer B (1994) Association between chronic cutaneous lupus erythematosus and HLA class II alleles. Hum Immunol 41:280–284

Fisher DA, Everett MA (1996) Violaceous rash of dorsal fingers in a woman. Diagnosis: chilblain lupus erythematosus (perniosis). Arch Dermatol 132:459–462

Franke W, Kuhn A, Megahed M, Krutmann J, Ruzicka T, Lehmann P (1999) Periorbital edema as the initial symptom of lupus erythematosus profundus. Case report and discussion of the literature. Hautarzt 50:889–892

Frith PA, Burge SM, Millard PR, Wojnarowska F (1990) External ocular findings in lupus erythematosus: a clinical and immunopathological study. Br J Ophthalmol 74:163–167

Gammon WR, Woodley DT, Dole KC, Briggaman RA (1985) Evidence that anti-basement membrane zone antibodies in bullous eruption of systemic lupus erythematosus recognize epidermolysis bullosa acquisita autoantigen. J Invest Dermatol 84:472–476

Gammon WR, Briggaman RA (1993) Bullous SLE: a phenotypically distinctive but immunologically heterogeneous bullous disorder. J Invest Dermatol 100:28S-34S

George R, Mathai R, Kurian S (1992) Cutaneous lupus erythematosus in India: immunofluorescence profile. Int J Dermatol 31:265–269

Gibson GE, McEvoy MT (1998) Coexistence of lupus erythematosus and porphyria cutanea tarda in fifteen patients. J Am Acad Dermatol 38:569–573

Gilliam JN (1977) The cutaneous signs of lupus erythematosus. Cont Educ Fam Phys 6:34–70

Gilliam JN, Sontheimer RD (1981) Distinctive cutaneous subsets in the spectrum of lupus erythematosus. J Am Acad Dermatol 4:471–475

Gilliam JN, Sontheimer RD (1982) Subacute cutaneous lupus erythematosus. Clin Rheum Dis 8:343–352

Gilliam JM, Cohen SB, Sontheimer RD, Moscella SL (1985) Connective tissue diseases. In: Moscella, SL, Hurley HJ (eds) Dermatology. WB Saunders, Philadelphia, pp 1087–1135

Goerz G, Lehmann P, Schuppe HC, Lakomek HJ, Kind P (1990) Lupus erythematosus. Z Hautkr 65:226–234

Gougerot H, Burnier R (1930) Lupus érythémateux tumidus. Bull Soc Fr Dermatol Syphil 37:1219–1292

Gougerot H, Burnier R (1931) Lupus érythémateux tumidus. Bull Soc Fr Dermatol Syphil 38:195–196

Gougerot H, Burnier R (1932) Lupus érythémateux tumidus. Bull Soc Fr Dermatol Syphil 39:21

Grant JM (1981) Annular vesicular lupus erythematosus. Cutis 28:90–92

Green S, Piette W (1987) Treatment of hypertrophic lupus erythematosus with isotretinoin. Cutis 17:364–368

Grossberg E, Scherschun L, Fivenson DP (2001) Lupus profundus: not a benign disease. Lupus 10:514–516

Hall RP, Lawley TJ, Smith HR, Katz SI (1982) Bullous eruption of systemic lupus erythematosus. Ann Intern Med 97:165–170

Heiligenhaus A, Dutt JE, Foster CS (1996) Histology and immunopathology of systemic lupus erythematosus affecting the conjunctiva. Eye 10:425–432

Helm TN, Jones CM (2002) Chilblain lupus erythematosus lesions precipitated by the cold. Cutis 69:183–184

Herrero C, Bielsa I, Font J, Lozano F, Ercilla G, Lecha M, Ingelmo M, Mascaro JM (1988) Subacute cutaneous lupus erythematosus: clinicopathologic findings in thirteen cases. J Am Acad Dermatol 19:1057–1062

Hoffmann E (1909) Demonstrationen: Lupus erythematodes tumidus. Derm Zeitschr 16:159–160

Holland NW, McKnight K, Challa VR, Agudelo CA (1995) Lupus panniculitis (profundus) involving the breast: report of 2 cases and review of the literature. J Rheumatol 22:344–346

Holzle E, Plewig G, Lehmann P (1987) Photodermatoses: diagnostic procedures and their interpretation. Photodermatol 4:109–114

Hsu S, Hwang Ly, Ruiz H (2002) Tumid lupus erythematosus. Cutis 69:227–230

Hutchinson J (1888) Harveian lectures on lupus. Lecture III. On the various form of lupus vulgaris and erythematosus. Br Med J 1:113–118

Hymes SR, Jordon RE (1989) Chronic cutaneous lupus erythematosus. Med Clin North Am 73:1055–1071

Hymes SR, Jordon RE, Arnett FC (1986) Lupus erythematosus. Dermatol Clin 4:267–276

Irgang S (1940) Lupus erythematosus profundus. Arch Dermatol Syph 42:97–108

James DG (1992) Lupus pernio. Lupus 1:129–131

Jessner M, Kanof NB (1953) Lymphocytic infiltration of the skin. Arch Dermatol Syph 68: 447–449

Jolly M, Laumann AE, Shea CR, Utset TO (2004) Lupus erythematosus tumidus in systemic lupus erythematosus: novel association and possible role of early treatment in prevention of discoid lupus erythematosus. Lupus 13:64–69

Kanwar J, Dhar S, Ghosh S (1993) Involvement of nails in discoid lupus erythematosus. J Assoc Physicians India 41:543

Kaposi MK (1883) Pathologie und Therapie der Hautkrankheiten. Urban and Schwarzenberg, Vienna, p 642

Kind P, Goerz G (1988) Der kutane Lupus erythematodes (LE). In: Jahrbuch der Dermatologie. Biermann Verlag, Zülpich, Germany, pp 85–103

Kind P, Lehmann P, Plewig G (1993) Phototesting in lupus erythematosus. J Invest Dermatol 100:53S–57S

Knop J, Bonsmann G, Kind P, Doxiadis I, Vogeler U, Doxiadis G, Goerz G, Grosse-Wilde H (1990) Antigens of the major histocompatibility complex in patients with chronic discoid lupus erythematosus. Br J Dermatol 122:723–728

Kossard S (2002) Lupus panniculitis clinically simulating alopecia areata. Australas J Dermatol 43:221–213

Kuhn A (2003) Neue klinische, photobiologische und immunhistologische Erkenntnisse zur Pathophysiologie des kutanen Lupus erythematodes. In: Hautklinik. Düsseldorf: Heinrich-Heine University, Habilitationsschrift

Kuhn A, Schuppe HC, Megahed M, Goerz G, Lehmann P (1997) Kutaner Lupus erythematodes im Kindesalter (Tumidus-Typ). Z Hautkr 72:299–300

Kuhn A, Richter-Hintz D, Oslislo C, Ruzicka T, Megahed M, Lehmann P (2000a) Lupus erythematosus tumidus – a neglected subset of cutaneous lupus erythematosus: report of 40 cases. Arch Dermatol 136:1033–1041

Kuhn A, Richter-Hintz D, Schuppe HC, Ruzicka T, Lehmann P (2000b) Annular erythema in Sjögren's syndrome. A variant of cutaneous lupus erythematosus? Hautarzt 51:270–275

Kuhn A, Schuppe HC, Ruzicka T, Lehmann P (2000 c) Seltene kutane Manifestationsformen des Lupus erythematodes. Hautarzt 51:818–825

Kuhn A, Becker-Wegerich PM, Ruzicka T, Lehmann P (2000d) Successful treatment of discoid lupus erythematosus with argon laser. Dermatology 201:175–177

Kuhn A, Sonntag M, Richter-Hintz D, Oslislo C, Megahed M, Ruzicka T, Lehmann P (2001a) Phototesting in lupus erythematosus: a 15-year experience. J Am Acad Dermatol 45:86–95

Kuhn A, Sonntag M, Richter-Hintz D, Oslislo C, Megahed M, Ruzicka T, Lehmann P (2001b) Phototesting in lupus erythematosus tumidus – review of 60 patients. Photochem Photobiol 73:532–536

Kuhn A, Sonntag M, Lehmann P, Megahed M, Vestweber D, Ruzicka T (2002a) Characterization of the inflammatory infiltrate and expression of endothelial cell adhesion molecules in lupus erythematosus tumidus. Arch Dermatol Res 294:6–13

Kuhn A, Sonntag M, Sunderkotter C, Lehmann P, Vestweber D, Ruzicka T (2002b) Upregulation of epidermal surface molecule expression in primary and ultraviolet-induced lesions of lupus erythematosus tumidus. Br J Dermatol 146:801–809

Kuhn A, Sonntag M, Ruzicka T, Lehmann P, Megahed M (2003) Histopathologic findings in lupus erythematosus tumidus: review of 80 patients. J Am Acad Dermatol 48:901–908

Kulick KB, Mogavero HJ, Provost TT, Reichlin M (1983) Serologic studies in patients with lupus erythematosus and psoriasis. J Am Acad Dermatol 8:631–634

Landry M, Sams WM (1974) Systemic lupus erythematosus: studies of autoantibodies bound to skin. J Clin Invest 52:1871

Lapiere JC, Woodley DT, Parente MG, Iwasaki T, Wynn KC, Christiano AM, Uitto J (1993) Epitope mapping of type VII collagen. Identification of discrete peptide sequences recognized by sera from patients with acquired epidermolysis bullosa. J Clin Invest 92:1831–1839

Lau M, Kaufmann-Grunzinger I, Raghunath M (1991) A case report of a patient with features of systemic lupus erythematosus and linear IgA disease. Br J Dermatol 124:498–502

Lehmann P, Holzle E, von Kries R, Plewig G (1986) Lichtdiagnostische Verfahren bei Patienten mit Verdacht auf Photodermatosen. Z Haut Geschlechtskr 152:667–682

Lehmann P, Holzle E, Kind P, Goerz G, Plewig G (1990) Experimental reproduction of skin lesions in lupus erythematosus by UVA and UVB radiation. J Am Acad Dermatol 22:181–187

Lehmann P (1996) Photosensitivität des Lupus erythematodes. Akt Dermatol 22:47–51

Lodi A, Pozzi M, Agostoni A, Betti R, Crosti C (1993) Unusual onset of lupus erythematosus profundus. Br J Dermatol 129:96–97

Lodin A (1963) Discoid lupus erythematosus and trauma. Acta Derm Venereol 43:142–146

Lupton GP (1987) Discoid lupus erythematosus occurring in a smallpox vaccination scar. J Am Acad Dermatol 17:688–690

Lyon CC, Blewitt R, Harrison PV (1998) Subacute cutaneous lupus erythematosus: two cases of delayed diagnosis. Acta Derm Venereol 78:57–59

Magee KL, Hymes SR, Rapini RP, Yeakley JW, Jordon RE (1991) Lupus erythematosus profundus with periorbital swelling and proptosis. J Am Acad Dermatol 24:288–290

Magro CM, Crowson AN, Harrist TJ (1997) Atypical lymphoid infiltrates arising in cutaneous lesions of connective tissue disease. Am J Dermatopathol 19:446–455

Malcangi G, Brandozzi G, Giangiacomi M, Zampetti M, Danieli MG (2003) Bullous SLE: response to methotrexate and relationship with disease activity. Lupus 12:63–66

Martens PB, Moder KG, Ahmed I (1999) Lupus panniculitis: clinical perspectives from a case series. J Rheumatol 26:68–72

Mascaro JM, Herrero C, Hausmann G (1997) Uncommon cutaneous manifestations of lupus erythematosus. Lupus 6:122–131

McCauliffe DP (2001) Cutaneous lupus erythematosus. Semin Cutan Med Surg 20:14–26

McFadden N, Larsen TE (1988) Reticular erythematous mucinosis and photosensitivity: a case study. Photodermatol 5:270–272

Megahed M (2004) Bullous systemic lupus erythematosus. In: Megahed M (ed) Histopathology of blistering diseases – with clinical, electron microscopic, immunological, and molecular biological correlations. Springer, Berlin, Heidelberg, New York, pp 236–237

Meiusi RS, Cameron JD, Holland EJ, Summers CG (1991) Discoid lupus erythematosus of the eyelid complicated by wound dehiscence. Am J Ophthalmol 111:108–109

Milde P, Goerz G (1994) Depigmentierung bei Lupus erythematodes (LE) – klinischer "Clue" zum subakut kutanen Lupus erythematodes (SCLE). Z Hautkr 69:123–126

Millard LG, Barker DJ (1978) Development of squamous cell carcinoma in chronic discoid lupus erythematosus. Clin Exp Dermatol 3:161–166

Millard LG, Rowell NR (1978) Chilblain lupus erythematosus (Hutchinson). A clinical laboratory study of 17 patients. Br J Dermatol 98:497–506

Millard TP, Hawk JL, McGregor JM (2000) Photosensitivity in lupus. Lupus 9:3–10

Miller JF, Downham TF, Chapel TA (1978) Coexistent bullous pemphigoid and systemic lupus erythematosus. Cutis 21:368–373

Miyagawa S, Minowa R, Yamashina Y, Ohi H, Shira T (1996) Development of squamous cell carcinoma in chronic discoid lupus erythematosus: a report of two patients with anti-Ro/SSA antibodies. Lupus 5:630–632

Moises-Alfaro C, Berron-Perez R, Carrasco-Daza D, Gutierrez-Castrellon P, Ruiz-Maldonado R (2003) Discoid lupus erythematosus in children: clinical, histopathologic, and follow-up features in 27 cases. Pediatr Dermatol 20:103–107

Molad Y, Weinberger A, David M, Garty B, Wysenbeek AJ, Pinkhas J (1987) Clinical manifestations and laboratory data of subacute cutaneous lupus erythematosus. Isr J Med Sci 23: 278–280

Mosquera Vieitez JC, de la Torre Fraga C, Cruces Prado MJ (1984) Gougerot's lupus erythematosus tumidus. Med Cutan Ibero Lat Am 12:425–429

Murphy GM, Hawk JL (1991) The prevalence of antinuclear antibodies in patients with apparent polymorphic light eruption. Br J Dermatol 125:448–451

Mutasim DF (2003) Severe subacute cutaneous lupus erythematosus presenting with generalized erythroderma and bullae. J Am Acad Dermatol 48:947–949

Nagai Y, Ishikawa O, Hattori T, Ogawa T (2003) Linear lupus erythematosus profundus on the scalp following the lines of Blaschko. Eur J Dermatol 13:294–296

Nagy E, Balogh E (1961) Bullous form of chronic discoid lupus erythematodes accompanied by LE-cell symptoms. Dermatologica 122:6–10

Ng PP, Tan SH, Koh ET (2000) Epidemiology of cutaneous lupus erythematosus in a tertiary referral centre in Singapore. Australas J Dermatol 41:229–233

Ng PP, Tan SH, Tan T (2002) Lupus erythematosus panniculitis: a clinicopathologic study. Int J Dermatol 41:488–490

Nicholas BK, Gilliam JM (1981) Isolation and characterization of an epidermal basement membrane zone antigen which may be involved in antibody binding at the dermal/epidermal junction in systemic lupus erythematosus. Fed Proc 40:198

Nicholas BK, Gilliam JM (1982) Computerimmunoelectrophoretic detection of epidermal basement membrane antibody in systemic lupus erythematosus serum. Clin Res 30:600

Nishikawa T, Provost TT (1991) Differences in clinical, serologic, and immunogenetic features of white versus Oriental anti-SS-A/Ro-positive patients. J Am Acad Dermatol 25:563–564

Nived O, Johansen PB, Sturfelt G (1993) Standardized ultraviolet-A exposure provokes skin reaction in systemic lupus erythematosus. Lupus 2:247–250

Norden D, Weinberg JM, Schumacher HR, Keenan G, Freundlich B (1993) Bilateral periorbital edema in systemic lupus erythematosus. J Rheumatol 20:2158–2160

O'Toole EA, Powell F, Barnes L (1999) Jessner's lymphocytic infiltrate and probable discoid lupus erythematosus occurring separately in two sisters. Clin Exp Dermatol 24:90–93

Olansky AJ, Briggaman RA, Gammon WR, Kelly TF, Sams WM (1982) Bullous systemic lupus erythematosus. J Am Acad Dermatol 7:511–520

Ortel B, Tanew A, Wolff K, Honigsmann H (1986) Polymorphous light eruption: action spectrum and photoprotection. J Am Acad Dermatol 14:748–753

Otani A (1977) Lupus erythematosus hypertrophicus et profundus. Br J Dermatol 96:75–78

Pacheco TR, Spates ST, Lee LA (2002) Unilateral tumid lupus erythematosus. Lupus 11: 388–391

Parodi A, Caproni M, Cardinali C, Bernacchi E, Fuligni A, De Panfilis G, Zane C, Papini M, Veller FC, Vaccaro M, Fabbri P (2000) Clinical, histological and immunopathological features of 58 patients with subacute cutaneous lupus erythematosus. A review by the Italian group of immunodermatology. Dermatology 200:6–10

Parrish LC, Kennedy RJ, Hurley HJ (1967) Palmar lesions in lupus erythematosus. Arch Dermatol 96:273

Patel P, Werth V (2002) Cutaneous lupus erythematosus: a review. Dermatol Clin 20:373–385

Penneys NS, Wiley HE (1979) Herpetiform blisters in systemic lupus erythematosus. Arch Dermatol 115:1427–1428

Perniciaro C, Randle HW, Perry HO (1995) Hypertrophic discoid lupus erythematosus resembling squamous cell carcinoma. J Rheumatol 21:255–257

Peters J (2000) Lupus erythematosus profundus of the breast. Zentralbl Gynakol 122:528–530

Peters MS, Su WP (1989) Lupus erythematosus panniculitis. Med Clin North Am 73:1113–1126

Petzelbauer P, Binder M, Nikolakis P, Ortel B, Honigsmann H (1992) Severe sun sensitivity and the presence of antinuclear antibodies in patients with polymorphous light eruption-like lesions. A form fruste of photosensitive lupus erythematosus? J Am Acad Dermatol 26: 68–74

Pistiner M, Wallace DJ, Nessim S, Metzger AL, Klinenberg JR (1991) Lupus erythematosus in the 1980 s: a survey of 570 patients. Semin Arthritis Rheum 21:55–64

Ploysangam T, Breneman DL, Mutasim DF (1998) Cutaneous pseudolymphomas. J Am Acad Dermatol 38:877–905

Pramatarov K (1998) Drug-induced lupus erythematosus. Clin Dermatol 16:367–377

Pramatarov K, Vassileva S, Miteva L (2000) Subacute cutaneous lupus erythematosus presenting with generalized poikiloderma. J Am Acad Dermatol 42:286–288

Provost TT, Talal N, Harley JB, Reichlin M, Alexander E (1988) The relationship between anti-Ro (SS-A) antibody-positive Sjögren's syndrome and anti-Ro (SS-A) antibody-positive lupus erythematosus. Arch Dermatol 124:63–71

Prystowsky SD, Gilliam JM (1975) Discoid lupus erythematosus as part of a larger disease spectrum. Correlation of clinical features with laboratory findings in lupus erythematosus. Arch Dermatol 111:1448–1452

Rahman P, Gladman DD, Urowitz MB (1999) Nasal-septal perforation in systemic lupus erythematosus – time for a closer look. J Rheumatol 26:1854–1855

Raizman MB, Baum J (1989) Discoid lupus keratitis. Arch Ophthalmol 107:545–547

Rao B, Coldiron B, Freemann RG, Sontheimer RD (1990) Subacute cutaneous lupus erythematosus lesions progressing morphea. J Am Acad Dermato l 23:1019–1022

Reed BR, Huff JC, Jones SK, Orton PW, Lee LA, Norris DA (1985) Subacute cutaneous lupus erythematosus associated with hydrochlorothiazide therapy. Ann Intern Med 103:49–51

Reichart PA (2003) Oral precancerous conditions – an overview. Mund Kiefer Gesichtschir 7:201–207

Romero RW, Nesbitt LTJ, Reed RJ (1977) Unusual variant of lupus erythematosus or lichen planus. Clinical, histopathologic, and immunofluorescent studies. Arch Dermatol 113: 741–748

Rothfield NF (1993) Lupus erythematosus. In: Fitzpatrick TB, Eisen AZ, Wolff K, Freedberg IM, Austen KF (eds) Dermatology and general medicine. McGraw, New York, pp 2138

Rowell NR, Swanson-Beck J, Anderson JP (1963) Lupus erythematosus and erythema multifirme-like lesions. Arch Dermatol 88:176–180

Rowell NR (1987) Chilblain lupus erythematosus responding to etretinate. Br J Dermatol 117:100–102

Rowell NR, Goodfield MJD (1992) The "connective tissue diseases". In: Chamion RH, Burton JL, Ebling FJG (eds) Textbook of dermatology. Blackwell Scientific, London, pp 2163–2194

Rubin RL (1999) Etiology and mechanisms of drug-induced lupus. Curr Opin Rheumatol 11:357–363

Ruhdorfer S, Hein R, Ring J (1998) Differenzialdiagnostische und pathogenetische Aspekte des Lupus erythematodes tumidus. Z Hautkr 73:602–606

Ruiz H, Sanchez JL (1999) Tumid lupus erythematosus. Am J Dermatopathol 21:356–360

Sanchez NP, Peters MS, Winkelmann RK (1981) The histopathology of lupus eyrthematosus panniculitis. J Am Acad Dermatol 122:576–582

Sanchez-Perez J, Fernandez-Herrera J, Sols M, Jones M, Garcia Diez A (1993) Leucocytoclastic vasculitis in subacute cutaneous lupus erythematosus. Br J Dermatol 128:469–470

Santa Cruz DJ, Uitto J, Eisen AZ, Prioleau PG (1983) Verrucous lupus erythematosus: ultrastructural studies on a distinct variant of chronic discoid lupus erythematosus. J Am Acad Dermatol 9:82–90

Scheinman PL (1994) Acral subacute cutaneous lupus erythematosus: an unusual variant. J Am Acad Dermato l 30:800–801

Seiger E, Roland S, Goldman S (1991) Cutaneous lupus treated with topical tretinoin: a case report. Cutis 47:351–355

Sherman RN, Lee CW, Flynn KJ (1993) Cutaneous squamous cell carcinoma in black patients with chronic discoid lupus erythematosus. Int J Dermatol 32:677–679

Shirahama S, Furukawa F, Yagi H, Tanaka T, Hashimoto T, Takigawa M (1998) Bullous systemic lupus erythematosus: detection of antibodies against noncollagenous domain of type VII collagen. J Am Acad Dermatol 38:844–848

Shou-yi S, Shu-fang F, Kang-huang L, Ke-fei K (1987) Clinical study of 30 cases of subacute cutaneous lupus erythematosus. Chin Med J 100:45–48

Sonntag M, Lehmann P, Megahed M, Ruzicka T, Kuhn A (2003) Lupus erythematosus tumidus in childhood. Report of 3 patients. Dermatology 207:188–192

Sontheimer RD, Thomas JR, Gilliam JN (1979) Subacute cutaneous lupus erythematosus: a cutaneous marker for a distinct lupus erythematosus subset. Arch Dermatol 115:1409–1415

Sontheimer RD, Stastny P, Gilliam JN (1981) Human histocompatibility antigen associations in subacute cutaneous lupus erythematosus. J Clin Invest 67:312–316

Sontheimer RD (1985a) Clinical significance of subacute cutaneous lupus erythematosus skin lesions. J Dermatol 12:205–212

Sontheimer RD (1985b) Subacute cutaneous lupus erythematosus. Clin Dermatol 3:58–68

Sontheimer RD (1989) Subacute cutaneous lupus erythematosus: a decade's perspective. Med Clin North Am 73:1073–1090

Sontheimer RD, Provost TT (1996) Lupus erythematosus. In: Sontheimer RD, Provost TT (eds) Cutaneous manifestations of rheumatic diseases. Williams & Wilkins, Baltimore, pp1–71

Sontheimer RD (1997) The lexicon of cutaneous lupus erythematosus – a review and personal perspective on the nomenclature and classification of the cutaneous manifestations of lupus erythematosus. Lupus 6:84–95

Sontheimer RD (2000) Questions answered and a $1 million question raised concerning lupus erythematosus tumidus: is routine laboratory surveillance testing during treatment with hydroxychloroquine for skin disease really necessary. Arch Dermatol 136:1044–1049

Spann CR, Callen JP, Klein JB, Kulick KB (1988) Clinical, serologic and immunogenetic studies in patients with chronic cutaneous (discoid) lupus erythematosus who have verrucous and/or hypertrophic skin lesions. J Rheumatol 15:256–261

Srivastava M, Rencic A, Diglio G, Santana H, Bonitz P, Watson R, Ha E, Anhalt GJ, Provost TT, Nousari CH (2003) Drug-induced, Ro/SSA-positive cutaneous lupus erythematosus. Arch Dermatol 139:45–49

Stainforth J, Goodfield MJ, Taylor PV (1993) Pregnancy-induced chilblain lupus erythematosus. Clin Exp Dermatol 18:449–451

Su WP, Perniciaro C, Rogers RS, White JW (1994) Chilblain lupus erythematosus (lupus pernio): clinical review of the Mayo Clinic experience and proposal of diagnostic criteria. Cutis 54:395–399

Suss R, Meurer M, Schirren CG, Lubke S, Ruzicka T (1994) Lupus erythematodes profundus Kaposi-Irgang. Hautarzt 45:38–41

Tada J, Arata J, Katayama H (1991) Linear lupus erythematosus profundus in a child. J Am Acad Dermatol 24:871–874

Tan EM, Cohen AS, Fries JF, Masi AT, McShane DJ, Rothfield NF, Schaller JG, Talal N, Winchester RJ (1982) The 1982 revised criteria for the classification of systemic lupus erythematosus. Arthritis Rheum 25:1271–1277

Tebbe B, Orfanos CE (1997) Epidemiology and socioeconomic impact of skin disease in lupus erythematosus. Lupus 6:96–104

Tebbe B, Mansmann U, Wollina U, Auer-Grumbach P, Licht-Mbalyohere A, Arsenmeier M, Orfanos CE (1997) Markers in cutaneous lupus erythematosus indicating systemic involvement. A multicenter study on 296 patients. Acta Derm Venereol 77:305–308

Tsutsui K, Imai T, Hatta N, Sakai H, Takata M, Takehara K (1996) Widespread pruritic plaques in a patient with subacute cutaneous lupus erythematosus and hypocomplementemia: response to dapsone therapy. J Am Acad Dermatol 35:313–315

Tuffanelli DL, Dubois EL (1964) Cutaneous manifestations of systemic lupus erythematosus. Arch Dermatol 90:377–386

Tuffanelli DL (1971) Lupus erythematosus panniculitis (profundus). Arch Dermatol 103: 231–242

Ueki H (1994) Koebner phenomenon in lupus erythematosus. Hautarzt 45:154–160

Urman JD, Lowenstein MB, Abeles M, Weinstein A (1978) Oral mucosal ulceration in systemic lupus erythematosus. Arthritis Rheum 21:58–62

Uter W, Proksch E, Schauder S (1988) Chilblain lupus erythematosus. Hautarzt 39:602–605

Uy HS, Pineda R 2nd, Shore JW, Polcharoen W, Jakobiec FA, Foster CS (1999) Hypertrophic discoid lupus erythematosus of the conjunctiva. Am J Ophthalmol 127:604–605

Vanuytrecht-Henderickx D, Dewolf-Peeters C, Degreef H (1984) Morphological study of the reticular erythematous mucinosis syndrome. Dermatologica 168:163–169

Viguier M, Pinquier L, Cavelier-Balloy B, de la Salmoniere P, Cordoliani F, Flageul B, Morel P, Dubertret L, Bachelez H (2001) Clinical and histopathologic features and immunologic variables in patients with severe chilblains. A study of the relationship to lupus erythematosus. Medicine (Baltimore) 80:180–188

Vinciullo C (1986) Hypertrophic lupus erythematosus: differentiation from squamous cell carcinoma. Australas J Dermatol 27:76–82

Voigtlander V, Boonen H (1990) Squamous cell carcinoma of the lower lip in discoid lupus erythematosus associated with hereditary deficiency of complement 2. Z Hautkr 65:836–837

Walchner M, Messer G, Kind P (1997) Phototesting and photoprotection in LE. Lupus 6:167–174

Watanabe T, Tsuchida T (1995) Classification of lupus erythematosus based upon cutaneous manifestations. Dermatological, systemic and laboratory findings in 191 patients. Dermatology 190:277–283

Weatherhead L, Adam J (1985) Discoid lupus erythematosus. Coexistence with porphyria cutanea tarda. Int J Dermatol 24:453–455

Weber F, Schmuth M, Fritsch P, Sepp N (2001) Lymphocytic infiltration of the skin is a photosensitive variant of lupus erythematosus: evidence by phototesting. Br J Dermatol 144: 292–296

Wechsler HL, Stavrides A (1982) Systemic lupus erythematosus with anti-Ro antibodies: clinical, histologic and immunologic findings. Report of three cases. J Am Acad Dermatol 6:73–83

Weinberg JM, Rook AH, Lessin SR (1993) Molecular diagnosis of lymphocytic infiltrates of the skin. Arch Dermatol 129:1491–1500

Werth VP, White WL, Sanchez MR, Franks AG (1992) Incidence of alopecia areata in lupus erythematosus. Arch Dermatol 128:368–371

Weyers W, Bonczkowitz M, Weyers I (1998) LE or not LE – that is the question: an unsuccessful attempt to separate lymphocytic infiltration from the spectrum of discoid lupus erythematosus. Am J Dermatopathol 20:225–232

Wilson CL, Burge SM, Dean D, Dawber RP (1992) Scarring alopecia in discoid lupus erythematosus. Br J Dermatol 126:307

Winkelmann RK (1970) Panniculitis and systemic lupus erythematosus. JAMA 211:472–475

Winkelmann RK (1983) Panniculitis in connective tissue disease. Arch Dermatol 119:336–344

Wolska H, Blaszczyk M, Jablonska S (1989) Phototests in patients with various forms of lupus erythematosus. Int J Dermatol 28:98–103

Wong KO (1969) Systemic lupus erythematosus: a report of forty-five cases with unusual clinical and immunological features. Br J Dermatol 81:186–190

Wysenbeek AJ, Block DA, Fries JF (1989) Prevalence and expression of photosensitivity in systemic lupus erythematosus. Ann Rheum Dis 48:461–463

Wysenbeek AJ, Guedj D, Amit M, Weinberger A (1992) Rash in systemic lupus erythematosus: prevalence and relation to cutaneous and non-cutaneous disease manifestations. Ann Rheum Dis 51:717–719

Yamazaki S, Katayama I, Kurumaji Y, Yokozeki H, Nishioka K (1999) Treatment of reticular erythematous mucinosis with a large dose of ultraviolet B radiation and steroid impregnated tape. J Dermatol 26:115–118

Yell JA, Allen J, Wojnarowska F, Kirtschig G, Burge SM (1995) Bullous systemic lupus erythematosus: revised criteria for diagnosis. Br J Dermatol 132:921–928

Yell JA, Mbuagbaw J, Burge SM (1996) Cutaneous manifestations of systemic lupus erythematosus. Br J Dermatol 135:355–362

Yell JA, Wojnarowska F (1997) Bullous skin disease in lupus erythematosus. Lupus 6:112–121

Yung A, Oakley A (2000) Bullous systemic lupus erythematodes. Australas J Dermatol 41:234–237

CHAPTER 7

Nonspecific Cutaneous Manifestations of Systemic Lupus Erythematosus

THOMAS T. PROVOST

Nonspecific cutaneous lesions in systemic lupus erythematosus (SLE) are morphologically varied (Table 7.1). Some lesions, such as urticarial-like vasculitis and livedo reticularis, are reflective of potentially serious complications. Others, however, such as hypopigmentation and hyperpigmentation and dermal mucinosis, have no prognostic significance.

Vasculitis

Vasculitis is probably the most common nonspecific cutaneous lesion occurring in patients with SLE. Frequencies have varied from 20% to 70% (Dubois and Tuffanelli 1964, Estes and Christian 1971, Pistiner et al. 1991). Our experience with 150 patients with SLE reported a 27% frequency (Hochberg et al. 1985). Although the cutaneous manifestations of vasculitis can vary from urticarial-like lesions to deep ulcerations,

Table 7.1. Nonspecific cutaneous lesions in systemic lupus erythematosus

Vasculitis
  Palpable and nonpalpable purpura
  Urticarial-like vasculitis
  Hypocomplementemic urticarial vasculitis
Livedo reticularis
Photosensitivity
Perniosis
Alopecia
Raynaud's phenomenon
Erythromelalgia
Bullous lesions
Arthritis
Sclerodermatous changes
Dermal mucinosis
Erythema multiforme-like lesions
Pigmentary changes
Nail changes
Cutis laxa
Lichen planus
Acanthosis nigricans
Angioedema

the most common presentation is palpable and nonpalpable purpura of the lower extremities.

The intensity of the inflammatory response and its location in the vasculature of the skin determines the morphologic presentation. For example, vasculitic lesions involving arterioles and venules in the papillary portion of the dermis commonly present as nonpalpable purpura, whereas vasculitic lesions involving blood vessels in the middle portion of the reticular dermis present as palpable purpuric lesions. If the inflammatory insult is minor, the vasculitis may present as urticarial-like lesions, whereas if the vasculitic inflammation is intense, ulceration may occur.

Intense inflammatory responses involving blood vessels in the upper portion of the papillary dermis may result in destruction of the integrity of the dermal-epidermal junction, producing vesicles and bullae.

Vasculitic lesions involving the venules and arterioles at the tips of the fingers can produce small tender nodules (Osler nodes). Vasculitic lesions involving the thenar and hypothenar eminences and characterized by erythematous, generally nontender lesions have been referred to as Janeway spots. Inflammation of the arterioles in the cuticle nail folds can present as infarcts.

A putative immune complex process is thought to be causative. The reason for predominance of vasculitic lesions on the lower extremities or on the back in bedridden patients is probably due to hydrostatic pressure as well as local constriction of blood vessels producing eddying, facilitating immune complex deposition. Vasculitic lesions may occur at sites of trauma (e. g., following shaving of the legs) or at pressure sites such as around the waist. These sites of trauma or pressure application may also cause alteration in blood flow or the local release of histamine, promoting the deposition of immune complexes.

Biopsy specimens of most vasculitic lesions in SLE demonstrate the presence of a leukocytoclastic vasculitis. On infrequent occasions, a mononuclear vasculopathy is present. Direct immunofluorescence examination generally demonstrates the deposition of immunoglobulin, complement components, and fibrin in the affected blood vessels.

Although the weight of scientific data indicate that immune complexes are involved in the pathogenesis of the vasculitic lesions, patients with SLE can produce antibodies reactive against blood vessel endothelial cell surface antigens. Thus, from a conceptual point of view, it is conceivable that antibodies directed against these endothelial surface antigens could activate the complement sequence, inducing a prominent neutrophilic chemotactic response to the area of antigen antibody reaction, producing a similar, if not identical, histopathologic picture as leukocytoclastic vasculitis. It is also conceivable that antigen-committed T cells could also be involved in the pathogenesis of the vasculitis.

Urticaria as a manifestation of vasculitis in SLE has been increasingly recognized (O'Laughlin et al. 1978, Provost et al. 1980). At the present time, two forms of urticarial-like vasculitis have been detected. The most common form, occurring in approximately 10% of patients with SLE, is associated with various autoantibodies (such as anti-double-stranded DNA, anti-Ro/SSA, anti-U1RNP antibodies). In general, these patients have clinical features of systemic disease, including glomerulonephritis and arthritis. Most patients demonstrate a leukocytoclastic angiitis, but, on a few occasions, a mononuclear vasculopathy has been described.

The second form of urticarial-like vasculitis seen in patients with SLE is characterized by the presence of anti-C1q antibodies and hypocomplementemia. This form of urticarial-like vasculitis (a leukocytoclastic angiitis) also can occur in patients without SLE and is termed "hypocomplementemic urticarial vasculitis (HUVS)" (Shu and Mannik 1988). Clinically, these patients frequently demonstrate arthralgias, arthritis, glomerulonephritis, angioedema, ocular inflammation (such as conjunctivitis, episcleritis, uveitis), and obstructive lung disease. Rarely, pericarditis is detected. Some patients with SLE have anti-C1q antibodies, and several patients initially presenting with HUVS subsequently develop SLE (Trendelenburg et al. 1999, Wisnieski and Jones 1992). These studies indicate that SLE and HUVS, once thought to be distinct entities, may be related, representing opposite ends of a spectrum of disease.

Clinically, the HUVS lesions and urticarial-like vasculitis are characterized by persistence, lasting 24 h or longer. The lesions, unlike those of classic urticaria (which are transient, lasting 6 h or less), are associated with a burning sensation rather than pruritus. The application of light touch to the individual lesions may produce hyperpathia. On occasion, careful examination of the urticarial-like vasculitic lesion will demonstrate petechae, indicating disruption of the blood vessel integrity.

Livedo Reticularis

In recent years, it has been recognized that livedo reticularis is the manifestation of the presence of antiphospholipid antibodies in patients with SLE [(secondary antiphospholipid syndrome (APS)]. One study indicates that 17% of 66 patients with SLE demonstrated the presence of livedo reticularis and that 81% of these patients demonstrated the presence of antiphospholipid antibodies (Yasue 1986). The APS can also occur in the absence of evidence of SLE and is termed "primary APS."

Patients with SLE possessing antiphospholipid antibodies have a disease process that is characterized by recurrent arterial and venous thrombosis, thrombocytopenia, increased fetal wastage late in the first trimester, valvular heart disease, Libman-Sachs endocarditis, and pulmonary hypertension. In addition to the livedo pattern on the skin, these patients may demonstrate acrocyanosis, small vessel infarction predominantly on the lower extremities producing atrophie blanche-like lesions. On unusual occasions, cutaneous infarction may occur, simulating Degos' disease.

The most common serious systemic sequelea associated with livedo reticularis is repeated central nervous system infarction producing neurologic defects and frequently resulting in postinfarction dementia (Sneddon's syndrome) (Levine et al. 1988, Sneddon 1965).

The APS is serologically characterized by a heterogeneous group of autoantibodies, which interfere with intrinsic anticoagulant macromolecules located on blood vessel endothelial cell surfaces (Levin 2002, Roubey 1996). These antibodies are most commonly directed at negatively charged phospholipids complexed with β_2 glycoprotein I (apolipoprotein H). Epitopes formed by this complex of negatively charged phospholipid-β_2 glycoprotein I or epitopes localized only to β_2 glycoprotein I are the pathologic antigens. Other possible pathophysiologic mechanisms occurring in the APS are listed in Table 7.2.

Table 7.2. Procoagulant effects of antiphospholipid antibodies on coagulation (see Levin 2002)

Inhibition of the activated protein C pathway
Up-regulation of the tissue factor pathway
Inhibition of antithrombin III activity
Disruption of annexin V shield on membranes
Inhibition of anticoagulant activity of β_2 glycoprotein I
Inhibition of fibrinolysis
Enhanced expression of adhesion molecules by endothelial cells and adherence of
   neutrophils and leukocytes to endothelial cells
Activation and degranulation of neutrophils
Potentiation of platelet activation
Enhanced platelet aggregation
Enhanced binding of β_2 glycoprotein I to membranes
Enhanced binding of prothrombin to membranes

It should be recognized that antiphospholipid antibodies occur in chronic infections such as syphilis and leprosy and with drugs such as chlorpromazine. These autoantibodies, however, are directed against the phospholipid protein alone and not β_2 glycoprotein I and are unassociated with a hypercoagulable state.

The antiphospholipid antibodies are detected by two techniques: lupus anticoagulant and anticardiolipin assays. Lupus anticoagulant activity is detected by the use of one of a variety of phospholipids-dependent in vitro coagulation assays. These assays include activated partial thromboplastin time, dilute activated thromboplastin time, colloidal silica clotting time, kaolin clotting time, and the Russel viper venom test. The anticoagulant activity detected in patients with the anti-APS is not corrected by mixing the patient's plasma with fresh normal plasma. However, the prolonged coagulation time is corrected by excess phospholipid or platelets that have been frozen and then thawed.

The second test commonly used to detect the APS measures anticardiolipin antibodies. Anticardiolipin antibodies are generally detected by a solid-phase assay in which cardiolipin-coated plates in the presence of bovine serum β_2 glycoprotein I are reacted with the patient's serum. In addition, recent assays to detect anti-β_2 glycoprotein I antibodies have been developed.

These two assays (lupus anticoagulant and anticardiolipin) are concordant in most cases. However, it has been recognized that the APS can occur in patients possessing antibodies directed against activated protein C, protein S, thrombin III, and annexin V (for a review, see Levine 2002). All these antibodies are capable of inducing a hypercoagulable state in patients with SLE. Each of these antibody systems produces a positive lupus anticoagulant assay, but each fails to demonstrate anticardiolipin or anti-β_2 glycoprotein I activity (anticardiolipin negative).

Treatment of APS has been successfully accomplished using Warfarin, maintaining an anticoagulant activity equal to or greater than an international normalization ratio of 3 (Khamashta et al. 1995).

Table 7.3. Provocative phototesting in lupus erythematosus (see Kuhn et al. 2001)

Diagnosis	Patients (n)	Positive phototesting results n (%)[a]
DLE	74	33 (45)
LET	62	47 (76)
SCLE	63	40 (63)
CLE	104	43 (41)
SLE	20	12 (60)

CLE, chronic lupus erythematosus (hypertrophic lupus erythematosus, lupus erythematosus profundus, chilblain lupus erythematosus); DLE, discoid lupus erythematosus; LET, lupus erythematosus tumidus; SCLE, subacute cutaneous lupus erythematosus; SLE, systemic lupus erythematosus.

[a] Cumulative positive results from ultraviolet (UV)A-positive, UVB-positive, and UVA- + UVB-positive patients.

Photosensitivity

Photosensitivity is commonly detected in patients with SLE. The frequency of photosensitivity varies with the geographical region and the specific lupus cohort studied. For example, our group reported a 45% frequency of photosensitivity in 150 patients with SLE evaluated in the Mid-Atlantic states in the United States (Hochberg et al. 1985). The late James Gilliam living in Dallas, Texas, believed that almost all of his patients with SLE were photosensitive (personal communication). Other studies have indicated that patients with subacute cutaneous LE (SCLE) possessing anti-Ro/SSA antibodies have an 80%–90% frequency of photosensitivity (Mond et al. 1989, Simmons-O'Brien et al. 1995). Indeed, many of these patients burn through window glass, indicating that low-energy long-wave ultraviolet (UV) light is capable of activating their disease.

Provocative phototesting has indicated that various subsets of lupus erythematosus (LE) have different frequencies of photosensitivity (Kuhn et al. 2001, Table 7.3); however, photosensitivity also occurs in patients with dermatomyositis (DM). Indeed, in recent years ours as well as other groups of investigators have become aware of a group of patients with DM without clinical evidence of muscle disease (amyopathic DM; DM sine myositis) who are frequently referred to a dermatologist because of the presence of a photosensitive erythematous dermatosis thought to be LE (Euwer and Sontheimer 1991, Stonecipher et al. 1993). We have evaluated 33 of these patients over the past 15 years. At least 75% of these patients have noted that their dermatitis is exacerbated by ultraviolet light exposure. At the present time, this author is unaware of any studies investigating the roles of UVA, UVB, or both wavelengths and provocative phototesting in these DM patients.

Perniosis (Chilblains)

Perniosis is an inflammatory disease process commonly occurring in patients living in cold, damp geographical regions. It typically consists of erythematous papules involving the fingers, toes, nose, or ears. In general, most cases resolve within a few days and are not related to SLE. However, some lesions persist and demonstrate blister or ulcer formation. French investigators have determined that one third of the patients with chilblain lupus having this disease process for greater than 1 month have evidence of LE (Viguier et al. 2001). Another one third are patients with atypical chilblains characterized by persistent perniosis lesions who possess one to three of the preliminary criteria of the American College of Rheumatology (ACR) for the diagnosis of SLE. Follow-up of the latter patients indicated that 2 of 10 (20%) developed SLE.

Those patients with chilblain LE demonstrated that 50% of the time the chilblain lesions persisted during spring and summer. In addition, chronic discoid lupus lesions were detected in approximately 60% of these patients, and 50% had arthralgias. Raynaud's phenomenon was detected in approximately one third. A comparison of the histopathologic features of chilblain LE and idiopathic chilblains is given in Table 7.4 (Cribier et al. 2001, Viguier et al. 2001).

Two subsequent studies have reported an association of chilblain lupus with the presence of anti-Ro/SSA antibodies (Aoki et al. 1996, Franceschini et al. 1999). These preliminary studies plus our own observations indicate that perniosis associated with LE is an unusual cutaneous finding, occurring in patients with SLE living in geographical areas with cold, damp winters (e. g., Great Britain and other European countries). For example, during a recent winter in Baltimore, Maryland, characterized by dampness and nonfreezing temperatures, the author personally saw two anti-Ro/SSA antibody-positive patients develop chilblain lupus. One had Sjögren's/LE overlap syndrome and the other had anti-Ro/SSA antibody-positive SLE.

Alopecia

Three types of alopecia can be detected in patients with LE (Sontheimer and Provost 1996). In addition to the permanent scarring alopecia associated with discoid lupus lesions, patients with SLE may experience transient alopecia with increased disease activity. Two types of transient hair loss, a result of the severe catabolic effect of the

Table 7.4. Comparative histologic findings in chilblain lupus erythematosus (LE) vs idiopathic chilblains (see Cribier et al. 2001, Viguier et al. 2001)

Histopathologic Findings	Patients (%)	
	Chilblain LE (n=7)	Idiopathic Chilblains (n=17)
Epidermal spongiosis	0	58
Basal vacuolation	43	6
Perieccrine infiltrate	57	76
Dermal edema	86	70

lupus disease flare, have been detected. One is classic telogen effluvium, in which the patient develops prominent and at times alarming loss of hair all over the scalp. If the patient's SLE is a chronic active disease process, the telogen effluvium may persist for a prolonged time. However, with quiescence of the lupus disease process, normal growth of hair resumes. The second form of alopecia, related to a flare of the SLE process, is termed "lupus hair" or "woolly hair". It is most likely a type of telogen effluvium characterized by the development of thin, weakened hairs most prominent at the periphery. These hairs easily fragment; the hair becomes unruly, giving a characteristic appearance. Conceptually, it is theorized that with the negative nitrogen balance of the lupus disease flare, normal hair growth is interrupted, leading to a reduced number of thin, weakened hairs, which easily fragment above the surface of the scalp.

Alopecia areata has also been seen in patients with SLE. In all probability, it probably reflects the occurrence of two autoimmune disease processes in the same individual.

Raynaud's Phenomenon

Raynaud's phenomenon is characterized by an initial vasopastic component producing blanching of digits (toes, fingers, or both). This initial blanching is followed by cyanosis discoloration and followed by reperfusion erythema with rewarming. Pain is commonly present.

Most patients who develop Raynaud's phenomenon do not have an associated connective tissue disease. It has been estimated that only 2%–10% of patients with Raynaud's phenomenon evaluated by rheumatologists have SLE. Raynaud's phenomenon, however, may predate the development of SLE by years (Diment et al. 1979, Kallenberg et al 1980). Patients with SLE possessing U1RNP antibodies seem to have an increased frequency of Raynaud's phenomenon. Our group, while in Buffalo, NY, detected that the frequency of Raynaud's phenomenon was twice the frequency of non-U1RNP antibody-positive patients with SLE (Maddison et al. 1978). We further have determined that the frequency of Raynaud's phenomenon in the anti-Ro/SSA antibody-positive patient population with SLE in Baltimore was 46% (23 of 50 patients) (Simmons-O'Brien et al. 1995). These studies also indicated that the frequency and severity of Raynaud's phenomenon is obviously environmentally dependent. For example, in Baltimore, a 44% frequency of Raynaud's phenomenon was detected in an SLE patient population (Hochberg et al. 1985). Dubois and Tuffanelli (Dubois and Tuffanelli 1964) reported an 18% frequency of Raynaud's phenomenon in patients with SLE seen in southern California.

Raynaud's phenomenon is due to severe vasospasm involving the digital arteries. In general, the severity of Raynaud's phenomenon does not correlate with SLE activity. One study claims that there is less renal disease and fewer deaths in patients with SLE and Raynaud's phenomenon than in unaffected patients (Diment et al. 1979).

In recent years, the calcium channel blocker nifedipine has been found to be effective in treating patients with Raynaud's phenomenon (10–30 mg/d or 30 mg/d in a sustained-release form of the drug preparation). Other vasodilators, such as nicardipine and nitroglycerin paste, have also been shown to be efficacious.

Erythromelalgia (Erythromalgia)

Erythromelalgia is a rare disease existing in two forms: primary and secondary (Cohen 2000). Primary erythromelalgia is the most common form and can begin at any age. Secondary erythromelalgia has been reported with many disorders, most commonly polycythemia and myelodysplastic disorders. It has also been associated with connective tissue disorders, most commonly SLE.

Erythromelalgia is characterized by prominent erythema and increased temperature involving predominantly the feet, but the hands also may be involved. Characteristically intense burning pain is present. The condition may be bilateral but at times may involve only one extremity. Exposure to warmth frequently triggers an attack. Ice water immersion of the affected extremity produces pain relief.

The etiology of erythromelalgia is unknown (Cohen 2000). However, recent research suggests an imbalance in limb perfusion characterized by some precapillary sphincter constriction while at the same time arteriovenous shunts remain open. It is theorized that this combination of vascular abnormalities produces the coexistence of hypoxia and hyperemia in the affected extremity.

This is a rare complication of SLE. Alarcon-Segovia et al. (Alarcon-Segovia et al. 1963) reviewed 51 cases of erythromelalgia at the Mayo Clinic between 1951 and 1960. Only one of these 51 cases had classic manifestations of SLE.

A recent study of chilblain LE indicated that 3 of 22 patients also had erythromelalgia (Viguier et al. 2001). Other vascular abnormalities, such as acrocyanosis and Raynaud's phenomenon, were prominent in this group of patients. This study also suggests that erythromelalgia in patients with SLE occurs in the setting of temperature-dependent vascular insults.

The treatment of erythromelalgia is problematic. Aspirin, prostaglandins, tetracycline, antidepression drugs inhibiting serotonin reuptake, calcium antagonists, nitroprusside infusions, lidocaine patches, and infusions have all been tried with varying degrees of success.

Bullous Lesions

Bullous lesions occur infrequently in patients with SLE. Blister formation may develop in some lupus lesions, especially at the periphery. This is generally associated with the presence of anti-Ro/SSA antibodies. On rare occasions, blister formation, in all probability an extension of the microscopic separation at the dermal-epidermal junction, may become very extensive, especially in anti-Ro/SSA antibody-positive photosensitive patients with SLE, producing cutaneous manifestations similar to toxic epidermal necrolysis (Bielsa et al. 1987).

In addition, to this type of blister formation, an acquired form of epidermolysis bullosa acquisita has been described (Gammon et al. 1985, Gammon and Briggaman 1993). These patients with SLE are HLA-DR2 positive and possess in their sera autoantibodies reactive against type VII collagen. Clinically, these patients have widespread vesiculobullous eruptions. Immunofluorescence studies detect a thick, linear deposit of IgA, IgG, and C_3 along the basement membrane zone. Using a 1 M NaCL split-skin technique, anti-basement membrane antibodies are found on the dermal side of the split. Immunoelectron microscopy studies demonstrate that the IgG deposits are below the lamina densa. These epidermolysis bullosa acquisita lesions may occur simultaneously with, or occur after the development of SLE.

A third pathophysiologic mechanism of blister formation in SLE has been described as a vesiculobullous eruption characterized histologically by the presence of neutrophilic microabscess formation in the dermal papillae reminiscent of dermatitis herpetiformis (Hall et al. 1982). Direct immunofluorescence of non-UV light-exposed normal-appearing skin revealed IgA, IgE, IgM, and C_3 deposition along the dermal-epidermal junction. Immune complexes were demonstrated in the sera of several of these patients.

It seems likely that these blisters were the result of an immune complex–mediated vasculitis involving small blood vessels at the dermal-epidermal junction. It is theorized that the inflammatory infiltrate destroyed the integrity of the dermal-epidermal junction promoting blister formation. It should be noted that all patients had a dramatic response to diaminodiphenylsulfone (Dapsone).

In addition to these forms of bullous lesions, bullous pemphigoid, dermatitis herpetiformis, and pemphigus erythematosus have occasionally been reported in association with LE. The Senear-Usher syndrome (pemphigus erythematosus) is a rare condition characterized by patients having a combination of pemphigus foliaceus and SLE (Chorzelski et al. 1968, Cruz et al. 1987). Clinically, these patients most commonly demonstrate seborrheic dermatitis-like distribution of their pemphigus disease process. Histologically, an acantholytic process at the level of the stratum malpighii has been demonstrated, and these patients demonstrate pemphigus antibodies directed against desmoglein I. Serologic studies generally demonstrate the presence of antinuclear antibodies, but the presence of other antibodies, such as anti-dsDNA and anti-RNP, are unusual.

Based on the author's personal experience and a review of the literature, it seems that the coexistence of LE with other punitive autoimmune bullous diseases most likely represents the occurrence of two autoimmune diseases in patients who are genetically susceptible.

Finally, a few words should be stated regarding porphyria cutanea tarda, which has been reported in association with SLE, discoid LE, and SCLE (Callen and Ross 1981, Clemmenson and Thomasen 1982, Cram et al. 1973, Weatherhead and Adam 1985). It also should be noted that in addition to porphyria cutanea tarda, acute intermittent porphyria and variegate porphyria have also been found in association with LE.

Although studies published in the 1970 s suggested that porphyria cutanea tarda was a common association with SLE, it is now believed that a causative relationship between the two diseases is unlikely. It is suspected that the use of antimalarials in the treatment of lupus precipitates or aggravates the underlying porphyrin abnormality, producing manifestations of porphyria cutanea tarda.

Arthritis

In general, the arthritis associated with SLE is a symmetrical nonerosive polyarthritis. However, it has been recognized on occasions that patients develop a rheumatoid-like arthritis that is reminiscent of Jaccoud's arthritis. The deformities associated with this arthritis are extra-articular, producing very striking ulnar hand deviation, which is corrected by applying pressure on a flat surface. In recent years, it has been recognized that these patients have SCLE, and this type of arthritis is frequently associated with the presence of anti-Ro/SSA antibodies (Boire and Menard 1988, Cohen et al. 1986, Dubois and Tuffanelli 1964, Simmons-O'Brien et al. 1995).

Occasionally, rheumatoid nodules have been detected in patients with SLE. For example, a recent study of 50 anti-Ro/SSA antibody-positive patients with SLE detected two patients with rheumatoid nodules (Simmons-O'Brien et al. 1995).

Further studies examining patients with rheumatoid arthritis have determined that approximately 5% possess anti-Ro/SSA antibodies and in general have a deforming arthritis corresponding to Jaccoud's type (Boire et al. 1993).

Sclerodermatous Changes

Sclerodermatous changes are an unusual feature of patients with SLE. In general, they occur in patients with SLE who possess anti-U1RNP antibodies. In addition to the sclerotic and swollen puffy hands, these patients with SLE frequently have Raynaud's phenomenon, pulmonary insufficiency, and esophageal dysmotility.

Many of these patients, because of the presence of anti-U1RNP antibodies, have been described under the rubric of the mixed connective tissue syndrome (Maddison et al. 1978, Sharp et al. 1976). This is a somewhat controversial designation, and many of these patients would be described by other investigators as having SLE. In one study of 100 anti-U1RNP antibody-positive patients with mixed connective tissue disease, 66% had swollen hands, 65% of 75 patients tested demonstrated esophageal dysmotility, and 67% of 43 tested had pulmonary diffusion abnormalities (Sharp et al. 1976).

Furthermore, cutaneous calcinosis is rare in SLE (Kabir and Malkinson 1969).

Dermal Mucinosis

Histologic demonstration of dermal mucin deposition is commonly detected in biopsy specimens of LE lesions. Sometimes, flesh-colored papulonodular cutaneous mucin deposition occurs. Rarely, massive mucin deposition has been reported in Japanese patients with SLE (Maruyama et al. 1997).

The author and other investigators have seen a group of Japanese patients possessing anti-Ro/SSA antibodies who have demonstrated a very peculiar "donut-like" erythematous plaque-like lesion (Nishikawa and Provost 1991, Teramato et al. 1989). They have been generally described under the rubric of Sjögren's syndrome, although some investigators have proposed that these lesions are similar to SCLE (Ruzicka et al. 1991, Watanabe et al. 1997). This author, based on his experience, believes that this is a very distinctive lesion. Histologically, mucin deposition is prominent, and this author believes that the mucin deposition, which is hydroscopic, is responsible for the prominent edematous features of the lesions.

In general, the papulonodular cutaneous mucin deposition detected in patients with SLE responds to prednisone or antimalarial drug therapy.

Erythema Multiforme-like Lesions

Rowell et al. (Rowell et al. 1963) described erythema multiforme–like lesions in patients with LE. Pernio has also been described in these patients (Millard and Rowell 1978). These patients were found to possess an antibody against the saline extract of human tissue termed "anti-SjT". This antibody was named for the original patient who had Sjögren's syndrome. It is now postulated that the SjT antibody system is identical to the anti-La/SSB antibody system. The absence of an anti-Ro/SSA antibody equivalent (SjD antibody) in this cohort of four patients is of interest. The author, in more than 25 years' experience dealing with these antibody systems, has never seen the occurrence of anti-La/SSB antibodies in the absence of anti-Ro/SSA. Furthermore, based on experience, this author suspects that these patients had Sjögren's syndrome/LE overlap syndrome.

In the evaluation of several patients with both anti-U1RNP and anti-Ro/SSA antibody-associated neonatal lupus, the author detected the presence of erythema multiforme-like targetoid-like lesions (Provost et al. 1987, 1996).

Pigmentary Changes

Both hypopigmentation and hyperpigmentation in sites of previous cutaneous lesions have been detected in patients with LE. On rare occasions, depigmentation and postinflammatory hyperpigmentation may be extensive. In the author's experience, cosmetically objectionable pigmentary changes are more commonly detected in African American patients.

Antimalarial therapy can cause altered pigmentation. Premature graying of scalp hair, eyelashes, eyebrows, and beard has been detected. Also, diffuse hyperpigmentation or linear horizontal bands of pigmentation can be detected in nails. A blue/black patchy hyperpigmentation has also been noted on the mucous membranes and over the anterior shins. These pigmentary alterations associated with antimalarial therapy disappear with discontinuation of therapy.

Nail Changes

Nail alterations have been detected in patients with SLE. One study detected nail alterations in 42 (31%) of 165 patients with SLE (Urowitz et al. 1978). The most common abnormality is onycholysis. These SLE patients also demonstrated pitting, horizontal and longitudinal ridging, and leukonychia. Atrophy and telangiectasia of the cuticle nail fold were also commonly detected.

Diffuse and linear nail dyschromia has been detected in 52% of African American patients with SLE (Vaughn et al. 1990). The pathogenesis of this abnormality is unknown but is not related to disease activity or antimalarial therapy.

Miscellaneous Cutaneous Lesions

Anetoderma (DeBracco et al. 1979) and generalized cutis laxa (Randle and Muller 1983) have been described in patients with SLE. Acanthosis nigricans has been reported in patients with SLE in association with type B insulin resistance (Rendon et al. 1989). Lichen planus, a putative T-cell autoaggressive disease, has been described in patients with LE (van der Horst et al. 1983)

Finally, angioedema has been seen on rare occasions in patients with SLE. This seems to represent the increased risk of SLE occurring in patients with a hereditary deficiency of the C_1 inhibitor (Collier and Lee 2000, Kohler et al. 1974).

References

Alarcon-Segovia D, Babb RR, Fairbairn JF (1963) Systemic lupus erythematosus and ery-thromyalgias. Ann Intern Med 112:102–106

Aoki T, Ishizawa T, Hozumi Y, Aso K, Kondo S (1996) Chilblain lupus erythematosus of Hutchin-son responding to surgical treatment: a report of two patients with anti Ro/SS-A antibodies. British J Dermatol 134:533–537

Bielsa I, Herrero C, Font J, Mascaro JM (1987) Lupus erythematosus and toxic epidermal necro-lysis. J Am Acad Dermatol 16:1265–1267

Boire G, Menard HA, Gendron M, Lussier A, Myhal D (1993) Rheumatoid arthritis: anti Ro anti-bodies define a non HLA-DR4 associated clinical serological cluster. J Rheumatol 20:1654–1660

Boire G, Menard HA (1988) Clinical significance of anti-Ro (SS-A) antibody in rheumatoid arthritis. J Rheumatol 15:391–394

Callen J, Ross L (1981) Subacute cutaneous lupus in porphyria cutanea tarda. J Am Acad Derma-tol 5:269–273

Chorzelski T, Jablonska S, Blasczyk M (1968) Immunopathological investigations in the Senear Usher syndrome (coexistence of pemphigus and lupus erythematosus). Br J Dermatol 80:211–217

Clemmenson O, Thomasen K (1982) Porphyria cutanea tarda in systemic lupus erythematosus. Arch Dermatol 118:160–162

Cohen JS (2000) Erythromelalgia: new theories and new therapies. J Am Acad Dermatol 43:841–847

Cohen S, Stastny P, Sontheimer RD (1986) Concurrence of subacute cutaneous lupus erythe-matosus and rheumatoid arthritis. Arthritis Rheum 29:421–425

Collier DH, Lee LA (2000) Three generations of patients with lupus erythematosus and heredi-tary angioedema. Am J Med 109:256–257

Cram DL, Epstein JH, Tuffanelli DL (1973) Lupus erythematosus in porphyria: coexistence in 7 patients. Arch Dermatol 108:779–784

Cribier B, Djeridi N, Peltre B, Grosshans E (2001) A histologic and immunohistochemical study of chilblains. J Am Acad Dermatol 45:924–929

Cruz PD Jr, Colison BM, Sontheimer RD (1987) Concurrent features of cutaneous lupus erythe-matosus following myosthenia gravis and thymoma. J Am Acad Dermatol 16:472–480

DeBracco MM, Bianchi CA, Bianchi O (1979) Hereditary complement (C2) deficiency with dis-coid lupus erythematosus and idiopathic anetoderma. Int J Dermatol 18:713–717

Diment J, Ginzler E, Schleisinger M, Sterba G, Diamond H, Kaplan D, Weiner M (1979) The clini-cal significance of Raynauds phenomenon in systemic lupus erythematosus. Arthritis 22:815–819

Dubois EL, Tuffanelli DL (1964) Clinical manifestations of systemic lupus erythematosus. JAMA 190:104–107

Estes D, Christian CL (1971) The natural history of systemic lupus erythematosus by prospective analysis. Medicine 50:85–95

Euwer RL, Sontheimer RD (1991) Amyopathic dermatomyositis (dermatomyositis sine myositis). J Am Acad Dermatol 24:959–966

Franceschini F, Calzavara-Pinton P, Quinzanini M, Cavazzana I, Bettoni L, Zane C, Faccheti F, Airo P, McCauliffe DP, Cattanes R (1999) Chilblain lupus erythematosus is associated with antibodies to SSA/Ro. Lupus 8:215–219

Gammon WR, Briggaman RA (1993) Bullous SLE: a phenotypically distinctive but immunologic heterogeneous bullous disorder. J Invest Dermatol 100:28S-34S

Gammon WR, Woodley D, Dole KC, Briggaman RA (1985) Evidence that anti-basement membrane zone antibodies in bullous eruption of systemic lupus erythematosus recognize epidermolysis bullosa acquisita autoantigen. J Invest Dermatol 84:472–476

Gilliam JM, Cohen SB, Sontheimer RD, Moscella SL (1985) Connective tissue diseases. In: Moscella SL, Hurley HJ (eds) Dermatology, WB Saunders, Philadelphia, 1087–1135

Hall RP, Lawley TJ, Smith HR, Katz SI (1982) Bullous eruption of systemic lupus erythematosus. Ann Intern Med 97:165–170

Hochberg MC, Boyd RB, Ahearn JM, Arnett FC, Bias WB, Provost TT, Stevens MB (1985) Systemic lupus erythematosus: a review of clinico-laboratory features and immunogenetic markers in 150 patients with emphasis on demographics subsets. Medicine 64:285–295

Kabir JDI, Malkinson FD (1969) Lupus erythematosus and calcinosis cutis. Arch Dermatol 100:17–22

Kallenberg CS, Wouda AA, The TH (1980) Systemic involvement and immunologic findings in patients presenting with Raynaud's phenomenon. Am J Med 69:675–680

Khamashta MA, Cuadrado MJ, Mujic F, Taub NA, Hunt BJ, Hughes GRV (1995) The management of thrombosis in the antiphospholipid antibody syndrome. N Engl J Med 332:993–997

Kohler PF, Percy J, Campion WM, Smyth CJ (1974) Hereditary angioedema and "familial" lupus erythematosus in identical twin bodies. Am J Med 56:406–411

Kuhn A, Sonntag M, Richter-Hintz D, Oslislo C, Megahed M, Ruzicka T, Lehmann P (2001) Phototesting in lupus erythematosus: a 15 year experience. J Am Acad Dermatol 45:86–95

Levine JS (2002) The antiphospholipid syndrome. N Eng J Med 346:752–763

Levine SR, Langer SL, Albers JW, Welch KMA (1988) Sneddon's syndrome: an antiphospholipid antibody syndrome. Neurology 38:798–800

Maddison PJ, Mogavero H, Reichlin M (1978) Patterns of clinical disease associated with antibodies to nuclear ribonucleo protein. J Rheumatol 5:407–411

Maruyama M, Miyaychi S, Hashimoto K (1997) Massive cutaneous mucinosis associated with systemic lupus erythematosus. Br J Dermatol 137:450–453

Millard LG, Rowell NR (1978) Chilblain lupus erythematosus (Hutchinson). Br J Dermatol 98:497–506

Mond CB, Peterson MGE, Rothfield NF (1989) Correlation of anti-Ro antibody with photosensitivity rash in systemic lupus erythematosus patients. Arthritis Rheum 32:202–204

Nishikawa T, Provost TT (1991) Difference in clinical serological and immunogenetic features of White versus Oriental anti-Ro (SS-A) antibody positive patients. J Am Acad Dermatol 25:563–564

O'Laughlin S, Schroeter AL, Jordon RE (1978) Chronic urticaria-like lesions in systemic lupus erythematosus. Arch Dermatol 114:879–883

Pistiner M, Wallace DJ, Nessim S, Metzger AL (1991) Lupus erythematosus in the 1980's: a survey of 570 patients. Semin Arthritis Rheum 21:55–64

Provost TT, Watson R, Simmons-O'Brien E (1996) Significance of the anti-Ro (SS-A) antibody in evaluation of patients with cutaneous manifestations of a connective tissue disease. J Am Acad Dermatol 35:147–169

Provost TT, Watson RM, Gammon WR, Reichlin M (1987) The neonatal lupus syndrome associated with U₁RNP antibodies. N Eng J Med 316:1135–1138

Provost TT, Zone JJ, Synkowski DL, Maddison PJ, Reichlin M (1980) Unusual cutaneous manifestation of systemic lupus erythematosus: urticarial-like lesions. J Invest Dermatol 75:495–499

Randle HW, Muller S (1983) Generalized elastolysis associated with systemic lupus erythematosus. J Am Acad Dermatol 8:869–873

Rendon MI, Cruz PD, Sontheimer RD, Bergstresser RD (1989) Acanthosis nigricans: a cutaneous marker of tissue resistance to insulin. J Am Acad Dermatol 21:461–469

Roubey RAS (1996) Immunology of antiphospholipid syndrome. Arthritis Rheum 39:1444–1454

Rowell NR, Swanson-Beck J, Anderson JR (1963) Lupus erythematosus and erythema multiforme-like lesions. Arch Dermatol 88:176–180

Ruzicka T, Faes J, Bergner T (1991) Annular erythema associated with Sjögren's syndrome: a variant of systemic lupus erythematosus. J Am Acad Dermatol 25:557–560

Sharp GC, Irvin WS, May CM (1976) Association of antibodies to ribonucleoprotein and Sm antigens with mixed connective tissue disease systemic lupus erythematosus and other rheumatic diseases. N Engl J Med 295:1149–1154

Shu U, Mannik M (1988) Low molecular weight C1q binding immunoglobulin G in patients with systemic lupus erythematosus consists of antibodies to collagen-like region of C1q. Clin Invest 82:816–820

Simmons-O'Brien E, Chen S, Watson R, Provost TT (1995) 100 anti-Ro (SS-A) antibody positive patients: a ten year follow up. Medicine 74:109–130

Sneddon IB (1965) Cerebro-vascular lesions and livedo reticularis. Br J Dermatol 77:180–185

Sontheimer RD, Provost TT (1996) Lupus erythematosus. In: Sontheimer RD, Provost TT (eds) Cutaneous manifestations of rheumatic diseases. Williams & Wilkins, Baltimore, pp 1–71

Stonecipher MR, Jorrigo JL, White WL, Walker FO (1993) Cutaneous changes of dermatomyositis in patients with normal enzymes: dermatomyositis sine myositis. J Am Acad Dermatol 28:951–956

Teramato N, Katayama A, Arai H (1989) Annular erythema: a possible association with primary Sjögren's syndrome. J Am Acad Dermatol 20:596–601

Trendelenburg M, Courvoisier S, Späth PJ, Moll S, Mihatsch M, Itin P, Schifferli JA (1999) Hypocomplementemic urticarial vasculitis or systemic lupus erythematosus. Am J Kidney Dis 34:745–751

Urowitz MB, Gladmann DD, Chalmers A, Ogryzlo MA (1978) Nail lesions in systemic lupus erythematosus. J Rheumatol 5:441–447

van der Horst JC, Cirkel PKS, Niebore C (1983) Mixed lichen planus – lupus erythematosus disease – a distinct entity? Clinical, histopathologic, and immunopathological studies in 6 patients. Clin Exp Dermatol 8:631–640

Vaughn RY, Bailey JP Jr, Field RS, Loebl DH, Mealing HG Jr, Jerath RS, Dorlon RE (1990) Diffuse nail dyschromia in black patients with systemic lupus erythematosus. J Rheumatol 16:640–643

Viguier M, Pinqirier L, Cavelier-Balloy B, Salmoniere P, Cordoliani F, Flageul B, Morel P, Dubertrt L, Bachelez H (2001) Clinical and histopathologic features and immunologic variables in patients with severe chilblains: a study of the relationship to lupus erythematosus. Medicine 80:180–188

Watanbe T, Tsuchida T, Ito Y, Kanda N, Ueda Y, Tamaki K (1997) Annular erythema associated with lupus erythematosus/Sjögren's syndrome. J Am Acad Dermatol 36:214–218

Weatherhead L, Adam J (1985) Discoid lupus erythematosus: coexistence with porphyria cutanea tarda. Int J Dermatol 108:453–455

Wisnieski JJ, Jones SM (1992) Comparison of autoantibodies to collagen-like region of C1q in hypcomplementemic urticarial vasculitis syndrome and systemic lupus erythematosus. J Immunol 148:1396–1403

Yasue T (1986) Lividoid vasculitis and central nervous system involvement in systemic lupus erythematosus. Arch Dermatol 122:66–70

CHAPTER 8

Cutaneous Lupus Erythematosus During the Neonatal and Childhood Periods

LELA A. LEE

Cutaneous Lupus Erythematosus in Neonates and Infants: Maternally Derived Autoimmunity and the Neonatal Lupus Syndrome

Introduction and Epidemiology

Neonates are not sufficiently immunologically competent to develop IgG autoantibody–mediated disease independently. However, IgG autoantibodies from the mother transmitted in utero can initiate disease in susceptible individuals. In a small percentage of fetuses and neonates exposed to maternal autoantibodies of the Ro/SSA family, an autoimmune disease called "neonatal lupus erythematosus (NLE)" will develop (Lee 1993, 2001). It may be argued that NLE is misnamed, as many of its clinical findings are not shared by systemic LE (SLE) of children or adults, but the name NLE remains in common use. The main features of the syndrome are cutaneous lupus lesions, cardiac disease (primarily complete congenital heart block), hepatobiliary disease, and hematologic cytopenias. Many affected individuals have only one manifestation of NLE, but any combination of these findings may occur.

NLE is an uncommon condition. Although approximately 1 in 200 pregnant women have anti-Ro/SSA autoantibodies, few have a child with NLE (Harmon et al. 1984). The incidence of NLE has been estimated as 1 in 20,000 live births (Lee and Weston 1996). Cardiac disease is reportedly the most common feature, but this may be due in part to its being more likely than the other manifestations to be detected and properly diagnosed. The sex distribution is approximately equal for children with cardiac NLE, but girls outnumber boys approximately 2:1 in cases of cutaneous NLE (Buyon et al. 1998, Neiman et al. 2000).

Cutaneous Neonatal Lupus Erythematosus

The skin lesions of NLE represent subacute cutaneous LE (SCLE), although with a distribution distinct from that of SCLE in adults. Cutaneous NLE is characterized by annular, erythematous, nonscarring, photosensitive plaques, sometimes associated with hypopigmentation (Weston et al. 1999). Occasionally, lesions reminiscent of cutis marmorata congenita occur. The onset is generally in the first few weeks of life, although lesions have been noted at birth in several cases. There is a predilection for the head, in particular the periorbital skin, but lesions may occur at any site. The affected periorbital skin has been described as having an "owl eye," "eye mask," or "raccoon eye" appearance. Disease activity resolves in a few weeks or months, but dyspigmentation may persist for several months, and in some cases there are residual telangiectasias (Thornton et al. 1995).

The risk for a child with cutaneous NLE to have extracutaneous features is not precisely known. It has been estimated that approximately 10% of children with cutaneous NLE also have cardiac disease (Lee 1993). An examination of records from a national NLE registry indicates that 23% of children with cutaneous NLE without cardiac disease have hepatobiliary or hematologic findings (Neimann et al. 2000). Thus, perhaps one third of the cases of cutaneous NLE have extracutaneous manifestations.

Extracutaneous Manifestations of Neonatal Lupus Erythematosus

Cardiac NLE is the most frequently reported manifestation of NLE. Cardiac NLE has significant morbidity and mortality: approximately two thirds of the children with cardiac NLE require permanent pacemaker implantation, and there is 15%–20% mortality (Buyon et al. 1998, Eronen et al. 2000). The most commonly occurring lesion is third-degree heart block. Heart block almost always begins in utero during the second or third trimester, often presenting as a lesser degree of block that relatively quickly advances to complete heart block. Complete heart block is almost always permanent. Autopsy studies have shown replacement of the atrioventricular nodal area by fibrosis and calcification (Lee et al. 1987, Lev et al. 1971). Assuming that the pathologic findings are similar in surviving children, it is easy to understand why heart block persists despite resolution of disease activity.

In some children with complete heart block, cardiac muscle is involved as well. This is often evident shortly after birth, when correction of the low heart rate with pacemaker implantation fails to correct heart failure. However, heart failure has developed later during infancy in a few individuals, demonstrating the importance of close monitoring in children with cardiac NLE (Taylor-Albert et al. 1997).

Hepatobiliary disease of NLE apparently may assume several phenotypes. In a review of data from a national research registry, approximately 10% (19/219) of the cases in the registry had evidence of hepatobiliary disease (Lee et al. 2002). The three types of presentations noted were as follows: (a) liver failure in utero or shortly after birth, often having the phenotype of neonatal iron storage disease (also known as "neonatal hemochromatosis"); (b) transient conjugated hyperbilirubinemia occurring in the first few weeks of life; and (c) transient aminotransferase elevations, occurring at 2–3 months of age. The latter two presentations eventuate in complete resolution, with no apparent residua. It has not been shown conclusively that each of these presentations truly represents a manifestation of NLE, but based on currently available information it seems likely.

The cytopenia most commonly associated with NLE has been thrombocytopenia (Watson et al. 1988). Remarkably, 5 of 57 children with cutaneous NLE in the national registry had neutropenia (Neiman et al. 2000). The cytopenias are transient and usually not associated with morbidity. One child had a nonfatal episode of gastrointestinal bleeding attributed to thrombocytopenia (Lee et al. 1993).

Laboratory Evaluation

Skin biopsy is not always performed owing to the age of the child and the predilection of lesions for the face. Biopsy findings for histologic examination and immunofluorescence are consistent with the findings of SCLE (David-Bajar et al. 1992). Notably, there is basal cell damage and a lymphocytic inflammatory infiltrate in the upper dermis. Histologic features more closely associated with discoid lupus, such as an intense deep dermal inflammatory infiltrate, an intense periadnexal infiltrate, follicular plugging, and basement membrane thickening, are not prominent in NLE. In the author's experience, the immunofluorescent finding characteristic of cutaneous NLE is epidermal particulate deposition of IgG. This finding can be reproduced in an animal model by infusion of anti-Ro/SSA antibodies (Lee et al. 1986, 1989).

Autoantibody testing of serum samples from the mother, the child, or both is important for diagnosis. The exact specificity or specificities responsible for NLE are debated, but there is no question that virtually all patients have autoantibodies of the Ro/SSA family. Autoantibodies reported to be associated with NLE include antibodies to 60-kDa Ro/SSA, 52-kDa Ro/SSA, La/SSB, calreticulin, alpha-fodrin, a 57-kDa protein, and a 75-kDa phosphoprotein (Buyon et al. 1994, Maddison et al. 1995, Miyagawa et al. 1998, Lee et al. 1994, Lieu et al. 1989, Wang et al. 1999, Weston et al. 1982). In a few cases of cutaneous NLE, antibodies to Ro/SSA were not detected but antibodies to U1RNP were (Provost et al. 1987). Many of the assays for autoantibodies associated with NLE are performed only in certain research laboratories. For the clinician, assays for antibodies to Ro/SSA, La/SSB, and U1RNP are commercially available and should suffice to confirm or, if negative, seriously question the diagnosis.

It is reasonable to evaluate children with cutaneous NLE for extracutaneous manifestations. Laboratory screening may include electrocardiography, liver function tests (transaminases and fractionated bilirubin), and a complete blood cell count with differential.

Pathogenesis

The available evidence points strongly to autoantibodies as the cause of NLE. Maternal autoantibodies are uniformly present in NLE, and they are of a distinct family of autoantibodies. Disease activity resolves as the maternal autoantibodies are metabolized. Antibody deposits in tissues have been shown to represent anti-Ro/SSA (Lee et al. 1989, Reichlin et al. 1994).

The autoantibodies most closely linked to NLE are antibodies to 60-kDa Ro/SSA and antibodies to 52-kDa Ro/SSA (Lee et al. 1994). Several investigators have attempted to reproduce disease using infused anti-Ro/SSA. Isolated rabbit cardiac muscle has been shown to develop abnormalities of repolarization when infused with anti-Ro/SSA-containing serum (likely representing a combination of anti-60-kDa Ro/SSA and anti-52-kDa Ro/SSA) (Alexander et al. 1992). Isolated rabbit hearts and isolated rat hearts perfused with anti-Ro-containing serum and anti-52-kDa Ro/SSA developed heart block (Boutjdir et al. 1998, Garcia et al. 1994, Viana et al. 1998). Some newborn mice whose mothers received anti-Ro/SSA and/or La/SSB-containing IgG during pregnancy experienced bradycardia and prolonged PR interval (Mazel et al. 1999). An interaction of NLE maternal IgG with human fetal cardiac sarcolemma and with human L-type calcium channel alpha (1C) protein has been demonstrated (Qu et al. 2001).

The 60- and 52-kDa Ro/SSA proteins are apparently expressed ubiquitously, and it has not been clear why the disease process in NLE is apparently limited to only a few organs. It has been proposed that tissue specificity may be conferred by cross-reactivity between 52-kDa Ro/SSA and the 5-HT4 serotoninergic receptor (Eftekhari et al. 2000). Pups from mice immunized with anti-5HT4 receptor peptides developed bradycardia, incomplete atrioventricular block, prolonged QT, skin lesions, and neuromotor problems (Eftekhari et al. 2001). One group reported that NLE serum samples contain, independent of anti-Ro, autoantibodies to neonatal heart M1 muscarinic acetylcholine receptor (Borda and Sterin-Borda 2001). The finding of expression of different isoforms of 52-kDa Ro/SSA at different times during cardiac development led to a proposed link between expression of specific 52-kDa Ro/SSA isoforms and the development of congenital heart block (Buyon et al. 1997). RNAs associated with 60-kDa Ro/SSA are also expressed differentially during development (Fraire-Velzquez et al. 1999).

Genetic factors that have been identified as contributors to NLE include genes of the major histocompatibility complex (MHC) and C4 (Lee et al. 1983, Miyagawa et al. 1997, 1999, Watson et al. 1992). These associations are noted in NLE mothers and may in part be related to increased risk for production of anti-Ro/SSA autoantibodies. Genetic factors that contribute to determining which babies exposed to maternal anti-Ro/SSA autoantibodies will be affected and which will not have not yet been completely established, but there is emerging evidence that tumor necrosis factor (TNF)-α and transforming growth factor (TGF)-β polymorphisms may contribute (Clancy et al. 2003).

Management

Cutaneous NLE is best managed conservatively. Low-potency topical corticosteroid therapy may aid in decreasing inflammation, and sun protection measures are advisable. Residual telangiectasia may be treated with a vascular laser such as a pulsed dye laser.

Optimal therapy for cardiac NLE has not been established. Pacemaker implantation and medications traditionally used to treat heart failure are used when indicated. Several other therapeutic interventions have been tried, including prophylactic therapy of the mother with corticosteroids during the first trimester, corticosteroid therapy during gestation for fetuses with heart block, plasma exchange for an infant with heart block and cardiomyopathy, and corticosteroid therapy for neonates and infants with progressive disease (Copel et al. 1995, Shinohara et al. 1999, Taylor-Albert et al. 1997, Yamada et al. 1999). Larger studies are needed before particular approaches may be accepted as standard care.

Long-Term Prognosis

Clearly, children with cutaneous NLE do well in the short run. For children with cardiac NLE, there is mortality of ca. 15%–20% (Buyon et al. 1998, Eronen et al. 2000). There is little mortality data concerning hepatobiliary NLE and hematologic NLE.

The finding of 6 deaths in 19 children with hepatobiliary disease in a survey of a national registry indicates that hepatobiliary disease may have a significant mortality rate as well, but more information is needed on this point (Lee et al. 2002).

A long-term concern is the possibility of the development of autoimmune disease later in life. It is to be expected that children with NLE have a slightly increased risk of autoimmunity because by definition they have a family history of autoimmunity. It is the magnitude of the risk that is in question. In a national registry study of 57 children with cutaneous NLE, one child developed Hashimoto's thyroiditis at age 7 years, two developed juvenile rheumatoid arthritis at ages 2 years and 5 years, one developed Raynaud's disease during childhood, and one had a persistently positive high-titer antinuclear antibody (Neiman et al. 2000). This high frequency of autoimmunity at an early age is of concern and points to the advisability of good patient and family education and continued follow-up.

The presence of NLE in a child is an indicator of autoimmunity in the mother. Many mothers are asymptomatic when the child is found to have NLE. With time, however, most mothers develop some symptoms of autoimmunity. Studies differ about which symptoms are most common, with some series indicating Sjögren's symptoms to be most common and others emphasizing LE or undifferentiated connective tissue disease (McCune et al. 1987, Press et al. 1996, Waltuck and Buyon 1994). One group found that mothers of babies with cutaneous NLE were more likely to have symptoms of an autoimmune disorder than were mothers of babies with cardiac NLE (Lawrence et al. 2000).

Mothers who have had one child with NLE are at a relatively high risk for having an affected child in a subsequent pregnancy. Several studies have examined the risk, with results ranging from approximately 1 in 6 pregnancies to 1 in 3 pregnancies resulting in another affected baby (Buyon et al. 1998, Julkunen et al. 1993, McCune et al. 1987, Neiman et al. 2000). It is not unusual for a woman who has had a baby with cutaneous NLE to have a baby with cardiac NLE in a subsequent pregnancy.

Cutaneous Lupus Erythematosus in Children

Introduction and Epidemiology

Cutaneous LE (CLE) developing later than 1 year of age is almost certainly not NLE but rather CLE in childhood. CLE in childhood is frequently seen in the context of systemic disease. SLE is a condition that affects females much more often than males, and sex steroids play a major role in initiating the disease. Thus, CLE is much more common in adolescent girls than in either prepubertal children or adolescent boys. Unfortunately, most reports of childhood LE do not discriminate between prepubertal and postpubertal LE.

The incidence of LE in childhood has been estimated to be 0.6 in 100 000 per year (Lehman 1993). The incidence of CLE in childhood is probably lower. Girls outnumber boys among adolescents with LE, but the effect of sex is not so strong in younger children (Schaller 1982). The prevalence of lupus in black, Asian, and Hispanic children has been reported to be three times that in white children (Siegel and Lee 1973).

Cutaneous Lesions

Malar erythema has been noted in up to four fifths of children with SLE (Font et al. 1998, Lehman 1993, Schaller 1982, Wananukul et al. 1998). Discoid lesions may occur in children with SLE, sometimes as a presenting sign. In a review of 16 cases of childhood discoid LE (DLE) with onset before age 10 years (10 boys and 6 girls), progression to systemic disease was common (George and Tunnessen 1993). Of the 16 cases, 10 were followed into adulthood, and 5 of the 10 developed SLE. SCLE, LE tumidus, LE panniculitis, and bullous LE have all been noted in children (Kettler et al. 1988, Kuhn et al. 2000, Provost et al. 1983, Siamopoulou et al. 1989, Taieb et al. 1986).

Extracutaneous Disease

Childhood-onset SLE has often been described as more severe than adult-onset disease, with a relatively high likelihood of nephritis (Font et al. 1998, Vlachoyianno-poulos et al. 1993). Studies of childhood-onset SLE are frequently limited by a small number of subjects and, often, a lack of distinction between prepubertal and postpubertal SLE. Effects of the disease and its treatment on growth and on emotional and intellectual development may be especially important considerations in the child and adolescent age groups.

Laboratory Evaluation

One study reported a correlation of childhood SLE with anti-Ro/SSA autoantibodies (Lehman et al. 1989). Complement deficiencies have also been reported in association with childhood SLE and in children with SCLE and lupus panniculitis (Meyer et al. 1985, Provost et al. 1983, Taieb et al. 1986).

Pathogenesis

LE is a complex genetic disease with environmental contributions. It may be that individuals who develop disease at an early age have a stronger genetic component through inheritance of more than the usual complement of lupus susceptibility genes.

Genes associated with childhood LE include MHC and complement genes. There are case reports of DLE occurring in association with chronic granulomatous disease (Manzi et al. 1991).

Management

Management of childhood CLE is similar to management of adulthood cutaneous LE, but special consideration must be given to the effects of therapy on growth, social and intellectual functioning, later ability to conceive, and later development of malignancy. Emphasis on conservative therapies such as sun protection and local corticosteroid therapy is advisable in most cases of childhood CLE. Cosmetic camouflage should not be overlooked as an integral part of management. Antimalarial therapy may be used if local measures are insufficient or if scarring in cosmetically sensitive areas is imminent. Education about the negative effects of tobacco use on the effectiveness of antimalarial drugs may be helpful (Jewell and McCauliffe 2000, Rahman et al. 1998). Systemic corticosteroids and immunosuppressive drugs are usually not indicated for cutaneous disease but may be indicated for severe systemic disease. Retinoids have been used in adults with CLE (Newton et al. 1986), but there is little information about the use of retinoids in children with CLE.

References

Alexander E, Buyon JP, Provost TT, Guarnieri T (1992) Anti-Ro/SS-A antibodies in the patho-physiology of congenital heart block in neonatal lupus syndrome, an experimental model. In vitro electrophysiologic and immunocytochemical studies. Arthritis Rheum 35:176–189

Borda E, Sterin-Borda L (2001) Autoantibodies against neonatal heart M1 muscarinic acetyl-choline receptor in children with congenital heart block. J Autoimmun 16:143–150

Boutjdir M, Chen L, Zhang ZH, Tseng CE, El-Sherif N, Buyon JP (1998) Serum and immu-noglobulin G from the mother of a child with congenital heart block induce conduc-tion abnormalities and inhibit L-type calcium channels in a rat heart model. Pediatr Res 44:11–19

Buyon JP, Slade SG, Reveille JD, Hamel JC, Chan EK (1994). Autoantibody responses to the "native" 52-kDa SS-A/Ro protein in neonatal lupus syndromes, systemic lupus erythemato-sus, and Sjögren's syndrome. J Immunol 152:3675–3684

Buyon JP, Tseng CE, Di Donato F, Rashbaum W, Morris A, Chan EKL (1997) Cardiac expression of 52 β, an alternative transcript of the congenital heart block-associated 52-kd SS-A/Ro autoantigen, is maximal during fetal development. Arthritis Rheum 40:655–660

Buyon JP, Hiebert R, Copel J, Craft J, Friedman D, Katholi M, Lee LA, Provost TT, Reichlin M, Rider L, Rupel A, Saleeb S, Weston WL, Skovron ML (1998) Autoimmune-associated congeni-tal heart block: demographics, mortality, morbidity and recurrence rates obtained from a national neonatal lupus registry. J Am Coll Cardiol 31:1658–1666

Clancy RM, Backer CB, Yin X, Kapur RP, Molad Y, Buyon JP (2003) Cytokine polymorphisms and histologic expression in autopsy studies: contribution of TNF-alpha and TGF-beta 1 to the pathogenesis of autoimmune-associated congenital heart block. J Immunol 171:3252–3261

Copel JA, Buyon JP, Kleinman CS (1995) Successful in utero therapy of fetal heart block. Am J Obstet Gynecol 17:1384–1390

David-Bajar KM, Bennion SD, DeSpain JD, Golitz LE, Lee LA (1992) Clinical, histologic, and immunofluorescent distinctions between subacute cutaneous lupus erythematosus and dis-coid lupus erythematosus. J Invest Dermatol 99:251–257

Eftekhari P, Salle L, Lezoualch F, Mialet J, Gastineau M, Briand JP, Isenberg DA, Fournie GJ, Argibay J, Fischmeister R, Muller S, Haebeke J (2000) Anti-SSA/Ro52 autoantibodies block-ing the cardiac 5-HT4 serotoninergic receptor could explain neonatal lupus congenital heart block. Eur J Immunol 30:2782–2790

Eftekhari P, Roegel JC, Lezoualc'h F, Fischmeister R, Imbs JL, Hoebeke J (2001) Induction of neonatal lupus in pups of mice immunized with synthetic peptides derived from amino acid sequences of the serotoninergic 5-HT4 receptor. Eur J Immunol 31:573–579

Eronen M, Siren MK, Ekblad H, Tikanoja T, Julkunen H, Paavilainen T (2000) Short- and long-term outcome of children with congenital complete heart block diagnosed in utero or as a newborn. Pediatrics 106:86–91

Font J, Cervera R, Espinosa G, Pallares L, Ramos-Casals M, Jimenez S, Garcio-Carrasco M, Seis-dedas L, Ingelmo M (1998) Systemic lupus erythematosus (SLE) in childhood: analysis of clinical and immunological findings in 34 patients and comparison with SLE characteristics in adults. Ann Rheum Dis 57:456–459

Fraire-Velazquez S, Herrera-Esparza R, Villalobos-Hurtado R, Avalos-Diaz E (1999) Ontogeny of Ro hYRNAs in human heart. Scand J Rheumatol 28:100–105

Garcia S, Nascimento JHM, Bonfa E, Levy R, Oliveria SF, Tavares AV, de Carvalho AC (1994) Cellular mechanism of the conduction abnormalities induced by serum from anti-Ro/SSA-positive patients in rabbit hearts. J Clin Invest 93:718–724

George PM, Tunnessen WW Jr (1993) Childhood discoid lupus erythematosus. Arch Dermatol 129:613–617

Harmon CE, Lee LA, Huff JC, Norris DA, Weston WL (1984) The frequency of antibodies to the SSA/Ro antigen in pregnancy sera. Arthritis Rheum 28:S20

Ho SY, Esscher E, Anderson RH, Michaëlsson M (1986) Anatomy of congenital complete heart block and relation to maternal anti-Ro antibodies. Am J Cardiol 58:291–294

Jewell ML, McCauliffe DP (2000) Patients with cutaneous lupus erythematosus who smoke are less responsive to antimalarial treatment. J Am Acad Dermatol 42:983–987

Julkunen H, Kaaja R, Wallgren E, Teramo K (1993) Isolated congenital heart block: fetal and infant outcome and familial incidence of heart block. Obstet Gynecol 82:11–16

Kettler AH, Bean SF, Duffy JO, Gammon WR (1988) Systemic lupus erythematosus presenting as a bullous eruption in a child. Arch Dermatol 124:1083–1087

Kuhn A, Richter-Hintz D, Oslislo C, Ruzicka T, Megahed M, Lehmann P (2000) Lupus erythematosus tumidus – a neglected subset of cutaneous lupus erythematosus: report of 40 cases. Arch Dermatol 136:1033–1041

Lawrence S, Luy L, Laxer R, Krafchik B, Silverman E (2000) The health of mothers of children with cutaneous neonatal lupus erythematosus differs from that of mothers of children with congenital heart block. Am J Med 108:705–709

Lee LA (1993) Neonatal lupus erythematosus. J Invest Dermatol 100:9S-13S

Lee LA (2001) Neonatal lupus: clinical features, therapy, and pathogenesis. Curr Rheumatol Rep 3:391–395

Lee LA, Weston WL (1996) Special considerations concerning the cutaneous manifestations of rheumatic diseases in children. In: Sontheimer RD, Provost TT (eds) Cutaneous manifestations of rheumatic diseases. Williams & Wilkins, Baltimore, pp 323–344

Lee LA, Bias WB, Arnett FC Jr, Huff JC, Norris DA, Harmon C, Provost TT, Weston WL (1983) Immunogenetics of the neonatal lupus syndrome. Ann Intern Med 99:592–596

Lee LA, Weston WL, Krueger GG, Emam M, Reichlin M, Stevens JO, Surbrugg SK, Vasil A, Norris DA (1986) An animal model of antibody binding in cutaneous lupus. Arthritis Rheum 29:782–788

Lee LA, Coulter S, Erner S, Chu H (1987) Cardiac immunoglobulin deposition in congenital heart block associated with maternal anti-Ro autoantibodies. Am J Med 83:793–796

Lee LA, Gaither KK, Coulter SN, Norris DA, Harley JB (1989) Pattern of cutaneous immunoglobulin G deposition in subacute cutaneous lupus erythematosus is reproduced by infusing purified anti-Ro (SSA) autoantibodies into human skin-grafted mice. J Clin Invest 83: 1556–1562

Lee LA, Reichlin M, Ruyle SZ, Weston WL (1993) Neonatal lupus liver disease. Lupus 2:333–338

Lee LA, Frank MB, McCubbin VR, Reichlin M (1994) The autoantibodies of neonatal lupus erythematosus. J Invest Dermatol 102:963–966

Lee LA, Sokol RJ, Buyon JP (2002) Hepatobiliary disease in neonatal lupus: prevalence and clinical characteristics in cases enrolled in a national registry. Pediatrics 109:E11

Lehman TJA, Reichlin M, Santner TJ, Silvermann E, Petty RE, Spencer CH, Harley JB (1989) Maternal antibodies to Ro (SS-A) are associated with both early onset of disease and male sex among children with systemic lupus erythematosus. Arthritis Rheum 32:1414–1420

Lehman TJA (1993) Systemic lupus erythematosus in childhood and adolescence. In: Wallace DJ, Hahn BH (eds) Dubois' lupus erythematosus. Lea & Febiger, Philadelphia, pp 431–441

Lev M, Silverman J, Fitzmaurice FM, Paul MH, Cassels DE, Miller RA (1971) Lack of connection between the atria and the more peripheral conduction system in congenital atrioventricular block. Am J Cardiol 27:481–488

Lieu TS, Newkirk MM, Arnett FC, Lee LA, Deng JS, Capro JD, Sontheimer RD (1989) A major autoepitope is present on the amino terminus of a human SS-A/Ro polypeptide. J Autoimmun 2:367–374

Maddison PJ, Lee L, Reichlin M, Sinclair A, Wasson C, Schemmer G, Reichlin M (1995) Anti-p57: a novel association with neonatal lupus. Clin Exp Immunol 99:42–48

Manzi S, Urbach AH, McCune A, Altman HA, Kaplan SS, Medsger TA Jr, Ramsey-Goldman R (1991) Systemic lupus erythematosus in a boy with chronic granulomatous disease: case report and review of the literature. Arthritis Rheum 34:101–105

Mazel JA, El-Sherif N, Buyon J, Boutjdir M (1999) Electrocardiographic abnormalities in a murine model injected with IgG from mothers of children with congenital heart block. Circulation 99:1914–1918

McCune AB, Weston WL, Lee LA (1987) Maternal and fetal outcome in neonatal lupus erythematosus. Ann Intern Med 106:518–523

Meyer O, Hauptmann G, Tappeiner G, Ochs HD, Mascart-Lemone F (1985) Genetic deficiency of C4, C2 or C1q and lupus syndromes. Association with anti-Ro (SS-A) antibodies. Clin Exp Immunol 62:678–684

Miyagawa S, Yanagi K, Yoshioka A, Kidoguchi K, Shirai T, Hayashi Y (1998) Neonatal lupus erythematosus: maternal IgG antibodies bind to a recombinant NH2-terminal fusion protein encoded by human alpha-fodrin cDNA. J Invest Dermatol 111:1189–1192

Miyagawa S, Shinohara K, Kidoguchi K, Fujita T, Fukumoto T, Hashimoto K, Yoshioko A, Shirai T (1997) Neonatal lupus erythematosus: studies on HLA class II genes and autoantibody profiles in Japanese mothers. Autoimmunity 26:95–101

Miyagawa S, Kidoguchi K, Kaneshige T, Shirai T (1999) Neonatal lupus erythematosus: analysis of HLA class I genes in Japanese child/mother pairs. Lupus 8:751–754

Neiman AR, Lee LA, Weston WL, Buyon JP (2000) Cutaneous manifestations of neonatal lupus without heart block: Characteristics of mothers and children enrolled in a national registry. J Pediatr 137:674–680

Newton RC, Jorizzo JL, Solomon AR Jr, Sanches RL, Daniels JC, Bell JD, Cavallo T (1986) Mechanism-oriented assessment of isotretinoin in chronic or subacute cutaneous lupus erythematosus. Arch Dermatol 122:170–176

Press J, Uziel Y, Laxer RM, Luy L, Hamilton RM, Silverman ED (1996) Long-term outcome of mothers of children with complete congenital heart block. Am J Med 100:328–332

Provost TT, Arnett FC, Reichlin M (1983) Homozygous C2 deficiency, lupus erythematosus and anti-Ro (SSA) antibodies. Arthritis Rheum 26:1279–1282

Provost TT, Watson R, Gammon WR, Radowsky M, Harley JB, Reichlin M (1987) The neonatal lupus syndrome associated with U1RNP (nRNP) antibodies. N Engl J Med 31:1135–1138

Qu Y, Xiao GQ, Chen L, Boutjdir M (2001) Autoantibodies from mothers of children with congenital heart block downregulate cardiac L-type Ca channels. J Mol Cell Cardiol 33: 1153–1163

Rahman P, Gladman DD, Urowitz MB (1998) Smoking interferes with efficacy of antimalarial therapy in cutaneous lupus. J Rheumatol 25: 1716–1719

Reichlin M, Brucato A, Frank MB, Maddison PJ, McCubbin VR, Wolfson-Reichlin M, Lee LA (1994) Concentration of autoantibodies to native 60 kd Ro/SS-A and denatured 52 kd Ro/SS-A in eluates from the heart of a child who died with congenital complete heart block. Arthritis Rheum 37:1698–1703

Schaller J (1982) Lupus in childhood. Clin Rheum Dis 8:219–228

Shinohara K, Miyagawa S, Fujita T, Aono T, Kidoguchi K (1999) Neonatal lupus erythematosus: results of maternal corticosteroid therapy. Obstet Gynecol 93:952–957

Siamopoulou MA, Stefanou D, Drosos AA (1989) Subacute cutaneous lupus-erythematosus in childhood. Clin Rheumatol 8:533–537

Siegel M, Lee SL (1973) The epidemiology of systemic lupus erythematosus. Semin Arthritis Rheum 3:1–54

Taieb A, Hehunstre JP, Goetz J, Surleve Bazeille JE, Fizet D, Hauptmann G, Maleville J (1986) Lupus erythematosus panniculitis with partial genetic deficiency of C2 and C4 in a child. Arch Dermatol 122:576–582

Taylor-Albert E, Reichlin M, Toews WH, Overholt ED, Lee LA (1997) Delayed dilated cardiomyopathy as a manifestation of neonatal lupus: case reports, autoantibody analysis, and management. Pediatrics 99:733–735

Thornton CM, Eichenfield LF, Shinall EA, Siegfried E, Rabinowitz LG, Esterly NB, Lucky AW, Friedlander SF (1995) Cutaneous telangiectases in neonatal lupus erythematosus. J Am Acad Dermatol 33:19–25

Viana VS, Garcia S, Nascimento JH, Elkon KB, Brot N, Campos de Carvalho AC, Bonfa E (1998) Induction of in vitro heart block is not restricted to affinity purified anti-52 kDa Ro/SSA antibody from mothers of children with neonatal lupus. Lupus 7:141–147

Vlachoyiannopoulos PG, Karassa FB, Karakostas KX, Drosos AA, Moutsopoulos HM (1993) Systemic lupus erythematosus in Greece. Clinical features, evolution and outcome: a descriptive analysis of 292 patients. Lupus 2:303–312

Waltuck J, Buyon JP (1994) Autoantibody-associated congenital heart block: outcome in mothers and children. Ann Intern Med 120:544–551

Wananukul S, Watana D, Pongprasit P (1998) Cutaneous manifestations of childhood systemic lupus erythematosus. Pediatr Dermatol 15:342–346

Wang D, Buyon JP, Zhu W, Chan EK (1999) Defining a novel 75-kDa phosphoprotein associated with SS-A/Ro and identification of distinct human autoantibodies. J Clin Invest 104: 1265–1275

Watson RM, Scheel JN, Petri M, Lee LA, Bias WB, McLean RH (1992) Neonatal lupus erythematosus syndrome: analysis of C4 allotypes and C4 genes in 18 families. Medicine 71:84–95

Watson R, Kang JE, May M, Hudak M, Kickler T, Provost TT (1988) Thrombocytopenia in the neonatal lupus syndrome. Arch Dermatol 124:560–563

Weston WL, Harmon C, Peebles C, Manchester D, Franco HL, Huff JC, Norris DA (1982) A serological marker for neonatal lupus erythematosus. Br J Dermatol 107:377–382

Weston WL, Morelli JG, Lee LA (1999) The clinical spectrum of anti-Ro-positive cutaneous neonatal lupus erythematosus. J Am Acad Dermatol 40:675–681

Yamada H, Kato EH, Ebina Y, Moriwaki M, Yamamoto R, Furuta J, Fujimoto S (1999) Fetal treatment of congenital heart block ascribed to anti-SSA antibody: case reports with observation of cardiohemodynamics and review of the literature. Am J Reprod Immunol 42:226–232

CHAPTER 9

Drug-Induced Lupus Erythematosus   9

JACK UETRECHT

Characteristics of Drug-Induced Lupus Erythematosus

Systemic lupus erythematosus, often abbreviated SLE, is a serious autoimmune syndrome that usually affects young women. Most lupus is idiopathic, which means that its cause is unknown, but approximately 10% is associated with the use of specific drugs (Adams and Hess 1991). The diagnosis of drug-induced lupus is made on the same basis as idiopathic lupus; in addition, the symptoms must have begun after initiation of treatment with a drug and must resolve on discontinuation of that drug treatment. Although the signs and symptoms of drug-induced lupus overlap with those of idiopathic lupus and the two syndromes cannot be differentiated on the basis of differences in signs and symptoms, the usual clinical picture is somewhat different. A significant difference is that drug-induced lupus is usually milder, and the most serious manifestations of idiopathic lupus are usually absent in the drug-induced variety. Despite the overlap in symptoms between idiopathic and drug-induced lupus, the differences suggest that their pathogenic mechanisms are different. In addition, drugs associated with the induction of lupus do not usually exacerbate idiopathic lupus (Reza et al. 1975), and the genetically associated risk factors are different for the two syndromes, as described below. Therefore, it is probably more accurate to call the drug-induced variety a drug-induced lupus-like syndrome. However, the pathogenic mechanisms of both are unknown, and even in idiopathic lupus the mechanisms may be significantly different in different patients. Therefore, until we know more about the mechanism of both syndromes, it is reasonable to use the term "drug-induced lupus".

Typical Symptoms and Manifestations

Most symptoms of drug-induced lupus are similar for all drugs that cause a lupus-like syndrome; however, the spectrum is somewhat different with each. The only two drugs for which a sufficient number of cases of a lupus-like syndrome have been accumulated to provide a clear picture are procainamide and hydralazine. The symptoms and laboratory characteristics associated with these two drugs are contrasted with those of idiopathic lupus in Table 9.1. As mentioned previously, although there is overlap with idiopathic lupus, the drug-induced syndrome is usually mild, and the most serious manifestations of idiopathic lupus, especially involvement of the central nervous system and the kidneys, are uncommon in most types of drug-induced lupus. Several reviews summarize the clinical syndrome, including the following:

Adams and Hess 1991, Lee and Chase 1975, Price and Venables 1995, Yung and Richardson 1994.

The syndrome of drug-induced lupus usually begins a month or more after drug therapy is initiated. In fact, unlike most idiosyncratic drug reactions, the symptoms of lupus usually begin more than a year after initiating use of the responsible drug. The most common symptoms are arthralgias, myalgias, pleurisy, pulmonary infiltrates, fever, and malaise. The arthralgias usually involve small joints and are symmetrical but can involve single joints. In some cases, frank arthritis can occur, but it rarely leads to destruction of the joints. Rashes are not uncommon, but they are usually maculopapular "drug rashes," and the classic malar rash associated with idiopathic lupus is rare in drug-induced lupus.

Table 9.1. Characteristics of idiopathic lupus and drug-induced lupus[a]

	Idiopathic lupus (Dubois and Wallace 1987)	Drug-induced lupus	
		Procainamide (Blomgren et al. 1972)	Hydralazine (Perry 1973)
Patient profile			
Age (years)	29	63	48
Sex (female)	89	41	64
Race (white)	72	95	95
Symptoms			
Arthralgias	92	95	93
Arthritis	35	18	70
Fever	84	45	52
Myalgias	48	48	NR
Pleurisy	45	52	25
Rash	72	5	34
Adenopathy	59	9	12
Pericarditis	31	14	NR
Splenomegaly	9	5	20
Renal involvement	46	0	5
Central nervous system involvement	26	2	0
Arthralgias	92	95	93
Laboratory findings			
Antinuclear antibodies	100	100	98
Antihistone antibodies (Yung and Richardson 1994)	70	>95	>95
Anti-double strand DNA (Yung and Richardson 1994)	44	<1	<1
Lupus cells	76	77	62
VDRL	11	0	5
Anemia	57	9	17
Leukopenia	43	2	24

[a] Data are given as percentages, except where otherwise indicated.
NR, not reported.

Typical Laboratory Findings

As in idiopathic lupus, antinuclear antibodies (ANAs) are almost always present, and the pattern is usually homogenous. Although antibodies against single-stranded DNA are common, unlike idiopathic lupus, antibodies against double-stranded DNA are uncommon. Antihistone antibodies are classic (Fritzler and Tan 1978); however, they are not diagnostic because they are often present in idiopathic lupus, and the exact specificity is even different for lupus caused by different drugs (Burlingame and Rubin 1991, Portanova et al. 1987). Antineutrophil cytoplasmic antibodies, many with specificity for myeloperoxidase, are common (Dunphy et al. 2000, Nassberger et al. 1990). These antibodies may activate neutrophils and increase inflammation (Falk et al. 1990). Mild anemia, leukopenia, and thrombocytopenia are common. Complement levels are usually normal, but they can be depressed (Rich 1996). When the offending drug is discontinued, manifestations such as anemia usually resolve with other symptoms. However, other laboratory manifestations of drug-induced lupus, such as ANAs, decrease with time but usually remain detectable for years.

Risk Factors

The incidence of idiopathic lupus is approximately 10-fold higher in females than in males. Although the incidence of drug-induced lupus is often said to be the same in males and females, as with many idiosyncratic drug reactions, it seems that the incidence is somewhat higher in females than in males. However, the issue is complicated by the fact that many categories of drugs are used more frequently by one sex than the other. For example, in Table 9.1, 41% of patients with procainamide-induced and 64% of patients with hydralazine-induced lupus were females, but many more males than females are treated with these drugs. In one study, the incidence in males treated with hydralazine was 2.8% and that in females was 11.6% (Cameron and Ramsay 1984). Unlike idiopathic lupus, drug-induced lupus usually occurs in an older age group, and it has been reported to be more common in caucasians, whereas idiopathic lupus is more common in blacks (Dubois and Wallace 1987). Specific HLA types have been associated with an increased risk of drug-induced lupus. For example, 73% of patients with hydralazine-induced lupus were HLA-DR4, which is significantly higher than the incidence of this HLA type in patients with idiopathic lupus (Batchelor et al. 1980). However, others have failed to find this association (Brand et al. 1984). HLA-DR4 was also found in 9 of 13 patients with minocycline-induced lupus, and the other 4 patients were HLA-DR2, whereas all of the patients had an HLA-DQB1 allele encoding for tyrosine at position 30 (Dunphy et al. 2000). In contrast, penicillamine-induced lupus is associated with HLA-DR6 (Chin et al. 1991), and chlorpromazine-induced lupus is associated with HLA-Bw44 (Canoso et al. 1982). These findings are in contrast to the HLA associations found in patients with idiopathic lupus.

Although all adverse drug reactions are dose dependent, idiosyncratic drug reactions are often referred to as independent of dose because they do not occur in most patients at any dose and the usual dose range is sufficiently narrow that the dependence on dose is not apparent. In the case of drug-induced lupus, the dose dependency is more obvious. The best-documented example is hydralazine-induced lupus, which is much less common if the dose is kept below 200 mg/d (Cameron and Ramsay 1984). Being of the slow acetylator phenotype is a risk factor for drug-induced lupus when the drug involved is an aromatic amine or hydrazine (Uetrecht and Woosley 1981). This is quite apparent in the case of hydralazine, where acetylation is the major metabolic pathway and rapid acetylators are at significantly decreased risk of hydralazine-induced lupus. It is also apparent for sulfasalazine-induced lupus (Gunnarsson et al. 1997). In contrast, the major mode of elimination of procainamide is renal excretion of unchanged drug; therefore, acetylation makes a much smaller contribution to the elimination of procainamide. Thus, although the time to onset of procainamide-induced lupus seems to be shorter in slow acetylators, the overall incidence is not significantly higher (Woosley et al. 1978). The formation of the reactive metabolite of procainamide in the liver is mediated by CYP 2D6 (Lessard et al. 1997); therefore, patients with the impaired metabolism phenotype may be protected from procainamide-induced lupus. However, if oxidation by leukocytes mediated by myeloperoxidase is the more important mode of activation, the CYP 2D6 phenotype should not be a factor (Uetrecht 1988).

Although drugs associated with the induction of lupus do not seem to exacerbate idiopathic lupus, the incidence of drug-induced lupus may be higher in patients with certain diseases. However, the use of specific drugs in specific diseases makes it very difficult to sort out this possible risk factor.

Management

As indicated previously, the incidence of laboratory abnormalities such as ANAs is much more common than the clinical syndrome, and, therefore, there is no reason to stop the drug treatment or to treat patients who have laboratory abnormalities without symptoms. When symptoms develop in a patient who is taking a drug that is known to induce a lupus-like syndrome, the primary treatment is discontinuation of the drug treatment. When use of the offending drug is discontinued, almost invariably the symptoms abate, usually over a period of weeks; however, the recovery can be relatively slow and may require a year. The speed of recovery seems to correlate with the acuteness of the onset of symptoms; so, if the onset of symptoms is insidious, recovery is usually slower. The symptoms can usually be controlled by administering simple nonsteroidal anti-inflammatory agents, and corticosteroids or other immunosuppressants usually should be reserved for patients with evidence of significant organ damage. If the symptoms do not decrease with time, the diagnosis must be reconsidered. In general, rechallenge with the offending drug results in a recurrence, and it is to be avoided unless the diagnosis is in question and the drug is essential to the patient. In one study, rechallenge with a single dose of minocycline in patients with a history of minocycline-induced lupus resulted in symptoms in most patients within 12 hours, and there was also a large increase in C-reactive protein (Lawson et al. 2001).

Specific Drugs Associated with the Induction of Lupus Erythematosus

Procainamide

Procainamide is associated with the highest incidence of lupus of any available drug. The incidence varies by study. This is probably because the incidence increases with time over a period of years. The average time to onset for slow acetylators is 12 months, but that for rapid acetylators is 48 months (Woosley et al. 1978). The incidence with prolonged therapy is close to 30% (Henningsen et al. 1975). The incidence of ANA development is even higher: more than 90% with chronic therapy (Woosley et al. 1978). However, most patients with procainamide-induced ANAs are asymptomatic, so there is no rationale for monitoring ANAs in asymptomatic patients. Pleurisy and pulmonary infiltrates seem to be somewhat more common in procainamide-induced lupus than in lupus associated with other drugs. Patients who develop procainamide-induced lupus can be treated with N-acetylprocainamide, a major metabolite of procainamide, although a small amount of this drug is converted back to procainamide (Stec et al. 1979).

Since the CAST study found that this class of antiarrhythmic agents actually increases mortality due to cardiac arrhythmias, the use of procainamide and many other antiarrhythmic agents has decreased significantly (CAST 1989). Procainamide use is also associated with a relatively high incidence of agranulocytosis, which further discourages its use. Therefore, procainamide-induced lupus is now less of an issue than it was a decade or two ago.

Quinidine

Quinidine is the other antiarrhythmic agent associated with a significant incidence of drug-induced lupus, and it can also cause a polymyalgia rheumatica-like illness (Alloway and Salata 1995). Quinidine-induced lupus seems to be associated with decreased levels of complement, which is unusual in drug-induced lupus associated with other drugs (Rich 1996). Quinidine therapy is also associated with a relatively high incidence of an immune-mediated thrombocytopenia (Christie et al. 1985).

Hydralazine

Hydralazine is also associated with a high incidence of drug-induced lupus. With chronic therapy, the incidence of ANA induction is approximately 50% and that of a symptomatic lupus-like syndrome is approximately 10%; however, it depends on the acetylator phenotype (Perry 1973, Perry et al. 1970). In addition, as mentioned previously, the incidence is dose dependent, and if the daily dose is kept below 200 mg, the incidence is lower. Unlike most drug-induced lupus, there have been several reports of significant kidney involvement with hydralazine-induced lupus (Shapiro et al. 1984). As with procainamide, the use of hydralazine has significantly declined because many effective alternative drugs have been developed.

Isoniazid

One of the few other drugs that contain a hydrazine group is isoniazid. The incidence of circulating ANAs in patients treated with isoniazid is approximately 20% (Rothfield et al. 1978). There are several reports of isoniazid-induced lupus; however, the incidence is significantly lower than that associated with hydralazine therapy, and it is difficult to estimate. Isoniazid therapy is also associated with a relatively high incidence of idiosyncratic liver toxicity (Maddrey and Boitnott 1973).

Minocycline

Minocycline is probably one of the more common drugs associated with the induction of lupus at the present time. It is interesting to note that although minocycline has been available for 30 years, its association with lupus has only recently been appreciated (Matsuura et al. 1992). There are three major idiosyncratic adverse reactions associated with minocycline therapy: a serum sickness-like syndrome, liver toxicity, and a lupus-like syndrome. The serum sickness-like syndrome occurs after only approximately 2 weeks of therapy. In contrast, liver toxicity occurs after a mean of 20 months of therapy, and lupus has a mean time to onset of 28 months (range, 10 days to 10 years) (Schaffer et al. 2001). Most of the reported cases have been in women. There is a large amount of overlap between liver toxicity and the lupus-like syndrome, and many patients with elevated liver enzymes also have fever and arthralgias. Some patients report impaired concentration and poor memory, which suggest central nervous system involvement, and one patient had a peripheral sensory neuropathy (Lawson et al. 2001). Minocycline seems to be the only tetracycline associated with the induction of lupus (Shapiro et al. 1997).

In one study of the lupus-like syndrome to minocycline, all 14 patients had antineutrophil cytoplasmic antibodies with a perinuclear pattern (p-ANCAs). P-ANCAs are usually against either myeloperoxidase or elastase, and 11 of the 14 patients had antimyeloperoxidase antibodies and 10 had antielastase antibodies. None of the minocycline-treated controls had detectable p-ANCAs, and this led to the suggestion that p-ANCAs could be used as a marker for the development of a lupus-like syndrome to minocycline (Dunphy et al. 2000).

β-Blockers

Although there have been case reports of a lupus-like syndrome associated with other β-blockers, the only two associated with a significant incidence are practolol and acebutolol. Practolol was one of the first β-blockers, and it was associated with a lupus-like syndrome and an unusual occulo-mucocutaneous syndrome that led to its withdrawal (Raftery and Denman 1973). This led some people to suspect that it might be a class effect, and this increased suspicion about other drugs in this class. In one study, ANAs were found in eight of nine patients treated with acebutolol, and there are also case reports of acebutolol-induced lupus (Booth et al. 1982). As mentioned in the "Involvement of Reactive Metabolites" subsection, practolol and acebutolol are the only β-blockers that are readily metabolized to aromatic amines.

Propylthiouracil

Propylthiouracil is one of the few drugs associated with the induction of a lupus-like syndrome that is given at a relatively low dose (Amrhein et al. 1970). Other antithyroid drugs, such as methimazole, have also been implicated in the induction of a lupus-like syndrome. Propylthiouracil is also associated with a relatively high incidence of agranulocytosis and liver necrosis, and it causes a lupus-like syndrome in cats (Aucoin et al. 1988).

Penicillamine

It is ironic that D-penicillamine is used to treat autoimmune diseases, such as rheumatoid arthritis, and yet it causes autoimmune syndromes such as lupus, myasthenia gravis, pemphigoid lesions, and dermatomyositis (Harkcom et al. 1978, Jaffe 1981, Knezevic et al. 1984). The kidneys are commonly involved, and anti-double-stranded DNA antibodies and hypocomplementemia are also common. Penicillamine also causes a lupus-like syndrome in Brown Norway rats (Donker et al. 1984).

Anticonvulsants

Several anticonvulsants, such as carbamazepine, phenytoin, and ethosuximide, are associated with a low but significant incidence of drug-induced lupus (Beernink and Miller 1973, Jain 1991). The incidence of circulating ANAs in patients treated with carbamazepine is reported to be 78% (Alarcon-Segovia et al. 1972). Patients are often taking more than one anticonvulsant, so it is often difficult to be certain what drug is responsible. The aromatic anticonvulsants are also associated with a hypersensitivity syndrome in which there is some overlap with the lupus-like syndrome, but it is more acute in onset (Shear and Spielberg 1988).

Phenothiazines

ANAs were found in more than 25% of patients being treated with chlorpromazine; however, the incidence of symptoms is much lower (Dubois et al. 1972, Zarrabi et al. 1979). Phenothiazine-induced lupus seems to be associated with a high incidence of antiphospholipid antibodies (Derksen and Kater 1985).

Sulfonamides and Sulfasalazine

The first report of drug-induced lupus involved a sulfonamide (Hoffman 1945), and yet the incidence of sulfonamide-induced lupus is very low. Sulfasalazine is associated with induction of a lupus-like syndrome, probably because it is metabolized to a sulfonamide and another aromatic amine. Consistent with this hypothesis is the observation that the slow acetylator genotype is a very strong risk factor for sulfasalazine-induced lupus (Laversuch et al. 1995, Gunnarsson et al. 1997). Such an association is usually related to metabolism of aromatic amines, but the parent drug is not an aromatic amine. Renal disease seems to be common in sulfasalazine-induced lupus (Gunnarsson et al. 1997).

Immune-Modulating Biological Agents

Agents such as interferon alfa (Fukuyama et al. 2000, Ronnblom et al. 1990, Schilling et al. 1991), interferon gamma (Graninger et al. 1991, Machold and Smolen 1990), and infliximab (anti–tumor necrosis factor α antibodies) (Charles et al. 2000, Markham and Lamb 2000, Rutgeerts et al. 1999) have been associated with lupus. Use of such immune-modulating agents is likely to increase, and, by their very nature, many are likely to cause autoimmune syndromes.

Other Drugs

The list of drugs that have been associated with induction of lupus is very long. Some drugs, such as methyldopa, were not mentioned in the interest of brevity. There is also a new antiangiogenesis agent, COL-3, with a structure similar to tetracyclines, that has been reported to cause a lupus-like syndrome (Ghate et al. 2001). Estrogens have been reported to be associated with lupus, but that association is more likely due to the potentiation of idiopathic lupus. In the case of most other drugs associated with lupus, the evidence is too weak to have confidence that the association is causal.

Environmental Agents

There is no intrinsic difference between drugs and other chemicals, and it has been suggested that some fraction of idiopathic lupus is caused by environmental agents, especially aromatic amines and hydrazines (Reidenberg 1983). Adulteration of rapeseed oil with aniline led to a large number of serious autoimmune reactions in Spain (Kammuller et al. 1988). Aniline is an aromatic amine that, when heated with vegetable oils, forms fatty acid anilides. However, it is still not clear exactly which component of the adulterated oil was responsible for the syndrome or what the mechanism of the syndrome was. Other agents that have been of concern are p-aminobenzoic acid (PABA) (Mackie and Mackie 1999) and paraphenylene diamine hair dyes (Steinberg et al. 1991). Although PABA and aniline-based hair dyes can be sensitizers, there is no clear association with the induction of lupus. Exposure to specific chemicals, such as hydrazine, has also been reported to induce lupus (Reidenberg et al. 1983). Administration of trichloroethylene led to a significant acceleration in a lupus-like autoimmune syndrome in female MRL+/+ mice, a strain that is predisposed to lupus (Khan et al. 1995). An epidemiologic link between trichloroethylene exposure and lupus-related symptoms has been reported (Kilburn and Warshaw 1992).

Although it is possible that some idiopathic lupus may be due to chemical exposure, it seems unlikely that this represents a significant cause of idiopathic lupus. The observation that large doses of pharmaceutical agents are required to induce a lupus-like syndrome may provide an explanation for this apparent failure of environmental agents to cause a significant incidence of lupus. Specifically, with the exception of natural food constituents, it would be extremely rare to be exposed to the same "dose" of environmental agents that are associated with drug-induced lupus. Ingesting large amounts of alfalfa sprouts, which contain relatively high levels of an unusual amino acid, L-canavanine, causes an autoimmune syndrome in monkeys (Malinow et al.

1982). The amount required is unlikely to be consumed by many humans, but consumption of alfalfa tablets from health food stores is a concern.

Possible Pathogenic Mechanisms of Drug-Induced Lupus Erythematosus

Involvement of Reactive Metabolites

The mechanism of drug-induced lupus is unknown; however, there is a large amount of circumstantial evidence to suggest that the mechanism involves a chemically reactive metabolite. In the case of procainamide, sulfonamides and sulfasalazine, acebutolol, and practolol, the reactive metabolite is formed by oxidation of the aromatic amine functional group (Uetrecht 1988). Acebutolol and practolol are the only two β-blockers that are metabolized to aromatic amines, and they are also the only two for which there are good data to support a causal relationship with a lupus-like syndrome (Wilson et al. 1978). In a similar vein, minocycline is the only tetracycline that is an aromatic amine, and it seems to be the only tetracycline that is associated with a significant incidence of a lupus-like syndrome. In the case of minocycline, the reactive metabolite seems to be a quinone imine rather than a hydroxylamine, but its formation still involves oxidation of the aromatic amine.

Hydralazine and isoniazid are hydrazine derivatives, which are readily oxidized to reactive metabolites. The exact structure of the reactive metabolite has not been proven, but it is most likely a diazonium ion intermediate (Hofstra and Uetrecht 1993). The reactive nature of propylthiouracil and penicillamine are due to the sulfur atoms. In the case of propylthiouracil, the sulfur is oxidized to several reactive species (Waldhauser and Uetrecht 1991), while the sulfhydryl group of penicillamine can react with protein without metabolic activation. The chemistry of quinidine reactive metabolite formation has not received much attention, but, on paper, it should be *o*-demethylated to a metabolite that is further converted to a quinone methide reactive metabolite. The phenothiazines are known to be oxidized to free radical intermediates (Kalyanaraman and Sohnle 1985), but the exact chemistry associated with the drug-induced lupus syndrome has not been demonstrated. The idiosyncratic reactions associated with anticonvulsants were believed to be due to arene oxide reactive intermediates (Spielberg et al. 1981); however, even anticonvulsants that do not have an aromatic ring have been associated with a lupus-like syndrome, and other types of reactive metabolites have been demonstrated (Ju and Uetrecht 1999).

Many other drugs are metabolized to reactive metabolites and yet are not associated with the induction of a lupus-like syndrome; however, in many cases, they do cause other types of idiosyncratic adverse reactions. There are several factors that are likely involved in determining the pattern of idiosyncratic reactions that a drug (or reactive metabolite) will be associated with. One is simply where the reactive metabolite is formed. By their very nature, most reactive metabolites will not reach significant concentrations at sites distant from where they are formed. Most drugs associated with lupus (or their hepatic metabolites) are oxidized by the myeloperoxidase system present in neutrophils and some macrophages (Uetrecht 1996). This may be an important factor because of the importance of these cells in the immune response.

The macromolecules that are modified by the reactive metabolite are also likely to be an important determinant of a drug's ability to cause lupus, and it is unlikely an accident that drug-induced lupus is often associated with antimyeloperoxidase antibodies (Shapiro et al. 2001). As mentioned earlier, there is a clear dose dependency to drug-induced lupus, and most drugs associated with the induction of lupus are given at dosages greater than 100 mg/d. In the case of procainamide, the dose can be several grams per day.

Many hypotheses have been proposed to link reactive metabolites with the pathogenesis of drug-induced lupus. It is likely that there are several different effects that contribute to the induction of lupus by drugs, and the pattern is probably different for different drugs.

Modification of Macromolecules

Modification of protein by a reactive metabolite (hapten) could lead to an immune response against the modified protein, including a response to the hapten. Antidrug antibodies have been reported in drug-induced lupus (Hahn et al. 1972); however, such antibodies are not a universal feature and are probably not pathogenic. Modification of a protein can also change the manner in which the protein is processed by antigen-presenting cells, and this can lead to the presentation of peptides that the immune system has not "seen" before and, therefore, have not been tolerized to. Such peptides are referred to as cryptic antigens. It has been suggested that an immune response against cryptic antigens could lead to an autoimmune response (Griem et al. 1998).

Drug-induced lupus has many of the characteristics of a graft-vs-host reaction (Gleichmann et al. 1984). Reactive metabolites presumably modify many different proteins, and there is no reason to believe that they would not also modify major histocompatibility complex II. In principle, modification of major histocompatibility complex II should induce a graft-vs-host reaction (Gleichmann 1982). However, this is a very difficult hypothesis to rigorously test.

Procainamide (Blomgren et al. 1972) and hydralazine (Dubroff et al. 1981) have been reported to induce a stable transition from the normal to the Z conformation of DNA. This form of DNA is immunogenic, and it has been proposed that this transition could be responsible for drug-induced lupus. However, these were test tube experiments, and there is no evidence that this transition occurs in vivo.

Inhibition of Tolerance

Kretz-Rommel and Rubin found that injection of the reactive metabolite of procainamide into the thymus of mice leads to autoantibodies against chromatin (Kretz-Rommel et al. 1997). Furthermore, transfer of T cells from one animal to another resulted in autoantibodies in the recipient mice (Kretz-Rommel and Rubin 1999). It has been proposed that this response is due to a failure in the normal development of tolerance in autoantigens. Although the amount of reactive metabolite was relatively small, the local concentration is likely to have been much higher than that produced in vivo and to kill cells in the area of injection. An important control experiment would be to inject some other caustic agent or even to use a hot needle to kill an area of cells in the thymus to see whether this would result in a similar syndrome that is unrelated to specific effects of procainamide.

Inhibition of DNA Methylation

Procainamide and hydralazine were found to inhibit DNA methylation (Cornacchia et al. 1988). DNA methylation inhibits gene transcription, and so inhibition of DNA methylation could lead to lymphocyte activation. This is an attractive mechanism for the induction of lupus, and it does not require the formation of a reactive metabolite. However, it is conceivable that it is a reactive metabolite that is responsible for inhibition of DNA methylation. Decreased DNA methylation has also been reported in idiopathic lupus (Richardson et al. 1990). In unpublished studies, we found other drugs that inhibited DNA methylation to the same extent as procainamide, and yet the drugs involved are not associated with drug-induced lupus. Even if inhibition of DNA methylation is not the exclusive mechanism of drug-induced lupus, it may make a significant contribution to the mechanism for some drugs.

Inhibition of Apoptosis

The first pathogenic mechanism of lupus that was discovered in an animal model was a defect in apoptosis that prevented the deletion of autoreactive T cells (Watanabe-Fukunaga et al. 1992). One article reported that chlorpromazine increased apoptosis in lymphoblasts (Hieronymus et al. 2000); however, the effects were studied in vitro, and it is unclear whether the effects seen in this system are representative of the effects that occur in vivo. Procainamide and hydralazine had no effect on apoptosis, but it is unlikely that significant amounts of reactive metabolite would be produced in this system. To my knowledge, no work has been done in vivo to determine the effects on apoptosis of drugs associated with the induction of lupus.

Inhibition of Complement

It is known that patients with genetic deficiencies in the complement system, especially C2 and C4, have a high incidence of lupus and other autoimmune diseases, presumably because this leads to defects in the clearance of immune complexes (Dubois and Wallace 1987). Hydralazine and several other drugs interact with C4 and inhibit binding of C4 to C2, and it was proposed that this could represent the mechanism of drug-induced lupus (Sim and Law 1985). The hydroxylamine of procainamide also binds to C4 (Sim et al. 1988), but the concentration of this metabolite in vivo is unlikely to be sufficient to have much of an effect.

Animal Models

It is interesting to note that although there are very few animal models of drug-induced idiosyncratic drug reactions, there seem to be more animal models of drug-induced lupus than other types of idiosyncratic drug reactions. As mentioned previously, these models include penicillamine- and mercury-induced autoimmunity in Brown Norway rats (Donker et al. 1984, Tournade et al. 1990), propylthiouracil-induced lupus in cats (Aucoin et al. 1985), and trichloroethylene-induced autoimmunity in MRL+/+ mice (Kilburn and Warshaw 1992).

Conclusions

In general, except for a few drugs, such as minocycline, use of drugs that induce a significant incidence of lupus seems to be decreasing, likely because of a trend in drug development to avoid drugs that form reactive metabolites and to develop more potent drugs so that the total dose is below the threshold required to induce a lupus-like syndrome. One type of drug associated with the induction of lupus that is likely to increase in importance is biological agents such as interferons.

Although the use of drugs that commonly cause lupus is, in general, decreasing, it is important to have a high index of suspicion because the diagnosis is often missed, likely because the onset of symptoms is often insidious and similar to that of other rheumatic diseases. In addition, the association of the adverse event with a drug is less obvious than for most adverse drug reactions because the patient has usually been taking the drug for a long time and the symptoms may take several months to completely resolve.

Although the differences between idiopathic and drug-induced lupus were highlighted at the beginning of this chapter, there are probably several common features in the pathogenesis of the two syndromes, and it is likely that a better understanding of drug-induced lupus could contribute to a better understanding of idiopathic lupus.

Acknowledgements. The author is supported by grants from the Canadian Institutes of Health Research and a Canada Research Chair in Adverse Drug Reactions.

References

Adams LE, Hess EV (1991) Drug-related lupus. Drug Safety 6:431–449
Alarcon-Segovia D, Fishbein E, Reyes PA, Dies H, Shwadsky S (1972) Antinuclear antibodies in patients on anticonvulsant therapy. Clin Exp Immunol 12:39–47
Alloway JA, Salata MP (1995) Quinidine-induced rheumatic syndromes. Semin Arthritis Rheum 24:315–322
Amrhein JA, Kenny FM, Ross D (1970) Granulocytopenia, lupus-like syndrome, and other complications of propylthiouracil therapy. J Pediatr 76:54–63
Aucoin DP, Peterson ME, Hurvitz AI, Drayer DE, Lahita RG, Quimby FW, Reidenberg M M (1985) Propylthiouracil-induced immune-mediated disease in the cat. J Pharmacol Exp Ther 234:13–18
Aucoin DP, Rubin RL, Peterson ME, Reidenberg MM, Drayer DE, Hurvitz AI, Lahita RG (1988) Dose-dependent induction of anti-native DNA antibodies in cats by propylthiouracil. Arthritis Rheum 31:688–692
Batchelor JR, Welsh KI, Tinoco RM, Dollery CT, Hughes GR, Bernstein R, Ryan P, Naish PF, Aber GM, Bing RF, Russel GI (1980) Hydralazine-induced systemic lupus erythematosus: influence of HLA-DR and sex on susceptibility. Lancet 1:1107–1109
Beernink DH, Miller JJ (1973) Anticonvulsant-induced antinuclear antibodies and lupus-like disease in children. J Pediatr 82:113–117
Blomgren SE, Condemi JJ, Vaughn JH (1972) Procainamide-induced lupus erythematosus: clinical and laboratory observations. Am J Med 52:338–348

Booth RJ, Wilson JD, Bullock JY (1982) β-Adrenergic-receptor blockers and antinuclear antibodies in hypertension. Clin Pharmacol Ther 31:555–558

Brand C, Davidson A, Littlejohn G, Ryan P (1984) Hydralazine-induced lupus: no association with HLA-DR4. Lancet 1:462

Burlingame RW, Rubin RL (1991) Drug-induced anti-histone autoantibodies display two patterns of reactivity with substructures of chromatin. J Clin Invest 88:680–690

Cameron HA, Ramsay LE (1984) The lupus syndrome induced by hydralazine: a common complication with low dose therapy. Br Med J 289:410–412

Canoso R, Lewis M, Yunis E (1982) Association of HLA-Bw44 with chlorpromazine-induced autoantibodies. Clin Immunol Immunopathol 25:278–282

CAST (1989) Preliminary report: Effect of encainide and flecainide on mortality in a randomized trial of arrhythmia suppression after myocardial infarction. N Engl J Med 321: 406–412

Charles PJ, Smeenk RJ, De Jong J, Feldmann M, Maini RN (2000) Assessment of antibodies to double-stranded DNA induced in rheumatoid arthritis patients following treatment with infliximab, a monoclonal antibody to tumor necrosis factor alpha: findings in open-label and randomized placebo-controlled trials. Arthritis Rheum 43:2383–2390

Chin G, Kong N, Lee B, Rose I (1991) Penicillamine induced lupus-like syndrome in a patient with classical rheumatoid arthritis. J Rheumatol 18:947–948

Christie DJ, Mullen PC, Aster RH (1985) Fab-mediated binding of drug-dependent antibodies to platelets in quinidine- and quinine-induced thrombocytopenia. J Clin Invest 75:310–314

Cornacchia E, Golbus J, Maybaum J, Strahler J, Hanash S, Richardson B (1988) Hydralazine and procainamide inhibit T cell DNA methylation and induce autoreactivity. J Immunol 140:2197–2200

Derksen R, Kater L (1985) Lupus anticoagulant: revival of an old phenomenon. Clin Exp Rheumatol 3:349–357

Donker AJ, Venuto RC, Vladutiu AO, Brentjens JR, Andres GA (1984) Effects of prolonged administration of D-penicillamine or captopril in various strains of rats. Clin Immunol Immunopath 30:142–155

Dubois EL, Wallace DJ (1987) Drugs that exacerbate and induce systemic lupus erythematosus In: Wallace DJ, Dubois EL (eds) Dubois' Lupus Erythematosus. Lea & Febiger, Philadelphia, pp 450–469

Dubois EL, Tallman E, Wonka RA (1972) Chlorpromazine-induced systemic lupus erythematosus: case report and review of the literature. J Am Med Assoc 221:595–596

Dubroff LM, Reid R Jr, Papalian M (1981) Molecular models for hydralazine-related systemic lupus erythematosus. Arthritis Rheum 24:1082–1085

Dunphy J, Oliver M, Rands AL, Lovell CR, McHugh NJ (2000) Antineutrophil cytoplasmic antibodies and HLA class II alleles in minocycline-induced lupus-like syndrome. Br J Dermatol 142:461–467

Falk RJ, Terrell RS, Charles LA, Jennette JC (1990) Anti-neutrophil cytoplasmic autoantibodies induce neutrophils to degranulate and produce oxygen radicals in vitro. Proc Natl Acad Sci USA 87:4115–4119

Fritzler MJ, Tan EM (1978) Antibodies to histones in drug-induced and idiopathic lupus erythematosus. J Clin Invest 62:560–567

Fukuyama S, Kajiwara E, Suzuki N, Miyazaki N, Sadoshima S, Onoyama K (2000) Systemic lupus erythematosus after alpha-interferon therapy for chronic hepatitis C: a case report and review of the literature. Am J Gastroenterol 95:310–312

Ghate J, Turner M, Rudek M, Figg W, Dahut W, Dyer V, Pluda J, Reed E (2001) Drug-induced lupus associated with COL-3: report of 3 cases. Arch Dermatol 137:471–474

Gleichmann E, Pals WT, Rolink AG, Radaszkiewicz T, Gleichmann H (1984) Graft-versus-host reactions: clues to the etiopathology of a spectrum of immunological diseases. Immunol Today 5:324–332

Gleichmann H (1982) Systemic lupus erythematosus triggered by diphenylhydantoin. Arthritis Rheum 25:1387–1388

Graninger WB, Hassfeld W, Pesau BB, Machold KP, Zielinski CC, Smolen JS (1991) Induction of systemic lupus erythematosus by interferon-gamma in a patient with rheumatoid arthritis. J Rheumatol 18:1621–1622

Griem P, Wulferink M, Sachs B, Gonzalez JB, Gleichmann E (1998) Allergic and autoimmune reactions to xenobiotics: how do they arise? Immunol Today 19:133–141

Gunnarsson I, Kanerud L, Pettersson E, Lundberg I, Lindblad S, Ringertz B (1997) Predisposing factors in sulphasalazine-induced systemic lupus erythematosus. Br J Rheumatol 36: 1089–1094

Hahn BH, Sharp GC, Irvin WS, Kantor OS, Gardner CA, Bagby MK, Perry HM Jr, Osterland CK (1972) Immune responses to hydralazine and nuclear antigens in hydralazine-induced lupus erythematosus. Ann Intern Med 76:365–374

Harkcom TM, Conn DL, Holley KE (1978) D-Penicillamine and lupus erythematosus-like syndrome. Ann Intern Med 89:1012

Henningsen NC, Cederberg A, Hanson A, Johansson BW (1975) Effects of long-term treatment with procaine amide. Acta Med Scand 198:475–482

Hieronymus T, Grotsch P, Blank N, Grunke M, Capraru D, Geiler T, Winkler S, Kalden JR, Lorenz HM (2000) Chlorpromazine induces apoptosis in activated human lymphoblasts: a mechanism supporting the induction of drug-induced lupus erythematosus? Arthritis Rheum 43:1994–2004

Hoffman BJ (1945) Sensitivity to sulfadiazine resembling acute lupus erythematosus. Arch Dermatol Syph 51:190–192

Hofstra A, Uetrecht JP (1993) Metabolism of hydralazine to a reactive intermediate by the oxidizing system of activated leukocytes. Chem Biol Interact 89:183–196

Jaffe IA (1981) Induction of auto-immune syndromes by penicillamine therapy in rheumatoid arthritis and other diseases. Springer Semin Immunopathol 4:193–207

Jain KK (1991) Systemic lupus erythematosus (SLE)-like syndromes associated with carbamazepine therapy. Drug Saf 6:350–360

Ju C, Uetrecht JP (1999) Detection of 2-hydroxyiminostilbene in the urine of patients taking carbamazepine and its oxidation to a reactive iminoquinone intermediate. J Pharmacol Exp Ther 288:51–56

Kalyanaraman B, Sohnle PG (1985) Generation of free radical intermediates from foreign compounds by neutrophil-derived oxidants. J Clin Invest 75:1618–1622

Kammuller ME, Bloksma N, Seinen W (1988) Chemical-induced autoimmune reactions and Spanish toxic oil syndrome. Focus on hydantoins and related compounds. J Toxicol Clin Toxicol 26:157–174

Khan MF, Kaphalia BS, Prabhakar BS, Kanz MF, Ansari GA (1995) Trichloroethene-induced autoimmune response in female MRL +/+ mice. Toxicol Appl Pharmacol 134:155–160

Kilburn KH, Warshaw RH (1992) Prevalence of symptoms of systemic lupus erythematosus (SLE) and of fluorescent antinuclear antibodies associated with chronic exposure to trichloroethylene and other chemicals in well water. Environ Res 57:1–9

Knezevic W, Mastaglia FL, Quintner J, Zilko PJ (1984) Guillain-Barré syndrome and pemphigus foliaceus associated with D-penicillamine therapy. Aust NZ J Med 14:50–52

Kretz-Rommel A, Duncan SR, Rubin RL (1997) Autoimmunity caused by disruption of central T cell tolerance. A murine model of drug-induced lupus. J Clin Invest 99:1888–1896

Kretz-Rommel A, Rubin RL (1999) Persistence of autoreactive T cell drive is required to elicit anti- chromatin antibodies in a murine model of drug-induced lupus. J Immunol 162: 813–820

Laversuch CJ, Collins DA, Charles PJ, Bourke BE (1995) Sulphasalazine-induced autoimmune abnormalities in patients with rheumatic disease. Br J Rheumatol 34:435–439

Lawson TM, Amos N, Bulgen D, Williams BD (2001) Minocycline-induced lupus: clinical features and response to rechallenge. Rheumatology (Oxford) 40:329–335

Lee SL, Chase PH (1975) Drug-induced systemic lupus erythematosus: a critical review. Semin Arthritis Rheum 5:83–103

Lessard E, Fortin A, Belanger PM, Beaune P, Hamelin BA, Turgeon J (1997) Role of CYP2D6 in the N-hydroxylation of procainamide. Pharmacogenetics 7:381–390

Machold KP, Smolen JS (1990) Interferon-gamma induced exacerbation of systemic lupus erythematosus. J Rheumatol 17:831–832

Mackie BS, Mackie LE (1999) The PABA story. Australas J Dermatol 40:51–53

Maddrey WC, Boitnott JK (1973) Isoniazid hepatitis. Ann Intern Med 79:1–12

Malinow MR, Bardana EJ, Pirofsky B, Craig S, McLaughlin P (1982) Systemic lupus erythematosus-like syndrome in monkeys fed alfalfa sprouts: role of a nonprotein amino acid. Science 216:415–417

Markham A, Lamb HM (2000) Infliximab: a review of its use in the management of rheumatoid arthritis. Drugs 59:1341–1359

Matsuura T, Shimizu Y, Fujimoto H, Miyazaki T, Kano S (1992) Minocycline-related lupus. Lancet 340:1553

Nassberger L, Sjoholm AG, Jonsson H, Sturfelt G, Akesson A (1990) Autoantibodies against neutrophil cytoplasm components in systemic lupus erythematosus and in hydralazine-induced lupus. Clin Exp Immunol 81:380–383

Perry HM (1973) Late toxicity to hydralazine resembling systemic lupus erythematosus or rheumatoid arthritis. Am J Med 54:58–72

Perry HM, Tan EM, Cordody S, Sahamato A (1970) Relationship of acetyl transferase activity to antinuclear antibodies and toxic symptoms on hypertensive patients treated with hydralazine. J Lab Clin Med 76:114–125

Portanova JP, Arndt RE, Tan EM, Kotzin BL (1987) Anti-histone antibodies in idiopathic and drug-induced lupus recognize distinct intrahistone regions. J Immunol 138:446–451

Price EJ, Venables PJ (1995) Drug-induced lupus. Drug Saf 12:283–290

Raftery EB, Denman AM (1973) Systemic lupus erythematosus syndrome induced by practolol. Br Med J 2:452–455

Reidenberg MM (1983) Aromatic amines and the pathogenesis of lupus erythematosus. Am J Med 75:1037–1042

Reidenberg MM, Durant PJ, Harris RA, De Boccardo G, Lahita R, Stenzel KH (1983) Lupus erythematosus-like disease due to hydrazine. Am J Med 75:365–370

Reza MJ, Dornfeld L, Goldberg LS (1975) Hydralazine therapy in hypertensive patients with idiopathic systemic lupus erythematosus. Arthritis Rheum 18:335–338

Rich MW (1996) Drug-induced lupus: the list of culprits grows. Postgrad Med 100:299–308

Richardson B, Scheinbart L, Strahler J, Gross L, Hanash S, Johnson M (1990) Evidence for impaired T cell methylation in systemic lupus erythematosus and rheumatoid arthritis. Arthritis Rheum 33:1665–1673

Ronnblom LE, Alm GV, Oberg KE (1990) Possible induction of systemic lupus erythematosus by interferon-alpha treatment in a patient with a malignant carcinoid tumour. J Intern Med 227:207–210

Rothfield NF, Bierer WF, Garfield JW (1978) Isoniazid induction of antinuclear antibodies: a prospective study. Ann Intern Med 88:650–652

Rutgeerts P, D'Haens G, Targan S, Vasiliaskas E, Hanauer SB, Present DH, Mayer L, Van Hogezand RA, Braakman T, DeWoody KL, Schaible TF, Van Deventer SJ (1999) Efficacy and safety of retreatment with anti-tumor necrosis factor antibody (infliximab) to maintain remission in Crohn's disease. Gastroenterology 117:761–769

Schaffer JV, Davidson DM, McNiff JM, Bolognia JL (2001) Perinuclear antineutrophilic cytoplasmic antibody-positive cutaneous polyarteritis nodosa associated with minocycline therapy for acne vulgaris. J Am Acad Dermatol 44:198–206

Schilling PJ, Kurzrock R, Kantarjian H, Gutterman JU, Talpaz M (1991) Development of systemic lupus erythematosus after interferon therapy for chronic myelogenous leukemia. Cancer 68:1536–1537

Shapiro KS, Pinn VW, Harrington JT, Levey AS (1984) Immune complex glomerulnephritis in hydralazine-induced SLE. Am J Kidney Dis 3:270–274

Shapiro LE, Knowles SR, Shear NH (1997) Comparative safety of tetracycline, minocycline, and doxycycline. Arch Dermatol 133:1224–1230

Shapiro LE, Uetrecht J, Shear NH (2001) Minocycline, perinuclear antineutrophilic cytoplasmic antibody, and pigment: the biochemical basis. J Am Acad Dermatol 45:787–789

Shear NH, Spielberg SP (1988) Anticonvulsant hypersensitivity syndrome. J Clin Invest 82:1826–1832

Sim E, Law SA (1985) Hydralazine binds covalently to complement component C4: different reactivity of C4A and C4B gene products. FEBS 184:323–327

Sim E, Stanley L, Gill EW, Jones A (1988) Metabolites of procainamide and practolol inhibit complement components C3 and C4. Biochem J 251:323–326

Spielberg SP, Gordon GB, Blake DA, Mellits ED, Bross DS (1981) Anticonvulsant toxicity in vitro: possible role of arene oxides. J Pharmacol Exp Ther 217:386–389

Stec GP, Lertora JJL, Atkinson AJ, Nevin MJ, Kushner W, Jones C, Schmid FR, Askenazi J (1979) Remission of procainamide-induced lupus erythematosus with N-acetylprocainamide therapy. Ann Intern Med 90:799–801

Steinberg AD, Gourley MF, Klinman DM, Tsokos GC, Scott DE, Krieg AM (1991) NIH conference. Systemic lupus erythematosus. Ann Intern Med 115:548–559

Tournade H, Pelletier L, Pasquier R, Vial M, Mandet C, Druet P (1990) D-Penicillamine-induced autoimmunity in Brown-Norway rats: similarities with $HgCl_2$-Induced autoimmunity. J Immunol 144:2985–2991

Uetrecht JP (1988) Mechanism of drug-induced lupus. Chem Res Toxicol 1:133–143

Uetrecht JP (1996) Drug-induced lupus: possible mechanisms and their implications for prediction of which new drugs may induce lupus. Expert Opinion on Invest Drugs 5:851–860

Uetrecht JP, Woosley RL (1981) Acetylator phenotype and lupus erythematosus. Clin Pharmacokin 6:118–134

Waldhauser L, Uetrecht J (1991) Oxidation of propylthiouracil to reactive metabolites by activated neutrophils: implications for agranulocytosis. Drug Metab Dispos 19:354–359

Watanabe-Fukunaga R, Brannan CI, Copeland NG, Jenkins NA, Nagata S (1992) Lymphoproliferation disorder in mice explained by defects in Fas antigen that mediates apoptosis. Nature 356:314–317

Wilson JD, Bullock JY, Sutherland DC, Main C, O'Brien KP (1978) Antinuclear antibodies in patients receiving non-practolol beta-blockers. Br Med J 1:14–16

Woosley RL, Drayer DE, Reidenberg MM, Nies AS, Carr K, Oates JA (1978) Effect of acetylator phenotype on the rate at which procainamide induces antinuclear antibodies and the lupus syndrome. N Engl J Med 298:1157–1159

Yung RL, Richardson BC (1994) Drug-induced lupus. Rheum Dis Clin North Am 20:61–86

Zarrabi MH, Zucker S, Miller F, Derman RM, Romano GS, Hartnett JA, Varma AO (1979) Imunologic and coagulation disorders in chlorpromazine-treated patients. Ann Intern Med 91:194–199.

CHAPTER 10

Association of Cutaneous Lupus Erythematosus with Other Dermatological Diseases

10

Kyrill Pramatarov, Nikolai Tsankov

Lupus erythematosus (LE) may be associated with various systemic and dermatologic diseases. In some cases, this association may be explained by autoimmune mechanisms or by the similarity of the clinical features; in other cases, the possible coexistence of diseases is coincidental.

Psoriasis and Lupus Erythematosus

The coincidence of LE and psoriasis seems to be rare. Based on their prevalence in the population, the coexistence of psoriasis with all forms of lupus seems to be less than expected. Dubois (Dubois 1974) reported that 0.6% of 520 patients with systemic LE (SLE) had concurrent psoriasis. Tumarkin et al. (Tumarkin et al. 1971) described 637 patients with discoid LE (DLE), and only 1 had coexistent psoriasis. In 1927, O'Leary (O'Leary 1927) described one of the first cases of coexistent psoriasis and LE. Throughout the years, several explanations concerning this coexistence have been developed. Schaumann (Schaumann 1928) postulated that the combination of LE and psoriasis – disorders with different "affinity" to the ground on which they appear – must be sought in the etiologic factors determining their pathogenesis. Louste et al. (Louste et al. 1939) focused on the "endocrine deficiency." Charpy et al. (Charpy et al. 1952) proposed that both disorders (in combination with arteriitis and hypertonia) be considered "disorders of adaptation." Kocsard (Kocsard 1974) considered the association of cutaneous LE and psoriasis vulgaris for a best explanation of the frequency of pseudopelade in patients with psoriasis. Millns and Muller (Millns and Muller 1980) think that LE and psoriasis could appear independently in the same patient without there being a causal relationship between the two disorders. Kulick et al. (Kulick et al. 1983) found that the frequency of antibodies to Ro/SSA is increased in patients with psoriasis and LE. They suggested that this might be a specific serologic marker for the LE-psoriasis overlap. It is well-known that the same antibodies occur in the antinuclear antibody (ANA)-negative, highly photosensitive group of patients with SLE. Accordingly, patients with psoriasis and LE may in fact have an increased risk for photosensitivity. Forty-three percent of all patients with SLE are photosensitive. On the contrary, the subset of "photosensitive psoriasis" is very small and comprises approximately 5.5% of all cases. These patients have a significantly higher prevalence of skin type I, and 50% have preceding polymorphous light eruption rising into psoriasis. Psoriasiform or annular lesions are also typical for patients with subacute cutaneous LE (SCLE). In such cases, histologic examination, immunofluorescence, and serology tests are necessary to distinguish SCLE from psoriasis.

Some of these patients, especially those with circulating anti-Ro/SSA antibodies, may be exclusively photosensitive. The action spectrum for LE is generally considered to be ultraviolet (UV)B, but some patients may flare after UVA exposures received in tanning salons or from sunlight filtered through window glass.

The control of SLE often requires systemic administration of steroids, especially for renal and central nervous system involvement. A rebound flare of psoriasis is always possible on withdrawal of steroid therapy. Administration of antimetabolites used as steroid-sparing agents may prevent this rebound flare and improve psoriasis. Phototherapy is contraindicated in patients with cutaneous LE. On the contrary, psoralen-UVA exposure is indicated in psoriatic individuals and in those with severe "photosensitive psoriasis." Screening for ANAs, including anti-Ro/SSA and anti-La/SSB antibodies, is necessary before treating any photosensitive patient with UV light. Psoriasis could coexist with other photosensitive disorders, such as vitiligo, porphyria, drug-induced photodermatitis, polymorphous light eruption, chronic actinic dermatitis, solar urticaria, actinic prurigo, and the so-called "fair skin type".

Some psoriasis patients develop LE (subacute cutaneous, chronic cutaneous, or systemic) after psoralen-UVA therapy (Dowdy et al. 1989). Zalla and Muller (Zalla and Muller 1996) studied 9420 patients with psoriasis, and 65 (0.69%) had concomitant photosensitive disorders. Of these, 23 (35%) had psoriasis and nonlupus-related photosensitivity and 42 (65%) had psoriasis and LE with or without photosensitivity. The conclusion is that the coexistence of psoriasis with LE or other photosensitive disorders is rare. These studies may explain the coexistence of LE in patients with psoriasis after UV therapy. However, this possibility does not help explain the coexistence of LE in patients with psoriasis who have not had significant exposure to UV light or in those in whom LE develops before the onset of psoriasis. The explanation probably resides in the multifactorial etiology of both diseases. The hypothesis that patients with LE and psoriasis have common serologic markers (anti-Ro/SSA antibodies) is not convincing (Baselga et al. 1994, Hays et al. 1984, Kobayashi et al. 1995, Kulick et al. 1983). Both disorders may appear independently in the same patient with no causal relationship between them (Millns and Muller 1980, Wlashev et al. 1986).

Antimalarials are now the drugs of choice for treatment of the cutaneous and joint manifestations of LE. It is well known that the use of chloroquine and hydroxychloroquine may aggravate or precipitate psoriasis (Nicolas et al. 1988). We suggest that in patients treated with antimalarials in which LE precedes the development of psoriasis, drug-induced psoriasis could be possible (Tsankov et al. 1990). Large-scale prospective studies of the general population for the coexistence of diseases such as LE and psoriasis aim at the same scientific goal: elucidation of the etiology and prescription of the the most appropriate therapy (Rongioletti et al. 1990a).

Erythema Multiforme and Lupus Erythematosus: Rowell's Syndrome

In 1963, Rowell et al. (Rowell et al. 1963) described four patients with the clinical picture of chronic DLE associated with erythema multiforme (EM). Besides the skin changes compatible with both diseases, the patients had characteristic immunologic findings consisting of the speckled type of ANAs, the anti-SjT type of precipitating antibody to saline extract of human tissues and rheumatoid factor. In some patients, perniotic-like lesions were also observed. Later it turned out that SjT is identical to anti-La/SSB or anti-Ro/SSA antibodies. Several cases with this unusual picture have been reported subsequently, and this distinctive subset of LE is called "Rowell's syndrome." Twenty-seven cases of the syndrome had been reported by 1989. Our group observed a 30-year-old man who had DLE, EM-like lesions, and ANAs in a low titer (Pramatarov et al. 1983). SjT antibodies were not studied. Four additional cases were reported later. Parodi et al. (Parodi et al. 1989), in 1989, described a 62-year-old man with DLE and EM. They reviewed the previous reported cases and suggested that most are cases of coincidental association of LE and EM. Their review revealed that none of the cases reported after that described by Rowell covered the diagnostic criteria of the syndrome. In 1995, Fiallo et al. (Fiallo et al. 1995) described a 19-year-old man with SLE and annular polycyclic lesions on the cheeks, upper trunk, back, and arms. They believed that Rowell's syndrome was a distinct entity and that their patient was additional evidence for its existence. In 1996, Fitzgerald et al. (Fitzgerald et al. 1996) described a 47-year-old woman with a long history of EM-like eruptions in association with LE. The patient had a speckled ANA pattern, and the authors believed that she met the criteria for Rowell's syndrome and that this syndrome is a distinct clinical and immunologic entity. In 1996, Chua et al. (Chua et al. 1996) described a 9-year-old girl with SLE and ANA titer of 1:640 who also had necrotizing lymphadenitis. In 1999, Shteyngarts et al. (Shteyngarts et al. 1999) described a 34-year-old woman with a history of SLE with concomitant EM lesions. The case was compared with other cases with Rowell's syndrome. Their belief is that the coexistence of LE and EM does not impart any unusual characteristics to either disease and that the immunologic disturbances in such patients are probably coincidental. In 2000, Roustan et al. (Roustan et al. 2000) described a 27-year-old woman with EM-like lesions. They also reviewed the cases of Rowell's syndrome reported previously and declared that the main clinical and immunologic findings are not distinctive and could be detected in various subtypes of LE. Roustan et al. believed that their patient might be included in so-called Rowell's syndrome but with the clinical picture of SCLE. In 1999, Marzano et al. (Marzano et al. 1999) described a woman with LE and long-standing vesiculobullous EM-like lesions and typical laboratory findings of the antiphospholipid syndrome. The case could be consistent with the diagnosis of Rowell's syndrome, if the latter is regarded as a clinical entity. In conclusion, the existence of Rowell's syndrome is still disputable since few, if any, cases met the criteria of the originally reported cases by Rowell, but coexistence of LE and EM is possible and well documented. EM-like lesions can appear in patients with DLE, as it was in the original article by Rowell, they can also appear in patients with SLE, and they might be a clinical picture of SCLE. Moreover, in 1989, Sontheimer (Sontheimer 1989) stressed that the annular polycyclic changes may resemble EM.

Lupus Erythematosus and Lichen Planus

LE and lichen planus (LP) possess different clinical and histologic pictures and immunologic findings. Copeman et al. (Copeman et al. 1970) reported first in 1970 the coexistence of both diseases in four patients. Additionally, several cases of the coexistence of both diseases have been reported (Baumann 1997, Camisa et al. 1984, Davies et al. 1977, Dimitrova et al. 1982, Piamphongsant et al. 1978, Plotnick and Burnham 1986, Razzaque et al. 1982, Romero et al. 1977). Most of the reported cases are patients with DLE and coexistent LP. In 1982, our group (Dimitrova et al. 1982) described a 55-year-old woman whose disease began with scarring alopecia. Two years later, discoid lesions appeared on her face. One year later, itching papules appeared on her back and wrists. The histologic and immunologic findings were compatible with both diseases. The case reported by Razzaque et al. (Razzaque et al. 1982) had LP associated with SLE. The diagnosis was based on the criteria of the American Rheumatism Association for SLE and on findings from histologic and immunofluorescence studies suggestive of LP. LE discoides and LP verrucosus in the same patient has also been reported (Baumann 1997), and this association is of great clinical importance since categorizing the verrucous forms of both diseases is some-times very difficult (Uitto et al. 1978). From the reported cases with the association of both diseases it could not be justified which of the diseases is usually preceding. In some reported cases, the clinical, histologic, and immunofluorescence features showed an overlap pattern between LE and LP, as it was in the 11 patients described by Romero et al. On the other hand, Davies et al. (Davies et al. 1977) in 1977, drew attention to the fact that despite the distinctive characteristic of both diseases, they share some common features. Both may show scarring alopecia and development of lesions at the site of trauma (Koebner's phenomenon), may cause atrophy or hyper-trophy, and may exhibit photosensitivity. Immunoglobulins, fibrin, and complement are found in LP papules, and colloid bodies are detected in both diseases. In sum-mary, Davies et al. suspected a common pathophysiologic pathway because of the similarities between LE and LP. Some authors use the term "LE-LP overlap syn-drome" for cases in which differentiation between the diseases is impossible. In such cases, Camisa et al. (Camisa et al. 1984) in 1984, recommended using the modern immunologic studies as a possible way to distinguish LE from LP in patients with the overlap syndrome. From six patients they described, intensive staining of stratum granulosum was found. The latter is consistent with LP. A third patient developed cri-teria for the diagnosis of SLE. This overlap syndrome is characterized by chronic livid atrophic patches and plaques, mostly on the extremities. Lichenoid flat papules are generally not observed, and telangiectasias are prominent. In the overlap syndrome, the palms, soles, and nails are involved. Histologically, either a hypocellular (LE) or a hypercellular (LP) type is seen (Shai and Halevy 1992). The immunofluorescence demonstrates ovoid or globular deposits of IgG, IgM, and C3 at the dermoepidermal junction. In addition, lichen actinicus, a distinctive variant of LP, is another point of relation of both diseases. Besides the typical LP papules and photosensitivity, a malar rash resembling LE can be also seen (Isaacson et al. 1981, Pramatarov et al. 1988).

Lupus Erythematosus and Cutaneous Mucinosis

Mucin is an acid mucopolysaccharide consisting of hyaluronic acid bound to small amounts of chondroitin sulphate and heparin. In 1991, Rongioletti and Rebora (Ron-gioletti and Rebora 1991) divided cutaneous mucinosis into two groups: the first has distinctive clinical characteristics, and the second appears in various diseases as an additional feature. In patients with LE and other connective tissue diseases, microscopic amounts of mucin in the dermis could be detected, but without clinical evidence (Choi et al. 1992). Gold (Gold 1954), in 1954, first reported an occurrence of mucinosis lesions in two patients with SLE. His patients had papular eruptions on the neck, the upper part of the trunk, and the extremities that preceded the development of SLE lesions. This condition, later named "papular and nodular mucinosis," (PNM) is a well-characterized cutaneous mucinosis predominantly associated with SLE. Rongioletti et al. (Rongioletti et al. 1990b) believed that PNM may herald a severe systemic disease. PNM typically presents as indolent, flesh-colored, centrally depressed papules and nodules on the neck, trunk, and extremities (Kanda et al. 1997, Rongioletti and Rebora 1986). Biopsies did not reveal the typical LE epidermal changes, but the immunofluorescence study detected immunoglobulin deposits and C3 at the dermoepidermal junction.

The temporal relationship with LE is different: in some cases PNM precedes LE and in others it appears with it. In 70% of patients, PNM appears in association with SLE, and in 30% it appears with DLE (Rongioletti et al. 1990b). DLE with dermal mucinosis has been reported by Weigand et al. (Weigand et al. 1981) in 1981 and Lowe et al. in 1992 (Lowe et al. 1992). In DLE, an acute periorbital mucinosis has been reported by Williams and Ramos-Caro (Williams and Ramos-Caro 1999) in 1999. Why cutaneous mucinosis appears in LE is still not known. In some patients, one could find a link between sun exposure and development of mucinosis. The two cases described by Weidner and Djawari (Weidner and Djawari 1982) in 1982 had DLE and dermal mucinosis, and both appeared after sun exposure. The patient described by Nishimoto et al. (Nishimoto et al. 1989) developed SLE and cutaneous mucinosis provoked by exposure to psoralen-UVA. Cutaneous mucinosis has been reported by Kuhn et al. (Kuhn et al. 1995) in association with SCLE. Several years later, Kuhn et al. (Kuhn et al. 2000) found deposits of mucin in patients with LE tumidus (LET). Both subtypes of LE, SCLE and LET, are recognized as being extremely photosensitive. Various clinical pictures of mucinosis in association with LE have been reported: massive cutaneous mucinosis (Maryama et al. 1997), plaque-like (Kobayashi et al. 1993), and atrophie blanche–like lesions (Egawa et al. 1994). In addition, lichen myxedematosus was described in two patients by Salomon et al. (Salomon et al. 1977) in 1977. The first patient had DLE and the other had SLE. Since in the most cases dermal mucinosis and especially PNM preceded LE, the early recognition of LE is important.

Lupus Erythematosus and Bullous Diseases

Vesiculobullous eruptions predominantly appear in patients with SLE. Loche et al. (Loche et al. 1998) divided vesiculobullous eruptions in SLE into three groups: in the first group, blistering may appear in patients with SLE owing to cutaneous fragility; in the second group, vesiculobullous eruptions are the main clinical features of a distinct clinical entity called bullous SLE; and in the third group, SLE may be primarily associated with bullous diseases.

Because the association between LE and pemphigus is considered generally to be pemphigus erythematosus only, a few cases of coexistence of both diseases have been reported. Fong et al. in 1985 described a 59-year-old Chinese woman with LE preceding pemphigus. Their patient met the criteria for both diagnoses. In the report by Kuchabal et al. (Kuchabal et al. 1998), pemphigus preceded the development of SLE in a 15-year-old Indian girl.

In 1998, Loche et al. (Loche et al. 1998) described a 52-year-old woman who had SLE according to the criteria of American Rheumatism Association (ARA) and who 6 years later developed localized bullous pemphigoid. Loche et al. reviewed the previously reported cases with the coexistence of SLE and bullous pemphigoid. Nine cases of bullous pemphigoid associated with SLE were reported by 1998. In four cases, SLE preceded the appearance of bullous pemphigoid. Not all of the reported cases had the typical clinical presentation. Direct immunofluorescence showed deposition of IgG only at the basement membrane zone (BMZ) in three patients and of IgG with complement in five. Indirect immunofluorescence revealed circulating anti-BMZ antibodies in four patients. The authors believed that since there is plenty of autoimmune antibodies in SLE, one of them can be directed against the bullous pemphigoid antigen. Huang et al. in 1997 described a 77-year-old patient with a history of vesiculobullous eruptions specified as bullous pemphigoid of 3 months' duration. Several months later, because of the patient's deteriorated condition, SLE was diagnosed. Several cases with this coexistence have been previously reported, but some were not convincing (Jordan et al. 1969, Kumar et al. 1978, Miler et al. 1978).

An association between SLE and dermatitis herpetiformis is rare. A few cases with this association have been reported, and two of them deserve attention. The patient described by Aronson et al. (Aronson et al. 1979) also had Marfan's syndrome. The patient described by Vandersteen et al. (Vandersteen et al. 1974) had dermatitis herpetiformis and later developed DLE, probably induced by sulfone.

A few cases of coexistent linear IgA disease and SLE have been reported. The first, described in 1983 by Thaipisuttikul et al. (Thaipisuttikul et al. 1983), was a patient with SLE who later developed linear IgA disease. Lau et al. (Lau et al. 1991), in 1991, described a 35-year-old woman with a history of SLE who developed linear IgA disease 22 years later. Both patients had gluten-dependent enteropathy and responded dramatically to treatment with dapsone. Epidermolysis bullosa acquisita in association with SLE also has been reported (Dotson et al. 1981)

Lupus Erythematosus and Porphyria Cutanea Tarda

Porphyria cutanea tarda (PCT) can occur in patients with all subtypes of the spectrum of LE (Moshella 1989). This association has been reported in patients with DLE (Wheatherhead and Adam 1985), SLE, and SCLE (Callen and Ross 1981, Cram et al. 1973). This fact is well known, and the first cases with this association appeared in the early 1960s. Unfortunately, not all of the cases have been investigated using modern immunologic studies, and these cases cannot be specified well. The study by Wolfram in 1952 (Wolfram 1952) is the first with this association. Patients with SLE dominate the reported cases. LE occurred first in most cases. In the series by Gibson and McEvoy (Gibson and McEvoy 1998), PCT occurred either before or simultaneous with LE in almost 50% of the patients. In this article, a patient with DLE was described and 15 patients with coexistent LE and PCT were reviewed. These 15 patients were found in a group of 6,179 patients with LE – all variants – and 676 cases with PCT. Nine patients had DLE, five had SLE, and one had SCLE. The initial diagnosis was LE in eight patients, PCT in five patients, and simultaneous LE and PCT in two patients.

Often, antimalarial therapy precipitates PCT. Alcohol and sometimes estrogens and iron were also contributing factors (Callen and Ross 1981). The pathogenic pathways of the coexistence of PCT and LE remain unclear. The possible mechanisms are a common genetic fault, an acquired metabolic fault resulting in porphyria with preexisting LE, porphyria causing an autoimmune response, and a genetically determined metabolic fault for porphyria that is precipitated as a consequence of LE (Cram et al. 1973, Gibson et al. 1991). The hypothesis that lupoid hepatitis is a causative factor in patients with preceding LE is not convincing. The coexistence of both diseases is of great clinical importance. A possible complication, postulated by Callen and Ross (1981), is the treatment of PCT by phlebotomy or with antimalarial agents: Since anemia may be present in some patients with LE, phlebotomy may be unwise; moreover, phlebotomy can be an exacerbating factor for some patients with combined disorders. Antimalarial agents used for the treatment of LE are usually used in much higher doses, and this therapy must be applied cautiously so that an acute toxic reaction does not occur. Estrogen-containing medicines and oral contraceptives should be avoided or applied with caution in both diseases. The appropriate choice of a sunscreen in patients with both diseases is also difficult. A total block must be used in patients with PCT because PCT is activated by a longer wavelength than LE.

Lupus Erythematosus and Alopecia Areata

Diffuse alopecia and especially frontal alopecia due to increased hair fragility is more typical for SLE. Scarring alopecia is a frequent clinical feature of DLE and SLE. Alopecia areata is rarely associated with LE. In a large study of 736 patients with alopecia areata, only 2 had DLE and 2 had SLE (Muller and Winkelmann 1963). In 1975, Lerchin et al. (Lerchin et al. 1975) reported a single case of DLE associated with alopecia areata. Werth et al. (Werth et al. 1992) found 4 patients with alopecia areata in a group of 39 patients with LE. Two of the patients had DLE and two had SLE. The first of the reported patients had scarring alopecia as well. In each patient, continuous granular deposits of IgG at the dermoepidermal junction were detected. The authors believed that the incidence of alopecia areata in patients with LE is increased because of the common lines of evidence of both diseases.

Lupus Erythematosus and Sjögren's Syndrome

Sjögren's syndrome (SS) can be associated with all connective tissue diseases. The overlap syndromes of SS and other dermatoses, LE included, form a distinct subtype in the classification of SS. The incidence of SS in connective tissue diseases is different. Mostly, this association appears in systemic sclerosis. Immunologic markers of SS, anti-Ro/SSA and anti-La/SSB antibodies, occur in all connective tissue diseases, sometimes without clinical evidence. Provost et al. (Provost et al. 1988) postulated that there is a relation between SS with anti-Ro/SSA and LE with anti-Ro/SSA antibodies. In SLE, anti-La/SSB occurs in approximately 15% of patients, and most have SS and may be diagnosed as having SS-SLE overlap syndromes. Anti-Ro/SSA (without anti-La/SSB) occurs in approximately 30% of patients with SLE without dry eyes or mouth. SS can precede LE by years, but LE can precede the appearance of SS also. Anti-Ro/SSA antibodies etc found in polymyositis, scleroderma, and primary biliary cirrhosis, and association with SS is invariably (Venables 1988). The skin changes associated with SS include dry eyes, dry mouth, and dry genitals as major clinical symptoms. Other clinical symptoms include annular erythema, Sweet's syndrome–like lesions, vitiligo-like changes, sarcoidosis, and LP-like and amyloidosis nodularis–like symptoms (Ueki 1994, personal communication). Annular erythema is one of the prominent clinical features of both SS and SLE. Katayama et al. (Katayama et al. 1991) subdivided annular erythema into three types. Type I is an isolated annular erythema with an elevated and exudative border. Sometimes slight scale occurs on the overlying erythema. This type may form a polycyclic lesion. Type II is a less exudative and marginally scaled erythema that resembles SCLE. Type III is a papular erythema that usually appears as multiple cutaneous lesions and that disappears in a short period compared with the other two types. Since annular erythema is a prominent clinical picture of SS and SCLE, the article by Ruzicka et al. (Ruzicka et al. 1991) deserves attention. They described a patient with annular erythema and SS but with characteristics of SLE.

Lupus Erythematosus and Neutrophilic Dermatosis (Sweet's Syndrome)

Neutrophilic dermatosis was first reported in association with SCLE by Goette in 1985. The next patient, described by Levenstein et al. (Levenstein et al. 1991), had a simultaneous appearance of both SCLE and Sweet's syndrome. The patient was later investigated for SS, and the latter was diagnosed in him. Therefore, the authors recommended that each patient with the clinical picture of both diseases be investigated for SS. Their suggestion is based on the article by Katayama et al. (Katayama et al. 1991), who found clinical evidence of annular erythema resembling Sweet's syndrome in 14 of 22 patients with SS. Choi and Chung (Choi and Chung 1999) described a patient with SLE, Sweet's syndrome and herpes zoster. SLE preceded for 3 months the appearance of Sweet's syndrome. Choi and Chung presumed that antibodies of SLE may have a role in the development of Sweet's syndrome because autoantibodies are incriminated in the pathogenesis of Sweet's syndrome. The patient described by Choi and Chung is probably the only one with SLE and Sweet's syndrome. Two articles published earlier described patients with hydralazine-induced LE and Sweet's syndrome (Ramsey-Goldman et al. 1990, Sequeira et al. 1986).

Miscellaneous

Pyoderma gangrenosum is associated with many systemic diseases, including SLE. The first reported case with coexisted pyoderma gangrenosum is the patient described by Olson in 1979. This association has been rarely reported, and all of the cases are not precise toward the condition of pyoderma gangrenosum (see Pinto et al.

1991). Among the several cases reported is one with hydralazine-induced SLE presenting as pyoderma gangrenosum–like ulcers (Peterson 1984). There are occasional studies about the association of LE with hereditary angioedema. All subtypes of LE have been reported to be coexistent with hereditary angioedema (see Gudat and Bork 1999). Duhra et al. (Duhra et al. 1990) reported in 1990 a female patient who developed DLE 6 years after the onset of hereditary angioedema. They tried to explain the coexistence of both diseases by C1 inhibitor deficiency, which can induce DLE. Duhra et al. believed that this association is rare, but its recognition is important because both diseases respond to danazol therapy. A single case showing an association between DLE and pseudoainhum has been reported (Sharma et al. 1998). Pseudoainhum is a rare dermatologic complication presenting as a constricting band around the digits. The reported patient was a 32-year-old male with 10 years duration of DLE. Pseudo-ainhum affected several digits of both hands. Vitiligo also has been reported predominantly in association with DLE. In most cases, vitiligo appeared first and DLE secondary into the lesions of vitiligo. DLE appeared in the vitiligo lesions usually (see Forestier et al. 1981). In some cases, vitiligo lesions appeared simultaneously with DLE (Wlotzke 1996). Calcinosis cutis appears in cutaneous LE rarely. Rothe et al. (Rothe et al. 1990), in 1990, described three patients with SLE and extensive calcinosis cutis. One patient had discoid lesions that ulcerated subsequently, but calcinosis was not apparent. LE and DLE is recognized as a facultative precancerosis. LE-associated skin cancers are observed usually on the face and scalp. The skin cancers observed most often are squamous cell carcinoma and keratoacanthomas, but basal cell carcinoma also has been reported (Stavropoulos et al. 1996)

References

Aronson AJ, Soltani K, Aronson IK, Ong RT (1979) Systemic lupus erythematosus and dermatitis herpetiformis. Concurrence with Marfan syndrome. Arch Dermatol 115:68–70

Baselga E, Puig L, Llobet J, Musulen E, de Moragas JM (1994) Linear psoriasis associated with systemic lupus erythematosus. J Am Acad Dermatol 30:130–133

Baumann A (1997) Lupus erythematodes discoides und Lichen ruber verrucosus. Z Hautkr 72:786–787

Callen JP, Ross L (1981) Subacute cutaneous lupus erythematosus and porphyria cutanea tarda. J Am Acad Dermatol 5:269–273

Camisa C, Neff JC, Olsen RG (1984) Use of indirect immunofluorescence in lupus erythematosus/lichen planus overlap syndrome. An additional diagnostic clue. J Am Acad Dermatol 11:1050–1059

Charpy J, Bonnet J, Tramier G (1952) Association de lupus eryhtemateux, psoriasis, arterite et hypertension. Bull Soc Fr Derm Syph 59:209–210

Choi EH, Hann SK, Chung KY, Park YK (1992) Papulonodular cutaneous mucinosis associated with systemic lupus erythematosus. Int J Dermatol 31:649–652

Choi JW, Chung KY (1999) Sweet syndrome with systemic lupus erythematosus and herpes zoster. Br J Dermatol 140:1174–1175

Chua SH, Giam YC, Sim CS (1996) Systemic lupus erythematosus with erythema multiforme-like lesions and histiocytic necrotizing lymphadenitis: a case report. Ann Acad Med 25:599–601

Clayton CA, Burnham TK (1982) Systemic lupus erythematosus and coexisting bullous pemphigoid: immunofluorescent investigation. J Am Acad Dermatol 72:236–245

Copeman PWM, Schroeter AL, Kierland RR (1970) An unusual variant of lupus erythematosus or lichen planus. Br J Dermatol 83:269–272

Cram DL, Epstein JH, Tuffaneli DL (1973) Lupus erythematosus and porphyria. Arch Dermatol 108:779–784

Cyran S, Douglas MC, Silverstein LE (1992) Chronic cutaneous lupus erythematosus presenting as periorbital edema and erythema. J Am Acad Dermatol 26:334–338

Davies MG, Gorkievicz A, Knight A, Marks R (1977) Is there a relationship between lupus erythematosus and lichen planus. Br J Dermatol 96:145–154

Davies MG, Marks R, Waddington E (1976) Simultaneous systemic lupus erythematosus and dermatitis herpetiformis. Arch Dermatol 112:1292–1294

Dimitrova J, Obreshkova E, Pramatarov K, Lankova I (1982) Lupus erythematodes discoides oder lichen planus. Z Hautkr 57:889–895

Domke HF, Ludwigsen E, Thormann J (1979) Discoid lupus erythematosus possibly due to photochemotherapy. Arch Dermatol 115:642

Dotson AD, Raimer SS, Pursley TV, Tschen J (1981) Systemic lupus erythematosus occurring in a patient with epidermolysis bullosa acquisita. Arch Dermatol 117:422–426

Dowdy MJ, Nigra TP, Barth WF (1989) Subacute cutaneous lupus erythematosus during PUVA therapy for psoriasis: case report and review of the literature. Arthritis Rheum 32:343–346

Dubois EL (1974) Lupus erythematosus (2nd ed). University of Southern California Press, Los Angeles, pp 559–564

Duhra P, Holmes J, Porter DI (1990) Discoid lupus erythematosus associated with hereditary angioneurotic edema. Br J Dermatol 123:241–244

Egawa H, Abe-Matsuura Y, Tada J (1994) Nodular cutaneous lupus mucinosis associated with atrophie blanche-like lesions in a patient with systemic lupus erythematosus. J Dermatol 21:674–679

Eyanson S, Greist MC, Brandt KD, Skinner B (1979) Systemic lupus erythematosus: association with psoralen-ultraviolet – a treatment of psoriasis. Arch Dermatol 115:54–56

Fiallo P, Tagliapietra AG, Santoro G, Venturino E (1995) Rowell syndrome. Int J Dermatol 34:635–636

Fitzgerald EA, Purcell SM, Kantor GR, Goldman HM (1996) Rowell syndrome: report of a case. J Am Acad Dermatol 35:801–803

Fong PH, Chan HL (1985) Systemic lupus erythematosus with pemphigus vulgaris. Arch Dermatol 121:26–27

Forestier JY, Ortonne JP, Thivolet J, Souteyrand P (1981) Lupus erythematéux et vitiligo. Ann Dermatol Venereol 108:33–38

Gibson GE, McEvoy M (1998) Coexistence of lupus erythematosus and porphyria cutanea tarda in fifteen patients. J Am Acad Dermatol 38:569–573

Goette DK (1985) Sweet syndrome in subacute lupus erythematosus. Arch Dermatol 121:789–791

Gold SC (1954) An unusual papular eruption associated with lupus erythematosus. Br J Dermatol 66:429–433

Green LS, Saperia D, Lowe NJ, David M (1989) Coexistent psoriasis and lupus erythematosus: successful therapy with etretinate. J Derm Treatment 1:19–22

Gudat W, Bork K (1989) Hereditary angioedema associated with subacute cutaneous lupus erythematosus. Dermatologica 179:211–213

Hall-Smith SP (1955) Psoriasis and lupus erythematosus. Br J Dermatol 67:227–229

Hays SB, Camisa C, Luzar M (1984) The coexistence of systemic lupus erythematosus and psoriasis. J Am Acad Dermatol 10:619–622

Huang CY, Chen TC (1997) Bullous pemphigoid associated with systemic lupus erythematosus. Int J Dermatol 36:37–58

Isaacson D, Turner M, Elgart M (1981) Summertime actinic lichenoid eruption (lichen planus actinicus). J Am Acad Dermatol 4:404–411

Jordon RE, Muller SA, Hale WL (1969) Bullous pemphigoid associated with systemic lupus erythematosus. Arch Dermatol 99:17–25

Kanda N, Tsuchida T, Watanabe T, Tamaki K (1997) Cutaneous lupus mucinosis: a review of our cases and the possible pathogenesis. J Cutan Pathol 24:553–558

Katayama I, Teramoto N, Arai H, Nishioka K, Nishiyama S (1991) Annular erythema: a comparative study of Sjogren syndrome with subacute cutaneous lupus erythematosus. Int J Dermatol 30:635–639

Katz F, Fakete Z (1959) Simultaneous evolution of a subacute lupus erythematosus and of psoriasis. Arch Dermatol 80:584–587

Kobayashi T, Naka W, Harada T, Nishikawa T (1995) Association of the acral type of pustular psoriasis, Sjogren's syndrome, systemic lupus erythematosus, and Hashimoto's thiroiditis. J Dermatol 22:125–128

Kobayashi T, Shimitzu H, Shimitzu S, Harada T, Nishikawa T (1993) Plaquelike cutaneous lupus mucinosis. Arch Dermatol 129:383–384

Kocsard E (1974) Associated dermatoses and triggering factors in psoriasis. Australas J Dermatol 15:64–76

Kuchabal DS, Kuchabal SD, Pandit AM, Nashi HK (1998) Pemphigus vulgaris associated with systemic lupus erythematosus. Int J Dermatol 37:636–637

Kuhn A, Lehmann P, Goerz G (1995) Papulöse Muzinose bei subakut kutanem Lupus erythematodes. Z Hautkr 70:295–297

Kuhn A, Richter-Hintz D, Oslislo C, Ruzicka T, Megahed M, Lehmann P (2000) Lupus erythematosus tumidus – a neglected subset of cutaneous lupus erythematosus: report of 40 cases. Arch Dermatol 136:1033–1041

Kulick KB, Mogavero H, Provost TT, Reichlin M (1983) Serologic studies in patients with lupus erythematosus and psoriasis. J Am Acad Dermatol 8:631–634

Kumar V, Binder WL, Schotland E (1978) Coexistence of bullous pemphigoid and systemic lupus erythematosus. Arch Dermatol 114:1187–1190

Lau M, Kaufmann-Grunzinger I, Raghunath M (1991) A case report of a patient with features of systemic lupus erythematosus and linear IgA disease. Br J Dermatol 124:498–502

Lerchin E, Schwiner B (1975) Alopecia areata associated with discoid lupus erythematosus. Cutis 15:87–88

Levenstein MM, Fisher BK, Fisher LL, Pruzanski V (1991) Simultaneous occurrence of subacute cutaneous lupus erythematosus and Sweet syndrome. Int J Dermatol 30:640–644

Loche F, Bernard P, Bazex J (1998) Bullous pemphigoid associated with systemic lupus erythematosus. Br J Dermatol 139:927–928

Louste AC, Levy-Francel A, Cailliau A (1939) Lupus eryhtematéux et psoriasis. Bull Soc Fr Derm Syph 40:249–252

Lowe L, Rapini R, Golitz LE, Johnson TM (1992) Papulonodular mucinosis in lupus erythematosus. J Am Acad Dermatol 27:312–315

Lynch WS, Roenigk HS (1978) Lupus erythematosus and psoriasis vulgaris. Cutis 21: 511–525

Maruyama M, Miyauchi S, Hashimoto K (1997) Massive cutaneous mucinosis associated with systemic lupus erythematosus. Br J Dermatol 137:450–453

Marzano AV, Berti E, Gasparini G, Caputo R (1999) Lupus erythematosus with antiphospholipid syndrome and erythema multiforme-like lesions. Br J Dermatol 141:720–724

Miler JF, Downham TF, Chapel TA (1978) Coexistent bullous pemphigoid and systemic lupus erythematosus. Cutis 21:368–373

Millns JR, Muller SA (1980) The coexistence of psoriasis and lupus erythematosus. Arch Dermatol 116:658–663

Moncada B (1974) Dermatitis herpetiformis in association with systemic lupus erythematosus. Arch Dermatol 109:723–725

Moshella S (1989) Dermatologic overview of lupus erythematosus and its subsets. J Dermatol 46:417–428

Muller SA, Winkelmann RK (1963) Alopecia areata. Arch Dermatol 88:290–297

Nicolas JF, Mauduit G, Haond J, Chouvet B, Thivolet J (1988) Psoriasis grave induit par la chloroquine (Nivaquine). Ann Dermatol Venereol 115:298–293

Nishimoto M, Takaiwa T, Kodama H, Nohara N (1989) Cutaneous mucinosis associated with systemic lupus erythematosus – a case provoked by PUVA. J Dermatol 16:374–378

O'Leary PA (1927) Chronic lupus erythematosus disseminatus and psoriasis vulgaris. Arch Dermatol Syphiol 15:92–96

Olson K (1979) Pyoderma gangrenosum with systemic lupus erythematosus. Acta Derm Venereol (Stockh) 51:233–234

Parodi A, Drago EF, Varaldo G, Rebora A (1989) Rowell's syndrome. J Am Acad Dermatol 21:374–377

Peterson LL (1984) Hydralazine-induced systemic lupus erythematosus presenting as pioderma gangrenosum-like ulcers. J Am Acad Dermatol 10:379–384

Piamphongsant T, Sawannapreecha S, Arangson PG (1978) Mixed lichen planus – lupus erythematosus disease. J Cutan Pathol 5:209–215

Pinto GM, Cabecas MA, Riscado M, Goncales H (1991) Pyoderma gangrenosum associated with systemic lupus erythematosus. J Am Acad Dermatol 24:818–821

Plotnick H, Burnham TK (1986) Lichen planus and coexisting lupus erythematosus versus lichen planus – like lupus erythematosus. J Am Acad Dermatol. 14:931–938

Pramatarov K, Popova L, Konstantinov K (1983) Unusual variants of cutaneous lupus erythematosus Dermatol Venereol (Bulg) 4:25–30

Pramatarov K, Nikolova E, Mintcheva A (1988) Lichen ruber actinicus. Dermatol Venereol (Bulg) 3:57–60

Provost TT, Talal N, Harley GB (1988) The relationship between anti-Ro (SS-A) antibody-positive Sjogren's syndrome and anti-Ro (SS-A) antibody-positive lupus erythematosus. Arch Dermatol 124:62–71

Ramsey-Goldman R, Franz T, Solano FX (1990) Hydralazine-induced lupus and Sweet's syndrome. J Rheumatol 17:682–684

Razzaque Ahmed A, Schreiber P, Abramovits P (1982) Coexistence of lichen planus and systemic lupus erythematosus. J Am Acad Dermatol 7:478–483

Romero RW, Nesbitt LT, Reed RJ (1977) Unusual variant of lupus erythematosus or lichen planus. Clinical, histopathologic and immunofluorescence studies. Arch Dermatol 113:741–748

Rongioletti F, Rebora A (1986) Papular and nodular mucinosis associated with lupus erythematosus. Br J Dermatol 115:631–636

Rongioletti F, Rebora A (1991) The new cutaneous mucinoses: a review with an up-to-date classification of cutaneous mucinoses. J Am Acad Dermatol 24:265–270

Rongioletti F, Casciaro S, Boccaccio P, Rebora A (1990a) Annular pustular psoriasis and systemic lupus erythematosus. Int J Dermatol 290–292

Rongioletti F, Parodi A, Rebora A (1990b) Papular and nodular mucinosis as a sign of lupus erythematosus. Dermatologica 180:221–223

Rothe MJ, Grant-Kels JM, Rothfield NF (1990) Extensive calcinosis cutis with systemic lupus erythematosus. Arch Dermatol 126:1060–1063

Roustan G, Salas C, Barbadillo C, Sanchez Yus E, Mulero J, Simon A (2000) Lupus erythematosus with erythema multiforme-like eruption. Eur J Dermatol 10:459–462

Rowell NR, Swanson-Beck J, Anderson JR (1963) Lupus erythematosus and erythema multiforme-like lesions. Arch Dermatol 88:176–80

Ruzicka T, Faes J, Bergner T, Peter RU, Braun-Falco O (1995) Annular erythema associated with Sjogren's syndrome: a variant of systemic lupus erythematosus. J Am Acad Dermatol 25:557–560

Salomon T, Radovanovic V, Lazovic O (1977) Lichen myxoedematosus und lupus erythematodes. Hautarzt 28:148–151

Schaumann J (1928) Psoriasis et lupus erythemateux associes. Bull Soc Fr Derm Syph 35:278–282

Sequeira WI, Polisky RB, Alrenga DP (1986) Neutrophilic dermatosis association with a hydralazine-induced lupus syndrome. Am J Med 81:558–564

Shai A, Halevy S (1992) Lichen planus and lichen planus-like eruptions: pathogenesis and associated diseases. Int J Dermatol 31:379–384

Sharma RC, Sharma AK, Sharma NL (1998) Pseudo-ainhum in discoid lupus erythematosus. J Dermatol 25:275–276

Shteyngarts AR, Warner MR, Camisa C (1999) Lupus erythematosus associated with erythema multiforme: does Rowell syndrome exist? J Am Acad Dermatol 40:773–777

Sontheimer RD (1989) Subacute cutaneous lupus erythematosus: a decade's perspective. Med Clin North Am 73:1073–1090

Stavropoulos P, Tebbe B, Tenorio S, Orfanos C (1996) LE-associated squamous cell carcinoma. Eur J Dermatol 6:48–50

Stoll DM, King LE (1984) Association of bullous pemphigoid and systemic lupus erythematosus. Arch Dermatol 120:362–366

Szabo E, Husz S, Kovacz I (1981) Coexistent atypical bullous pemphigoid and systemic lupus erythematosus. Br J Dermatol 104:71–75

Thaipisuttikul Y, Piamphongsant T, Suwanela N (1983) Coexistence of linear IgA dermatitis herpetiformis and systemic lupus erythematosus. J Dermatol 10:161–166

Tsankov N, Stoimenov A, Lazarova A (1990) Psoriasis induit par la chloroquine chez un malade ayant un lupus erythemateux discoide. Rev Eur Dermatol MST 2:453–458

Tumarkin BM, Menshikova AK, Glavinskaya TA (1971) Some data on clinical pattern and course of discoid lupus erythematosus and of psoriasis when they occur simultaneously in patients. Vestn Dermatol Venerol Moskow 2:43–47

Ueki H (1994) Sjogren's Syndrome (personal communication)

Uitto J, Santa-Cruz DJ, Eisen AZ, Leone P (1978) Verrucous lesions in patients with discoid lupus erythematosus: clinical, histopathological and immunofluorescence studies. Br J Dermatol 98:507–520

Vandersteen PR, Fargo ND, Jordan RE (1974) Dermatitis herpetiformis with discoid lupus erythematosus. Occurrence of sulfone-induced discoid lupus erythematosus. Arch Dermatol 110:95–98

Venables P (1988) Sjogren's syndrome: differential diagnosis, immunopathology and genetics. Reports of rheumatic diseases (Series 2), N 10

Weatherhead L, Adam J (1985) Discoid lupus erythematosus: coexistence with porphyria cutanea tarda. Int J Dermatol 24:453–455

Weidner F, Djawari D (1982) Mucinosis papulosa bei Lupus erythematodes integumentalis. Hautarzt 33:286–288

Weigand DA, Burgdorf WHC, Gregg LJ (1981) Dermal mucinosis in discoid lupus erythematosus. Arch Dermatol 117:735–788

Werth VP, White WL, Sanchez MR, Franks AG (1992) Incidence of alopecia areata in lupus erythematosus. Arch Dermatol 128:368–371

Williams WL, Ramos-Caro F (1999) Acute periorbital mucinosis in discoid lupus erythematosus. J Am Acad Dermatol 41:871–873

Wlashev D, Pramatarov K, Tonev S, Abadjieva D, Marina S (1986) Psoriasis vulgaris et lupus erythematosus chronicus discoides. Dermatol Venereol (Sofia) 25:46–48

Wlotzke U (1996) Kutaner Lupus erythematodes mit Vitiligo. Z Hautkr 71:806–807

Wolfram S (1952) Über Porphyrinkolik: ein Beitrag zur Symptomatologie des Lupus erythematodes acutus. Hautarzt 3:298–300

Zalla MJ, Muller SA (1996). The coexistence of psoriasis with lupus erythematosus and other photosensitive disorders. Acta Derm Venereol (Suppl) 195:1–15

CHAPTER 11

Clinical Differential Diagnosis of Cutaneous Lupus Erythematosus

Florian Weber, Peter Fritsch

The cutaneous manifestations of lupus erythematosus (LE) are notoriously diverse and may mimic a broad range of unrelated skin disorders, although many of its skin symptoms are straightforward and pose few diagnostic problems. Clinical differential diagnosis has a place in directing the dermatologist toward the correct diagnosis in the primary screening process. This chapter summarizes the diagnostic considerations at this point, before additional diagnostic procedures are carried out. Of course, a definite diagnosis of LE must be based on the whole of the clinical appearance, history, and the histopathologic, immunofluorescent, laboratory, and, occasionally, phototesting findings (see the respective sections of this book). Obviously, no reference to these investigational procedures are made in this chapter.

The main building blocks that make up the cutaneous lesions of LE are the classic triad of erythema, scaling, and atrophy. The relative weight of these elements, however, is subject to variation according to the type of LE (chronic cutaneous, subacute cutaneous, and systemic), the age and location of the lesions, and the presence of additional morphologic features (e. g., hypertrophy, adipose tissue involvement, and mucopolysaccharide accumulation). Erythema, epidermal thickening and scaling, and atrophy and scarring represent a clinical and dynamic continuum along which all lesions of cutaneous LE (CLE) develop; only the chronic discoid type, however, may go all the way, whereas the other types hold in earlier stages. For this reason, there is a considerable morphological overlap between all types of CLE, and many differential diagnostic considerations pertain to more than one or all types of LE, as will be seen below.

According to an old saying, LE and syphilis are the "great imitators" among the skin diseases. We tried to list only reasonable and practically useful differential diagnoses and may have missed a few less appropriate ones. It must also be borne in mind that erythema, scaling, and atrophy are fairly common cutaneous features. Single LE lesions, particularly fresh ones, may thus be totally indistinguishable from single lesions of a score of other dermatoses; only in the frame of the clinical appearance as a whole does the diagnosis appear obvious and unmistakable. We tried to satisfy both aspects in this chapter.

As the structural framework for differential diagnoses, we used the accepted classification of LE as laid down in the textbooks of dermatology (Braun-Falco et al. 1997, Champion et al. 1998, Fitzpatrick et al. 1999, Fritsch 1998).

Discoid Lupus Erythematosus

Classic Appearance

Discoid LE (DLE) (Kaposi 1872) is the most common variant of CLE. It typically (but not exclusively) evolves at light-exposed skin: face, ears, extensor aspects of the forearms, scalp, trunk, and, more rarely, the oral mucosa. Lesions are single or sparse in most cases; if numerous disseminated lesions are present, they are haphazardly distributed at the predilection sites without striking symmetry. Among multiple lesions, many are found in the butterfly area (see later herein), and some tend to appear in unusual places, for example, the "niches" of the external ear, the eyelids, the lips, or the vestibule of the nose; there is a tendency not to transgress natural border lines, for example, the vermilion border of the lip or the areola mammae.

Lesions evolve according to a characteristic time course. Fresh lesions first present as small, round, well-defined, slightly raised erythemas with dull surfaces that soon become rough to the touch and scaly. Scales are adherent and are often attached to the hair follicles ("carpet tack" phenomenon). Follicular orifices are first widened with keratotic plugs and may then disappear completely; there is a gradual loss of hair in the lesions, leading to irreversible scarring alopecia. Lesions spread slowly and regress at the centers, which become smooth and sunken. Intermediate lesions become elevated and indurated at variable degrees and develop atrophy and loss of normal skin texture in their centers. At the periphery, rests of the active lesion remain as ring-like, arcuate, or polycyclic scaly erythemas that continue to spread. Old (burnt-out) lesions may be disfiguring: they are large, with irregular borders, sharply demarcated, depigmented (porcelain white in dark skin), hairless, flat, thin, and with a scarring appearance. Pitted scars and crateriform indentations may occur. In acral location (e. g., nose and ears), there may be a loss of tissue (mutilation).

It is important to note that the lesions differ in their individual ages; fresh lesions will thus be seen alongside intermediate and burnt-out ones. Activity of lesions may spontaneously cease at all stages; fresh lesions may heal with restitutio ad integrum, older ones result in atrophy.

Differential Diagnosis

Fresh Discoid Lupus Erythematosus Lesions
Before central atrophy develops, fresh lesions present as homogenous scaly erythemas. As such, they may resemble a wide spectrum of unrelated disorders.

Actinic keratoses (Fig. 11.1A), as individual lesions, may mimic DLE, especially if flat and inflamed; as a distinguishing mark, they are rougher than DLE lesions and hyperkeratotic rather than scaly (keratotic masses do not detach). At the clinical overview, however, actinic keratoses differ from DLE lesions by their usually smaller size, greater number, and more regular distribution owing to their tendency to concentrate at the sites of the highest cumulative UV damage (forehead, nose, bald head, etc). In addition, patients with actinic keratoses are usually much older than those with DLE (25–45 years), and their facial skin shows signs of chronic actinic damage.

Bowen's disease (Fig. 11.1B) is most often a solitary lesion that may be located anywhere on the body, including light-exposed areas. It may look similar to a DLE lesion;

it is less inflamed, however, and its surface is velvety and occasionally hyperkeratotic. There is no scaling.

In *psoriasis vulgaris,* again, individual psoriatic plaques may be similar to DLE, especially fresh lesions and those of the photosensitive type. Psoriatic plaques are round and well demarcated; their scales, however, are large, silvery, and easily detachable. They do not lead to hair loss or epidermal atrophy. At the clinical overview, psoriasis differs from DLE by its exanthematic distribution and its totally different predilection sites. Also, psoriatic plaques of the face are rare. As antimalarials can aggravate psoriasis, psoriasis should be ruled out before treatment of DLE is started.

Again, individual patches of *seborrheic dermatitis* may resemble fresh DLE lesion because they are well-demarcated, scaly erythemas most often on the face. They differ, however, by their color (light yellow–red) and the type of scaling (small, branny, easily detachable, greasy). At the clinical overview, seborrheic dermatitis is strikingly symmetrical (lesions on and bordering the eyebrows, glabella, nasolabial folds, and V-shaped areas of the chest and the back). Also, it is usually accompanied by seborrheic dermatitis of the scalp. History usually reveals that the condition is chronic, with exacerbations in winter and improvement in the warm season. Importantly, sun exposure can aggravate seborrheic dermatitis, as is also the case in DLE.

Discoid Lupus Erythematosus Lesions of Intermediate Age

At this stage, central atrophy becomes apparent, and active sectors of the lesion appear as annular or semicircular peripheral erythemas (Fig. 11.1C). *DLE lesions of the scalp* usually belong to this category (see below).

Superficial dermatophytic infections typically present as nummular lesions with raised erythematous, scaly borders and central clearing. Annular and semicircular lesions are often found. In contrast to DLE, there is no atrophy. In adults, superficial mycoses are mainly found in the context of tinea pedis and in the inguinal folds and only exceptionally on the trunk or face. Children are much more prone to develop superficial mycoses of the face, but they only rarely develop DLE. Potassium hydroxide examination of scales will quickly reveal the etiology.

Erythema arcuatum, the superficial variant of granuloma annulare, is characterized by stable, erythematous, slightly infiltrated annular lesions predominantly of the upper trunk. In contrast to DLE, the lesions are quite large, the erythematous rings display no scaling, and the centers are nonatrophic.

Erythema annulare centrifugum lesions may be somewhat reminiscent of DLE but they are predominantly located at the trunk and do not exhibit central atrophy, and their elevated borders typically show collerette-like scaling that is nonadherent and localized to the interior slope of the margin. Also, erythema annulare is not stable but is characterized by slow migration.

Superficial basal cell carcinoma may occasionally somewhat resemble DLE. It is usually located on the trunk, may display an atrophic center, and is reddish owing to the presence of telangiectasias. In contrast to DLE lesions, it is not too well defined and has a raised border of translucent peripheral papules (which may be not very conspicuous). Scaling, if present, is scant.

Old (burnt-out) Lesions of Discoid Lupus Erythematosus

Long lasting DLE lesions are dominated by atrophy, scarring, and depigmentation.

Atrophic scars may be indistinguishable from burnt-out DLE, lacking any signs of inflammation, particularly depigmented scars after superficial third-degree burns. Atrophic acne scars differ by their multiplicity and characteristic distribution. They are not accompanied by pigmentary changes in white skin. The characteristically depressed scars after cutaneous leishmaniosis, in contrast, are hyperpigmented. In all instances, the borders of the scars must be carefully inspected to detect residual rims of scaling erythemas, which would be a clue for DLE.

Lesions of vitiligo may closely resemble burnt-out DLE, with regular and only mildly altered surface texture because of its round shape and circular outlines. Lesions must be carefully examined for minimal signs of scarring. At the clinical overview, vitiligo is characterized by its larger lesions and its predilection for periorificial location.

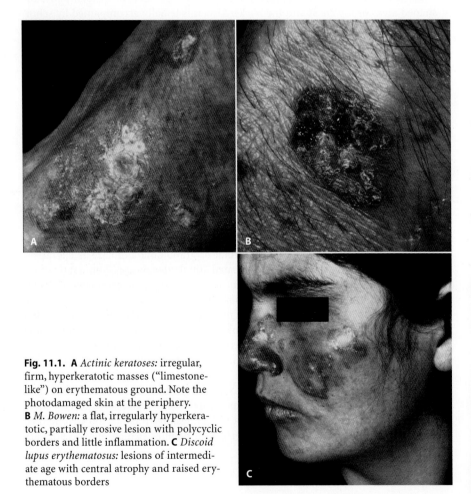

Fig. 11.1. A *Actinic keratoses:* irregular, firm, hyperkeratotic masses ("limestone-like") on erythematous ground. Note the photodamaged skin at the periphery.
B *M. Bowen:* a flat, irregularly hyperkeratotic, partially erosive lesion with polycyclic borders and little inflammation. **C** *Discoid lupus erythematosus:* lesions of intermediate age with central atrophy and raised erythematous borders

Hypopigmented lesions of tuberculous leprosy differ by their ill-defined borders; the presence of residual pigmentation, scaling, and faint erythema; and loss of sensory function.

Lupus vulgaris in advanced stages may show similarity with scarring lesions of DLE. Whereas fresh lesions of lupus vulgaris are characterized by reddish brown macules and patches of soft and friable consistency that display a typical "apple-jelly" color on diascopy, more advanced lesions may exhibit considerable atrophy and scarring. As a distinguishing mark, remnants of tuberculous granulation tissue are often found at the periphery and in the centers; if probed, the instrument tends to break through the overlying skin. Moreover, lupus vulgaris has a tendency to ulcerate, which is very uncommon in DLE, and depigmentation is absent. A common feature of lupus vulgaris and DLE is mutilation of acral sites, for example, ear lobes or nose, which was the historical reason to apply the term "lupus" to both.

Coral reef keratoakanthomas may imitate old DLE lesions, with pronounced scarring and irregular, "moth-eaten" change of the surface texture. These low-grade malignancies are characterized by their large and round size, their location in sun-exposed skin areas, and their elevated borders. In their early stage, they display multiple keratotic plugs that are larger than the follicular plugs of DLE.

Differential Diagnosis at Particular Sites

Discoid Lupus Erythematosus of the Scalp

DLE of the scalp (Fig. 11.2A) typically arises as one or a few roundish erythematous plaques identical to DLE lesions elsewhere on the skin. When atrophy develops, they gradually transform into patches of scarring alopecia that may be surrounded by rims of scaly erythema. In the early phase, it must be distinguished from psoriasis and seborrheic dermatitis (see previously herein). In advanced stages, DLE may

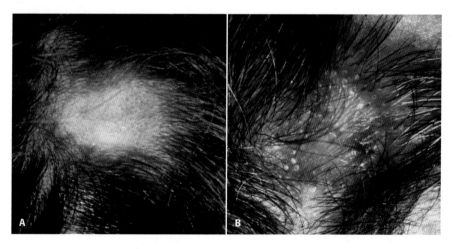

Fig. 11.2. A Atrophic alopecia in *discoid lupus erythematosus*. Note the widened erythematous follicular openings between flattened atrophic areas. **B** *Lichen ruber planopilaris*: confluent small areas of atrophic skin with interspersed unaffected hair-bearing follicles

resemble all other instances of scarring alopecia. One important mark is that DLE of the scalp is often accompanied by analogous lesions of the face.

Lichen planopilaris (Fig. 11.2B) of the scalp is characterized by very small (2–3 mm) hairless atrophic areas that, by partial confluence, may occupy larger areas, particularly in the central scalp regions, a distribution pattern reminiscent of lichen planus lesions of the skin. The atrophic areas are smooth, devoid of follicular orifices, and skin colored (because the inflammatory infiltrate is not located at the interfollicular epidermis but around the hair follicles) but may display a subtle violaceous hue at the periphery. Characteristically, tufts of normal hairs emerge from between the alopecic areas, resulting in an irregular, "moth-eaten" appearance.

Linear morphea (coup de sabre) is an easy clinical diagnosis. It is characterized by a single linear paramedian band of depressed sclerodermatous skin that adheres to the deep fascia and even the bone. Erythema and scaling is usually absent, and hair loss develops as a late event.

Folliculitis decalvans, which in its active stages can hardly be confused with DLE because of its pustules and crusts, eventually leads to cicatricial alopecia, which is morphologically similar to that of lichen planopilaris (small areas of alopecia intermingled with tufts of normal hair, most often in the parietal and occipital areas). Similar hairless scars, although less extensive, may arise from furuncles and *trichophytic infections* (*Kerion Celsi* type).

Noninflammatory and *epidemic types of tinea capitis* (*microsporia*) begin with small erythemas or erythematous papules around hair follicles that subsequently spread centrifugally like DLE lesions of the scalp. In contrast to DLE, these lesions tend to be multiple, show little inflammation at early stages, and occur almost exclusively in children. Typically, hairs do not fall out but break close to the skin surface, and residual scarring is minimal. In contrast, scarring is pronounced in the favus type of tinea capitis. This rare type of mycosis can be distinguished from DLE by its typical focal crusting and scaling ("scutula").

Discoid Lupus Erythematosus of the Oral Mucosa

DLE of the oral mucosa is not an infrequent finding. It begins as one or a few round, well-demarcated erythematous plaques with patchy and streaky white hyperkeratosis, most often of the buccal mucosa, the (lower) lips, and the hard palate, that often turn into erosions and even ulcers. Lesions tend to be symptomless. Involvement of the conjunctival mucosa occurs much less often and may lead to ectropium and scarring (differential diagnoses: *cicatricial pemphigoid, chlamydial conjunctivitis, and basal cell carcinoma*).

Lichen planus is set apart from mucosal DLE by its greater extent, its symmetrical distribution, and its (at least in part) reticulated appearance. Patients with mucosal lichen planus commonly exhibit lichen planus of the skin as well. *Erosive lichen planus* is usually accompanied by lesions of classic oral lichen planus. Erosions are often extensive, superficial, covered with fibrin, with irregular outlines, and painful. The sites most often involved are the buccal mucosa, the lateral aspects of the tongue, and the lip mucosa.

Plane leukoplakias are hyperkeratotic plaques of the mucosa, with regular outlines and a tylotic appearance, that are most often caused by chronic frictional trauma. The cause of the lesion is usually obvious, for example, ill-fitting dentures. Plane leukoplakias are not or are only minimally inflamed. *Premalignant leukoplakias* have an irregular outline and an irregular, at times verrucous, surface; they progress to squamous cell carcinomas, which may first appear as irregular red erosions (often localized to the floor of the oral cavity).

Recurrent aphthous ulcers of the oral mucosa have a typical morphology: they represent most often small, round, and multiple ulcers covered by a white slough of fibrin and debris, usually bounded by an erythematous rim. Clinical differential diagnosis of a single lesion from DLE may be difficult, but the history of frequent recurrences, painfulness, and spontaneous clearing within days facilitate the diagnosis.

Discoid Lupus Erythematosus of the Palms and Soles

DLE of the palms and soles is a rare occurrence characterized by sharply demarcated erythemas and adherent scaling; the lesions tend to be painful and may become erosive. Atrophy and scarring are the features that allow a distinction from the following:

Palmoplantar psoriasis has no signs of atrophy. Note that palmoplantar psoriasis is only rarely an isolated finding.

Keratoderma blennorhagicum in patients with Reiter's disease presents with psoriasiform palmoplantar lesions composed of erythemas, erosions, crusting, and hyperkeratosis. In contrast to DLE, hyperkeratosis and inflammation may be marked and extend over the whole surface of the palms and soles.

Porokeratosis plantaris and palmaris may be similar to palmoplantar DLE because it presents as relatively small, multiple, sharply demarcated annular lesions with a hyperkeratotic peripheral ridge (cornoid lamella) and central atrophy. Palmoplantar porokeratosis is transmitted as an autosomal-dominant trait.

Special Manifestations

Hypertrophic Discoid Lupus Erythematosus

Hypertrophic DLE usually presents as a solitary, raised, indurated, hyperkeratotic lesion, most often of the face or the extensor surfaces of the extremities. It is not a very characteristic type of lesion, and the diagnosis is often made histologically. Clinical differential diagnoses include hypertrophic lichen planus (usually multiple lesions, location on the extremities, often accompanied by classic lichen planus, extremely itchy), hypertrophic psoriasis (usually exanthematic), nodular prurigo (which is also intensively pruritic), with multiple lesions in a characteristic distribution (trunk and shoulders; only those regions are involved that can be reached by the scratching finger). Particularly in elderly people, squamous cell carcinoma and keratoacanthoma must be considered.

Lupus Erythematosus Profundus

LE profundus (LEP) is an inflammatory condition involving the subcutaneous adipose tissue (lupus panniculitis) and presenting with deep cutaneous and subcutaneous nodules (Kaposi 1883, Irgang 1940). Lesions are usually multiple and symmetrically distributed on the upper arms and face. Lupus panniculitis may arise in association with both DLE and SLE. In the first, lesions tend to be few in number, noninflammatory, firm, attached to the skin, and not painful; they resolve by forming deeply indented atrophic scars, calcification, and lipoatrophy. The epidermis above these lesions may be normal or show DLE lesions (Kaposi-Irgang type of LE profundus). If associated with SLE, panniculitis lesions are more numerous, inflamed, and tender; there are systemic symptoms; and the lesions are clinically indistinguishable from other instances of *lobular panniculitis* (*idiopathic lobular panniculitis, pancreatic panniculitis, panniculitis of alpha1 antitrypsin deficiency*); they end up in similar deeply indented lipoatrophic scars.

Firm, deep-seated nodules of LEP must be distinguished from benign subcutaneous tumors such as *schwannoma* and *pilomatrixoma* (calcifying epithelioma of Malherbe). Both usually occur in childhood and as solitary lesions (ultrasound investigation allows differentiation of these and LEP). *Insulin- or corticosteroid-induced fat atrophy* may resemble burnt-out LE profundus (history).

Lupus Erythematosus Tumidus

LE tumidus (LET) is a probably not so infrequent variety of CLE that is defined histopathologically by LE-type dermal inflammation, accumulation of mucin, and the absence of epidermal involvement (Kuhn et al. 2003). Clinically, it corresponds to erythematous discoid lesions most often of the face (zygomatic area) that are persistent and without a tendency for atrophy and scarring (Kuhn et al. 2000). Lymphocytic infiltration Jessner-Kanof is defined practically in the same way (Jessner and Kanof, 1953), and many authors argue that these conditions are identical (Ackerman 1997, Weber et al. 2001). Phototesting revealed a high incidence of photosensitivity with a distinct time course profile that was common to both conditions but different from polymorphous light eruption (Kuhn et al. 2001).

Plaque-type sarcoidosis may be clinically similar to LET because it features elevated, smooth-surfaced discoid lesions most often located on the face, scalp, upper trunk, and arms. In contrast to LET, they exhibit a brownish "apple-jelly" color under diascopy.

Plaque-like lesions of *polymorphous light eruption (PLE)* are both clinically and histopathologically similar to LET, and in both a history of photosensitivity is typically found. There are clinical differences, however: LET presents as a solitary or a few persistent nonitchy lesions, especially of the zygomatic area; polymorphous light eruption, in contrast, with multiple itchy lesions, particularly of the sun-exposed areas of the upper extremities, and decolleté, which regress spontaneously within a few days. In the same line, PLE usually arises within 24 hours of sun exposure, whereas LET appears 2–5 days after phototesting (Weber et al. 2001). One should keep in mind, however, that photosensitivity of the PLE type is also found in SLE.

Granuloma faciale is another skin disorder that closely resembles LET. It presents as well-demarcated, elevated, asymptomatic, and persistent nodules and plaques, mostly in the faces of middle-aged patients. Granuloma faciale is usually a solitary lesion.

Subacute Cutaneos Lupus Erythematosus

Differential Diagnosis

Subacute CLE (SCLE) is an exanthematic skin condition with a typical clinical appearance (diagnosis can often be made before the presence of Ro/SSA antibodies is documented) that is localized at the trunk and the extensor aspects of the upper extremities, more rarely in the face and neck (Sontheimer et al. 1979). Lesions have an intermediate morphology between DLE and SLE: they are erythematous flat plaques, much thinner than DLE, with some dry scaling but without adherent scales and hyperkeratotic follicular plaques. There is a tendency for central regression (which often results in annular lesions), but there is no full-blown atrophy or scarring and depigmentation (Fig. 11.3A). Patients with SCLE only rarely have systemic symptoms, but there is a clear history of photosensitivity.

Psoriasis (Fig. 11.3B) is the skin disorder that most closely resembles SCLE. The size, nummular shape, and color of the individual lesions may be quite comparable, but the predilection sites are different (SCLE has no lesions on the knees, elbows, scalp, and sacral areas), as are the types of scaling (psoriasiform vs small and thin lamellar) and the presence of slight (mostly central) atrophy in SCLE.

Fig. 11.3. A Annular *subacute cutaneous lupus erythematosus* lesions. Except for their slight central atrophy, almost indistinguishable from annular psoriasis (**B**). **C** *Erythema annulare centrifugum:* no epidermal involvement (scaling and atrophy)

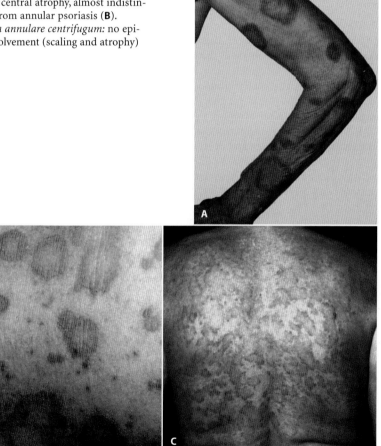

Pityriasis rosea differs from SCLE by its acute onset, its more inflammatory character, its typical distribution on the trunk ("christmas tree-like"), and its peripheral collerette-like scaling.

Tinea corporis and *superficial trichomycosis* may be confused with SCLE because they represent annular lesions with a peripheral erythematous scaly margin. Differences are in that the mycotic infections rarely arise in an exanthematic fashion on the trunk (except in immunodeficient individuals), and they are pruritic. Potassium hydroxide preparations quickly resolve diagnostic problems.

Erythema annulare centrifugum (Fig. 11.3C; see above) and other figurated erythemas may clinically (and histopathologically) look similar to SCLE, and indeed they have been equated with this disorder by some authors (Ruzicka et al. 1991). They lack epidermal involvement, however, except of some cases of erythema annulare centrifugum that exhibit a distinctive pattern of scaling at the inner slope of the erythematous margin.

Granuloma annulare, especially the superficial generalized variant (see previously herein) may show some similarity to SCLE; likewise, there is no epidermal involvement.

Neonatal LE (NLE) is caused by maternal Ro/SSA antibodies and therefore shares many features with SCLE: well-demarcated, annular skin lesions with little tendency for atrophy arising in mainly light-exposed areas (photosensitivity) and combined with anemia and heart block. This transient LE syndrome must be distinguished from *seborrheic dermatitis,* which is also found in the first months of life but shows a predilection for the scalp (where it is more desquamative than NLE) and the intertriginous regions (where it is more inflammatory and at times oozing). NLE is further distinguished by larger, stable polycyclic lesions with moderate central atrophy.

Differential diagnosis of neonatal NLE also includes *atopic dermatitis,* which usually sets in at a later time and presents as a more widespread eruption with predilection of the face, extremities, and intertriginous areas. There is pruritus and skin irritability. Neonatal *psoriasis* may look similar to neonatal LE, but it lacks annular patterns and central atrophy.

Systemic Lupus Erythematosus

Differential Diagnosis

Skin lesions of SLE are manifold and often quite characteristic. Most of the cutaneous symptoms are erythematous lesions without or with only mild epidermal involvement (scaling, atrophy, etc): malar erythema (butterfly rash), morbilliform macular rashes, circumscribed erythemas. A second and less frequent morphologic component consists of bullous or ulcerative lesions. Differential diagnosis in SLE is not dominated by the morphology of the cutaneous lesions but by systemic symptoms and laboratory data.

Butterfly Rash
The "butterfly rash" or "malar rash", a proverbial "diagnostic" lesion of SLE, is most often seen in early SLE (Dubois et al. 1964). It is composed of (at least partially) well-

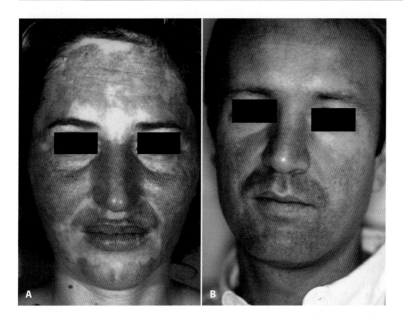

Fig. 11.4. A Butterfly rash in *systemic lupus erythematosus.* A well-demarcated, symmetrical erythema of the malar areas and the back of the nose that has progressed to the forehead and perioral skin. Note the sparing of the nasolabial folds. **B** *Seborrheic dermatitis:* note the yellowish color and involvement of the nasolabial folds

demarcated symmetrical erythemas (and edema) of the malar areas that are connected over the bridge of the nose and thus result in a butterfly-like shape. The forehead and chin may be affected, and the nasolabial folds are characteristically spared (Fig. 11.4A). If the malar rash persists for some time, scales and mild atrophy may develop.

Dermatomyositis may show an analogous erythema of the face ("heliotropic erythema") that may be difficult to distinguish (an encompassing term, "erysipelas perstans," has therefore been coined by the old dermatologists). Typically, the heliotropic erythema is more pronounced in the upper portions of the face (forehead and eyelids), is more edematous, is of a more violaceous color, and not well demarcated. Differential diagnosis may be complicated by muscle weakness and elevated serum muscle enzyme levels, which may be seen in both entities.

Erysipelas of the face is a classic differential diagnosis of the butterfly rash. The main distinguishing marks are its acute onset, asymmetrical distribution pattern, more intensive inflammatory character, regional lymphadenitis, and systemic signs.

Drug-induced phototoxic reactions may be indistinguishable from the butterfly rash of SLE, but they are accompanied by analogous lesions of other exposed body sites in most instances. A history of potentially photosensitizing drugs must be taken (tetracyclines, nonsteroidal anti-inflammatory drugs, amiodarone, phenothiazines, diuretics, sulfonamides, and psoralens).

Seborrheic dermatitis (Fig. 11.4B), *rosacea,* and *perioral dermatitis* are trivial dermatoses that are not always easy to distinguish from facial lesions of SLE; this is less true for the butterfly rash than for cases of advanced SLE. In these, indistinct erythema and erythematous papules of the face may develop (more often with female patients who more generously apply various ointments on their facial lesions). Distinguishing criteria are the absence of prominent telangiectasias and pustules; absence of inflammatory papules in the perioral regions; absence of seborrhea of the scalp and face; and absence of the yellowish color of seborrheic dermatitis.

DLE lesions may be arranged in the butterfly area, mimicking a chronic butterfly rash.

Maculopapular Exanthemas

Generalized exanthemas of SLE may appear as transitory indistinct morbilliform macular rashes that regress after hours or days and may wax and wane parallel to disease activity; they may persist, however, and transform into more stable macular lesions that are well demarcated, are slightly hypertrophic and scaly, and somewhat resemble the lesions of SCLE. Some may acquire annular shapes or a tylotic morphology (e. g., chilblain lupus). All exanthemas of SLE, except the morbilliform rashes, are situated in the light-exposed areas (face, V region of the neck, extensor surfaces of the arms, wrists, and dorsa of the fingers). Following regression, they leave no atrophy or depigmentation (rather, hyperpigmentation in dark skin). Macular eruptions are clinically much less characteristic than the stable lesions.

Macular drug eruptions and *viral exanthemas* may be morphologically indistinguishable except for the clear predilection of SLE exanthemas for light-exposed areas. Also, SLE exanthemas lack the characteristic symptoms associated with some viral eruptions (such as lymphadenopathy, "catarrhalic" rhinitis and conjunctivitis in rubella, Koplik spots in measles). Constitutional symptoms (fever, malaise, and arthralgias) are little contributory for differential diagnosis because they may occur in all; moreover, episodes of SLE may be precipitated by viral infections, and the respective symptoms may occur simultaneously or in short succession.

Erythema annulare centrifugum may mimic stable lesions of SLE (see previously herein).

Acral maculopapular lesions of dermatomyositis resemble acral maculopapular lesions of SLE. Both appear as reddish and slightly elevated scaly papules of the dorsa of the fingers; there is a peculiar and unexplained difference, however, in that the lesions of dermatomyositis are localized over the interphalangeal joints and spare the skin in between, whereas the opposite is true for the lesions of SLE. Also, those of dermatomyositis are more elevated and hyperkeratotic; nailfold erythemas, telangiectasias, and hemorrhage may occur in both conditions but are more pronounced in dermatomyositis.

Acral vasculitic skin lesions in SLE present as flat, erythematous palmoplantar painful plaques or nodules and resemble *chilblains* ("chilblain lupus"). These lesions are also typically found in LE-like syndromes of *C2* or *C4 deficiency*.

Bullous and Ulcerative Lesions of Systemic Lupus Erythematosus

Vesicle formation and erosions or ulcers are infrequent manifestations of severe SLE (Thivolet et al. 1969). They occur most often as ulcers of the oral mucosa in the course of acute SLE; differential diagnosis includes aphthous stomatitis and erosive lichen planus (see previously herein). Ulcers may arise in the nasal vestible and potentially lead to perforations of the nasal septum (differential diagnosis: *Wegener´s granulomatosis*).

Nonspecific Skin Lesions in Patients with Systemic Lupus Erythematosus

A spectrum of other skin symptoms that are not LE proper may accompany SLE. By definition, these lesions can be found in other diseases as well, but they do have diagnostic significance.

Vascular lesions play a dominant role. *Raynaud's phenomenon* occurs frequently in SLE, as it does in other collagen vascular diseases. *Leukocytoclastic vasculitis* may arise, often associated with periods of increased disease activity; it may present as cutaneous necrotizing vasculitis (palpable purpura) or as urticarial vasculitis, less often as arteritis, with symptoms similar to polyarteritis nodosa. Thrombophlebitis and thrombotic vessel damage is seen particularly in patients with secondary antiphospholipid syndrome, leading to *livedo reticularis* or *acral cyanosis* or *necrosis*. Thrombocytopenia may cause *thrombocytopenic purpura*. Similar to patients with dermatomyositis, patients with SLE often show *nailfold erythema, telangiectasia, or hemorrhage*. Characteristic nonspecific signs are thin, brittle hair with an "uncombed" appearance, referred to as *woolly* or *lupus hair,* and *telogen effluvium*.

References

Ackerman AB (1997) Tumid lupus erythematosus. In: Ackerman AB, Congchitnant N, Sanchez J, Guo Y (eds) Histologic diagnosis of inflammatory skin diseases. Williams & Wilkins, Baltimore, p 529

Braun-Falco O, Plewig G, Wolf HH (1997) Dermatologie und Venerologie. Springer, Berlin, Heidelberg, New York

Champion RH, Burton JL, Ebling FJG (1998) Textbook of dermatology. Blackwell Science, Oxford

Dubois EL, Tuffanelli DL (1964) Clinical manifestations of systemic lupus erythemosus. JAMA 190:104–111

Fitzpatrick TB (1999) Dermatology in general medicine. In: Freedberg IM, Eisen AZ, Wolff K, Austen KF, Goldsmith LA, Katz SE, Fitzpatrick TB (eds) Dermatology in general medicine. McGraw-Hill, New York

Fritsch P (1998) Dermatologie und Venerologie. Springer-Verlag, Berlin

Irgang S (1940) Lupus erythematosus profundus: report of an example with clinical resemblance to Darier-Roussy sarcoid. Arch Dermatol Syph 42:97–108

Jessner M, Kanof NB (1953) Lymphocytic infiltration of the skin. Arch Dermatol 68:447–449

Kaposi M (1872) Neue Beiträge zur Kenntnis des Lupus erythematodes. Arch Dermatol Syphil 4:36–78

Kaposi M (1883) Pathologie und Therapie der Hautkrankheiten. Urban & Schwarzenberg, Vienna, p 642

Kuhn A, Richter-Hintz D, Oslislo C, Ruzicka T, Megahed M, Lehmann P (2000) Lupus erythematosus tumidus – a neglected subset of cutaneous lupus erythematosus: report of 40 cases. Arch Dermatol 136:1033–1041

Kuhn A, Sonntag M, Richter-Hintz D, Oslislo C, Megahed M, Ruzicka T, Lehmann P (2001) Phototesting in lupus erythematosus tumidus: review of 60 patients. Photochem Photobiol 73:532–536

Kuhn A, Sonntag M, Ruzicka T, Lehmann P, Megahed M (2003) Histopathologic findings in lupus erythematosus tumidus: review of 80 patients. J Am Acad Dermatol 48:901–908

Ruzicka T, Faes J, Bergner T, Peter RU, Braun-Falco O (1991) Annular erythema associated with Sjogren's syndrome: a variant of systemic lupus erythematosus. J Am Acad Dermatol 25:557–560

Sontheimer RD, Thomas JR, Gillilam JN (1979) Subacute cutaneous lupus erythematosus: a cutaneous marker for a distinct lupus erythematosus subset. Arch Dermatol 115:1409–1415

Thivolet J, Perrot H, Beyvin AJ, Preumy H, Storch J (1969) Cutaneous bullous evolution during acute disseminated lupus erythematosus. Bull Soc Fr Dermatol Syphil 76:374–377

Weber F, Schmuth M, Fritsch P, Sepp N (2001) Lymphocytic infiltration of the skin is a photo-sensitive variant of lupus erythematosus: evidence by phototesting. Br J Dermatol 144: 292–296

CHAPTER 12

Photosensitivity in Lupus Erythematosus 12

Percy Lehmann, Annegret Kuhn

Photosensitivity is a characteristic feature of all forms and subsets of lupus erythematosus (LE) that has been recognized since the first phenomenologic descriptions of this complex disease. In 1881, Cazénave (Cazénave 1881) described exacerbations of the disease related to "cold, heat, fire, and direct action of the air", and Hutchinson (Hutchinson 1888) reported in 1888 that patients with LE did not tolerate the sun well. At the beginning of the 19th century, several physicians had already realized that environmental factors, such as sun exposure, play a role in the induction of LE (Pusey 1915, Macleod 1924, Freund 1929). Pusey (Pusey 1915) described in 1915 a young lady who had her first outbreak of cutaneous LE (CLE) a few days after extensive golfing in the summertime. The lesions disappeared after strict avoidance of the sun, but another exacerbation occurred during the next summer, again after a golf tournament. In 1929, Freund (Freund 1929) could clearly demonstrate in a large series of patients with LE ($n=507$), which he followed between 1920 and 1927, that inductions and exacerbations of this disease showed significant clustering in the spring and summer months. In agreement with earlier observations by Haxthausen from Kopenhagen, he concluded that the increasing intensity of ultraviolet (UV) irradiation in spring and summer was responsible for the deterioration and outbreak of LE. In the same year, Fuhs (Fuhs 1929) described a specifically sun-sensitive form of LE, which occurred in a 27-year-old woman. For 10 years he had regularly observed a subacute onset of the erythematosquamous lesions in the springtime subsequent to the first periods of sunny weather, and he termed this exquisitely photosensitive subset "LE subacutus".

Whereas these and other observations delineated natural physical agents as triggering factors in LE, artificial light sources were also already recognized as causative inductors of specific LE symptoms by the second decade of the 20th century. Jesionek (Jesionek 1916), a German pioneer of phototherapy, wrote in 1916 the "guidelines for the modern applications of phototherapy". He enthusiastically described several skin diseases that responded excellently to phototherapy. In contrast, he cautioned not to irradiate patients with LE, since he had observed deterioration of the disease on irradiation, and he even described two patients with discoid LE (DLE) who developed systemic manifestations of the disease after having been irradiated with therapeutic artificial lamps. Subsequently, the induction of skin lesions by artificial lamps in patients with LE was reported in a lecture delivered to the Royal Danish Medical Association. In 1929, Fuhs (Fuhs 1929) was the first to perform experimental light testing with different wavelengths to characterize the UV sensitivity in a patient with a photosensitive form of LE. He could demonstrate a high sensitivity toward unfiltered quartz lamps but was unable to determine further wavelength-dependent sensitivity by using different filters in these early phototesting experiments.

The appearance of suntanning parlors in the past decades led to the occurrence of inductions and exacerbations of LE by artificial irradiation units that were not medically controlled but run by commercially oriented individuals. Several reports on such events have been published, such as by Stern and Drocken (Stern and Drocken 1986) and Tronnier et al. (Tronnier et al. 1988), who described the outbreak of severe systemic LE (SLE) after the visits to suntanning parlors. Today it is generally accepted that natural and artificial UV irradiation can induce and exacerbate LE and, furthermore, that it may exert specific effects on the complex pathophysiology of this disease.

Pathophysiology of Photosensitivity in Lupus Erythematosus

Since clinical data, phototesting procedures, and experimental evidence have demonstrated the detrimental effects of sun irradiation on patients with LE, research on pathogenetic mechanisms of UV-induced LE has become an increasingly dynamic field; this research was additionally fueled by the immense progress of the relatively young discipline of photoimmunology. Initiation and perpetuation of autoimmune responses by UV irradiation have been the subjects of extensive in vivo and in vitro studies (Norris 1993, Orteu et al. 2001, Sontheimer 1996). In summary, UV irradiation may cause the formation of molecules by different epidermal and dermal cells. These molecules have the capacity to up-regulate (prostaglandin E_2, reactive oxygen species [ROS], tumor necrosis factor [TNF]-α, interleukin [IL]-1, intercellular adhesion molecule-1) or down-regulate (IL-10, IL-1 receptor antagonist) inflammatory processes. Since genetic regulation is crucial for the induction of these molecules, a putative genetic polymorphism in LE may play an important role in the specific photosensitivity of LE (Ollier et al. 1996, von Schmiedeberg et al. 1996).

Despite these general possibilities of UV-induced autoimmunity, more specific pathogenetic pathways have been experimentally demonstrated. Thus, Furukawa et al. (Furukawa et al. 1990) could show in the absence of apoptosis the cellular redistribution of the Ro/SSA antigen on UV irradiation, which enables its presentation to the immune system as a possible first step in the autoimmune response cascade. Although the four-step model for the pathogenesis of UV-induced LE based on the translocation of the Ro/SSA antigen, which was developed by Norris and Lee (Norris and Lee 1985), has been widely referred to and agreed on, it is limited to the Ro/SSA-positive forms of LE, such as subacute CLE (SCLE) and neonatal LE (NLE).

Bennion and Norris (Bennion and Norris 1997) have also discussed in depth the role of UV irradiation in the induction of cytokine mediator release and adhesion molecules in the epidermis and dermal vessels. Recent studies have demonstrated that adhesion molecules are not only induced secondary to cytokines (TNF-α, IL-1) but also directly through transcriptional activation. This activation occurs by formation of transcriptional factors such as activator protein-2 in a single oxygen-dependent mechanism (Grether-Beck et al. 1996). Growing evidence suggests the link between UVA sensitivity and free oxygen radical formation (Krutmann 2000). Chemicals with the ability to scavenge free radicals may, therefore, be of special potential value, that is, as additives in sunscreen products to prevent UV-induced LE lesions (McVean and Liebler 1997, Steenvorden and Beijersbergen van Henegouwen 1999, Tebbe et al. 1997, Trevithick et al. 1992). A potentially crucial role in the initiation of the autoimmune reaction cascade has been attributed to UV-induced keratinocyte apoptosis in several studies and reviews (Norris 1993, Orteu et al. 2001, Sontheimer 1996). Casciola-Rosen et al. (Casciola-Rosen et al. 1994) have demonstrated the clustering of autoantigens at the cell surface of cultured keratinocytes with apoptotic changes due to UV irradiation. These autoantigens were found within two distinct forms of blebs, the smaller ones containing Ro/SSA, calreticulin, ribosomes, and endoplasmatic reticulum and the larger ones containing Ro/SSA, La/SSB, and nucleosomal DNA. This localized concentration of autoantigens may be able to break self-tolerance, thus leading to autoimmunity (Sontheimer 1996). Using a standardized photoprovocation test protocol, our group was able to detect increased numbers of apoptotic keratinocytes in CLE after UVA and UVB irradiation compared with control subjects (Kuhn et al. 1998a). Since the cytokine-inducible nitric oxide synthase (iNOS) is believed to play an important role in the course of various autoimmune diseases and in the regulation of apoptosis (Kolb and Kolb-Bachofen 1998), we studied in further experiments, using this photoprovocation test model, the expression of iNOS at the messenger RNA and protein levels in UV-induced LE (Kuhn et al. 1998b). The results of this study demonstrated a delayed iNOS-specific signal after UV irradiation in patients with LE compared with controls, suggesting that the kinetics of iNOS induction and abnormalities in the apoptotic pathway seem to play an important role in the pathogenesis of UV-induced LE. Further elucidation of the various factors that contribute to the UV initiation and perpetuation of the autoimmune response may lead to the future development of effective strategies to prevent induction and exacerbation of LE (Furukawa 1997, Gil and Kim 2000, Golan et al. 1994, LeFeber et al. 1984, Lehmann and Ruzicka 2001, Nyberg et al. 1998). It is conceivable that the prevention of sunburn cell formation (apoptotic keratinocytes) by simple photoprotection measures and strategies significantly reduces disease activity (Sontheimer 1996, Orteu et al. 2001). According to the presented evidence, a further beneficial effect could be achieved by additional use of oxygen scavengers, that is, nitric oxide via chemical donors. Since DNA is a primary target for UV insults, leading to DNA damage with higher antigenicity, a very interesting and elegant photoprotection concept includes the addition of DNA repair enzymes into sunscreens (Stege et al. 2000, Yarosh et al. 2000). However, clinical data on this hypothetical treatment strategy are still lacking.

Clinical Photosensitivity in Lupus Erythematosus

Despite the numerous anecdotal reports and the overwhelming clinical evidence demonstrating the clear relationship between sunlight exposure and the manifestations of LE, almost no systematic studies on photobiologic reactivity in patients with this disease existed until the early 1960s (Hasan et al. 1997, Millard et al. 2000, Leenutaphong and Boonchai 1999, Walchner et al. 1997). The first group to phototest a larger number (n=25) of patients with LE was Epstein et al. (Epstein et al. 1965). They introduced the repeated exposure technique, which made it possible to induce specific lesions of LE in the test area in 5 of the 25 tested patients. The eliciting wavelengths were in the UVB range. In the same year, Everett and Olson (Everett and Olson 1965) demonstrated that 1 minimal erythema dose (MED) of hot quartz UV light exposure produced an increase in the size of skin lesions in patients with DLE. Baer and Harber (Baer and Harber 1965) administered phototests to 29 patients with LE by applying one to six times the MED of UVB in single exposures to multiple test sites. An abnormal reaction was detected in only one patient with SCLE, and it consisted of a markedly decreased erythema threshold dose and persistence of the erythema for 4 weeks. Wavelengths longer than 315 nm were not evaluated in this study. Freeman et al. (Freeman et al. 1969) used monochromatic light to determine the wavelength dependency of phototest reactions in 15 patients with LE by also applying the repeated UV exposure technique, which became a valuable tool later on for photoprovocation tests in several photosensitive disorders, such as polymorphous light eruption (PLE) (Lehmann et al. 1986). However, the UVA doses used in only a few patients with LE were probably too low for positive photoprovocation reactions. Cripps and Rankin (Cripps and Rankin 1973) also used monochromatic light between 250 and 330 nm in an attempt to determine the erythema action spectrum; specific lesions of LE were reproduced in the UVB range by applying 8–13 times the MED. At 330 nm (UVA), only a persistent erythematous response but no LE lesions could be detected. Because of these studies, the action spectrum of LE was ascribed to the UVB range despite experimental evidence from in vitro and animal studies indicating that UVA irradiation also had specific detrimental effects in LE (Doria et al. 1996, Friou 1957, Sontheimer 1996, Zamansky et al. 1980). However, the clinical phototesting experiments had shortcomings in that either only a very limited number of patients had been tested or the UVA testing was insufficient (Cripps et al. 1973, Epstein et al. 1965, Freeman et al. 1969, van Weelden 1989).

The description by Sontheimer et al. (Sontheimer et al. 1979) of SCLE as a very photosensitive subset marked a major step forward in the photobiology of this disease. Evidence of a role for UV irradiation in the pathogenesis of SCLE came from the observations of patients that sun exposure resulted in lesion formation, the limitation of SCLE lesions to sun-exposed skin, and the predilection for fair-skinned individuals with skin type I or II (David-Bajar et al. 1992, Sontheimer 1989). The observation that certain photosensitizing drugs, such as thiazide diuretics and sulfonylureas, can induce SCLE is also an indication that sun exposure plays an important role in the pathogenesis of this disease (Reed et al. 1985). Further experiments evolving from these clinical results have led to the concept that keratinocytes damaged by antibody-dependent cellular cytotoxicity might be a mechanism in photosensitive LE (Lee et al. 1986, LeFeber et al. 1984, Norris and Lee 1985).

In 1986, our group (Kind et al. 1993, Lehmann et al. 1986, 1990) was the first to demonstrate experimental reproduction of skin lesions by UVB and UVA irradiation using a standardized test protocol on a large number of patients with the disease. A total of 128 patients with different forms of LE underwent phototesting with polychromatic UVB and long-wave UVA irradiation, and characteristic skin lesions clinically and histologically resembling LE were induced in 43% of patients (Fig. 12.1). Subsequent investigators confirmed UVA reactivity in LE by phototesting (Nived et al. 1993, Wolska et al. 1989). In the following years, this testing regimen received much attention because the reproduction of skin lesions in patients with LE by UVB and

Fig. 12.1. Photoprovocation of subacute cutaneous lupus erythematosus (SCLE) with UVA (left test field) and UVB (right test field). Picture taken 10 days after the last irradiation. Characteristic genuine annular SCLE lesions on the shoulder of the patient.

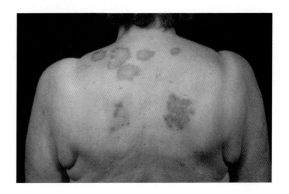

UVA irradiation is an optimal model for clinical and experimental studies (Beutner et al. 1991, Hasan et al. 1997, Kind et al. 1993, Kuhn et al. 1998a, b, Leenutaphong and Boonchai 1999, van Weelden et al. 1989, Walchner et al. 1997). Meanwhile, provocative phototesting in patients with LE has become routine at our department, and protocols for phototesting have become optimized by taking into account multiple factors (Table 12.1). Nonlesional, non-sun-exposed areas of the upper back or extensor aspects of the arms were used for performance of the phototest reactions because other parts of the skin might not react to the same extent, probably owing to some kind of local predisposition of unknown nature other than UV irradiation, such as thickness of the stratum corneum, vascularization, presence of antigens, or distribution of antigen-presenting cells (Walchner et al. 1997). Furthermore, it is important to use a defined test area, which should be sufficiently large to provide reactions. The initial observable response following exposure to UV irradiation is an erythema reaction that most commonly arises with the normal time course. Although the duration of the erythema was not studied in particular, a prolonged erythematous response was not a conspicuous feature. In contrast to other photodermatoses, such as PLE, the development of skin lesions in patients with LE is characterized by a latency of several days to 3 weeks or even longer, and it might persist in some cases for several months (Kuhn et al. 2001a, Lehmann 1996). In addition, phototesting has been crucial in further characterizing a highly photosensitive form of CLE, namely, LE tumidus (LET) (Kuhn et al. 2000, 2001b). LET was first described by Gougerot and Bournier (Gougerot and Bournier 1930) and has since been somewhat "forgotten" or rarely described and diagnosed. In 1990, Goerz et al. (Goerz et al. 1990) emphasized for the first time that extreme photosensitivity is a major characteristic of LET, and a few further case reports of this disease followed from groups other than our own (Alexiades-Armenakas et al. 2003, Dekle et al. 1999). According to our experience, we regard LET to be an unusual clinical variant of CLE, and skin lesions of LET consist of sharply demarcated, smooth, red-violet, infiltrated plaques with hardly any scaling and no scarring. The lesions usually disappear on therapy with antimalarials and sun avoidance. It could be shown that this form is even more UV sensitive than SCLE, which, until recently, was believed to be the most photosensitive LE subset (Sontheimer et al. 1979). Using a standardized protocol, reproduction of characteristic skin lesions occurred in 76% of patients with LET, 63% with SCLE, 45% with DLE, and 41% with other forms of CLE, such as LE profundus and Chilblain LE (Kuhn et al. 2001a).

Table 12.1. Provocative phototesting in patients with lupus erythematosus (LE): optimized protocol (modified from Kuhn et al. 2001a)

Criteria	Protocol	Comments
Test site	Non-sun-exposed, unaffected areas of the upper back or extensor aspects of the arms	Other parts of the skin might not react to the same extent
Size of test field	Defined test areas that should be sufficiently large to provide reactions (4×5 cm)	Test areas that are too small or different in size might not show reproducible results
Pretesting	MED, IPD, MTD	Testing of the MED is necessary to make data comparable; a prolonged erythematous response is not a conspicuous feature
Dosage	60–100 J/cm^2 UVA and/or 1.5 MED UVB on 3 consecutive days	Single UV exposure is unlikely to induce positive reactions in all possible patients
Light sources	UVA: UVASUN 3000 (330–460 nm), Mutzhas or UVA1 Sellas 2000 (340–440 nm), Sellas UVB: UV-800 with fluorescent bulbs, Philipps TL 20 W/12 (285–350 nm), Waldmann	Different light sources with a different action spectrum can result in different numbers of positive phototests
Pretreatment	No pretreatment	Any topical or systemic pretreatment might affect the phototesting procedure
Medication	If possible, no systemic medication for skin disease	Systemic medications, such as antimalarial agents, corticosteroids, and immunosuppressive drugs, might lead to false-negative results
Evaluation	24, 48, 72 h up to 4 weeks after last irradiation	Follow-up shorter than 3 weeks might miss positive provocative phototest results in some patients
Criteria for positive photoprovocation	Induced skin lesions clinically resemble LE Skin lesions develop slowly over several days or weeks Skin lesions persist up to several months Clinical diagnosis is confirmed by histologic analysis	Positive phototest reactions are considerably slower and persist longer than other photodermatoses, such as polymorphous light eruption, persistent light reaction, photoallergy, hydroa vacciniforme, and solar urticaria

Table 12.1. Provocative phototesting in patients with lupus erythematosus (LE): optimized protocol (modified from Kuhn et al. 2001a) (continued)

Criteria	Protocol	Comments
Results of phototesting (different wavelengths)	UVA and UVB: 20%–53% UVB: 25%–72% UVA: 0%–55%	Differences in phototest results are found because of different protocols and the age of the patients at onset of disease
Results of phototesting (different LE subtypes)	LET: 70%–81% SCLE: 50%–100% DLE: 10%–64% SLE: 25%–85%	Differences in phototest results are found because of different protocols; in our studies, LET patients are the most photosensitive patients
Local side effects	Persistence of hyperpigmentation and hypopigmentation for several months after irradiation	Patients should be reminded of these possible side effects because they might lead to cosmetic problems
Induction of disease	Exacerbation of cutaneous lesions in a few patients, no provocation of systemic disease in our studies	Follow-up of SLE patients after phototesting is very important because reports in the literature describe exacerbation of systemic disease under phototesting
History of photosensitivity	LET: 43%–50% SCLE: 27%–100% DLE: 25%–90% SLE: 6%–94%	Positive phototesting results are not always associated with a positive history of photosensitivity; it might be difficult for patients to recognize the association between sun exposure and induction of skin lesions

DLE, discoid LE; IPD, immediate pigment darkening; LET, LE tumidus; MED, minimal erythema dose; MTD, minimal tanning dose; SCLE, subacute cutaneous LE; SLE, systemic LE.

Results of reported phototesting in patients with LE often differ between various groups because there are numerous technical differences between the studies that could explain the different findings (Beutner et al. 1991, Hasan et al. 1997, Kind et al. 1993, Kuhn et al. 2001a, Lehmann et al. 1990, Nived et al. 1993, Van Weelden et al. 1989, Sanders et al. 2003, Walchner et al. 1997, Wolska et al. 1989). Varying factors are light source, energy dose, wavelength, time points of provocation and evaluation, and location and size of the test area. Most studies were conducted in white patients; however, there is one recent article on phototesting in 15 oriental patients with LE using exactly the same test protocol as our group (Leenutaphong and Boonchai 1999). The incidence of positive phototest reactions in these patients seemed to be similar to or a little lower than that in white patients, and there was no correlation between a positive history of UV sensitivity and phototest reactions. However, classification of positive test results might be difficult in some patients because persistent erythema can develop, which is even histologically hard to interpret. It is also unclear why skin lesions cannot always be reproduced under the same conditions several months after the initial phototest and why phototesting results are not positive in all patients with LE tested, providing indirect evidence for variant factors in the pathophysiology of this disease (Higuchi et al. 1991).

Furthermore, a history of photosensitivity in patients with LE does not necessarily predict positive reactions on phototesting, and results of reported photosensitivity often differ between various groups (Beutner et al. 1991, Callen 1985, Callen and Klein 1988, Doria et al. 1996, Drosos et al. 1990, Grigor et al. 1978, Harvey et al. 1954, Herrero et al. 1988, Hymes et al. 1986, Kuhn et al. 2001a, Lee et al. 1977, Millard et al. 2000, Mond et al. 1989, O'Loughlin et al. 1978, Pande et al. 1993, Pistiner et al. 1991, Sontheimer et al. 1979, Sontheimer 1989, Tan et al. 1982, Tuffanelli and Dubois 1964, Vila et al. 1999, Walchner et al. 1997, Wilson and Hughes 1979, Wilson et al. 1984, Wysenbeek et al. 1989). This might be because skin lesions after UV irradiation do not develop rapidly after sun exposure, and, therefore, a relationship between sun exposure and exacerbation of LE does not seem obvious to the patient. An additional factor might be age at onset of disease, as observed by Walchner et al. (Walchner et al. 1997), demonstrating that mainly patients younger than 40 years reported photosensitivity. Furthermore, the occurrence of photosensitivity varies among different types of LE, and some ethnic groups, such as African blacks, seem to be less photosensitive than others (Mody et al. 1994, Petri et al. 1992, Shi et al. 1987, Sutej et al. 1989, Taylor and Stein 1986, Ward and Studenski 1990). Nevertheless, the term "photosensitivity" (skin rash as a result of unusual reaction to sunlight by patient history or physician observation) is poorly defined (Lee and Farris 1999), although it is listed as one of the American Rheumatism Association (ARA) criteria for the classification of SLE (Tan et al. 1982). In 1996, a large discrepancy between a personal history of photosensitivity and a decreased MED was documented by Doria et al. (Doria et al. 1996), concluding that the use of photosensitivity as a classification criterion for SLE remains questionable, at least when it is assessed according to the ARA criteria. Therefore, a detailed clinical history is important to the diagnosis and assessment of photosensitivity in patients with LE. There are several key components to a history of photosensitivity, including the morphology of the rash, duration, distribution, and the relationship to sun exposure and specific symptoms (such as pain, pruritus, burning, blistering, and swelling). Each of these symptoms may provide clues to the nature of the photosensitive eruption and thus the diagnosis. Differentiating between the morphology and the time course of CLE and, for instance, PLE, in terms of history alone can be difficult; clinically, PLE tends to consist of an acute eruption of tiny, pruritic plaques and vesicles that lasts several days, in contrast to SCLE, which usually involves larger, nonpruritic annular or psoriasiform lesions that persist for weeks to months after UV exposure. In contrast, LET may, in some cases, be clinically very similar to PLE. A past medical history should also include a detailed drug history, particularly in temporal relation to a suspected phototoxic eruption.

Physical examination may reveal a distribution suggestive of a photosensitive condition in the absence of a history of photosensitivity. The most common areas for skin lesions in LE include sun-exposed areas such as the face, the V-area and posterior aspect of the neck, the ears, the dorsa of the hands, and the forearms. Equally helpful may be areas that are specifically spared from sun exposure, including the upper eyelids, submental areas, finger web spaces, and general creases within skin folds, where a photosensitive eruption is noticeably absent. Furthermore, investigation of patients with photosensitivity includes routine tests to establish the diagnosis and extent of disease activity, including hematology, biochemistry, serology, and complement studies. Skin biopsies and immunofluorescence may also be appropriate. Provocative phototesting is an objective means of demonstrating whether a patient has an abnormal response to UV exposure; however, phototesting does not play a role in the routine assessment or diagnosis of a patient with CLE. Indications for phototesting in patients with LE include (a) the objective demonstration of photosensitivity where there is doubt about the history and where such demonstration would support a diagnosis of LE; (b) the exclusion of other causes of photosensitivity, such as PLE, chronic dermatitis, solar urticaria, and drug-induced phototoxicity; and (c) use of the photoprovocation test as a useful research tool with which to study the immunopathology of evolving lesions of LE-specific skin disease (Millard et al. 2000).

Results of histopathologic and immunopathologic examination of UV-induced LE lesions are similar to the findings of spontaneously developing primary skin lesions but can give further insight into the earliest pathologic events of CLE lesions. Kind et al. (Kind et al. 1993) demonstrated that histopathologic examination of early UV-induced lesions (up to 10 days) in patients with CLE and SLE shows nonspecific changes such as superficial perivascular lymphocytic infiltration. On the other hand, late UV-induced lesions (more than 10 days) were characterized by parakeratosis, few necrotic basal keratinocytes, and vacuolar degeneration of the dermoepidermal zone. Furthermore, under experimental conditions, the appearance of immunoglobulins in UV-induced LE lesions has been reported as a late phenomenon, and in our study, direct immunofluorescence findings were negative in all skin lesions investigated up to 3 weeks after UV exposure. This is in accordance with Cripps and Rankin (Cripps and Rankin 1973), who detected the first immunoglobulin deposits 6 weeks after irradiation and mainly along the basement membrane. In contrast, Velthuis et al. (Velthuis et al. 1990) demonstrated that in UV-induced lesions of patients with LE, immunohistochemical changes can be induced similar to those in spontaneously evolved lesions. Furthermore, Nyberg et al. (Nyberg et al. 1998) observed that in experimentally UV-induced lesions of patients with LE, dust-like particles, a specific fine-speckled, epidermosubepidermal direct immunofluorescence staining pattern, can be detected within 2 weeks of UV exposure.

A potential interplay of UV irradiation with specific autoantibodies, particularly anti-Ro/SSA and anti-La/SSB antibodies, has been previously reported, and, in different subtypes of LE, such as SCLE and NLE, photosensitivity has been found to be strongly associated with the presence of such antibodies (for review see Lee and Farris 1999). Results of an early study by LeFeber et al. (LeFeber et al. 1984) indicated that UV irradiation of cultured keratinocytes led to increased immunoglobulin G binding to the cell surface of keratinocytes; several years later, Norris (Norris 1993) noted increased antibody binding as a result of in vivo UV irradiation to human skin. Golan et al. (Golan et al. 1992) independently observed UV-induced binding of antibodies from Ro/SSA-positive sera to a small percentage of cultured keratinocytes. Nevertheless, the strongest evidence supporting the possibility that these antibodies play a role in the pathogenesis of LE comes from patients with NLE (Lee 1993). These infants have maternally acquired anti-Ro/SSA antibodies and develop SCLE-like skin lesions, and because these antibodies are cleared from the infant's circulation several months after birth, the skin lesions resolve spontaneously (Lee et al. 1989). In DLE, the association of skin disease with antibodies is much less clear, and in previous studies, a clear association between the presence of anti-Ro/SSA antibodies and the clinical finding of photosensitivity was not found (Lee and Farris 1999). However, because similar levels of anti-Ro/SSA antibodies are seen in other disorders, such as Sjögren's syndrome, that are not usually associated with specific LE lesions, other factors must be involved in the production of LE inflammation.

In conclusion, photoprovocation tests are an objective tool for evaluating possible photosensitivity in patients with different forms of LE and are even required for diagnosis in some cases. A very important and practically relevant feature of LE photosensitivity, which became evident on routine phototesting, is the delayed and slow UV reactivity in these patients. This conspicuous feature may explain the negligence of many patients with LE as to the negative effects of the sun's radiation on their disease. Therefore, education on photoprotection measures seems to be especially important in this group. Recently, our group demonstrated with the aforementioned test protocol that broadband sunscreens were able to suppress the induction of LE lesions on UV irradiation (Kuhn et al. 2002). Consequent protection against UV light and also other physical and mechanical injuries may be of significant value for the course and prognosis of LE, especially since such injuries may even initiate systemic manifestations of the disease, which was previously limited to the skin. Further steps in the future will consider the pathogenetic mechanisms in LE photosensitivity to develop more specific pharmaceuticals beyond UV filters, such as antioxidants or DNA repair enzymes, which will be able to counteract the detrimental effects of UV irradiation on the disease.

References

Alexiades-Armenakas MR, Baldassano M, Bince B, Werth V, Bystryn JC, Kamino H, Soter NA, Franks AG Jr (2003) Tumid lupus erythematosus: criteria for classification with immunohistochemical analysis. Arthritis Rheum 15:494–500

Baer RL, Harber LC (1965) Photobiology of lupus erythematosus. Arch Dermatol 92: 124–128

Bennion SD, Norris DA (1997) Ultraviolet light modulation of autoantigens, epidermal cytokines and adhesive molecules as contributing factors of the pathogenesis of cutaneous LE. Lupus 6:181–192

Beutner EH, Blaszczyk M, Jablonska S, Chorzelski TP, Kumar V, Wolska H (1991) Studies on criteria of the European Academy of Dermatology and Venerology for the classification of cutaneous lupus erythematosus. 1. Selection of clinical groups and study factors. Int J Dermatol 30:411–417

Callen JP (1985) Discoid lupus erythematosus – variants and clinical associations. Clin Dermatol 3:49–57

Callen JP, Klein J (1988) Subacute cutaneous lupus erythematosus. Clinical, serologic, immunogenetic, and therapeutic considerations in seventy-two patients. Arthritis Rheum 31: 1007–1013

Casciola-Rosen LA, Anhalt G, Rosen A (1994) Autoantigens targeted in systemic lupus erythematosus are clustered in two populations of surface structures on apoptotic keratinocytes. J Exp Med 179:1317–1330

Cazénave PLA (1881) Lupus érythémateux (érythéme centrifuge) Ann Mal Peau Syph 3:297–299

Cripps DJ, Rankin J (1973) Action spectra of lupus erythematosus and experimental immunofluorescence. Arch Dermatol 107:563–567

David-Bajar KM, Bennion SD, Despain JD, Golitz LE, Lee LA (1992) Clinical, histologic, and immunofluorescent distinctions between subacute cutaneous lupus erythematosus and discoid lupus erythematosus. J Invest Dermatol 99:251–257

Dekle CL, Mannes KD, Davis LS, Sangueza OP (1999) Lupus tumidus. J Am Acad Dermatol 41:250–253

Doria A, Biasinutto C, Ghirardello A, Sartori E, Rondinone R, Piccvoli A, Veller Fornasa C, Gambari PE (1996) Photosensitivity in systemic lupus erythematosus: laboratory testing of ARA/ ACR definition. Lupus 5:263–268

Drosos AA, Dimou GS, Siamopoulou-Mavridou A, Hatzis J, Moutsopoulos HM (1990) Subacute cutaneous lupus erythematosus in Greece. A clinical, serological and genetic study. Ann Med Interne 141:421–424

Epstein JH, Tuffanelli DL, Dubois EL (1965) Light sensitivity and lupus erythematosus. Arch Dermal 91:483–485

Everett MA, Olson RL (1965) Response of cutaneous lupus erythematosus to ultraviolet light. J Invest Dermatol 44:133–134

Freeman RG, Knox JM, Owens DW (1969) Cutaneous lesions of lupus erythematosus induced by monochromatic light. Arch Dermatol 100:677–682

Freund H (1929) Inwieweit ist der Lupus erythematosus von allgemeinen Faktoren abhängig? Dermatol Wochenschr 89:1939–1946

Friou GJ (1957) Clinical application of lupus serum: nucleoprotein reaction using fluorescent antibody technique. J Clin Invest 36:890 –896

Fuhs E (1929) Lupus erythematosus subacutus mit ausgesprochener Überempfindlichkeit gegen Quarzlicht. Z Hautkr 30:308–309

Furukawa F, Kashihara-Sawami M, Lyons MB, Norris DA (1990) Binding of antibodies to the extractable nuclear antigens SS-A/Ro and SS-B/La is induced on the surface of human keratinocytes by ultraviolet light (UVL): implications for the pathogenesis of photosensitive cutaneous lupus. J Invest Dermatol 94:77–85

Furukawa F (1997) Animal models of cutaneous lupus erythematosus and lupus erythematosus photosensitivity. Lupus 6:193–202

Gil EM, Kim TH (2000) UV-induced immune suppression and sunscreen. Photodermatol Photoimmunol Photomed 16:101–110

Goerz G, Lehmann P, Schuppe HC, Lakomek HJ, Kind P (1990) Lupus erythematodes (LE). Z Hautkr 65:226–234

Golan TD, Elkon KB, Gharavi AE, Krueger JG (1992) Enhanced membrane binding of autoantibodies to cultured keratinocytes of systemic lupus erythematosus patients after ultraviolet B/ultraviolet A irradiation. J Clin Invest 90:1067–1076

Golan TD, Dan S, Haim H, Varda G, Sol K (1994) Solar ultraviolet radiation induces enhanced accumulation of oxygen radicals in murine SLE-derived splenocytes in vitro. Lupus 3:103–106

Gougerot H, Burnier R (1930) Lupus érythémateux "tumidus". Bull Soc Fr Derm Syphil 37: 1291–1292

Grether-Beck S, Olaizola-Horn S, Shmitt H, Grewe M, Jahnke A, Johnson JP, Briviba K, Sies H, Krutmann J (1996) Activation of transcription factor AP-2 mediates UVA radiation and singlet oxygen-induced expression of the human intercellular adhesion molecule 1 gene. Proc Natl Acad Sci USA 93:14586–14591

Grigor R, Edmonds J, Lewkonia R, Bresnihan B, Hughes GRV (1978) Systemic lupus erythematosus – a prospective analysis. Ann Rheum Dis 37:121–128

Harvey AM, Shulman LE, Tumulty PA, Conley CL, Schoenrich EH (1954) Systemic lupus erythematosus: review of the literature and clinical analysis of 138 cases. Medicine 33:291–437

Hasan T, Nyberg F, Stephansson E, Puska P, Hakkinen M, Sarna S, Ros AM, Ranki A (1997) Photosensitivity in lupus erythematosus, UV photoprovocation results compared with history of photosensitivity and clinical findings. Br J Dermatol 136:699–705

Herrero C, Bielsa I, Font J, Lozano F, Ercilla G, Lecha M, Ingelmo M, Mascaro JM (1988) Subacute cutaneous lupus erythematosus: clinicopathologic findings in thirteen cases. J Am Acad Dermatol 19:1057–1062

Higuchi D, Ogura Y, Watanabe H, Takiuchi I (1991) Experimental production of DLE lesion with a single exposure to UVB (2.7 MEDs) radiation. J Dermatol 18:545–548

Hutchinson J (1888) Harveian lectures on lupus. Lecture III. On the various form of lupus vulgaris and erythematosus. Br Med J 1:113–118

Hymes SR, Russell TJ, Jordon RE (1986) The anti-Ro antibody system. Int J Dermatol 25:1–7

Jesionek A (1919) Richtlinien der modernen Lichttherapie. Strahlentherapie 7:41–45

Kind P, Lehmann P, Plewig G (1993) Phototesting in lupus erythematosus. J Invest Dermatol 100:53S–57S

Kolb H, Kolb-Bachofen V (1998) NO in autoimmune disease: cytotoxic or regulatory mediator? Immunol Today 1912:556–561

Krutmann J (2000) Ultraviolet A radiation-induces biological effects in human skin: relevance for photoaging and photodermatosis. J Dermatol Sci 23:S22–S26

Kuhn A, Fehsel K, Lehmann P, Ruzicka T, Kolb-Bachofen V (1998a) Detection of apoptosis in human epidermis after ultraviolet radiation in cutaneous lupus erythematosus. Arch Dermatol Res 290:82

Kuhn A, Fehsel K, Lehmann P, Krutmann J, Ruzicka T, Kolb-Bachofen V (1998b) Aberrant timing in epidermal expression of inducible nitric oxide synthase after UV irradiation in cutaneous lupus erythematosus. J Invest Dermatol 111:149–153

Kuhn A, Richter-Hintz D, Oslislo C, Ruzicka T, Megahed M, Lehmann P (2000) Lupus erythematosus tumidus: a neglected subset of cutaneous lupus erythematosus: report of 40 cases. Arch Dermatol 136:1033–1041

Kuhn A, Sonntag M, Richter-Hintz D, Oslislo C, Megahed M, Ruzicka T, Lehmann P (2001a) Phototesting in lupus erythematosus: a 15-year experience. J Am Acad Dermatol 45:86–95

Kuhn A, Sonntag M, Richter-Hintz D, Oslislo C, Megahed M, Ruzicka T, Lehmann P (2001b) Phototesting in lupus erythematosus tumidus. Review of 60 patients. Photochem Photobiol 73:532–536

Kuhn A, Sonntag M, Boyer F, Lehmann P, Dupuy P (2002) Evaluation of photoprotective effects of a broadspectrum highly protective sunscreen in photoinduced cutaneous lupus erythematosus. Ann Dermatol Venereol 129:1S726–1S727

Lee PL, Urowitz MB, Bookman AM, Koehler BE, Smythe HA, Gordon DA, Ogryzlo MA (1977) Systemic lupus erythematosus. A review of 110 cases with reference to nephritis, the nervous system, infections, aseptic necrosis and prognosis. Q J Med 46:1–32

Lee LA, Weston WL, Krueger GG, Emam M, Reichlin M, Stevens JO, Surbrugg SK, Vasil A, Norris DA (1986) An animal model of antibody binding in cutaneous lupus. Arthritis Rheum 29:782–788

Lee LA, Gaither JK, Coulter SN, Norris DA, Harley JB (1989) Pattern of cutaneous immunoglobulin G deposition in subacute cutaneous lupus erythematosus is reproduced by infusing purified anti-Ro (SSA) autoantibodies into human skin-graft mice. J Clin Invest 83: 1556–1562

Lee LA (1993) Neonatal lupus erythematosus. J Invest Dermatol 100:9S-13S

Lee LA, Farris AD (1999) Photosensitivity diseases: cutaneous lupus erythematosus. J Invest Dermatol Symp Proc 4:73-78

Leenutaphong V, Boonchai W (1999) Phototesting in oriental patients with lupus erythematosus. Photodermatol Photoimmunol Photomed 15:7-12

LeFeber WP, Norris DA, Ran SR, Lee LA, Huff JC, Kubo M, Boyce ST, Kotzin BL, Weston WL (1984) Ultraviolet light induces binding of antibodies to selected nuclear antigens on cultures human keratinocytes. J Clin Invest 74:1545-1551

Lehmann P (1996) Photosensitivität des Lupus erythematodes. Akt Dermatol 22:52-56

Lehmann P, Ruzicka T (2001) Sunscreens and photoprotection in lupus erythematosus. Dermatologic Therapy 14:167-173

Lehmann P, Holzle E, von Kries R, Plewig G (1986) Lichtdiagnostische Verfahren bei Patienten mit Verdacht auf Photodermatosen. Z Haut Geschlechtskr 152:667-682

Lehmann P, Holzle E, Kind P, Goerz G, Plewig G (1990) Experimental reproduction of skin lesions in lupus erythematosus by UVA and UVB radiation. J Am Acad Dermatol 22:181-187

Macleod JMH (1924) Lupus erythematosus: some observations on its etiology. Arch Dermatol Syphil 9:1-12

McVean M, Liebler DC (1997) Inhibition of UVB-induced DNA damage in mouse epidermis by topically applied α-tocopherol. Carcinogenesis 18:1617-1622

Mody GM, Parag KB, Nathoo BC, Pudifin DJ, Duursma J, Seedat YK (1994) High mortality with systemic lupus erythematosus in hospitalized African blacks. Br J Rheumatol 33:1151-1153

Millard TP, Hawk JL, McGregor JM (2000) Photosensitivity in lupus. Lupus 9:3-10

Mond CB, Peterson MG, Rothfield NF (1989) Correlation of anti-Ro antibody with photosensitivity rash in systemic lupus erythematosus patients. Arthritis Rheum 32:202-204

Nived O, Johansen PB, Sturfelt G (1993) Standardized ultraviolet-A exposure provokes skin reaction in systemic lupus erythematosus. Lupus 2:247-250

Norris DA, Lee LA (1985) Antibody-dependent cellular cytotoxicity and skin disease. J Invest Dermatol 85:165S-175S

Norris DA (1993) Pathomechanisms of photosensitive lupus erythematosus. J Invest Dermatol 100:58S-68S

Nyberg F, Skoglund C, Stephansson E (1998) Early detection of epidermal dust-like particles in experimentally UV-induced lesions in patients with photosensitivity and lupus erythematosus. Acta Derm Venereol 78:177-179

Ollier W, Davies E, Snowden N, Alldersea J, Fryer A, Jones P, Strange R (1996) Association of homozygosity for glutatione S-transferase GSTM1 null alleles with the Ro+/La- autoantibody profile in patients with systemic lupus erythematosus. Arthritis Rheum 39:1763-1764

O'Loughlin S, Schroeter AL, Jordon RE (1978) A study of lupus erythematosus with particular reference to generalized discoid lupus. Br J Dermatol 99:1-11

Orteu CH, Sontheimer RD, Dutz JP (2001) The pathophysiology of photosensitivity in lupus erythematosus. Photodermatol Photoimmunol Photomed 17:95-113

Pande I, Sekharan NG, Kailash S, Uppal SS, Singh RR, Kumar A, Malavivya AN (1993) Analysis of clinical and laboratory profile in Indian childhood systemic lupus erythematosus and its comparison with SLE in adults. Lupus 2:83-87

Petri M, Perez-Gutthann S, Craig Longenecker J, Hochberg M (1992) Morbidity of systemic lupus erythematosus: role of race and socioeconomic status. Am J Med 91:345-353

Pistiner M, Wallace DJ, Nessim S, Metzger AL, Klinenberg JR (1991) Lupus erythematosus in the 1980s: a survey of 570 patients. Semin Arthritis Rheum 21:55-64

Pusey WA (1915) Attacks of lupus erythematosus following exposure to sunlight or other weather factors. Arch Derm Syph 34:388

Reed BR, Huff JC, Jones SK, Orton PW, Lee LA, Norris DA (1985) Subacute cutaneous lupus erythematosus associated with hydrochlorothiazide therapy. Ann Intern Med 103:49-51

Sanders CJ, Van Weelden H, Kazzaz GA, Sigurdsson V, Toonstra J, Bruijnzeel-Koomen CA (2003) Photosensitivity in patients with lupus erythematosus: a clinical and photobiological study of 100 patients using a prolonged phototest protocol. Br J Dermatol 149:131-137

Shi SY, Feng SF, Liao KH, Fang L, Kang KF (1987) Clinical study of 30 cases of subacute cutaneous lupus erythematosus. Chin Med J 100:45–48

Sontheimer RD, Thomas JR, Gilliam JN (1979) Subacute cutaneous lupus erythematosus. Arch Dermatol 115:1409–1415

Sontheimer RD (1989) Subacute cutaneous lupus erythematosus: a decade's perspective. Med Clin North Am 73:1073–1090

Sontheimer RD (1996) Photoimmunology of lupus erythematosus and dermatomyositis: a speculative review. Photochem Photobiol 63:583–594

Steenvorden DP, Beijersbergen van Henegouwen G (1999) Protection against UV-induced systemic immunosuppression in mice by a single topical application of the antioxidant vitamins C and E. Int J Radiat Biol 747–755

Stege H, Roza L, Viink AA, Grewe M, Ruzicka T, Grether-Beck S, Krutmann J (2000) Enzyme plus light therapy to repair DNA damage in ultraviolet-B-irradiated human skin. Proc Natl Acad Sci USA 97:1790–1795

Stern RS, Drocken W (1986) An exacerbation of SLE after visiting a tanning salon. JAMA 155:3120

Sutej PG, Gear AJ, Morrison RC, Tikly M, de Beer M, Dos Santos L, Sher R (1989) Photosensitivity and anti-Ro (SS-A) antibodies in black patients with systemic lupus erythematosus (SLE). Br J Rheumatol 28:321–324

Tan EM, Cohen AS, Fries JF, Masi AT, McShane DJ, Rothfield NF, Schaller JC, Talal N, Winchester RJ (1982) The 1982 revised criteria for the classification of systemic lupus erythematosus. Arthritis Rheum 25:1271–1277

Taylor HG, Stein CM (1986) Systemic lupus erythematosus in Zimbabwe. Ann Rheum Dis 45:645–648

Tebbe B, Wu S, Geilen CC, Eberle J, Kodelja V, Orfanos CE (1997) L-ascorbic acid inhibits UVA-induced lipid peroxidation and secretion of IL-1alpha and IL-6 in cultured human keratinocytes in vitro. J Invest Dermatol 108:302–306

Trevithick JR, Xiong H, Lee S, Shum DT, Sanford SE, Karlik SJ, Norley C, Dilworth GR (1992) Tropical tocopherol acetate reduces post-UVB, sunburn-associated erythema, edema, and skin sensitivity in hairless mice. Arch Biochem Biophys 296:575–582

Tronnier H, Petri H, Pierchalla P (1988) UV-provozierte bullöse Hautveränderungen bei systemischem Lupus erythematodes. Z Hautkr 154:617A

Tuffanelli DL, Dubois EL (1964) Cutaneous manifestations of systemic lupus erythematosus. Arch Dermatol 90:377–386

Van Weelden H, Velthuis PJ, Baart de la Faille H (1989) Light-induced skin lesions in lupus erythematosus: photobiological studies. Arch Dermatol Res 281:470–474

Velthuis PJ, van Weelden H, van Wichen D, Baart de la Faille H (1990) Immunohistopathology of light-induced skin lesions in lupus erythematosus. Acta Derm Venereol 70:93–98

Vila LM, Mayor AM, Valentin AH, Rodriguez SI, Reyes ML, Acosta E, Vila S (1999) Association of sunlight exposure and photoprotection measures with clinical outcome in systemic lupus erythematosus. P R Health Sci J 18:89–94

Von Schmiedeberg S, Fritsche E, Rönnau AC, Specker C, Golka K, Richter-Hintz D, Schuppe HC, Lehmann P, Ruzicka T, Esser C, Abel J, Gleichmann E (1996) Polymorphisms of drug-metabolizing enzymes in patients with idiopathic systemic autoimmune diseases. Exp Toxic Patho 48:349–353

Walchner M, Messer G, Kind P (1997) Phototesting and photoprotection in LE. Lupus 6:167–174

Ward MM, Studenski S (1990) Clinical manifestations of systemic lupus erythematosus. Identification of racial and socioeconomic influences. Arch Intern Med 150:849–853

Wilson WA, Scopelitis E, Michalski JP (1984) Association of HLA-DR7 with both antibody to SSA(Ro) and disease susceptibility in blacks with systemic lupus erythematosus. J Rheumatol 11:653–657

Wolska H, Blazczyk M, Jablonska S (1989) Phototests in patients with various forms of lupus erythematosus. Int J Dermatol 28:98–103

Wysenbeek AJ, Block DA, Fries JF (1989) Prevalence and expression of photosensitivity in systemic lupus erythematosus. Ann Rheum Dis 48:461–463

Yarosh DB, O'Connor A, Alas L, Potten C, Wolf P (2000) Photoprotection by topical DNA repair enzymes: molecular correlates of clinical studies. Photochem Photobiol 69:136–140

Zamansky GB, Kleinmann LF, Kaplan JC (1980) Effect of UV light irradiation on the survival of NZB mouse cells. Arthritis Rheum 23:866–867

CHAPTER 13

Relationship Between Cutaneous and Systemic Lupus Erythematosus

13

Christof Specker, Matthias Schneider

Systemic lupus erythematosus (SLE) is a multisystem inflammatory autoimmune disease characterized by highly varied clinical manifestations in association with autoantibody production (antinuclear antibodies [ANAs], anti-double-stranded DNA [ds-DNA] antibodies, and anti-extractable nuclear antigen antibodies). Next to, for instance, kidneys, brain, heart, and joints, the skin is one of the organs typically affected in lupus. Cutaneous manifestations of lupus erythematosus (LE) appear frequently at the beginning or in the course of SLE, but they may also occur without systemic involvement. This book deals with a broad spectrum of cutaneous forms of lupus with respect to the clinic, pathophysiology, and treatment. The aim of this chapter is to analyze what the skin is telling us about the autoimmune process below the surface. Several analyses tried to predict the clinical situation of the patients by their antibody profile or their genetic background, but as every patient with lupus is writing his or her own chapter in the book of lupus, the value of these attempts are limited. Even if we can read the disease activity in some cases from the cutaneous manifestations only, the pages in this chapter describing the skin lesions of an individual patient outline the whole disease.

According to the "Düsseldorf Classification 2003," the cutaneous manifestations of LE are subclassified in four lupus-specific types (Kuhn 2003):
- Acute cutaneous lupus erythematosus (ACLE)
- Subacute cutaneous lupus erythematosus (SCLE)
- Chronic cutaneous lupus erythematosus (CCLE)
  - Discoid lupus erythematosus (DLE)
  - Lupus erythematosus profundus (LEP)
  - Lupus erythematosus hypertrophicus/verrucous (HVLE)
  - Chilblain lupus erythematosus (CHLE)
- Intermittent cutaneous lupus erythematosus (ICLE)
  - Lupus erythematosus tumidus (LET)

ACLE and SCLE are clearly related to a specific picture of SLE. CCLE lesions may occur in both cutaneous LE (CLE) and SLE. In addition to these classes, a variety of unspecific cutaneous symptoms like alopecia and vasculitis may reflect lupus activity (Wysenbeek et al. 1991) or may indicate specific associated syndromes such as purpura in Sjögren's syndrome or livedo reticularis in antiphospholipid syndrome. The nonspecific LE skin lesions are detected only in patients with SLE, not in those with DLE or SCLE (Cardinali et al. 2000).

Acute Cutaneous Lupus Erythematosus

ACLE manifestations indicate SLE. Acute skin lesions include "butterfly" rash, generalized erythema, and bullous lesions. Butterfly rash is the most common acute skin
lesion of SLE, developing as an erythematous, sometimes raised, lesion most often in
a malar distribution. It lasts from days to weeks and often is painful or pruritic. A
temporal association with sun exposure is common.

ACLE is reported to occur in about 50%–60% of patients at the onset of SLE, and
during follow-up, the frequency of skin involvement reaches about 80% (Table 13.1).
Butterfly rash is present in less than 50% of patients at disease onset, a reminder not
to exclude SLE when this diagnostic clue is missing. Because no other symptom is
100% specific for SLE and sensitivity varies for the different manifestations, classification of SLE is made using classification criteria (Table 13.2). The specificity of the
cutaneous scoring items is very high (96%–99%), and the sensitivity ranges from 18%
for discoid lesions to 57% for butterfly rash (photosensitivity, 43%; oral ulcers, 27%)
(Tan et al. 1982).

The prevalence of SLE is higher than that of CCLE, and it varies from 12 cases per
100,000 population in Britain to 39 cases per 100,000 population in Sweden. Although
African-Americans have a high prevalence of this disease, SLE is exceedingly rare
among blacks living in Africa (Hart et al. 1983). The disease occurs primarily in young
women and ranges in severity from a mild disease to a devastating illness with multiorgan involvement (Gladman and Urowitz 1998).

Indicators of SLE are constitutional symptoms, which mostly occur in patients
during the course of active disease and often are the earliest symptoms. Fatigue, fever,

Table 13.1. Frequency of lupus manifestations[a]

Manifestation	Number of patients (%) [n=108]	Number of patients (%) [n=605]	Number of patients (%) [n=520]
Arthralgia	77	85	92
Constitutional	73	84	86
Skin	57	81	72
Arthritis	56	63	92
Renal	44	77	46
Raynaud's phenomenon	33	58	18
Lymphadenopathy	25	32	59
Central nervous system	24	54	26
Pleurisy	23	37	45
Pericarditis	20	29	31
Mucous membranes	18	54	9
Vasculitis	10	37	21
Lung	9	17	0
Myositis	7	5	0
Nephrotic syndrome	5	11	23
Myocarditis	1	4	8

[a] The frequency of lupus manifestations at onset is based on 108 patients and at any time for
605 patients (before 1990) and 520 patients (after 1990) (Gladman and Urowitz 1998).

Table 13.2. The 1982 revised American College of Rheumatology (ACR) criteria for classification of systemic lupus erythematosusa

Criterion	Definition
1. Malar rash	Fixed erythema, flat or raised, over the malar eminences, tending to spare the nasolabial folds
2. Discoid rash	Erythematous raised patches with adherent keratotic scaling and follicular plugging; atrophic scarring may occur in older lesions
3. Photosensitivity	Skin rash as a result of unusual reaction to sunlight, by patient history or physician observation
4. Oral ulcers	Oral or nasopharyngeal ulceration, usually painless, observed by a physician
5. Arthritis	Nonerosive arthritis involving 2 peripheral joints, characterized by tenderness, swelling, or effusion
6. Serositis	Pleuritis – convincing history of pleuritic pain or rubbing heard by a physician or evidence of pleural effusion
	Pericarditis – documented by electrocardiographic or rub or evidence of pericardial effusion
7. Renal disorder	Persistent proteinuria – >0.5 g/d or >3+ if quantitation is not performed
	Cellular casts – may be red blood cells, hemoglobin, granular, tubular, or mixed
8. Neurologic disorder	Seizures – in the absence of offending drugs or known metabolic derangements, e. g., uremia, ketoacidosis, or electrolyte imbalance
	Psychosis – in the absence of offending drugs or known metabolic derangements, e. g., uremia, ketoacidosis, or electrolyte imbalance
9. Hematologic disorder	Hemolytic anemia – with reticulocytosis
	Leukopenia – <4,000/mm total on 2 occasions
	Lymphopenia – <1,500/mm on 2 occasions
	Thrombocytopenia – <100,000/mm in the absence of offending drugs
10. Immunologic disorder	Anti-DNA – antibody to native DNA in abnormal titer
	Anti-Sm – presence of antibody to Sm nuclear antigen
	Antiphospholipid antibodies (positive reaction at 2 time points with at least 6 weeks' separation):
	– Increased IgG or highly increased IgM anti-cardiolipin antibodies or
	– Positive lupus anticoagulants using a standard method or
	– Positive serologic test results for syphilis
11. Antinuclear antibody	An abnormal titer of antinuclear antibody by immunofluorescence or an equivalent assay at any point in time and in the absence of drugs known to be associated with "drug-induced lupus" syndrome

[a] The proposed classification is based on 11 criteria. For the purpose of identifying patients in clinical studies, a person shall be said to have systemic lupus erythematosus if any four or more of the 11 criteria are present, serially or simultaneously, during any interval of observation (Tan et al. 1982).

arthralgia and myalgia, and weight changes are the most common of these complaints (Hildebrand and Muller 2002).

Fever due to active disease, infection (favored by immunosuppression), and drug use is another common and nonspecific symptom that occurs in more than 50% of patients with SLE.

Musculoskeletal Symptoms

Arthralgia, myalgia, and arthritis represent the most common presenting complaints in SLE. Arthritis tends to be migratory and asymmetrical. It can affect any joint, but the small joints of the hands, wrists, and knees are involved most frequently. Arthritis classically is nonerosive and usually nondeforming. Soft-tissue swelling is common, and effusions, when they occur, are usually mildly inflammatory. However, as many as 10% of patients develop hand deformities due to chronic arthritis and tendinitis, called "Jaccoud arthropathy", which mimic the changes observed in rheumatoid arthritis but lack erosions.

Renal Involvement

The kidney is the most commonly involved visceral organ in SLE, although involvement is asymptomatic in its earliest stages. Although only approximately 50% of patients develop clinically evident renal disease, results of kidney biopsy demonstrate some degree of renal involvement in almost all patients with SLE. Nephritis usually develops within the first few years after onset of disease. Clinically, patients may present with an acute nephritic picture, nephrotic syndrome, acute renal failure, or chronic renal insufficiency. Rarely, acute renal pain can be present secondary to an associated pyelonephritis or to vasculitis with renal infarction. Signs of nephropathy was the variable with the highest statistical relevance for distinguishing between patients with CLE (DLE/SCLE) and SLE in the European Centres of Dermatology (Tebbe et al. 1997).

Central Nervous System Symptoms

Neuropsychiatric symptoms are common manifestations of SLE. The multiple central nervous system manifestations can be divided into inflammatory and thrombotic processes, the latter most commonly presenting as thrombotic or thromboembolic stroke and often associated with the presence of antiphospholipid antibodies. Other central nervous system manifestations, some of which are related to a vasculitic lupus cerebritis, include headache, seizures (focal or generalized), organic brain syndrome, and psychosis.

A high percentage of patients with SLE have evidence of faint cognitive impairment by neurocognitive testing, but whether this represents true encephalopathy, a feature of previous neurologic damage, medication-induced effects, some other process, or some combination of the above is unclear.

Pulmonary Involvement

Pulmonary manifestations of SLE include acute and chronic processes. Pleurisy with pleuritic chest pain with or without pleural effusions is the most common feature of acute pulmonary involvement. Acute lupus pneumonitis and chronic lupus interstitial disease are unusual causes of shortness of breath in SLE. Other conditions, especially infection, should be considered. Diffuse alveolar hemorrhage is an acute, life-threatening pulmonary process in SLE, often occurring with other evidence of active lupus.

Cardiac Manifestations

Pericarditis (serositis), verrucous endocarditis (Libman-Sacks), myocarditis, and accelerated development of coronary artery disease occur at higher rates in patients with SLE. The most common cardiac manifestation is chest pain due to pericarditis, with or without pericardial effusion. Whereas atherosclerotic coronary artery disease is associated with inactive SLE and is thought to be in part secondary to chronic steroid therapy, pericarditis and myocarditis occur in patients with active SLE. Coronary vasculitis occurs only very rarely, and coronary thrombosis related to antiphospholipid antibodies also is a rare event.

Prognosis

An improvement in the survival rate has occurred during the past few years: the 10-year survival rate now approaches 90%, compared with a 5-year survival rate of less than 50% in the 1950s (Urowitz and Gladman 2000). The decrease in mortality can be attributed to facilitated diagnosis by feasibility of serologic markers, leading to identification of milder forms and cases at earlier stages and allowing for swift disease-specific treatment.

Death due to complications of SLE itself, such as nephritis, occurs at a higher rate within 5 years of onset of symptoms. Infectious complications coincident with active SLE and its treatment with immunosuppressives, cardiovascular complications, and malignancy are now the most common causes of death in patients with SLE and chronic damage due to long-lasting disease and therapy (Manger et al. 2002, Urowitz and Gladman 2000). This is explained by a variety of factors, including endothelial cell injury during active SLE, premature atherosclerosis, and dyslipidemia related to renal disease or long-term administration of corticosteroids (Urowitz and Gladman 2000a, Urowitz et al. 2000). Despite the improvement in the overall survival rate, patients with SLE still have a death rate three times higher than that of the general population, and patients with isolated skin and musculoskeletal involvement have higher survival rates than those with renal and CNS disease (Gladman and Urowitz 1998).

Subsets of Systemic Lupus Erythematosus

In the wide spectrum of clinical manifestations, different subsets of systemic lupus and clusters can be defined by clinical or serologic items. Relevant and established

Table 13.3. Typical autoantibodies in patients with systemic lupus erythematosus (SLE)

Autoantibody	Incidence (%)	Antigen Detected	Clinical Importance
Antinuclear antibodies	98	Multiple nuclear	Repeatedly negative test results make SLE unlikely
Anti-DNA	70	DNA (double stranded)	Anti-double-stranded DNA is disease specific, anti-single-stranded DNA is not; high titers are associated with clinical activity
Anti-Sm	30	Protein complexed to six species of small nuclear RNA	Specific for SLE
Anti-RNP	40	Protein complexed to U1RNA	High titer in syndromes with features of polymyositis, lupus, scleroderma, and mixed connective tissue disease; if present in SLE without anti-DNA, risk of nephritis is low
Anti-Ro/SSA	30	Protein complexed to y1-y5 RNA	Former "antinuclear antibody- negative" lupus, SLE, SCLE, Sjögren's syndrome, Sjögren/lupus overlap, neonatal lupus, congenital heart block; can be associated with nephritis (+ double-stranded DNA antibodies)
Anti-La/SSB	10	Phosphoprotein	Always associated with anti-Ro/SSA (risk for nephritis is low if present)
Antihistone	70	Histones	More frequent in drug-induced LE (95%)
Antiphospholipid	50	Phospholipids	Lupus anticoagulant, anticardiolipin, and false-positive test result for syphilis; the two former (particularly high-titer IgG) are associated with thrombembolic complications (such as strokes) and fetal losses

autoantibodies of SLE are given in Table 13.3 (see also Chap. 24) (Elkon 1998). They can be divided into marker antibodies for diagnosis, for different subsets, and for disease activity. Clear positive ANAs in a standardized test (immunofluorescence) using the proper substrate (HEp-2 cells) are suitable as serologic screening for SLE, reaching a sensitivity of nearly 100%. However, as ANAs are also found in many other connective tissue diseases, their specificity is considerable low. Antibodies against ds-DNA are highly specific for SLE and have a rather strong (at least intraindividual) correlation with disease activity and in high titers of high avid antibodies with lupus nephritis. Antibodies against different extractable nuclear antigens, like Ro/SSA-, La/SSB-, Sm-, and U1RNP, alone or in different combinations, seem to define more homogeneous disease entities. Their concentration proved not to be of considerable additional value for monitoring of the disease.

U1RNP Antibody-Positive Lupus

In 1972, Sharp et al. (Sharp et al. 1972) described a "mixed connective tissue disease" subset with clinical features of SLE, scleroderma, and polymyositis. Serologically, this group is defined by the occurrence of ANAs, with a coarse speckled pattern revealing anti-U1RNP specificity (without anti-Sm antibodies). Rheumatoid factors and hyper-gammaglobulinemia are often present. Nearly all patients demonstrate Raynaud's phenomenon, acrocyanosis, edematous sclerodactyly, telangiectasias, and other erythematous skin lesions (Schneider and Fischer 2000). Dysphagia due to disturbance of esophageal motility is a frequent symptom, and microstomia and pulmonary basal fibrosis are also indicative of overlapping scleroderma as inflammatory myopathy for polymyositis. Renal or cerebral involvement is very rare, but transition into SLE (with development of anti-Sm and anti-ds-DNA antibodies) is reported. The overall activity of disease and prognosis are rather favorable compared with full-blown lupus or a diffuse form of systemic sclerosis.

Sm Antibody-Positive Lupus

Anti-Sm antibodies are regarded as the most specific marker autoantibodies for SLE, indicating in addition severe forms of it. As such, it is part of the American College of Rheumatology (ACR) classification criteria, even though prevalence in SLE is about 10% in whites (and higher in blacks). Cerebral vasculitis and lupus nephritis are reported to be more frequent in patients with LE and anti-Sm antibodies (Craft 1992). Skin manifestations are from the ACLE type, with the classic butterfly rash, photosensitive erythematous skin lesions, and severe acral vasculitis with a tendency to atrophic scarring.

Subacute Cutaneous Lupus Erythematosus

Subacute skin lesions begin as erythematous papules or plaques and can evolve either into annular lesions similar to erythema annular centrifugum or into scaling that resembles psoriasis or lichen planus. They tend to occur on sun-exposed areas of the body but can have a generalized distribution, they are nonfixed and nonscarring, and they follow a waxing and waning course. This lupus subset was first described by Sontheimer et al. (Sontheimer et al. 1979) in 1979. Two thirds of these patients show antibodies to Ro/SSA, mostly as anti-60-kDa Ro/SSA and annular lesions, with an HLA-A1, -B8, -DR3 association (Bielsa et al. 1991). Seven percent to 21% of patients with lupus present these cutaneous eruptions (McCauliffe 1997).

Comparing anti-Ro/SSA-positive with anti-Ro/SSA-negative patients with SLE, there is a correlation between anti-Ro/SSA-positive and photosensitivity and anti-

Ro/SSA-negative and nephritis (Mond et al. 1989). The typical presentation of a patient with anti-Ro/SSA antibodies covers features of Sjögren's syndrome with xerostomia, xerophthalmia, a history of parotid swelling, and arthralgias. Beyond ANAs (sometimes only weakly positive) and anti-Ro/SSA antibodies (often together with anti-La/SSB antibodies), many of these patients prove to have high titers of rheumatoid factors (>80%), elevated erythrocyte sedimentation rates, and hypergammaglobulinemia, which may be associated with purpura. Clinically, a polyadenopathy of lymph nodes, subfebrile states, and a tendency toward leukopenia marks the transition to SLE (also classified as Sjögren's/lupus overlap syndrome). When those patients develop additional features of systemic disease (i. e., arthritis, serositis, hemolytic anemia, and renal or cerebral involvement), anti-ds-DNA antibodies are usually present. Other typical associations with anti-Ro/SSA antibodies are C2 or C4 complement deficiency, interstitial pneumonitis, and late-onset lupus.

Anti-Ro/SSA antibodies are also related to congenital heart block and neonatal lupus, which has to be kept in mind in patients with SCLE. Half of these patients fulfill the ACR criteria for SLE (Callen and Klein 1988) but in general have a more favorable long-term prognosis.

Discoid Lupus Erythematosus

Discoid LE (DLE) lesions also begin as erythematous papules or plaques with scaling but progress to follicular plugging with central atrophy and scarring. Similar to the other cutaneous lesions of SLE, these develop primarily in sun-exposed regions, including the malar area. When present on the scalp, they can result in permanent alopecia. Generalized and localized forms exist, the former being associated more often with systemic symptoms and laboratory abnormalities.

DLE is the most common form of chronic CLE; 15%–30% of patients with SLE have DLE, about 5% as an initial symptom (Cervera et al. 1993). Of patients with localized DLE, 90%–95% express a disease that is limited to the skin. A few patients with DLE may develop other skin lesions, and systemic features like fever are rare, but half of them will exhibit arthritis/arthralgia (Wallace et al. 1992). ANA in low titers is detected in about half of the patients, and other autoantibodies are rarely seen (Bielsa et al. 1991, Wallace et al. 1992). About one third of the patients exhibit some leukopenia and an elevated erythrocyte sedimentation rate.

Less common clinical forms of DLE are seldom described in larger cohorts. LE profundus may show more frequently systemic signs of lupus than DLE: one third of the patients develop serositis and about one quarter a lupus nephritis. More often, unspecific findings like fatigue and musculoskeletal complaints exist, but overall the disease is milder than SLE (Sontheimer 1999).

Conclusion

Skin changes are one of the hallmarks of SLE and often the initial symptom the patient is aware of. Their kind and severity indicate certain disease subsets, serologic patterns, other organ involvements, and inflammatory activity of the systemic disease.

Since SLE might show many features of skin disease and must only have the potential to involve sites other than the skin to be classified as systemic, it will always be of substantial value for a given patient with SLE when the dermatologist is aware of and familiar with systemic features and the rheumatologist is able to recognize the different skin manifestations of the disease.

References

Bielsa I, Herrero C, Ercilla G, Collado A, Font J, Ingelmo M, Mascaró JM (1991) Immunogenetic findings in cutaneous erythematosus. J Am Acad Dermatol 25:251–257

Callen JR, Klein J (1988) Subacute cutaneous lupus erythematosus. Arthritis Rheum 31:1007–1013

Cardinali C, Caproni M, Bernacchi E, Amato L, Fabbri P (2000) The spectrum of cutaneous manifestations in lupus erythematosus – the Italian experience. Lupus 9: 417–423

Cervera R, Khamashta MA, Font J, Sebastiani GD, Gil A, Lavilla P, Doménech I, Aydintug A, Jedryka-Góral A, de Rámon E, Galeazzi M, Haga HJ, Mathieu A, Houssiau F, Ingelmo M, Hughes GRV (1993) European Working Party on SLE. Systemic lupus erythematosus: Clinical and immunological patterns of disease expression in a cohort of 1,000 patients. Medicine 72:113–124

Craft J (1992) Antibodies to snRNPs in systemic lupus erythematosus. Rheum Dis Clin North Am 18:311–335

Elkon KB (1998) Systemic lupus erythematosus: autoantibodies in SLE. In: Klippel JH, Dieppe PA (eds) Rheumatology, 2nd ed. Mosby, St. Louis

Gladman DD, Urowitz MB (1998) Systemic lupus erythematosus: clinical features. In: Klippel JH, Dieppe PA (eds) Rheumatology, 2nd ed. Mosby, St. Louis

Hart HH, Grigor RR, Caughey DE (1983) Ethnic difference in the prevalence of systemic lupus erythematosus. Ann Rheum Dis 42:529–532

Hildebrand J, Muller D (2002) Systemic lupus erythematosus. emedicine.com. http://www.emedicine.com/med/topic2228.htm

Kuhn A (2003) Neue klinische, photobiologische und immunhistologische Erkenntnisse zur Pathophysiologie des kutanen Lupus erythematodes. In: Hautklinik. Düsseldorf: Heinrich-Heine University, Habilitationsschrift

Manger K, Manger B, Repp R, Geisselbrecht M, Geiger A, Pfahlberg A, Harrer T, Kalden JR (2002) Definition of risk factors for death, end stage renal disease, and thromboembolic events in a monocentric cohort of 338 patients with systemic lupus erythematosus. Ann Rheum Dis 61:1065–1070

McCauliffe DP (1997) Cutaneous diseases in adults associated with anti-Ro/SS-A autoantibody production. Lupus 6:158–166

Mond CB, Peterson MGE, Rothfield NF (1989) Correlation of anti-Ro antibody with photosensitivity rash in systemic lupus erythematosus patients. Arthritis Rheum 32:202–204

Schneider M, Fischer R (2000) Mischkollagenose. In: Miehle W, Fehr K, Schattenkirchner M, Tillmann K (eds) Rheumatologie in Praxis und Klinik. Thieme Verlag, Stuttgart, pp 995–1002

Sharp GC, Irwin WS, Tan EM, Gould RG, Holman MR (1972) MCTD – an apparently distinct rheumatic disease syndrome associated with a specific antibody to an extractable nuclear antigen (ENA). Am J Med 2:148–159

Sontheimer RD (1999) Systemic lupus erythematosus and skin. In: Lahita RG (ed) Systemic lupus erythematosus, 3rd ed. Academic Press, San Diego, pp 631–656

Sontheimer RD, Thomas JR, Gilliam JN (1979) Subacute cutaneous lupus erythematosus: a cutaneous marker for a distinct lupus erythematosus subset. Arch Dermatol 115:1409–1415

Tan EM, Cohen AS, Fries JF, Masi AT, McShane DJ, Rothfield NF, Schaller JG, Talal N, Winchester RJ (1982) The 1982 revised criteria for the classification of system lupus erythematosus. Arthritis Rheum 25:1271–1277

Tebbe B, Mansmann U, Wollina U, Auer-Grumbach P, Licht-Mbalyohere A, Arensmeier M, Orfanos CE (1997) Markers of cutaneous lupus erythematosus indicating systemic involvement. A multicenter study on 296 patients. Acta Derm Venereol 77:305–308

Urowitz MB, Gladman DD (2000) How to improve morbidity and mortality in systemic lupus erythematosus. Rheumatology (Oxford) 39:238–244

Urowitz MB, Gladman DD, Bruce I (2000) Atherosclerosis and systemic lupus erythematosus. Curr Rheumatol Rep 2:19–23

Wallace DJ, Pistiner M, Nessim S, Metzger AL, Klinenberg JR (1992) Cutaneous lupus erythematosus without systemic lupus erythematosus: clinical and laboratory features. Semin Arthritis Rheum 21:221–226

Wysenbeek AJ, Leibovici L, Amit M, Weinberger A (1991) Alopecia in systemic lupus erythematosus. Relation to disease manifestations. J Rheumatol 18:1185–1186

CHAPTER 14

Prognosis of Cutaneous Lupus Erythematosus 14

Beate Tebbe, Constantin E. Orfanos

Systemic lupus erythematosus (SLE) is one of the most frequently seen autoimmune disorders. Prevalence rates vary between 14 and 50 per 100,000 population (Hochberg 1997). Cutaneous LE (CLE) presumably occurs two to three times more frequently than SLE. However, exact population-based epidemiologic data are not available. In selected groups of patients with LE cared for in dermatology departments, the prevalence of patients with chronic discoid LE (DLE) varies between 42% and 72% (Kind and Goerz 1987, Tebbe and Orfanos 1987), and subacute cutaneous LE (SCLE) is found in 7%–32% of the entire collective (Molad 1987, Sontheimer et al. 1979, Tebbe and Orfanos 1987).

The prognosis of SLE depends on the severity and extent of visceral involvement. Most fatalities among patients with SLE are attributable to active disease, especially to renal and central nervous system involvement, and to various infections. However, the 10-year survival rate today exceeds 80% owing to treatment with oral corticosteroids and potent immunosuppressive drugs (Drenkard and Alarcón-Segovia 2000, Gladman 1996, Swaak 1989). In general, the prognosis of CLE is regarded as more favorable than that of SLE, although prospective studies in large groups are rare.

Classic variants of specific CLE lesions are DLE and SCLE. Other typical CLE subsets, such as LE profundus/panniculitis, LE tumidus, urticaria vasculitis, hypertrophic LE, and bullous LE, are rather rare variants. Butterfly rash and macular exanthema are characteristic skin lesions of SLE rarely found in patients with CLE. DLE and SCLE may appear at any age, but the most common age at onset is 20–40 years in females and males, with a female predominance of 3:1 in DLE and 3:1 to 6:1 in SCLE. Nonspecific LE skin lesions such as generalized or acrolocalized vasculitis (4%–30%), livedo reticularis (22%–35%), and alopecia (38%–78%) are frequently seen in patients with CLE (Beutner et al. 1991, Callen 1985, 1986, Molad 1987, Moschella 1989, Sontheimer 1979, Tebbe and Orfanos 1992).

DLE and SCLE are generally regarded as disease variants with a better prognosis than that of SLE, and severe courses of cutaneous variants with a lethal outcome are rare. However, if mild signs of systemic manifestations, such as proteinuria and arthralgia, were registered in CLE, 14%–27% of patients with DLE and 67%–70% of patients with SCLE had extracutaneous involvement (Sontheimer 1989, Tebbe et al. 1997, Watanabe and Tsuchida 1995).

It seems that ca. 5%–10% of patients with DLE will experience transition to SLE during long-term disease (Healy et al. 1995, Le Bozec et al. 1994, Millard and Rowell 1979, Rowell 1984, Schiodt 1984). In most cases, transition to SLE requires more than 5 years (Healy et al. 1995, Le Bozec et al. 1994). However, severe life-threatening man-

Table 14.1. Prognostic factors of cutaneous lupus erythematosus (LE): discoid LE and subacute cutaneous LE

Genetic predisposition:	HLA associations, complement deficiencies
Race and sex:	Annular erythema as Asian counterpart of SCLE, female predominance
Clinical presentation:	Systemic involvement
Autoantibodies:	ANA titer (≥1:320), anti-Ro/SSA antibodies
Photosensitivity:	Family or personal history of PLE
Drugs and hormones:	Thiazides, calcium channel blockers, angiotensin-converting enzyme inhibitors, estrogens and others
Association with tumors:	Skin tumors on DLE scars, internal tumors in SCLE

ifestations such as renal or neurologic involvement may occur in patients with DLE (Le Bozec et al. 1994). Up to 50%–60% of all patients with SCLE may develop systemic involvement in just a few years, in addition to their cutaneous manifestations, that may require systemic immunosuppressive treatment (Callen and Klein 1988, Cohen and Crosby 1994, Johansson-Stephansson et al. 1989, Sontheimer 1989).

The prognosis of CLE depends of the clinical variant of the cutaneous disease and the severity of associated extracutaneous manifestations. Several risk factors may influence the course and prognosis of CLE: genetic predisposition, race and sex, clinical presentation, age at disease onset, and triggering factors such as exposure to ultraviolet (UV) light and oral medications (Table 14.1).

Genetic Predisposition

LE is a multifactorial systemic disease. A genetic background has been suggested by familial aggregation and twin studies (Shai et al. 1999). Several studies have found human leukocyte antigen (HLA) associations in DLE with the A1, B7, B8, DR2, and DR3 haplotypes (Fowler et al. 1985, Knop et al. 1990, Millard et al. 1977). However, other studies have not confirmed these findings (Bielsa et al. 1991, Tongio et al. 1982). In SCLE, associations to HLA A1, B8, DR2, DR3, DQ2, and DRw52 are described (Callen and Klein 1988, Herrereo et al. 1988, Johansson-Stephansson et al. 1989, Provost et al. 1988, Sontheimer et al. 1981). It has been suggested that the HLA-DR antigen associations of SCLE relate more to the anti-Ro/SSA antibody response than to the specific SCLE lesions (Watson et al. 1991). Patients with CLE who generate anti-Ro/SSA antibodies show immunogenetic association with the HLA A1, B8, DRB1*0301 extended haplotype (Meyer et al. 1985, Watson et al. 1991) and a significant negative association with DRB*04 (Stephens et al. 1991). SCLE has also been independently associated with the rare tumor necrosis factor 308A allele, part of the same A1, B8, DRB*0301 extended haplotype (Werth et al. 2000, Wilson et al. 1993).

Genetic deficiencies (e. g., homozygous deficiency of C2, C3, C4, and C5) and C1-esterase inhibitor deficiency have been found in association with SCLE and DLE (Asghar et al. 1991, Meyer et al. 1985, Partanen et al. 1988, Perkins et al. 1994, Provost et al. 1983). Deficiencies in early components of the complement system are significantly associated with LE (Schur 1978, Sullivan 1998). The prevalence of homozygous

C4A deficiency is approximately 10 times higher in patients with LE than in controls (Howard et al. 1986, Petri et al. 1993). Interestingly, patients with LE associated with complement C2 and C4 deficiencies are said to have a better prognosis than individuals with LE without inherited complement deficiencies (Petri et al. 1993, Ratnoff et al. 1996, Sullivan 1998). Cutaneous and articular involvement is prominent, but pleuropericardial, neurologic, and renal involvement is absent or mild. The prevalence of anti-Ro/SSA antibodies is reported to be much higher than in non-C2-deficient patients with LE (Meyer et al. 1985, Provost et al. 1983). Comparison between LE patients with C2 deficiency and a large cohort of unselected patients revealed that photosensitivity, SCLE lesions, and anti-Ro/SSA antibodies are more frequent among C2-deficient patients (Lipsker et al. 2000).

Race and Sex

Differences concerning the clinical presentation of CLE in various ethnic groups are not a frequent finding. However, a peculiar variant of CLE is annular erythema frequently associated with Sjögren's syndrome in Japan. It is regarded as the counterpart of SCLE in whites, except for the paucity of LE-specific histopathologic findings and HLA-DR3 tissue type (Miyagawa 1994, Watanabe et al. 1997). Japanese annular erythema of Sjögren's syndrome sera and American SCLE sera share several types of anti-52-kDa and anti-60-kDa Ro/SSA autoantibodies (McCauliffe et al. 1996).

In CLE, it seems likely that sex differences exist concerning the course and prognosis of the disease. In one study, 28 males and 111 females with SLE were examined. Widespread DLE and papular and nodular mucinosis occur significantly more commonly in men than in women with SLE and serum sex hormone levels within the reference range in male patients with LE (Kanda et al. 1996). However, other groups reported that men with SLE showed hyperestrogenemia and hypotestosteronemia and suggested that estrogens may facilitate the development of SLE and that testosterone may have protective properties (Miller et al. 1983, Sequeira et al. 1993). In a series of 261 patients with SLE, only 12% were male. Follow-up of these patients for a mean of 64 months showed that discoid skin lesions and deeply localized subcutaneous LE skin lesions occur more frequently in men than in women (Font et al. 1992). However, in another series of patients with SLE including 61 males and 86 females, no significant difference in CLE manifestations was found between the two groups (Kaufman et al. 1989, Koh et al. 1994).

Clinical Presentation and Systemic Involvement

Although DLE and SCLE can be easily diagnosed using clinical and histologic criteria, it is still difficult to predict which cases will develop systemic involvement and transition to SLE. The criteria established by the American Rheumatism Association (ARA) (Tan et al. 1982) characterize an inhomogeneous group of patients with cutaneous manifestations of LE. A maximum of 20% of all patients with DLE and 30%–50% of all patients with SCLE have four or more positive ARA criteria, whereas only two to three criteria are fulfilled in most cases of CLE (Beutner et al. 1991,

Higuchi et al. 1978, Parodi et al. 2000). In addition, typical skin lesions for differentiating DLE from SCLE are not included in the ARA list. Using that list, correct diagnosis and proper evaluation of the course of CLE is difficult, if not impossible. There is a need, therefore, to establish suitable diagnostic criteria for CLE.

Univariate statistical analysis comparing a wide panel of clinical and serologic data in patients with either SLE ($n=464$) or CLE ($n=67$), mainly DLE, showed that the following parameters were significantly more frequent in SLE than in CLE: female predominance, fever, arthralgia/arthritis, pericarditis, hypertension, pleurisy, oral ulcers, Raynaud's phenomenon, severe headaches, nephritis, proteinuria, anemia, leukopenia, positive antinuclear antibody (ANA) titer, high anti-DNA antibody titer, low complement C3, and elevated erythrocyte sedimentation rate (Wallace et al. 1992).

SCLE is believed to be associated with extracutaneous manifestations in a large proportion of patients. A cohort of 79 patients with SCLE and 58 with SLE was studied and compared concerning clinical presentation, histopathologic findings, and immunserologic data. SCLE differed from SLE by cutaneous changes, significantly less frequent kidney involvement (2.5% vs 48%), serositis (4% vs 17%), and arthritis (47% vs 88%), together with the rare presence of anti-double-stranded (ds) DNA antibodies (1.2% vs 34%) and U1RNP antibodies (1.2% vs 17%) (Chlebus et al. 1995).

If patients with SCLE fulfilling four or more ARA criteria were compared with patients with SLE without these LE-specific skin lesions, remarkable differences would be noted. Photosensitivity was more frequent in patients with SCLE (82%) than in patients without these cutaneous lesions (45%), whereas arthritis, Raynaud's phenomenon, pleurisy, central nervous system disorder, renal disease, anemia, hypocomplementemia, and anti-ds-DNA antibodies were significantly more frequent in patients without SCLE (Lopez-Longo et al. 1997).

From the dermatologic point of view, it is necessary to develop criteria for recognizing patients with CLE at risk to develop SLE. For elucidating this subject, several studies were performed. Classification criteria for CLE have been published by the European Academy of Dermatology and Venereology (EADV) to obtain more reliable parameters for classifying these patients (Beutner et al. 1991). EADV criteria include ARA criteria and other parameters that are more suitable for the evaluation of patients with CLE, such as vasculitis of the fingers, muscle weakness, lupus band test, elevated erythrocyte sedimentation rate, and anti-Ro/SSA and anti-La/SSB antibodies. In one study, 207 patients with chronic CLE and SCLE were comparatively classified according to ARA and EADV criteria. ARA criteria showed a sensitivity of 88%, a specificity of 79%, a positive predictive value of 56%, and a negative predictive value of 96%. EADV criteria showed a sensitivity of only 64% but a specificity of 93%, a positive predictive value of 61%, and a negative predictive value of 94% (Parodi and Rebora 1997). These data support the view that ARA criteria are less useful for evaluating patients with CLE and that selection of EADV criteria has to be improved to obtain a greater rate of sensitivity.

In a prospective multicenter study of 296 patients with LE performed in five cooperating dermatology departments in Germany and Austria, many variables were collected for each patient (Tebbe et al. 1997). The selected variables were most relevant for disease progression. Univariate and multivariate analysis of the data showed that mild signs of nephropathy (proteinuria and hematuria) had the highest statistical relevance for distinguishing patients with CLE (DLE/SCLE) from those with SLE

Table 14.2. Criteria for differentiation between cutaneous and systemic lupus erythematosus (LE)

	CLE (n=464) vs SLE[a] (n=67)	SCLE (n=79) vs SLE[b] (n=58)	DLE/SCLE (n=245) vs SLE[c] (n=51)
Clinical symptoms and immunserologic findings more frequently occurring in SLE than in CLE	Oral ulcers Raynaud's phenomenon Fever Arthralgia/arthritis Nephritis, proteinuria Hypertension Headaches Pericarditis Pleurisy Anemia, leukopenia ESR elevation ANA, anti-ds-DNA antibodies Low complement C3	Arthritis Kidney involvement Serositis Anti-ds-DNA antibodies U1RNP antibodies	Mild signs of nephropathy (proteinuria, hematuria) Arthralgias ANA titer ($\geq$1:320) ESR elevation

[a] Wallace et al. 1992, [b] Chlebus et al. 1998, [c] Tebbe et al. 1997.

(odds ratio [OR], 4.21; confidence interval [CI], 1.88–9.38), followed by high ANA titer ($\geq$1:320) (OR, 3.11; CI, 1.49–6.48), the presence of arthralgias (OR, 3.58; CI, 1.49–8.60), and erythrocyte sedimentation rate elevation (OR, 2.57; CI, 0.97–6.78). In contrast, low ANA titers as well as anti-ds-DNA antibodies had little or no statistical relevance for differentiation (Tebbe et al. 1997). Thus, patients with CLE and signs of nephropathy, arthralgias, and elevated ANA titers ($\geq$1:320) should be carefully monitored because they may be at risk for transition to SLE. The individual risk of developing a severe course of the disease increases with the number of positive variables, as calculated by multiplication of the ORs (Table 14.2).

Course and Activity Scores

A few studies have been performed applying well-established SLE disease activity scores in cohorts of patients with CLE. Evaluation of 176 patients with CLE by the Systemic Lupus Activity Measure (SLAM) and follow-up for more than 5 years (mean, 9 years) showed that most had mildly to moderately active disease. Ninety-seven patients had localized discoid LE, 59 had disseminated DLE, and 20 had SCLE. With SLAM criteria, 85 patients (48%) had low-activity disease, 72 (41%) had mild-activity disease, 15 (9%) had moderate-activity disease, and only 4 (2%) had very active disease. Photosensitivity, alopecia, oral ulcers, and Raynaud's phenomenon may indicate a worse prognosis (Parodi et al. 2000). Among the 50 patients followed up, SLAM scores decreased in 27, remained the same in 14, and increased in 9. The systemic manifestations at follow-up were arthritis, elevated erythrocyte sedimentation rate, and lymphopenia. These data indicate a good prognosis for CLE. However, the SLAM is far from being fully satisfactory. LE-specific skin lesions are not subdivided into different categories, but malar rash, DLE, lupus profundus, and bullous LE are all placed in the same group. However, these specific LE skin lesions are not equivalent regarding prognosis. Disease activity measured by the Systemic Lupus Erythematosus Disease Activity Index (SLEDAI) demonstrated that cases of SLE with nonspecific skin lesions have higher disease activity than those with specific skin lesions, supporting the fact that the latter group has a more benign course, including patients with DLE/SCLE (Zecevic et al. 2001).

Well-documented follow-up studies in patients with CLE are rare. However, continuous follow-up in 34 patients with SCLE documenting a wide panel of clinical and immunserologic data revealed that none of these patients developed severe LE crisis or died during 3 years of observation. Remarkably, the clinical symptoms, which occurred significantly more often, were acrolocalized vasculitis and arthralgias, being regarded as markers indicating mild progression of the disease (Tebbe et al. 1994). Nevertheless, a lethal outcome of CLE seems to be rare; in 10 years of follow-up, 10% of the patients with SCLE died, but only one from LE complications (Sontheimer 1989).

Prognosis of Rare Variants of Cutaneous Lupus Erythematosus

A few studies have been reported concerning the disease courses in rare CLE variants. LE profundus/panniculitis is regarded to have a more benign prognosis than SLE. In 10 years of follow-up, only 4 (25%) of 16 patients were classified as having SLE according to ARA criteria (Watanabe and Tsuchida 1996). In other case series, only 4 of 40 patients fulfilled the criteria for SLE. The major morbidity in this series resulted from disfigurement and occasional disability related to pain; 7 (18%) of 40 patients had applied for disability. Death related to active panniculitis did not occur. The disease course was chronic, with symptoms reported for an average of 6 years, and characterized by periods of remission and exacerbation (Martens et al. 1999).

LE tumidus (LET) is a subtype of CLE with some peculiarities. Clinically, LET is characterized by erythematous, succulent, urticaria-like, nonscarring plaques with a smooth surface in sun-exposed areas. Reproduction of skin lesions after UVA or UVB irradiation is possible in 70% of the cases. The sex ratio shows an equal distribution between males and females. Nonspecific LE skin lesions are uncommon, and, usually, none of the patients can be classified as SLE, reflecting that LET is a CLE variant with a more benign course (Kuhn et al. 2000) (Table 14.3).

Prognosis of Neonatal, Childhood, and Late-Onset Lupus Erythematosus

Neonatal LE (NLE) may occur in children of anti-Ro/SSA antibody-positive mothers owing to placental passage of these autoantibodies. The clinical characteristics of NLE include cutaneous lupus lesions, congenital heart block, cholestatic liver disease, and thrombocytopenia. Of these, cutaneous lupus and congenital complete heart block are the most common. The prevalence of NLE is not known but is probably at least 1 in 20,000 live births. The skin is affected in approximately half of the cases of

Table 14.3. Prognosis in rare variants of cutaneous lupus erythematosus

LE profundus/panniculitis (Martens et al. 1999, Watanabe and Tsuchida 1996)	Chronic disease course with disfigurement
LET (Kuhn et al. 2000)	Cutaneous variant without characteristics of SLE
NLE (Lee and Weston 1997, Neimann et al. 2000)	Skin is affected in 50%; skin lesions are SCLE-like; in most cases, resolution is by age of 6 months
Childhood LE (Lo et al. 1999, Wananukul et al. 1998)	
SLE	Malar rash is frequently found in SLE, 10-year-survival of 65%
DLE	Lack of female predominance, low incidence of photosensitivity, high rate of progression to systemic disease
Late-onset LE (Domenech et al. 1992, Fomiga et al. 1999, Ho et al. 1998, Ward and Polisson 1989)	Reduction of female predominance, cutaneous symptoms less frequent, but prognosis better than in early-onset LE

NLE. The skin lesions of NLE typically appear during the first few weeks of life, although in a few cases they have been reported to be present at birth. The skin lesions are similar to those of SCLE in adults (Lee and Weston 1997).

The expected outcome of cutaneous NLE is spontaneous resolution by a few months of life. Most babies have resolution of active skin lesions by age 6 months (Lee and Weston 1997). In 57 infants with NLE, mean age at diagnosis of the cutaneous manifestations was 6 weeks, and mean duration was 17 weeks. In 37 infants, the rash resolved without sequelae; 43% of which were untreated. A quarter of the patients had residual sequelae with telangiectasia and dyspigmentation (Neiman et al. 2000). Long-term rheumatologic outcome of children is good in general. However, rare cases of NLE are described with the development of autoimmune disorder in adulthood (Brucato et al. 1997).

CLE of childhood is identical morphologically and histologically to CLE in adults. CLE may occur in association with SLE or in children who have no evidence of internal involvement. In children who have SLE, malar rash of acute CLE is present in 30%–80% (Font et al. 1998, Lehmann 1995, Schaller 1982). Cutaneous manifestations are a prominent finding in children with SLE. In a group of 57 children followed for 6 years, 77% had cutaneous findings, followed by renal involvement (74%). The skin changes noted were malar rash (74%), oral ulcers (46%), vasculitis (42%), photosensitivity (40%), alopecia (32%), and discoid LE (19%). The ANA reaction was positive in 93% of patients, and anti-ds-DNA was positive in 46%. Eight patients died, six of severe infection and two of renal failure (Wanakul et al. 1998). Comparison of the disease course in childhood-onset SLE and adulthood-onset SLE reveals that malar rash, anemia, leukopenia, and anti-ds-DNA antibodies were significantly higher in childhood-onset SLE (Rood et al. 1999). The presence of arthritis, anemia, and seizures at onset of the disease resulted in a 2.6–3.9 times higher chance of a severe disease course (Rood et al. 1999). In a large study of 135 pediatric SLE cases, cumulative 5- and 10-year survival was 80.2% and 65%, respectively, without a sex difference (Lo et al. 1999).

DLE may occur in children who have SLE or as an isolated finding. In a study of 16 children with discoid lesions, it was noted that DLE is similar to its adult counterpart concerning its presentation and chronic course. Important differences are a lack of female predominance, a low incidence of photosensitivity, and a high rate of progression to systemic disease. Five of the 10 children followed into adulthood developed SLE (George and Tunnessen 1993). SCLE has rarely been noted in children (Wanakul et al. 1998).

Lupus profundus/panniculitis is also described in pediatric cases. Its main characteristics are a female predominance and the location of the skin lesions, electively on the face and the lateral aspect of the shoulders. Usually the lesions regress, leaving a characteristic atrophic scar (Bachmeyer et al. 1992).

Onset of SLE in later life, usually defined as after age 50 years, constitutes 6%–18% of the lupus population. Characteristic findings are a reduction of the female predominance from 9:1 in early-onset disease to 6–7:1 in late-onset SLE (Kammer and Mishra 2000, Pu et al. 2000). The interval from onset to diagnosis is usually longer in older patients with LE than in the younger ones. The mean interval between onset of symptoms and signs for diagnosis is approximately 32.5 months (Font et al. 1991, Kammer and Mishra 2000, Maddisin 1987). Racial differences are reported, with a higher proportion of blacks having early-onset LE than late onset (Domenech et al. 1992). Although rash and arthritis/arthralgia remain the most frequent signs in both early- and late-onset SLE, there is an increase in the frequency of interstitial pneumonitis, serositis, and hematocytopenias in late-onset LE (Kammer and Mishra 2000). In contrast, malar rash, livedo reticularis, alopecia, photosensitivity, oral and nasal ulcers, glomerulonephritis, and lymphadenopathy have a lower prevalence in late-onset compared with early-onset SLE (Domenech et al. 1992, Kammer and Mishra 2000, Ward and Polisson 1989). Late-onset LE has been associated with a milder clinical course and a better prognosis compared with earlier onset (Formiga et al. 1999, Ho et al. 1998, Koh and Boey 1994, Shaikh and Wang 1995). However, comparative retrospective and prospective studies have provided conflicting data on the pattern of presentation and the relationship of serologic abnormalities and disease expression (Baker et al. 1979, Kammer and Mishra 2000, Mak et al. 1998).

Prognostic Relevance of Circulating Autoantibodies

ANAs are frequently found in patients with CLE (DLE or SCLE). Using sensitive techniques, ANAs can be detected in 25%–80% of these patients (Millard et al. 1979, O'Loughlin et al. 1978, Sontheimer 1989, Wallace et al. 1992). ANAs are useful diagnostic markers in CLE. However, the relevance of positive ANA titers as a prognostic marker is limited. Only high levels of ANA ($\geq$1:320) in patients with CLE (DLE or SCLE) indicate patients at risk for developing a severe disease course (Tebbe et al. 1997). Anti-ds-DNA antibodies are highly sensitive for the diagnosis of LE, but widely used enzyme-linked immunosorbent assay (ELISA) tests for the detection of anti-DNA antibodies detect not only high-affinity antibodies of the IgG type but also less specific, low-affinity antibodies of the IgM type (Egner 2000). Therefore, a considerable number of patients with CLE have positive test results. In a study comparing a wide panel of clinical and serologic data from patients, anti-ds-DNA antibodies tested with a highly sensitive ELISA were not identified as a factor indicating the risk of transition from CLE to SLE (Tebbe et al. 1997).

Anti-Ro/SSA is a diagnostic marker for SCLE occurring in 60%–70% of all cases (Provost et al. 1993). Prognostic relevance was analyzed in a 10-year follow-up study including 100 anti-Ro/SSA antibody-positive patients. Sixty-five percent of the anti-Ro/SSA-positive patients revealed chronic progressive disease when followed for 10 years and more. At least 25% of these positive patients demonstrated a dynamic change in clinical presentation with development of Sjögren's syndrome and/or progressive rheumatoid-like arthritis (Simmons-O'Brien et al. 1995). Anti-Ro/SSA-positive patients should be routinely evaluated to recognize early transition to systemic disease. Anti-La/SSB antibodies can be found in 12%–42% of patients with SCLE, mostly associated with anti-Ro/SSA antibodies (Callen et al. 1986, Herrero et al. 1988, Mooney and Wade 1989).

Other autoantibodies are rarely found in CLE, with the exception of anticardiolipin antibodies (ACAs). ACAs of the IgG or IgM type could be detected in 16%–50% of the patients with CLE, being only slightly elevated in most cases (Fonesca et al. 1992, Tebbe and Orfanos 1992). However, according to different study populations or techniques, lower prevalence rates of positive ACA tests were reported in other studies (Kind et al. 1992, Wallace et al. 1992). The relevance of elevated ACAs in CLE concerning the prognostic outcome of the disease is still unclear because follow-up studies are missing.

Significance of Photosensitivity

Photosensitivity is a common feature in various subsets of CLE. LE-specific skin lesions often develop on sun-exposed skin and may be provoked by UV light irradiation. The reported prevalence of photosensitivity varies in the different types of CLE. Photosensitivity has been reported in 69%–90% of patients with DLE and in 52%–100% of patients with SCLE (Beutner et al. 1991, Callen 1985, Callen et al. 1986, Sontheimer et al. 1979). The lack of uniform criteria for photosensitivity may explain the broad scale of differences in prevalence. A pathologic photoprovocation test with UVA and UVB was found in 60%–70% of patients with CLE (DLE or SCLE) (Hasan et al. 1997, Kuhn et al. 2001, Lehmann et al. 1990, van Weelden et al. 1989). The presence of anti-Ro/SSA antibodies and of positive photoprovocation test results was found strongly associated (Hasan et al. 1997).

However, it seems likely that a personal history of polymorphous light eruption (PLE) is of predictive value for the development of CLE. Murphy and Hawk (Murphy and Hawk 1991) first suggested a possible relationship between PLE and LE in 1991, when they reported that 10% of their series of 142 patients with PLE had raised titers of ANAs or anti-Ro/SSA antibodies. PLE and lupus symptoms consistent with PLE were reported in 50%–61% of patients with DLE and in 33%–55% of patients with SCLE. In most cases, PLE preceded the development of CLE by several years (Millard et al. 2001, Nyberg et al. 1997). A significantly higher PLE prevalence was found in relatives of patients with LE than in the general population (Millard et al. 2001).

Therefore, patients with PLE should be carefully monitored for the development of CLE, especially those with positive ANA titer and anti-Ro/SSA antibodies.

Significance of Drugs and Hormones

SCLE has been linked to a variety of drugs, although it seems that thiazides are the most commonly reported agents (Callen 2001, Reed et al. 1985). Other drug classes frequently associated with the development of LE are calcium channel blockers and angiotensin-converting enzyme inhibitors (Crowson and Magro 1997, Fernandez-Diaz et al. 1995). More recently, terbinafine was mentioned as a causative agent for SCLE (Bonsmann et al. 2001). Several case reports mention a variety of drugs responsible for the induction of SCLE, including griseofulvin, interferon beta-1α, cimetidine, cinnarizine, thiethylperazine, and eternacept (Bleumink et al. 2001, Davidson et al. 1982, Miyagawa et al. 1989, Nousari et al. 1998, Toll et al. 1998). In most reported cases drug-induced SCLE had a good prognosis and skin lesions resolved after discontinuation of the responsible drug.

Because CLE clearly shows a female predominance, with disease onset mainly during the childbearing years, it has to be considered that hormones are a triggering factor for the disease or influence its course in genetically determined susceptible women. Empiric observations are that premenstrual flares occur in 20% of 57 women (Yell and Burge 1992). Perimenopausal flares occur in 35% of patients with CLE, whereas postmenopausal disease manifestations are rare (Yell and Burge 1992). SCLE-like disease can be induced by estrogen-containing contraceptives (Furukawa et al. 1991). Females taking postmenopausal estrogen replacement therapy for 2 or more years had a significantly increased risk of developing DLE (Meier et al. 1998).

Association with Tumors

In rare cases of DLE, the development of skin tumors is reported. Basal cell carcinoma, keratoacanthoma, and squamous cell carcinoma may develop on atrophic scars as a long-term complication of DLE lesions (Dabski et al. 1986, Fanti et al. 1989, Halder and Bridgeman-Shah 1995, Stavropoulo et al. 1996). Cutaneous squamous cell carcinoma rarely shows distant metastasis, however, the tendency for LE-associated carcinoma to metastasize has been observed more frequently, with the rates varying from 0.5% to 2% (Millard and Barker 1978).

SCLE is regarded as a facultative paraneoplastic syndrome by some authors, and cases have been described in association with various malignant tumors. In nearly 20 patients described, lung cancer and breast cancer were most frequently found. However, malignant tumors in other organ systems (stomach, liver, uterus, and brain) have been also reported. The patients described did not differ in clinical presentation, histopathologic findings, and serologic profile from other patients with SCLE except for a higher age at onset (Castanet et al. 1995, Ho et al. 2001, Kuhn and Kaufmann 1986, Richardson and Cohen 2000, Trueb and Trueb 1999). First disease manifestation of SCLE in older patients (>50 years) may possibly indicate the occurrence of the disease as a paraneoplastic syndrome.

References

Asghar SS, Venneker GT, Van Meegen M, Meinardi MM, Hulsmans RF, de Waal LP (1991). Hereditary deficiency of C5 in association with discoid lupus erythematosus. J Am Acad Dermatol 24:376–378

Bachmeyer C, Aractingi S, Blanc F, Verola O, Dubertret L (1992) Deep lupus erythematosus in children. Ann Dermatol Venereol 119:535–541

Baker SB, Rovira JR, Campion EW, Mills JA (1979) Late onset systemic lupus erythematosus. Am J Med 66:727–732

Ballou SP, Khan MA, Jushner I (1982) Clinical features of systemic lupus erythematosus-differences related to race and age of onset. Arthritis Rheum 25:55–60

Beutner EH, Blazczyk M, Jablonska S, Chorzelski TP, Kumar V, Wolska H (1991) Studies on criteria of the European Academy of Dermatology and Venerology for the classification of cutaneous lupus erythematosus. Int J Dermatol 30:411–417

Bielsa I, Herrero C, Ercilla G, Collado A, Font J, Ingelmo M, Mascaro JM (1991) Immunogenetic findings in cutaneous lupus erythematosus. J Am Acad Dermatol 25:251–257

Bleumink GS, ter Borg EJ, Ramselaar CG, Stricker BHCh (2001) Etanercept-induced subacute cutaneous lupus erythematosus. Rheumatology 40:1317–1319

Bonsmann G, Schiller M, Luger TA, Ständer S (2001) Terbinafine-induced subacute cutaneous lupus erythematosus. J Am Acad Dermatol 44:925–931

Brucato A, Franceschini F, Buyon JP (1997) Neonatal lupus: long term outcomes of mothers and children and recurrence rate. Clin Exp Rheumatol 15:467–473

Callen JP (1982) Chronic cutaneous lupus erythematosus. Clinical, laboratory, therapeutic and prognostic examination of 62 patients. Arch Dermatol 118:412–416

Callen JP (1985) Discoid lupus erythematosus: variants and clinical associations. Clin Dermatol 3:49–57

Callen JP, Kulick KB, Stelzer G, Fowler JF (1986) Subacute cutaneous lupus erythematosus. Clinical, serologic, and immunogenetic studies of 49 patients seen in a nonreferral setting. J Am Acad Dermatol 15:1227–1237

Callen JP, Klein J (1988) Subacute cutaneous lupus erythematosus. Clinical serologic, immunogenetic, and therapeutic considerations in seventy-two patients. Arthritis Rheum 31: 1007–1013

Callen JP (2001) Drug-induced cutaneous lupus erythematosus, a distinct syndrome that is frequently unrecognized. J Am Acad Dermatol 45:315–316

Castanet J, Taillan B, Lacour JP, Garnier G, Perrin C, Ortonne JP (1995) Subacute cutaneous lupus erthymatosus associated with Hodgkin's disease. Clin Rheumatol 14:692–694

Chlebus E, Wolska H, Blaszczyk M, Jablonska S (1998) Subacute cutaneous lupus erythematosus versus systemic lupus erythematosus: diagnostic criteria and therapeutic implications. J Am Acad Dermatol 38:405–412

Cohen MR, Crosby D (1994) Systemic disease in subacute cutaneous lupus erythematosus: a controlled comparison with systemic lupus erythematosus. J Rheumatol 21:1665–1669

Crowson AN, Magro CM (1997) Subacute cutaneous lupus erythematosus arising in the setting of calcium channel blocker therapy. Hum Pathol 28:67–73

Dabski K, Stoll H, Milgrom H (1986) Squamous cell carcinoma complicating late chronic discoid lupus erythematosus. J Surg Oncol 32:233–237

Davidson BL, Gilliam JN, Lipsky PE (1982) Cimetidine-associated exacerbation of cutaneous lupus erythematosus. Arch Intern Med 142:166–167

Domenech I, Aydintug O, Cervera R, Khamashta M, Jedryka-Goral A (1992) Systemic lupus erythematosus in 50 years old. Postgrad Med J 68:440–444

Drenkard C, Alarcón-Segovia D (2000) The new prognosis of systemic lupus erythematosus: treatment-free remission and decreased mortality and morbidity. Irs Med Assoc J 2:382–387

Egner W (2000) The use of laboratory tests in the diagnosis of SLE. J Clin Pathol 53:424–432

Fanti PA, Tosti A, Peluso AM, Bonelli U (1989) Multiple keratoacanthoma in discoid lupus erythematosus. J Am Acad Dermatol 21:809–810

Fernandez-Diaz ML, Herranz P, Suarez-Marrero MC, Vorbujo J, Manzano R, Casado M (1995) Subacute lupus erythematosus associated with cilazapril. Lancet 345:398

Fonseca E, Alvarez R, Gonzalez MR, Pascual D (1992) Prevalence of anticardiolipin antibodies in subacute cutaneous lupus erythematosus. Lupus 1:265–268

Font J, Pallares L, Cervera R, Lopez-Soto A, Navarro M, Bosch X, Ingelmo M (1991) Systemic lupus erythematosus in the elderly: clinical and immunological characteristics. Ann Rheum Dis 50:702–705

Font J, Cervera R, Navarro M, Pallares L, Lopez-Soto A, Vivancos J, Ingelmo M (1992) Systemic lupus erythematosus in men: clinical and immunological characteristics. Ann Rheum Dis 51:1050–1052

Font J, Cervera R, Espinosa G, Pallares L, Ramos-Casals M, Jimenez S, Garcia-Carrasco M, Seisdedos L, Ingelmo M (1998) Systemic lupus erythematosus (SLE) in childhood: analysis of clinical and immunological findings in 34 patients and comparison with SLE characteristics in adults. Ann Rheum Dis 57:456–459

Formiga F, Moga I, Pac M, Mitjavila F, Rivera A, Pujol R (1999) Mild presentation of systemic lupus erythematosus in elderly patients assessed by SLEDAI. Lupus 8:462–465

Fowler JF, Callen JP, Stelzer GT, Cotter PK (1985) Human histocompatibility antigen associations in patients with chronic cutaneous lupus erythematosus. J Am Acad Dermatol 12:73–77

Furukawa F, Tachibana T, Imamura S, Tamura T (1991) Oral contraceptives induced lupus erythematosus in a Japanese woman. J Dermatol 18:56–58

George PM, Tunnessen WW Jr (1993) Childhood discoid lupus erythematosus. Arch Dermatol 129:613–617

Gladman DD (1996) Prognosis and treatment of systemic lupus erythematosus. Curr Opin Rheum 8:430–437

Halder RM, Bridgeman-Shah S (1995) Skin cancer in African Americans. Cancer 75:667–673

Hasan T, Nyberg F, Stephansson E, Puska P, Häkkinen M, Sarna S, Ros AM, Ranki A (1997) Photosensitivity in lupus erythematosus, UV photoprovocation results compared with history of photosensitivity and clinical findings. Br J Dermatol 136:699–705

Healy E, Kieran E, Rogers S (1995) Cutaneous lupus erythematosus – a study of clinical and laboratory prognostic factors in 65 patients. Israel J Med Sci 164:113–113

Herrero C, Bielsa I, Font J, Lozano F, Ericilla G, Lecha M, Ingelmo M, Mascaro JM (1988) Subacute cutaneous lupus erythematosus: clinical pathologic findings in 13 cases. J Am Acad Dermatol 19:1057–1062

Higuchi T, Imamura S, Danno K (1978) Prognosis of discoid lupus erythematosus. Acta Derm 73:197–204

Ho CC, Mok CC, Lau CS, Wong RWS (1998) Late onset systemic lupus erythematosus in southern Chinese. Ann Rheum Dis 57:437–440

Ho C, Shumack SP, Morris D (2001) Subacute cutaneous lupus erythematosus associated with hepatocellular carcinoma. Austral J Dermatol 42:110–113

Hochberg MC (1997) The epidemiology of systemic lupus erythematosus. In: Wallace DJ, Hahn BH (eds) Dubois' lupus erythematosus. Lea & Febiger, Philadelphia, pp 49–65

Howard PF, Hochberg MC, Bias WB, Arnett FC, McLean RH (1986) Relationship between C4 null genes, HLA D region antigens, and genetic susceptibility to lupus erythematosus in Caucasians and black Americans. Am J Med 81:187–193

Johansson-Stephansson E, Koskimies S, Partanen J, Kariniemi AL (1989) Subacute cutaneous lupus erythematosus. Genetic markers and clinical and immunological findings in patients. Arch Dermatol 125:791–796

Kammer GM, Mishra N (2000) Systemic lupus erythematosus in the elderly. Rheum Dis Clin North Am 26:475–492

Kanda N, Tsuchida T, Watanabe T, Tamaki K (1996) Clinical features of systemic lupus erythematosus in men. Dermatology 193:6–10

Kaufman LD, Gomez-Reino JJ, Mark H, Heinicke MH, Gorevic PD (1989) Male lupus: retrospective analysis of the clinical and laboratory features of 52 patients, with a review of the literature. Semin Arthritis Rheum 18:189–197

Kind P, Goerz G (1987) Klinische Aspekte und Differentialdiagnose des kutanen Lupus erythematodes. Z Hautkr 62:1337–1347

Kind P, Schuppe HC, Jung KP, Degitz K, Lakomek HJ, Goerz G (1992) Kutaner Lupus erythematodes und Kardiolipin-Antikörper. Vorkommen und klinische Bedeutung. Hautarzt 43:126–129

Knop J, Bonsmann G, Kind P, Doxiadis I, Vogeler U, Goerz G, Grosse-Wilde H (1990) Antigens of the major histocompatibility complex in patients with chronic discoid lupus erythematosus. Br J Dermatol 122:723–728

Koh ET, Boey ML (1994) Late onset lupus: a clinical and immunological study in a predominantly Chinese population. J Rheumatol 21:1463–1467

Koh WH, Fong KY, Boey ML, Feng PH (1994) Systemic lupus erythematosus in 61 oriental males. A study of clinical and laboratory manifestations. Br J Rheumatol 33:339–342

Kuhn A, Kaufmann I (1986) Subakut kutaner Lupus erythematodes als paraneoplastisches Syndrom. Z Hautkr 61:581–583

Kuhn A, Richter-Hintz D, Oslislo C, Ruzicka T, Megahed M, Lehmann P (2000) Lupus erythematosus tumidus – a neglected subset of cutaneous lupus erythematosus: report of 40 cases. Arch Dermatol 136:1033–1041

Kuhn A, Sonntag M, Richter-Hintz D, Oslislo C, Megahed M, Ruzicka T, Lehmann P (2001) Phototesting in lupus erythematosus: a 15-year experience. J Am Acad Dermatol 45:86–95

Le Bozec P, La Guyadec T, Crickx B, Grossin M, Belaich S (1994) Chronic lupus erythematosus in lupus disease. Retrospective study in 136 cases. Presse Med 23:1598–1602

Lee LA, Weston WL (1997) Cutaneous lupus erythematosus during the neonatal and childhood periods. Lupus 6:132–138

Lehman TJ (1995) A practical guide to systemic lupus erythematosus. Pediatr Clin North Am 42:1223–1238

Lehmann P, Holzle E, Kind P, Goerz, Plewig G (1990) Experimental reproduction of skin lesions in lupus erythematosus by UVA and UVB radiation. J Am Acad Dermatol 22:181–187

Lipsker DM, Schreckenberg-Gilliot C, Uring-Lambert B, Meyer A, Hartmann D, Grosshans EM, Hauptmann G (2000) Lupus erythematosus associated with genetically determined deficiency of the second component of the complement. Arch Dermatol 136:1508–1514

Lo JT, Tsai MJ, Wang LH, Huang MT, Yang YH, Lin YT, Liu J, Chiang BL (1999) Sex differences in pediatric systemic lupus erythematosus: a retrospective analysis of 135 cases. J Microbiol Immunol Infect 32:173–178

López-Longo FJ, Monteagudo I, González CM, Grau R, Carreno L (1997) Systemic lupus erythematosus: clinical expression and anti-Ro/SS-A response in patients with and without lesions of subacute cutaneous lupus erythematosus. Lupus 6:32–39

Maddison PJ (1987) Systemic lupus erythematosus in the elderly. J Rheumatol 14 (Suppl 13): 182–187

Mak SK, Lam EKM, Wong AKM (1998) Clinical profile of patients with late-onset SLE: not a benign subgroup. Lupus 7:23–28

Martens PB, Moder KG, Ahmed I (1999) Lupus panniculitis: clinical perspectives from a case series. J Rheumatol 26:68–72

McCauliffe DP, Faircloth E, Wang L, Hashimoto T, Hoshino Y, Nishikawa T (1996) Similar Ro/SS-A autoantibody epitope and titer responses in annular erythema of Sjogren's syndrome and subacute cutaneous lupus erythematosus. Arch Dermatol 132:528–531

Meier CR, Sturkenboom MCJM, Cohen AS, Jick H (1998) Postmenopausal estrogen replacement therapy and the risk of developing systemic lupus erythematosus or discoid lupus. J Rheumatol 25:1515–1519

Meyer O, Hauptmann G, Tappeiner G, Ochs HD, Mascart-Lemone F (1985) Genetic deficiency of C4, C2 or C1q and lupus syndromes. Association with anti-Ro (SS-A) antibodies. Clin Exp Immunol 62:678–684

Millard LG, Rowell NR, Rajah SM (1977) Histocompatibility antigens in discoid and systemic lupus erythematosus. Br J Dermatol 96:139–144

Millard LG, Barker DJ (1978) Development of squamous cell carcinoma in chronic discoid lupus erythematosus. Clin Exp Dermatol 3:161–166

Millard LG, Rowell NR (1979) Abnormal laboratory test results and their relationship to prognosis in discoid lupus erythematosus: a longterm follow-up study of 92 patients. Arch Dermatol 115:1055–1058

Millard TP, Kondeatis E, Vaughan RW, Lewis CM, Khamashta MA, Hughes GR, Hawk JL, McGregor JM (2001) Polymorphic light eruption and the HLA DRB1*0301 extended haplotype are independent risk factors for cutaneous lupus erythematosus. Lupus 10: 473–479

Millard TP, Lewis CM, Khamashta MA, Hughes GRV, Hawk JLM, McGregor JM (2001) Familial clustering of polymorphic light eruption in relatives of patients with lupus erythematosus: evidence of a shared pathogenesis. Br J Dermatol 144:334–338

Miller MH, Urowitz MB, Gladman DD, Killinger DW (1983) Systemic lupus erythematosus in males. Medicine 62:327–334

Miyagawa S, Okuchi T, Shiomi Y, Sakamoto K (1989) Subacute cutaneous lupus erythematosus lesions precipitated by griseofulvin. J Am Acad Dermatol 21:343–346

Miyagawa S. Clinical, serological and immunogenetic features of Japanese anti-Ro/SS-A-positive patients with annular erythema. Dermatology 189 (Suppl 1):11–13

Molad Y (1987) Clinical manifestations and laboratory data of subacute cutaneous lupus erythematosus. Israel J Med Sci 23:278–280

Mooney E, Wade TR (1989) Subacute cutaneous lupus erythematosus in Iceland. Int J Dermatol 28:104–106

Moschella SL (1989) Dermatologic overview of lupus erythematosus and its subsets. J Dermatol 16:417–428

Murphy GM, Hawk JL (1991) The prevalence of antinuclear antibodies in patients with apparent polymorphic light eruption. Br J Dermatol 125:448–451

Neiman AR, Lee LA, Weston WL, Buyon JP (2000) Cutaneous manifestations of neonatal lupus without heart block: characteristics of mothers and children enrolled in a national registry. J Pediatr 137:674–680

Nousari HC, Kimyai-Asadi A, Tausk FA (1998) Subacute cutaneous lupus erythematosus associated with interferon beta-1α. Lancet 352:1825–1826

Nyberg F, Hasan T, Puska P, Stephansson E, Hakkinen M, Ranki A, Ros AM (1997) Occurrence of polymorphous light eruption in lupus erythematosus. Br J Dermatol 136:217–221

O'Loughlin S, Schroeter AL, Jordan RE (1978) A study of lupus erythematosus with particular reference to generalized discoid lupus. Br J Dermatol 99:1–11

Parodi A, Rebora A (1997) ARA and EADV criteria for classification of systemic lupus erythematosus in patients with cutaneous lupus erythematosus. Dermatology 194:217–220

Parodi A, Caproni M, Cardinali C, Bernacchi E, Fuligni A, De Panfilis G, Zane C, Papini M, Veller FC, Vaccaro M, Fabbri P (2000) Clinical, histological and immunopathological features of 58 patients with subacute cutaneous lupus erythematosus. Dermatology 200: 6–10

Parodi A, Massone C, Cacciapuoti M, Aragone MG, Bondavalli P, Cattarini G, Rebora A (2000) Measuring the activity of the disease in patients with cutaneous lupus erythematosus. Br J Dermatol 142:457–460

Partanen J, Koskimies S, Johansson E (1988) C4 null phenotypes among lupus erythematosus patients are predominantly the result of deletions covering C4 and closely linked C21-hydroxylase A genes. J Med Genet 25:387–391

Perkins W, Stables GI, Lever RS (1994) Protein S deficiency in lupus erythematosus secondary to hereditary angio-oedema. Br J Dermatol 130:381–384

Petri M, McLean RH, Watson R, Winckelstein JA (1993) Clinical expression of systemic lupus erythematosus in patients with C4A deficiency. Medicine 72:236–244

Provost TT, Arnett FC, Reichlin M (1983) Homozygous C2 deficiency, lupus erythematosus and anti-Ro (SSA) antibodies. Arthritis Rheum 26:1279–1283

Provost TT, Talal N, Bias W, Harley JB, Reichlin M, Alexander EL (1988) Ro/SS-A (SS-A) positive Sjogren's/lupus erythematosus overlap patients are associated with the HLA-DR3 and/or DRW6 phenotypes. J Invest Dermatol 91:369–371

Provost TT, Watson R, Simmons-O'Brien E (1996) Significance of the anti-Ro(SS-A) antibody in evaluation of patients with cutaneous manifestations of a connective tissue disease. J Am Acad Dermatol 35:147–169

Pu SJ, Luo SF, Wu YJJ, Cheng HS, Ho HH (2000) The clinical features and prognosis of lupus with disease onset at age 65 and older. Lupus 9:96–100

Ratnoff WD (1996) Inherited C2 deficiency of complement in rheumatic diseases. Rheum Dis Clin North Am 22:75–94

Reed BR, Huff JC, Jones SK, Orton PW, Lee LA, Norris DA (1985) Subacute cutaneous lupus erythematosus associated with hydrochlorothiazide therapy. Ann Intern Med 103:49–51

Richardson TT, Cohen PR (2000) Subacute cutaneous lupus erythematosus: report of a patient who subsequently developed a meningioma and whose skin lesions were treated with isotretinoin. Cutis 66:183–188

Rood MJ, ten Cate R, ven Suijlekom-Smit LW, den Ouden EJ, Ouwerkerk FE, Breedveld FC, Huizinga TW (1999) Childhood-onset systemic lupus erythematosus: clinical presentation and prognosis in 31 patients. Scand J Rheumatol 28:222–226

Rowell NR (1984) The natural history of lupus erythematosus. Clin Exp Dermatol 9:217–231

Schaller J (1982) Lupus in childhood. Clin Rheum Dis 8:219–228

Schiodt M (1984) Oral discoid lupus erythematosus. 2. Skin lesions and systemic lupus erythematosus in sixty-six patients with 6-year follow up. Oral Surg 57:177–180

Schur PH (1978) Genetics of complement deficiencies associated with lupus-like syndromes. Arthritis Rheum 21(Suppl 5):S153–S160

Sequeira JF, Keser G, Greenstein B, Wheeler MJ, Duarte PC, Khamashta MA, Hughes GR (1993) Systemic lupus erythematosus: Sex hormones in male patients. Lupus 2:315–317

Shai R, Quismorio FP Jr, Li L, Kwon OJ, Morrison J, Wallace DJ, Neuwelt CM, Brautbar C, Gauderman WJ, Jacob CO (1999) Genome-wide screen for systemic lupus erythematosus susceptibility gene in multiplex families. Hum Mol Genet 8:639–644

Shaikh SK, Wang F (1995) Late-onset systemic lupus erythematosus: clinical and immunological characteristics. Med J Malaysia 50:25–31

Simmons-O'Brien E, Chen S, Watson R, Antoni C, Petri M, Hochberg M, Stevens MB, Provost TT (1995) One hundred anti-Ro (SS-A) antibody positive patients: a 10-year follow-up. Medicine (Baltimore) 74:109–130

Sontheimer RD, Thomas JR, Gilliam JN (1979) Subacute cutaneous lupus erythematosus: a cutaneous marker for a distinct lupus erythematosus subset. Arch Dermatol 115:1409–1415

Sontheimer RD, Stastny P, Gilliam JN (1981) Human histocompatibility antigen associations in subacute cutaneous lupus erythematosus. J Clin Invest 67:312–316

Sontheimer RD (1989) Subacute cutaneous lupus erythematosus: a decade's perspective. Med Clin North Am 73:1073–1090

Stavropoulos PG, Tebbe B, Tenorio S, Orfanos CE (1996) LE-associated squamous cell carcinoma. Eur J Dermatol 6:48–50

Stephens HA, McHugh NJ, Maddison PJ, Isenberg DA, Welsh KI, Panayi GS (1991) HLA class II restriction of autoantibody production in patients with systemic lupus erythematosus Immunogenetics 33:276–280

Sullivan KE (1998) Complement deficiency and autoimmunity. Curr Opin Pediatr 10:600–606

Swaak AJG (1989) Systemic lupus erythematosus. I. Outcome and survival: Dutch experience with 110 patients studied prospectively. Ann Rheum Dis 48:447–454

Tan EM, Cohen AS, Fries JF, Masi AT, McShane DJ, Rothfield NF, Schaller JG, Talal N, Winchester RJ (1982) The 1982 revised criteria for the classification of systemic lupus erythematosus. Arthritis Rheum 25:1271–1277

Tebbe B, Orfanos CE (1987) Lupus erythematodes der Haut. Eine Analyse von 97 Patienten. Z Hautkr 62:1563–1584

Tebbe B, Orfanos CE (1992) Anticardiolipin-Antikörper beim kutanen Lupus erythematodes. Hautarzt 43:130–133

Tebbe B, Hoffmann S, Orfanos CE (1994) Verlauf und Prognose des subakut kutanen Lupus erythematodes. Hautarzt 45:690–695

Tebbe B, Mansmann U, Wollina U, Auer-Grumbach P, Licht-Mbalyohere A, Arensmeier M, Orfanos CE (1997) Markers in cutaneous lupus erythematosus indicating systemic involvement. A multicenter study on 296 patients. Acta Derm Venereol 77:305–308

Toll A, Campo-Pisa P, Gonzalez-Castro J, Campo-Voegeli A, Azon A, Iranzo P, Lecha M, Herrero C (1998) Subacute cutaneous lupus erythematosus associated with cinnarizine and thiethylperazine therapy. Lupus 7364–366

Tongio MM, Fersing J, Hauptmann G, Mayer S, Grange D, Samsoen M, Groshans E (1982) HLA antigens in discoid lupus erythematosus. Acta Derm Venereol 62:155–157

Trueb RF, Trueb RM (1999) Kutane Paraneoplasie als immunologisches Phänomen am Beispiel des paraneoplastischen subakut kutanen Lupus erythematodes. Schweiz Rundsch Med Prax 88:1803–1810

van Weelden H, Velthuis PJ, Baart de la Faille H (1989) Light-induced skin lesions in lupus erythematosus: photobiological studies. Arch Dermatol Res 28:1470–474

Wallace DJ, Pistiner M, Nessim S, Metzger AL, Klinenberg JR (1992) Cutaneous lupus erythematosus without systemic lupus erythematosus. Clinical and laboratory features. Semin Arthritis Rheum 21:221–226

Wananukul S, Watana D, Pongprasit P (1998) Cutaneous manifestations of childhood systemic lupus erythematosus. Pediatr Dermatol 15:342–346

Ward MM, Polisson RP (1989) A meta-analysis of the clinical manifestations of older-onset systemic lupus erythematosus. Arthritis Rheum 32:1226–1232

Watanabe T, Tsuchida T (1995) Classification of lupus erythematosus based upon cutaneous manifestations. Dermatology 190:277–283

Watanabe T, Tsuchida T (1996) Lupus erythematosus profundus: a cutaneous marker for a distinct clinical subset? Br J Dermatol 134:123–125

Watanabe T, Tsuchida T, Ito Y, Kanda N, Ueda Y, Tamaki K (1997) Annular erythema associated with lupus erythematosus/Sjogren's syndrome. J Am Acad Dermatol 36:214–218

Watson RM, Talwar P, Alexander E, Bias WB, Provost TT (1991) Subacute cutaneous lupus erythematosus-immunogenetic associations. J Autoimmun 4:73–85

Werth VP, Zhang W, Dortzbach K, Sullivan K (2000) Association of a promoter polymorphism of tumour necrosis factor-alpha (TNF-alpha) with subacute cutaneous lupus erythematosus. J Invest Dermatol 115:726–730

Wilson AG, de Vries N, Pociot F, diGiovine FS, van der Putte LB, Duff GW (1993) An allelic polymorphism within the human tumor necrosis factor alpha promoter region is strongly associated with HLA A1, B8, and DR3 alleles. J Exp Med 177:557–560

Yell JA, Burge SM (1993) The effect of hormonal changes on cutaneous disease in lupus erythematosus. Br J Dermatol 129:18–22

Zecevic RD, Vojvodvic D, Ristic B, Pavlovic MD, Stefanovic D, Karadaglic D (2001) Skin lesions – an indicator of disease activity in systemic lupus erythematosus? Lupus 10:364–367

Part III
Pathogenesis and Pathologic Features of Cutaneous Lupus Erythematosus

CHAPTER 15

Molecular Genetics of Cutaneous Lupus Erythematosus

15

Thomas P. Millard

This article examines the evidence of a genetic basis for cutaneous forms of lupus erythematosus (LE), namely, subacute cutaneous LE (SCLE) and discoid LE (DLE). The current theory is that multiple genes, including particular allelic polymorphisms, may confer susceptibility to these LE-specific skin diseases (Sontheimer 1996) and that perhaps some of these alleles may be shared with polymorphous light eruption (PLE), a common condition that is clinically related to lupus (Nyberg et al. 1997).

Sequeira (Sequeira 1903) described two pairs of sisters (not twins) affected by cutaneous LE (CLE), raising the possibility that it might be a familial condition. Since then, several studies have reported the occurrence of CLE, particularly DLE, in monozygotic twins (Steagall et al. 1962, Wojnarowska 1983) and first-degree relatives of lupus probands (Beckett and Lewis 1959, Leonhardt 1957). Gallo and Forde (Gallo and Forde 1966) suggested that inheritance of a "dominant gene," with or without common environmental factors, may explain the observation of DLE across three generations of one family. A mathematical analysis of the age and sex distribution of DLE incidence in the population was also used in the 1960s by Rowell to support a genetic basis for DLE (Burch and Rowell 1968).

More recently, Lawrence et al. (Lawrence et al. 1987) investigated first-degree relatives of 37 patients with DLE in a case-control study. They found a significantly increased prevalence of DLE (3.5%) in 255 first-degree relatives of DLE probands compared with 0.5% in 664 controls. Heritability analysis suggested a polygenic inheritance, with 44% heritability. Several recent genome-wide marker scans for systemic LE (SLE) have subsequently been performed in families with multiple affected individuals to identify regions of the genome that may be linked to the disease phenotype (Gaffney et al. 1998, 2000, Gray-McGuire et al. 2000, Lindqvist et al. 2000, Moser et al. 1998, Nath et al. 2001, Shai et al. 1999). These scans confirm that susceptibility to lupus is likely to be determined by multiple genetic regions, with different susceptibility loci in different ethnic groups.

It has long been known that certain conditions predispose to CLE. For example, DLE has been described in patients and carriers of X-linked and autosomal-recessive chronic granulomatous disease (Arnett 1997, Yeaman et al. 1992) and is also associated with non-X-linked hyper-immunoglobulin M syndrome (Wolpert et al. 1998). We and others have found a higher prevalence of PLE in patients with both SCLE and DLE than in controls (Millard et al. 2001a, Nyberg et al. 1997), suggesting that they may share a common genetic background. The study of these conditions may help shed light on the genetic basis of LE in the future.

Techniques to Examine Susceptibility Genes in Cutaneous Lupus Erythematosus

There are several major approaches to the study of genetic susceptibility in any given complex (multifactorial) disease, including twin pair analysis, association analysis, family linkage studies (including "genome scans"), and transmission disequilibrium testing. *Twin pair analysis* is probably the best approach to investigate the relative importance of genetic and environmental factors in disease susceptibility; however, the prevalence of CLE is too low for a formal concordance study even in a large population-based twin sample. *Association studies* (case-control) examine the relationship between the disease and a given candidate gene in the population. They assume that the candidate gene is involved in the pathogenesis of the disease and that a specified allelic variant (polymorphism) of this gene will be overrepresented in patients compared with unaffected controls. For example, this approach has been used to support a role for corneodesmosin in psoriasis (Enerback et al. 2000). This technique requires careful phenotype selection and is vulnerable to the problem of matching the ethnic background of cases and controls ("population stratification"). Another potential problem is that the association between a candidate gene polymorphism and disease may exist only because the polymorphism is a marker for the real disease-causing allele, either at the same gene locus or at a nearby gene, with the marker and the disease alleles being in "linkage disequilibrium" (Ralston 1998).

Family linkage analysis has the advantage that it does not require a candidate locus and also avoids the problem of population stratification. However, it requires a large set of several hundred molecular markers to type polymorphisms throughout the entire genome to identify regions that are linked within the family to the disease. These genome-wide scans, used in human SLE, have identified high "logarithm of odds" (lod) scores for several regions, including *FcγRIIA* at band 1q23, the major histocompatibility complex (MHC) at 6p21.3, and 1q31, which includes the genes encoding interleukin (IL) 10 and Ro60 (Moser et al. 1998, Gaffney et al. 1998, Shai et al. 1999). No genome-wide searches have so far been performed in CLE, although DLE families with multiple affected individuals are probably sufficiently common for such an analysis in the future.

Transmission disequilibrium testing (TDT) assumes that a heterozygous parent should transmit the disease-associated allele to an affected child more often than the 50% expected from standard Mendelian inheritance (Lewis 2000). TDT therefore tests family linkage in the presence of association, avoiding the problem of population stratification, and may be used to narrow candidate regions identified through genome-wide searches. We are currently using TDT to investigate susceptibility genes for SCLE and DLE.

Candidate Genes in Cutaneous Lupus Erythematosus

Selection of candidate genes for analysis in complex multifactorial traits such as CLE draws on multiple sources of information. In the case of LE, these include family linkage studies in human and animal models of lupus, immunohistochemical analysis of skin samples, and studies of alleles identified as possible candidates in other (related) autoimmune diseases. For example, at least 10 loci have been found to predispose to LE in New Zealand lupus-prone mice (Kono et al. 1994), in addition to the previously mentioned loci that are linked to human lupus. In the murine model, genetic susceptibility seems to confer different levels of pathogenesis, including separate loci for autoantibody production, specific organ destruction, and mortality. Only one locus, the MHC (H-2 in mice), is linked to all three levels of disease.

Immunohistochemical analysis may be used to localize the expression of specific proteins within the skin of patients with lupus, perhaps implying abnormal regulation of the underlying genes that encode these proteins. For example, increased keratinocyte expression of intercellular adhesion molecule-1 (ICAM-1) has been demonstrated in evolving ultraviolet (UV)-induced lesions of CLE and PLE, but not in healthy controls (Nyberg et al. 1999). Thus, ICAM-1, its ligand, and upstream regulators may be deemed possible candidates to study (Norris et al. 1992).

Association in other autoimmune disorders is reported for various loci encoding cytokines, cytokine receptors, antioxidant enzymes, and adhesion molecules in rheumatoid arthritis, dermatomyositis, and SLE. It is therefore possible that the polymorphisms at these loci may be candidates for the related autoimmune CLE.

Finally, a candidate gene may be inferred from knowing the therapeutic action of drugs used to treat the disease. For example, thalidomide, which inhibits tumor necrosis factor (TNF)-α, is particularly effective for treating SCLE and DLE (Wallace 1997). This suggests that TNF (or possibly one of its common polymorphisms) may contribute to the pathogenesis of CLE.

The Major Histocompatibility Complex

From such studies, a variety of candidate gene loci have emerged that may prove important in the pathogenesis of CLE. The most important of these loci to date are found within the MHC. The human MHC (Fig. 15.1) is a diverse genetic region that plays a crucial role in control of the immune response and that has recently been sequenced by the MHC Sequencing Consortium (1999). The human MHC genes, clustered together in a segment of chromosome 6 (6p21.3), are organized into three regions (I, II, and III) and encode three major classes of proteins: class I human leukocyte antigens (HLAs) (including the classical antigens A, B, and Cw), HLA class II antigens (DP, DQ, and DR), and class III molecules, including complement components, TNF (α and β), and heat shock proteins.

HLA Genes and Cutaneous Lupus Erythematosus
In several serologic studies of the class I and class II HLA regions in patients with SCLE (mainly Caucasian), the HLA A1, B8, DR3, DQ2, DRw52, C4null ancestral haplotype has been consistently identified as a susceptibility haplotype for SCLE, particularly in patients seropositive for anti-Ro/SSA (Bielsa et al. 1991, Herrero et al. 1988, Johansson-Stephansson et al. 1989, Provost et al. 1988, Sontheimer et al. 1981, 1982, Vazquez-Doval et al. 1992, Watson et al. 1991), confirmed by our recent analysis of HLA genes in 36 patients with SCLE (Millard et al. 2001b). This ancestral haplotype is associated with susceptibility to a variety of other autoimmune diseases, including insulin-dependent diabetes mellitus, dermatitis herpetiformis, and myasthenia gravis (Price et al. 1999).

Fig. 15.1. Abbreviated gene map of the human MHC at 6p21.3 illustrating the major loci to which the text refers. The illustrated class II loci are, themselves, composed of multiple genes that contribute to the class II antigen structure. HSP, heat shock protein; TNF, tumor necrosis factor

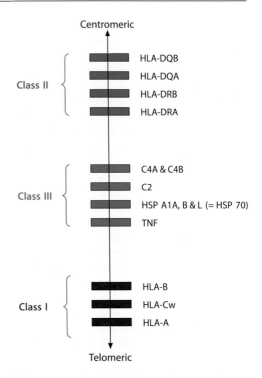

Watson et al. (Provost and Watson 1993, Watson et al. 1991) found that this association was only present in SCLE, SLE, and Sjögren's syndrome in the presence of anti-Ro/SSA, suggesting that the immunogenetic association is primarily with the production of antibody. There is substantial evidence to support the pathogenic role of the anti-Ro/SSA antibody in SCLE (Ben-Chetrit 1993), where circulating anti-Ro/SSA binds keratinocytes expressing surface Ro/SSA antigen, leading to the destruction of basal keratinocytes (Norris 1993) (Fig. 15.2). In addition to controlling the presence or absence of the anti-Ro/SSA response, the MHC may also determine the *level* of the response; Harley et al. (Harley et al. 1986) found that possession of both HLA DQ1 and DQ2 led to the highest titers of anti-Ro/SSA. This MHC specificity suggests that class II HLA antigens may determine whether the individual can present fragments of Ro/SSA antigen to their lymphocytes.

The Ro/SSA 60-kDa protein (Ro60 or SSA2) is the major component of the Ro ribonucleoprotein (RNP) complex [in stable association with a human cytoplasmic RNA (hY RNA) and the La/SSB protein, Fig. 15.3], to which an immune response is a specific feature of several autoimmune diseases, including SCLE and SLE. We recently characterized the *Ro60* gene structure (Fig. 15.4) and examined whether any observed sequence alterations were associated with serum anti-Ro/SSA antibody in SCLE and could therefore be of pathogenic significance (Millard et al. 2002). Heteroduplex analysis of polymerase chain reaction (PCR) products from patients and controls spanning all *Ro60* exons (1 to 8) revealed a common bandshift in the PCR products spanning exon 7. Sequencing of the corresponding PCR products demon-

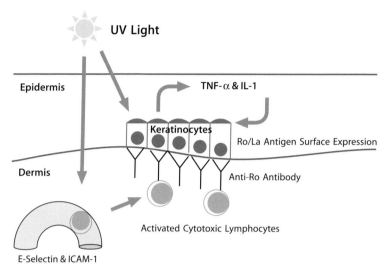

Fig. 15.2. Probable pathogenic mechanism of photosensitive skin lesions in LE. Ultraviolet radiation (UVR) stimulates the cell surface expression of nuclear antigens, including Ro/SSA, on the surface of keratinocytes and induces E-selectin and intercellular adhesion molecule-1 (ICAM-1) expression on dermal endothelial cells, which leads to the margination and local migration of lymphocytes. Norris (Norris 1993) proposed this model of photosensitive LE, whereby circulating anti-Ro/SSA antibody binds keratinocytes that express this surface Ro/SSA antigen, leading to antibody-dependent cellular cytotoxicity by the infiltrating cytotoxic lymphocytes and the subsequent destruction of basal keratinocytes. Casciola-Rosen and Rosen (Casciola-Rosen and Rosen 1997) have added to this model by describing the expression of Ro/SSA antigen in "surface blebs" of UVB-irradiated apoptotic keratinocytes, which may contribute to induction of autoimmunity to Ro/SSA. IL-1, interleukin-1; TNF, tumor necrosis factor

Fig. 15.3. Organization of the Ro/SSA RNP complex (Gordon et al. 1994). hY RNA, human cytoplasmic RNA

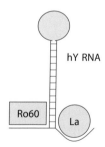

strated an A>G substitution at nucleotide position 1318-7, within the consensus acceptor splice site of exon 7 (GenBank XM001901). The allele frequencies were major allele A (0.71) and minor allele G (0.29) in 72 control chromosomes, with no significant differences among patients with SCLE (anti-Ro/SSA positive), patients with DLE (anti-Ro/SSA negative), and healthy controls, suggesting no relationship between this nucleotide substitution and generation of anti-Ro/SSA.

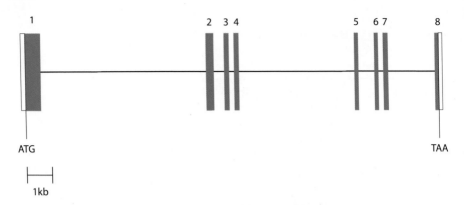

Fig. 15.4. Structural organization of the *Ro60* gene. The coding region of the gene contains 8 exons spanning more than 16 kB of genomic DNA and ranging in size from 114 to greater than 580 bp. Exons are depicted by the *vertical black shaded areas*, and the start of the 5' and 3' untranslated regions are in *white*. The exons are *numbered above*; introns are represented by *horizontal lines*

A relatively small number of studies have examined HLA associations in Caucasian patients with DLE. The major associations include the A1, B8, DR3 and also the B7, DR2 haplotypes (Fowler et al. 1985, Knop et al. 1990, Millard et al. 1977), although other studies have found no HLA associations with DLE (Bielsa et al. 1991, Tongio et al. 1982). Our own data indicate a significant association with the previously mentioned haplotypes and DLE (Millard et al. 2001b). Finally, the photosensitive "butterfly rash" of lupus (acute CLE) rarely occurs outside the context of active SLE, so little effort has been made to determine any specific HLA associations (Sontheimer and Provost 1997).

Complement Genes

The MHC also includes genes for various complement components (C2, C4A, C4B, and factor B) in the class III region (Meo et al. 1977), between class I and class II, which have been implicated in the pathogenesis of CLE. Inherited deficiencies of components C2 and C4 are associated with DLE (Braathen et al. 1986, Provost et al. 1983), SCLE (Callen et al. 1987, Levy et al. 1979, Provost et al. 1983), and the presence of anti-Ro/SSA (Meyer et al. 1985, Provost et al. 1983). In addition, lupus profundus has been reported in patients with partial deficiency of both C4 allotypes (Burrows et al. 1991, Nousari et al. 1999). The proposed basis for these associations includes either a failure to clear immune complexes and apoptotic cells or linkage disequilibrium with the real disease-predisposing locus (Levy et al. 1979, Sullivan 1998).

TNF Genes

TNF is encoded by a class III gene of the MHC (Carroll et al. 1987, MHC Sequencing Consortium 1999). TNF has been implicated in the pathogenesis of CLE following UVR (Kock 1990, Norris 1993) (Fig. 15.2) since it stimulates expression of the Ro antigen on the keratinocyte surface. The rare *–308A* polymorphic form of TNF (TNF2)

(Abraham et al. 1999) is associated with increased UVB-induced TNF production in keratinocytes (Silverberg et al. 1999) and has demonstrated a strong association with SCLE (Werth and Sullivan 1999). *TNF –308A* does, however, lie on the A1, B8, DR3 extended haplotype in Caucasians (Wilson et al. 1993) and may therefore demonstrate association only because of linkage disequilibrium. However, a recent analysis in patients with SLE suggests that both *TNF –308A* and HLA-DR3 contribute independently to lupus susceptibility (Rood et al. 2000).

Heat Shock Protein Genes

The three *heat shock protein 70* (*Hsp70*) genes are located within the class III MHC region, and linkage disequilibrium with other HLA genes has led several authors to investigate the role of *Hsp70* genes in susceptibility to autoimmune and allergic disease (Aron et al. 1999). The activation of *Hsp* gene expression (the "stress response") is a cellular mechanism that protects cells against stresses such as heat, UVR, cytokines, and chemicals (Muramatsu et al. 1992, Stephanou et al. 1997). Ghoreishi et al. (Ghoreishi et al. 1993) used immunohistologic analysis to demonstrate diffusely increased Hsp70 expression in the lesional skin of patients with SLE vs controls and DLE samples. Furukawa et al. (Furukawa et al. 1993) observed increased binding of anti-Ro/SSA antibodies to keratinocytes after incubation with a prostaglandin stressor that is known to induce Hsp formation, suggesting that heat shock proteins may be involved in the expression of Ro antigen at the cell surface. Various polymorphisms exist for the *Hsp70* genes (Bolla et al. 1998, Esaki et al. 1999), although none have yet been examined for association in CLE.

Candidate Loci Outside the MHC

Several genetic regions outside the MHC seem to confer susceptibility to cutaneous forms of LE or demonstrate association or linkage with the anti-Ro/SSA response, including loci encoding cytokines, cytokine receptors, molecules involved in antigen recognition, and antioxidant enzymes, all of which are plausible candidates and are summarized in Table 15.1.

IL-1 Gene Cluster

The primary cytokine IL-1 is a major proinflammatory cytokine, encoded by a gene cluster at band 2q13, comprising IL-1α and IL-1β (synthesized by keratinocytes and Langerhans' cells, respectively) and the IL-1 receptor antagonist gene (*IL-1RN*), which has been associated with photosensitivity in LE and with DLE by two separate teams in case-control studies (Blakemore et al. 1994, Suzuki et al. 1997). In our association analysis, we found that *IL1B +3954 T* was significantly less frequent in patients with SCLE (28%) compared with controls (47%; *P*=0.039), although this was lost on correction for multiple testing (Millard et al. 2001c).

IL-10

Linkage in human lupus has been shown for band 1q31 (Moser et al. 1998), within which lies the gene encoding IL-10 (Eskdale et al. 1997, Kim et al. 1992). IL-10 is expressed by UVB-stimulated keratinocytes and is chemotactic for CD8[+] T cells. It promotes an inflammatory response through its effects on B cells in lupus, whose produc-

Table 15.1. Genes outside the MHC[a] that seem to confer susceptibility to cutaneous forms of lupus erythematosus (LE) or demonstrate association or linkage with the anti-Ro/SSA response

Gene	Locus	Evidence
1. *Cytokine genes*		
Interleukin-1 gene cluster (IL-1A, B, and RA)	2q13	Association of an IL-1 RA allele with DLE and with photosensitivity in SLE.
Interleukin-10 (IL-10)	1q31	Linkage of 1q31 to human LE. Association of three IL-10 SNPs with anti-Ro production in SLE.
2. *Adhesion molecule/ receptor genes*		
Intercellular adhesion molecule-1 (ICAM1)	19p13.3-p13.2	Increased keratinocyte expression of ICAM-1 in CLE.
E-selectin (SELE)	1q23–25	Up-regulated endothelial expression in the skin of patients with cutaneous LE vs controls.
Fc gamma receptor II (FCGR2A)	1q23	Linkage of 1q23 to human systemic LE. Necessary for ADCC (Fig. 15.4).
T-cell receptor (TCR) Cβ1 and Cβ2	7q35	Association of two RFLPs, for TCRs Cb1 and Cb2, with anti-Ro/SSA production in SLE.
3. *Antioxidant enzyme genes*		
Glutathione S-transferase M1 (GSTM1)	1p13	Association of GSTM1 null status and anti-Ro/SSA production in SLE.
4. *Apoptosis genes*		
Fas (TNFRSF6)	10q24.1	Association of an SNP with photosensitivity in SLE

[a] Genes within the MHC are illustrated in Fig. 15.1.
ADCC, antibody-dependent cellular cytotoxicity; CLE, cutaneous lupus erythematosus; DLE, discoid LE; MHC, major histocompatibility complex; RA, receptor antagonist; RFLP, restriction fragment length polymorphism; SLE, systemic LE; SNP, single nucleotide polymorphism.

tion of immunoglobulin is largely IL-10 dependent (Llorente et al. 1995). It also up-regulates the expression of ICAM-1 and E-selectin on human dermal endothelial cells (Palmetshofer et al. 1994). Three functional single nucleotide polymorphisms (SNPs) of the IL-10 gene promoter were reported by Turner et al. (Turner et al. 1997), including –1082 G/A, –819 C/T, and –592 C/A, who showed that they influenced in vitro production of IL-10 by mononuclear cells. Comparing the overall haplotype combinations at these three loci, significant distortion was demonstrated between anti-Ro/SSA-positive and anti-Ro/SSA-negative SLE cases ($P=0.005$), with overrepresentation of the GCC and ACC haplotypes in the former group (Lazarus et al. 1997). This suggests that

IL-10 may be important in generation of the immune response to Ro and, therefore, potentially relevant to SCLE, although our initial study found no association with SCLE or DLE for either the −819 or −1082 SNPs (Millard et al. 2001c).

T-Cell Receptor C_β Gene

Genes encoding the T-cell receptor (TCR) have demonstrated an association with the generation of anti-Ro/SSA. Frank et al. (Frank et al. 1990) reported an association between a set of restriction fragment length polymorphisms (RFLPs) for TCRs $C_\beta 1$ and $C_\beta 2$ (Bgl II 9.8-kb and Kpn I 1.75-kb) that was present in 76% of patients with SLE and anti-Ro/SSA but in only 41% of patients with SLE without anti-Ro/SSA (P=0.002). The same group found that certain HLA DQ types, in combination with the TCR C_β RFLPs, increased the strength of this association (Scofield et al. 1994). This molecular specificity was cited as evidence that the breaking of tolerance to the Ro proteins in lupus requires the association of a class II HLA molecule with a fragment of Ro peptide and a particular TCR form.

Glutathione S-Transferase

The antioxidant enzymes encoded by the glutathione S-transferase (GST) genes are widely expressed in mammalian tissues. Ollier et al. (Ollier et al. 1996) examined the role of the GSTM1 null polymorphisms in the production of anti-Ro/SSA and anti-La/SSB in SLE using PCR to identify GSTM1 [chromosome band 1p13 (Pearson et al. 1993)] null homozygotes. A significant association was demonstrated between the Ro^{+ve}/La^{-ve} phenotype in SLE and GSTM1 null status, implicating oxidant stress in the loss of immunologic tolerance to Ro/SSA antigen.

Adhesion Molecules

ICAM-1 and E-selectin are potential candidate genes for CLE. ICAM-1 is usually expressed at very low levels on keratinocytes, but increased keratinocyte expression has been demonstrated in evolving lesions of CLE and PLE (Nyberg et al. 1999, Norris et al. 1992). Two functional polymorphisms of the ICAM-1 gene (ICAM1) were reported by Vora et al. (Vora et al. 1994), including G/R at codon 241 and K/E at codon 469, which therefore represent plausible candidates for CLE. The endothelial adhesion molecule E-selectin is also up-regulated in the skin of patients with CLE and patients with PLE compared with controls (Nyberg et al. 1999); elevated serum levels of soluble E-selectin have also been described in patients with DLE (Nyberg and Stephansson 1999). The E-selectin gene at band 1q23–25 (Collins et al. 1991) contains an A/C SNP at position 561, coding for serine or arginine at codon 128 (Wenzel et al. 1994a), which, so far, has demonstrated clinical association with atheromatous vascular disease (Wenzel et al. 1994b).

Fcγ Receptor II

The Fcγ receptor II genes, at chromosome band 1q23 (Qiu et al. 1990), lie within an area that has demonstrated strong linkage to SLE in humans, with an lod score of 3.37 (Moser et al. 1998). The Fc receptor is required by cytotoxic cells to initiate antibody-dependent cellular cytotoxicity of keratinocytes, which is up-regulated in CLE (Furukawa et al. 1999), and possibly directed against the Ro/SSA antigen (Norris 1993). The FcγRIIa gene (FCGR2A) possesses an SNP (G/A) coding for arginine or histidine at codon 131 (R/H131) in the EC2 domain of FcγRIIa, which alters the ability of the receptor to bind immunoglobulin G (Clark et al. 1989, Warmerdam et al. 1990).

Apoptosis Genes and Photosensitivity in Lupus

Apoptosis is a form of programmed cell death, over 6–48 h, that is characterized by cell shrinkage and nuclear condensation in response to the activation of the enzyme caspase 3 (Elkon 1997, Salmon and Gordon 1999). On early apoptotic keratinocytes, Casciola-Rosen (1997) reported the formation of surface blebs, which are highly enriched with several lupus autoantigens, including Ro/SSA; in genetically susceptible individuals, expression of this autoantigen is proposed to initiate an autoantibody response. Multiple stimuli, including UVR, cytokines, cytotoxic T cells, and cytotoxic drugs, are capable of inducing apoptosis (Arnold et al. 1999, Danno and Horio 1982, Elkon 1997, Haake and Polakowska 1993, Stone et al. 1998). The Fas transmembrane glycoprotein receptor (Fas, encoded by *TNFRSF6*) has an intracellular death domain that initiates a cascade of events when Fas binds external Fas ligand, leading to death of the cell by apoptosis. In normal human skin, Fas is found mainly in the basal layer of the epidermis; expression then gradually diminishes toward the stratum granulosum. The specific role of Fas and Fas ligand in human CLE is still a matter of debate, but both molecules are expressed on infiltrating cells around blood vessels and hair follicles (Fushimi et al. 1998, Nakajima et al. 1997). Consistent with this co-expression of Fas and Fas ligand around hair follicles, apoptotic cells in this region were found (Nakajima et al. 1997).

In murine models, the Fas/Fas ligand axis may be involved in LE. Mice that are homozygous for the *lpr* (lymphoproliferation) recessive mutation accumulate large numbers of CD3[+] CD4[-] CD8[-] T cells, which lead to the induction or acceleration of systemic autoimmunity (Kono and Theofilopoulos 1997, Takahashi et al. 1994). The *lpr* mutation on mouse chromosome 19 causes a point mutation in *Fas* that abolishes its ability to transduce the apoptotic signal. A recent study of MRL/n (control) mice found that they develop LE-like skin lesions later in life than the closely related MRL/lpr (homozygous) mice (Furukawa et al. 1996). In humans, the Fas gene is located on chromosome band 10q24.1 (Inazawa et al. 1992). Huang et al. (Huang et al. 1999) examined a Fas polymorphism, the MvaI RFLP (MvaI*1/ MvaI*2, caused by an A/G SNP at the -670 nucleotide position) in 103 Caucasian patients with SLE and found that MvaI*2 homozygosity was significantly higher in patients with *photosensitive* SLE, but polymorphic Fas loci have not yet been examined by association or linkage in CLE.

Summary

The genetic architecture of LE is far from understood. The most significant immunogenetic associations to date have been found in the presence of anti-Ro/SSA and/or anti-La/SSB in CLE and SLE, where HLA, TNF, complement, IL-10, TCR, and GST genes may be involved. However, other LE-specific associations, outside the context of anti-Ro/SSA, have been less well characterized to date. For CLE, where the phenotype can be accurately characterized, there are still numerous candidate gene loci in the wings.

Acknowledgements. This article is adapted (with written permission from Blackwell Science) from a review article of the same title (Millard and McGregor 2001d).

References

Abraham LJ, Kroeger KM (1999) Impact of the −308 TNF promoter polymorphism on the transcriptional regulation of the TNF gene: relevance to disease. J Leukoc Biol 66:562–566

Arnett FC (1997) The Genetics of human lupus. In: Wallace DJ, Hahn BH (eds) Dubois' lupus erythematosus. Williams & Wilkins, Baltimore, pp 77–117

Arnold R, Seifert M, Asadullah K, Volk HD (1999) Crosstalk between keratinocytes and T lymphocytes via Fas/Fas ligand interaction: modulation by cytokines. J Immunol 162: 7140–7147

Aron Y, Busson M, Polla BS, Dusser D, Lockhart A, Swierczewski E, Favatier F (1999) Analysis of hsp70 gene polymorphism in allergic asthma. Allergy 54:165–170

Beckett AG, Lewis JG (1959) Familial lupus erythematosus: a report of two cases. Br J Dermatol 71:360–363

Ben-Chetrit E (1993) The molecular basis of the SSA/Ro antigens and the clinical significance of their autoantibodies. Br J Rheumatol 32:396–402

Bielsa I, Herrero C, Ercilla G, Collado A, Font J, Ingelmo M, Mascaro JM (1991) Immunogenetic findings in cutaneous lupus erythematosus. J Am Acad Dermatol 25:251–257

Blakemore AI, Tarlow JK, Cork MJ, Gordon C, Emery P, Duff GW (1994) Interleukin-1 receptor antagonist gene polymorphism as a disease severity factor in systemic lupus erythematosus. Arthritis Rheum 37:1380–1385

Bolla MK, Miller GJ, Yellon DM, Evans A, Luc G, Cambou JP, Arveiler D, Cambien F, Latchman DS, Humphries SE, Day IN (1998) Analysis of the association of a heat shock protein 70–1 gene promoter polymorphism with myocardial infarction and coronary risk traits. Dis Markers 13:227–235

Braathen LR, Bratlie A, Teisberg P (1986) HLA genotypes in a family with a case of homozygous C2 deficiency and discoid lupus erythematosus. Acta Derm Venereol 66:419–422

Burch PR, Rowell NR (1968) The sex- and age-distributions of chronic discoid lupus erythematosus in four countries. Possible aetiological and pathogenetic significance. Acta Derm Venereol 48:33–46

Burrows NP, Walport MJ, Hammond AH, Davey N, Jones RR (1991) Lupus erythematosus profundus with partial C4 deficiency responding to thalidomide. Br J Dermatol 1991 125:62–67

Callen JP, Hodge SJ, Kulick K, Stelzer G, Buchino JJ (1987) Subacute cutaneous lupus erythematosus in multiple members of a family with C2 deficiency. Arch Dermatol 123:66–70

Carroll MC, Katzman P, Alicot EM, Koller BH, Geraghty DE, Orr HT, Strominger JL, Spies T (1987) Linkage map of the human major histocompatibility complex including the tumor necrosis factor genes. Proc Natl Acad Sci USA 84:8535–8539

Casciola-Rosen L, Rosen A (1997) Ultraviolet light-induced keratinocyte apoptosis: a potential mechanism for the induction of skin lesions and autoantibody production in LE. Lupus 6:175–180

Clark MR, Clarkson SB, Ory PA, Stolman N, Goldstein JM (1989) Molecular basis for a polymorphism involving Fc receptor II on human monocytes. J Immunol 143:1731–1734

Collins T, Williams A, Johnston GI, Kim J, Eddy R, Shows T, Giml MA Jr, Bevilacqua MP (1991) Structure and chromosomal location of the gene for endothelial-leukocyte adhesion molecule 1. J Biol Chem 266:2466–2473

Danno K, Horio T (1982) Formation of UV-induced apoptosis relates to the cell cycle. Br J Dermatol 107:423–428

Elkon KB (1997) Apoptosis. In: Wallace DJ, Hahn BH (eds) Dubois' lupus erythematosus. Williams & Wilkins, Baltimore, pp 133–142

Enerback C, Enlund F, Inerot A, Samuelsson L, Wahlstrom J, Martinsson T (2000) S gene (Corneodesmosin) diversity and its relationship to psoriasis; high content of cSNP in the HLA-linked S gene. J Invest Dermatol 114:1158–1163

Esaki M, Furuse M, Matsumoto T, Aoyagi K, Jo Y, Yamagata H, Nakano H, Fujima M (1999) Polymorphism of heat-shock protein gene HSP70-2 in Crohn disease: possible genetic marker for two forms of Crohn disease. Scand J Gastroenterol 34:703–707

Eskdale J, Kube D, Tesch H, Gallagher G (1997) Mapping of the human IL10 gene and further characterization of the 5' flanking sequence. Immunogenetics 46:120–128

Fowler JF, Callen JP, Stelzer GT, Cotter PK (1985) Human histocompatibility antigen associations in patients with chronic cutaneous lupus erythematosus. J Am Acad Dermatol 12:73–77

Frank MB, McArthur R, Harley JB, Fujisaku A (1990) Anti-Ro(SSA) autoantibodies are associated with T cell receptor beta genes in systemic lupus erythematosus patients. J Clin Invest 85:33–39

Furukawa F, Ikai K, Matsuyoshi N, Shimizu K, Imamura S (1993) Relationship between heat shock protein induction and the binding of antibodies to the extractable nuclear antigens on cultured human keratinocytes. J Invest Dermatol 101:191–195

Furukawa F, Kanauchi H, Wakita H, Tokura Y, Tachibana T, Horiguchi Y, Imamura S, Ozaki S, Takigawa M (1996) Spontaneous autoimmune skin lesions of MRL/n mice: autoimmune disease-prone genetic background in relation to Fas-defect MRL/1pr mice. J Invest Dermatol 107:95–100

Furukawa F, Itoh T, Wakita H, Yagi H, Tokura Y, Norris DA, Takigawa M (1999) Keratinocytes from patients with lupus erythematosus show enhanced cytotoxicity to ultraviolet radiation and to antibody-mediated cytotoxicity. Clin Exp Immunol 118:164–170

Fushimi M, Furukawa F, Tokura Y, Itoh T, Shirahama S, Wakita H, Takigawa M (1998) Membranous and soluble forms of Fas antigen in cutaneous lupus erythematosus. J Dermatol 25:302–308

Gaffney PM, Kearns GM, Shark KB, Ortmann WA, Selby SA, Malmgren ML, Rohlf KE, OckendenTC, Messner RP, King RA, Rich SS, Behrens TW (1998) A genome-wide search for susceptibility genes in human systemic lupus erythematosus sib-pair families. Proc Natl Acad Sci USA 95:14875–14879

Gaffney PM, Ortmann WA, Selby, Shark KB, Ockenden TC, Rohlf KE, Walgrave NL, Boyum WP, Malmgren ML, Miller ME, Kearns GM, Mesner RP, King RA, Rich SS, Behrens TW (2000) Genome screening in human systemic lupus erythematosus: results from a second Minnesota cohort and combined analyses of 187 sib-pair families. Am J Hum Genet 66:547–556

Gallo RC, Forde DL (1966) Familial chronic discoid lupus erythematosus and hypergammaglobulinemia. Arch Intern Med 117:627–631

Ghoreishi M, Katayama I, Yokozeki H, Nishioka K (1993) Analysis of 70 KD heat shock protein (HSP70) expression in the lesional skin of lupus erythematosus (LE) and LE related diseases. J Dermatol 20:400–405

Gordon T, Topfer F, Keech C, Reynolds P, Chen W, Rischmueller M, McCluskey J (1994) How does autoimmunity to La and Ro initiate and spread? Autoimmunity 18:87–92

Gray-McGuire C, Moser KL, Gaffney PM, Kelly J, Yu H, Olson JM, Jedrey CM, Jacobs KB, Kimberly RP, Neas BR, Rich SS, Behrens TW, Harley JB (2000) Genome scan of human systemic lupus erythematosus by regression modeling: evidence of linkage and epistasis at 4p16-15.2. Am J Hum Genet 67:1460–1469

Haake AR, Polakowska RR (1993) Cell death by apoptosis in epidermal biology. J Invest Dermatol 101:107–112

Harley JB, Reichlin M, Arnett FC, Alexander EL, Bias WB, Provost TT (1986) Gene interaction at HLA-DQ enhances autoantibody production in primary Sjogren's syndrome. Science 232:1145–1147

Herrero C, Bielsa I, Font J, Lozano F, Ercilla G, Lecha M, Ingelmo M, Mascaro JM (1988) Subacute cutaneous lupus erythematosus: clinicopathologic findings in thirteen cases. J Am Acad Dermatol 19:1057–1062

Huang QR, Danis V, Lassere M, Edmonds J, Manolios N (1999) Evaluation of a new Apo-1/Fas promoter polymorphism in rheumatoid arthritis and systemic lupus erythematosus patients. Rheumatol (Oxford) 38:645-651

Inazawa J, Itoh N, Abe T, Nagata S (1992) Assignment of the human Fas antigen gene (Fas) to 10q24.1. Genomics 14:821-822

Johansson-Stephansson E, Koskimies S, Partanen J, Kariniemi AL (1989) Subacute cutaneous lupus erythematosus. Genetic markers and clinical and immunological findings in patients. Arch Dermatol 125:791-796

Kim JM, Brannan CI, Copeland NG, Jenkins NA, Khan TA, Moore KW (1992) Structure of the mouse IL-10 gene and chromosomal localization of the mouse and human genes. J Immunol 148:3618-3623

Knop J, Bonsmann G, Kind P, Doxiadis I, Vogeler U, Doxiadis G, Goerz G, Grosse-Wilde H (1990) Antigens of the major histocompatibility complex in patients with chronic discoid lupus erythematosus. Br J Dermatol 122:723-728

Kock A, Schwarz T, Kirnbauer R, Urbanski A, Perry P, Ansel JC (1990) Human keratinocytes are a source for tumor necrosis factor alpha: evidence for synthesis and release upon stimulation with endotoxin or ultraviolet light. J Exp Med 172:1609-1614

Kono DH, Burlingame RW, Owens DG, Kuramochi A, Balderas RS, Balomenos D, Theofilopoulos AN (1994) Lupus susceptibility loci in New Zealand mice. Proc Natl Acad Sci USA 91: 10168-10172

Kono DH, Theofilopoulos AN (1997) The Genetics of Murine Systemic Lupus Erythematosus. In: Wallace DJ, Hahn BH (eds) Dubois' lupus erythematosus. Williams & Wilkins, Baltimore, pp 119-132

Lawrence JS, Martins CL, Drake GL (1987) A family survey of lupus erythematosus. 1. Heritability. J Rheumatol 14:913-921

Lazarus M, Hajeer AH, Turner D, Sinnott P, Worthington J, Ollier WE, Hutchinson IV (1997) Genetic variation in the interleukin 10 gene promoter and systemic lupus erythematosus. J Rheumatol 24:2314-2317

Leonhardt T (1957) Familial hypergammaglobulinaemia and systemic lupus erythematosus. Lancet 2:1200-1203

Levy SB, Pinnell SR, Meadows L, Snyderman R, Ward FE (1979) Hereditary C2 deficiency associated with cutaneous lupus erythematosus: clinical, laboratory, and genetic studies. Arch Dermatol 115:57-61

Lewis CM (2000) Using sib-pairs and parent-child trios in association studies. In: Spector TD, Snieder H, MacGregor AJ (eds) Advances in twin and sib-pair analysis. Greenwich Medical Media, London, pp 167-179

Lindqvist AK, Steinsson K, Johaneson B, Kristjansdottir H, Arnasson A, Grondal G, Jonasson I, Magnusson V, Sturfelt G, Truedsson L, Svenungsson E, Lundberg I, Terwilliger JD, Gyllensten UB, Alarcon-Riquelme ME (2000) A susceptibility locus for human systemic lupus erythematosus (hSLE1) on chromosome 2q. J Autoimmun 14:169-178

Llorente L, Zou W, Levy Y, Richaud-Patin Y, Wijdenes J, Alcocer-Varela J, Morel-Fourrier B, Brouet JC, Alarcon-Segovia D, Galanaud P, Emilie D (1995) Role of interleukin 10 in the B lymphocyte hyperactivity and autoantibody production of human systemic lupus erythematosus. J Exp Med 181:839-844

Meo T, Atkinson JP, Bernoco M, Bernoco D, Ceppellini R (1977) Structural heterogeneity of C2 Complement protein and its genetic variants in man: a new polymorphism of the HLA region. Proc Natl Acad Sci USA 74:1672-1675

Meyer O, Hauptmann G, Tappeiner G, Ochs HD, Mascart-Lemone F (1985) Genetic deficiency of C4, C2 or C1q and lupus syndromes. Association with anti-Ro (SS-A) antibodies. Clin Exp Immunol 1985 62:678-684

MHC Sequencing Consortium (1999) Complete sequence and gene map of a human major histocompatibility complex. Nature 401:921-923

Millard LG, Rowell NR, Rajah SM (1977) Histocompatibility antigens in discoid and systemic lupus erythematosus. Br J Dermatol 96:139-144

Millard TP, Lewis CM, Khamashta MA, Hughes GR, Hawk JL, McGregor JM (2001a) Familial clustering of polymorphic light eruption in relatives of lupus patients – evidence of a shared pathogenesis. Br J Dermatol 144:334–338

Millard TP, Kondeatis E, Vaughan RW, Lewis CM, Khamashta MA, Hughes GR, Hawk JL, McGregor JM (2001b) Polymorphic light eruption and the HLA DRB1*0301 extended haplotype are independent risk factors for cutaneous lupus erythematosus. Lupus 10: 473–479

Millard TP, Kondeatis E, Cox A, Wilson AG, Grabczynska SA, Carey BS, Lewis CM, Khamashta MA, Duff GM, Hughes GR, Hawk JL, Vaughan RW, McGregor JM (2001c) A candidate gene analysis of three related photosensitivity disorders: cutaneous lupus erythematosus, polymorphic light eruption and actinic prurigo. Br J Dermatol 145:229–236

Millard TP, McGregor JM (2001d) Molecular genetics of cutaneous lupus erythematosus. Clin Exp Dermatol 26:184–191

Millard TP, Ashton GHS, Kondeatis E, Vaughan RW, Hughes GR, Khamashta MA, Hawk JL, McGrath JA (2002) Human Ro60 genomic organization and sequence alterations in cutaneous lupus erythematosus. Br J Dermatol 146:210–215

Moser KL, Neas BR, Salmon JE, Yu H, Gray-McGuire C, Asundi N, Bruner GR, Fox J, Kelly J, Henshall S, Bacino D, Dietz M, Hogue R, Koelsch G, Nightingale L, Shaver T, Abdou NI, Albert DA, Carson C, Petri M, Treadwell EL, James JA, Harley JB (1998) Genome scan of human systemic lupus erythematosus: evidence for linkage on chromosome 1q in African-American pedigrees. Proc Natl Acad Sci USA 95:14869–14874

Muramatsu T, Tada H, Kobayashi N, Yamji M, Shirai T, Ohnishi T (1992) Induction of the 72-kD heat shock protein in organ-cultured normal human skin. J Invest Dermatol 98:786–790

Nakajima M, Nakajima A, Kayagaki N, Honda M, Yagita H, Okumura K (1997) Expression of Fas ligand and its receptor in cutaneous lupus: implication in tissue injury. Clin Immunol Immunopathol 1997 83:223–229

Nath SK, Kelly JA, Namjou B, Lam T, Bruner GR, Scofield RH, Aston CE, Harley JB (2001) Evidence for a susceptibility gene, SLEV1, on chromosome 17p13 in families with vitiligo-related systemic lupus erythematosus. Am J Hum Genet 69:1401–1406

Norris DA (1993) Pathomechanisms of photosensitive lupus erythematosus. J Invest Dermatol 100:58S–68S

Norris PG, Barker JN, Allen MH, Leiferman KM, MacDonald DM, Haskard DO, Hawk JL (1992) Adhesion molecule expression in polymorphic light eruption. J Invest Dermatol 99:504–508

Nousari HC, Kimyai-Asadi A, Provost TT (1999) Generalized lupus erythematosus profundus in a patient with genetic partial deficiency of C4. J Am Acad Dermatol 41:362–364

Nyberg F, Hasan T, Puska P, Stephansson E, Hakkinen M, Ranki A, Ros AM (1997) Occurrence of polymorphous light eruption in lupus erythematosus. Br J Dermatol 136:217–221

Nyberg F, Hasan T, Skoglund C, Stephansson E (1999) Early events in ultraviolet light-induced skin lesions in lupus erythematosus: expression patterns of adhesion molecules ICAM-1, VCAM-1 and E-selectin. Acta Derm Venereol 79:431–436

Nyberg F, Stephansson E (1999) Elevated soluble E-selectin in cutaneous lupus erythematosus. Adv Exp Med Biol 455:153–159

Ollier W, Davies E, Snowden N, Alldersea J, Fryer A, Jones P, Strange R (1996) Association of homozygosity for glutathione-S-transferase GSTM1 null alleles with the Ro+/La- autoantibody profile in patients with systemic lupus erythematosus. Arthritis Rheum 39:1763–1764

Palmetshofer A, Schwarz K, Mahnke R, Bhardway R, Luger TA, Schwarz T (1994) Interleukin-10 affects the expression of adhesion molecules on human dermal microvascular endothelial cells. Exp Dermatol 3:138 (Abstract)

Pearson WR, Vorachek WR, Xu SJ, Berger R, Hart I, Vannais D, Patterson D (1993) Identification of class-mu glutathione transferase genes GSTM1-GSTM5 on human chromosome 1p13. Am J Hum Genet 53:220–233

Price P, Witt C, Allcock R, Sayer D, Garlepp M, Kok CC, French M, Mallal S, Christiansen F (1999) The genetic basis for the association of the 8.1 ancestral haplotype (A1, B8, DR3) with multiple immunopathological diseases. Immunol Rev 167:257–274

Provost TT, Arnett FC, Reichlin M (1983) Homozygous C2 deficiency, lupus erythematosus, and anti-Ro (SSA) antibodies. Arthritis Rheum 26:1279–1282

Provost TT, Talal N, Bias W, Harley JB, Reichlin M, Alexander EL (1988) Ro(SS-A) positive Sjogren's/lupus erythematosus (SC/LE) overlap patients are associated with the HLA-DR3 and/or DRw6 phenotypes. J Invest Dermatol 91:369–371

Provost TT, Watson R (1993) Anti-Ro(SS-A) HLA-DR3-positive women: the interrelationship between some ANA negative, SS, SCLE, and NLE mothers and SS/LE overlap female patients. J Invest Dermatol 100:14S-20S

Qiu WQ, de Bruin D, Brownstein BH, Pearse R, Ravetch JV (1990) Organization of the human and mouse low-affinity Fc gamma R genes: duplication and recombination. Science 248:732–735

Ralston SH (1998) Do genetic markers aid in risk assessment? Osteoporos Int 8 (Suppl 1):S37–S42

Rood MJ, van Krugten MV, Zanelli E, van der Linden MW, Keijsers V, Schreuder GM, Verduyn W, Westendorp RG, de Vries RR, Breedveld FC, Verweij CL, Huizinga TW (2000) TNF-308A and HLA-DR3 alleles contribute independently to susceptibility to systemic lupus erythematosus. Arthritis Rheum 43:129–134

Salmon M, Gordon C (1999) The role of apoptosis in systemic lupus erythematosus. Rheumatol (Oxford) 38:1177–1183

Scofield RH, Frank MB, Neas BR, Horowitz RM, Hardgrave KL, Fujisaku A, McArthur R, Harley JB (1994) Cooperative association of T cell beta receptor and HLA-DQ alleles in the production of anti-Ro in systemic lupus erythematosus. Clin Immunol Immunopathol 72:335–341

Sequira JH (1903) Lupus erythematosus in two sisters. Br J Dermatol 15:171

Shai R, Quismorio FP, Li L, Kwon OJ, Morrison J, Wallace DJ, Neuwelt CM, Brautbar C, Gauderman WJ, Jacob CO (1999) Genome-wide screen for systemic lupus erythematosus susceptibility genes in multiplex families. Hum Mol Genet 8:639–644

Silverberg NB, Liotta M, Paller AS, Pachman LM (1999) TNF-alpha –308 polymorphism (AA, GA) is associated with increased UVB induced keratinocyte TNF-alpha production in vitro. Arthritis Rheum 42:S93(Abstract)

Sontheimer RD, Stastny P, Gilliam JN (1981) Human histocompatibility antigen associations in subacute cutaneous lupus erythematosus. J Clin Invest 67:312–316

Sontheimer RD, Maddison PJ, Reichlin M, Jordon RE, Stastny P, Gilliam JN (1982) Serologic and HLA associations in subacute cutaneous lupus erythematosus, a clinical subset of lupus erythematosus. Ann Intern Med 97:664–671

Sontheimer RD (1996) Photoimmunology of lupus erythematosus and dermatomyositis: a speculative review. Photochem Photobiol 63:583–594

Sontheimer RD, Provost TT (1997) Cutaneous manifestations of lupus erythematosus. In: Wallace DJ, Hahn BH (eds) Dubois' lupus erythemtosus. Williams & Wilkins, Baltimore, pp 569–623

Steagall RW, Ash HT, Fentanes LB (1962) Familial lupus erythematosus. Arch Dermatol 1962 85:394–396

Stephanou A, Amin V, Isenberg DA, Akira S, Kishimoto T, Latchman DS (1997) Interleukin 6 activates heat-shock protein 90 beta gene expression. Biochem J 321:103–106

Stone MS, Robson KJ, LeBoit PE (1998) Subacute radiation dermatitis from fluoroscopy during coronary artery stenting: evidence for cytotoxic lymphocyte mediated apoptosis. J Am Acad Dermatol 38:333–336

Sullivan KE (1998) Complement deficiency and autoimmunity. Curr Opin Ped 10:600–606

Suzuki H, Matsui Y, Kashiwagi H (1997) Interleukin-1 receptor antagonist gene polymorphism in Japanese patients with systemic lupus erythematosus. Arthritis Rheum 40:389–390

Takahashi T, Tanaka M, Brannan CI, Jenkins NA, Copeland NG, Suda T, Nagata S (1994) Generalized lymphoproliferative disease in mice, caused by a point mutation in the Fas ligand. Cell 76:969–976

Tongio MM, Fersing J, Hauptmann G, Mayer S, Grange D, Samsoen M, Groshans E (1982) HLA antigens in discoid lupus erythematosus. Acta Derm Venereol 62:155–157

Turner DM, Williams DM, Sankaran D, Lazarus M, Sinnott PJ, Hutchinsin IV (1997) An investigation of polymorphism in the interleukin-10 gene promoter. Eur J Immunogenet 24:1–8

Vazquez-Doval J, Ruiz E, Sanchez-Ibarrola A, Contreras F, Soto de Delas J, Quintanilla E (1992) Subacute cutaneous lupus erythematosus–clinical, histopathological and immunophenotypical study of five cases. J Investig Allergol Clin Immunol 2:27–32

Vora DK, Rosenbloom CL, Beaudet AL, Cottingham RW (1994) Polymorphisms and linkage analysis for ICAM-1 and the selectin gene cluster. Genomics 21:473–477

Wallace DJ (1997) Occasional, innovative and experimental therapies. In: Wallace DJ and Hahn BH (eds) Dubois' lupus erythemtosus. Williams & Wilkins, Baltimore, pp 1191–1202

Warmerdam PA, van de Winkel JG, Gosselin EJ, Capel PJ (1990) Molecular basis for a polymorphism of human Fc gamma receptor II (CD32). J Exp Med 172:19–25

Watson RM, Talwar P, Alexander E, Bias WB, Provost TT (1991) Subacute cutaneous lupus erythematosus-immunogenetic associations. J Autoimmun 4:73–85

Wenzel K, Hanke R, Speer A (1994a) Polymorphism in the human E-selectin gene detected by PCR-SSCP. Hum Gen 94:452–453

Wenzel K, Felix S, Kleber FX, Brachold R, Menke T, Schattke S, Schulte KL, Glaser C, Rohde K, Baumann G, Speer A (1994b) E-selectin polymorphism and atherosclerosis: an association study. Hum Mol Genet 3:1935–1937

Werth VP, Sullivan KE (1999) Strong association of a promoter polymorphism of tumour necrosis factor-alpha (TNF-alpha) with a photosensitive form of cutaneous lupus erythematosus. Arthritis Rheum 42:S105 (Abstract)

Wilson AG, de Vries N, Pociot F, di Giovine FS, van der Putte LB, Duff GW (1993) An allelic polymorphism within the human tumor necrosis factor alpha promoter region is strongly associated with HLA A1, B8, and DR3 alleles. J Exp Med 177:557–560

Wojnarowska F (1983) Simultaneous occurrence in identical twins of discoid lupus erythematosus and polymorphic light eruption. J R Soc Med 76:791–792

Wolpert KA, Webster AD, Whittaker SJ (1998) Discoid lupus erythematosus associated with a primary immunodeficiency syndrome showing features of non-X-linked hyper-IgM syndrome. Br J Dermatol 138:1053–1057

Yeaman GR, Froebel K, Galea G, Ormerod A, Urbaniak SJ (1992) Discoid lupus erythematosus in an X-linked cytochrome-positive carrier of chronic granulomatous disease. Br J Dermatol 126:60–65

CHAPTER 16

Experimental Models of Lupus Erythematosus 16

FUKUMI FURUKAWA

The etiology and pathogenesis of autoimmune diseases cannot be readily analyzed without appropriate animal models, although no single animal model perfectly mimics a human disease. Animal models are commonly used to study the genetic, environmental, and pathogenic aspects of autoimmune diseases. Regarding experimental autoimmune diseases, these models can be divided into several broad groups: (a) inbred mice that spontaneously develop a disease similar to human systemic lupus erythematosus (SLE); (b) chronic graft-vs-host diseases induced in F1 hybrid mice injected with lymphoid parental cells; (c) ultraviolet (UV) light-irradiated mice immunized with some components of DNA; (d) immunodeficient mice such as severe combined immunodeficient (SCID) mice and nude mice inoculated or engrafted with immunocompetent cells or tissues; and (e) gene-manipulated mice such as transgenic or knockout mice.

There are many inbred strains of SLE-prone mice, including New Zealand Black (NZB), F1 hybrids of NZB × New Zealand White (NZW) (B/W F1), MRL/Mp-lpr/lpr (MRL/lpr), and BXSB mice. The postulated etiologic factors of these murine diseases include retroviruses, thymic abnormalities, antithymocyte antibodies, polyclonal B-cell activation, an impaired balance of T-cell interaction, and abnormalities of phagocytic cells (Andrews et al. 1978). Such abnormalities described in SLE now span the spectrum from cellular immunology to immunoglobulin idiotypes, cytokines, apoptosis, DNA repair, and endogenous retroviruses (Steinberg 1995). Immunologic tolerance is now revisited to study the systemic and organ-specific autoimmune diseases (Nishimura and Honjo 2001, Shimizu et al. 2002). Based on these trends, several new and important studies on the pathogenesis of lupus have been reported in the field of internal organ biology, including the kidney, lung, and salivary glands. In this review, based on historical review, we focus on skin lesions from the well-studied MRL/lpr and B/W F1 mice and discuss how SLE-prone mice can contribute to a better understanding of the pathogenesis of cutaneous LE (CLE).

Autoimmune-Prone Mouse

The serologic characteristics of these mice are hyper-γ-globulinemia, a high titer of antinuclear antibodies, and the presence of anti-double-stranded DNA, anti-single-stranded DNA, and antihapten antibodies, high levels of retroviral gp70, circulating immune complexes, and reduced complement levels. Lupus nephritis, such as proteinuria and immune complex glomerulonephritis, is also common in SLE-prone

Table 16.1. Characteristics of systemic lupus erythematosus-prone mouse strains

Strain	Dermatitis	Photosensitivity	Histopathologic Features IGs at DEJ	IC-GN	Arteritis	Arthritis
NZB	0	+	+ (IgM)	+	0	0
NZB/KN	+ (alopecia)	unknown	+ (IgM)	+	0	+
B/W F1	0	+	++ (IgG)	+++	0	0
MRL/lpr	++	+++	+ (IgG)	+++	+	+
MRL/n	++ (aged)	–	+ (ANA)	+	+	+
BXSB	0	++	+ (IgG)	+++	0	0

IGs at DEJ, immunoglobulins deposits at the dermoepidermal junction; IC-GN, immune complex glomerulonephritis; ANA, antinuclear antibody.

mice. In addition, thymic atrophy and lymphoid hyperplasia (T cells in MRL/lpr mice and B cells in NZB mice and BXSB mice) are frequently observed (Theofilopoulos and Dixon 1981). Because these lymphocyte subsets are responsible for the development of murine lupus, MRL/lpr mice have been described as T lupus, and NZ and BXSB mice as B lupus. In these mouse models, common genes or genetic pathways may contribute to immune dysregulation and to susceptibility to multiple autoimmune diseases, such as SLE and rheumatoid arthritis (Wandstract and Wakeland 2002). Compared with B-lupus strains, such as NZB, B/W F1, and BXSB mice, the MRL/lpr mouse has some unique features, such as rheumatoid arthritis, inflammatory changes in their salivary glands (e.g., Sjögren's syndrome), and arteritis (Table 16.1). Macroscopic skin lesions are also observed in MRL/lpr mice (Murphy and Roths 1978). A common dermatologic finding in SLE-prone mouse strains is the deposition of immunoglobulins, complement components, or both at the dermoepidermal junction (DEJ) (Table 16.1). Immunoglobulin deposits at the DEJ are associated with the occurrence of anti-DNA antibodies and proteinuria (Furukawa et al. 1985a), and eluates from these skin lesions contain the binding ability to DNA components (Furukawa 1986b).

These autoimmune traits are regulated under multigenetic factors (Izui et al. 1994, Table 16.2). Although the precise nature and number of genes involved in the development of SLE remains unclear, several major histocompatibility complex (MHC) and non-MHC genes have been investigated as candidate genes to be implicated in SLE (Wandstract and Wakeland 2002), including immounglobulin variable (V) region genes encoding autoantibodies with pathogenic specificity, T-cell receptor (TCR) genes, and the MHC genes (Wandstract and Wakeland 2002). With respect to skin lesions, the immounglobulin deposition seen in NZB mice and MRL/lpr mice are regulated by the *Lbt*-1 gene on chromosome 17 (Furukawa et al. 1985b) and *lpr* gene on chromosome 19 (Furukawa et al. 1984, 1996), respectively.

Table 16.2. Possible genetic factors involved in murine systemic lupus erythematosus[a]

1. Immunoglobulin variable region genes
2. T-cell receptor genes
3. Major histocompatibility complex class II genes
4. Genes regulating apoptosis:
   Fas apoptosis gene: the *lpr* mutation
   gld gene: the Fas ligand
5. *Yaa* gene
6. Genes for the expression of nephritogenic autoantigens
   Genes encoding and/or regulating the expression of serum retroviral gp70 antigen
7. Genes regulating immunoglobulin class switching
   Genes for cytokines or their receptors
   xid gene: Bruton's tyrosine kinase

[a] This table is based on the report of Izui et al. 1994.
lpr, lymphoproliferation; *gld*, generalized lymphoproliferative disease; *Yaa*, Y chromosome-linked autoimmune acceleration; *xid*, X chromosome-linked immunodeficiency.

MRL Mouse

Fas-Defect MRL Mice as a Model of Systemic Lupus Erythematosus

MRL mice were originally developed by Murphy and Roths at Jackson Laboratories (Murphy and Roths 1978). Two substrains of MRL mice were developed: the MRL/lpr and the MRL/n mouse. These substrains were derived mainly from the LG/J strain with contributions from AKR/J, C3H/Di, and C57BL/6J mouse strains. The spontaneous autosomal recessive mutation *lpr* (lymphoproliferation) was first observed at the 12th generation of inbreeding. The lupus-like syndrome is earlier in onset and more acute in females than in males. Virgin female MRL/lpr mice have a 50% mortality rate at 6 months of age, whereas virgin female MRL/n mice have a 50% mortality rate at 18 months of age (Furukawa et al. 1996). The autosomal recessive *lpr* gene induces massive CD3+CD4−CD8− cell (double-negative T cell) proliferation. This striking proliferation of double-negative T cells is caused by a defect in the Fas antigen, which has been reported to mediate apoptosis (Watanabe-Fukunaga et al. 1992). The Fas defect is believed to accelerate the autoimmunity of MRL/lpr mice, and it results in lupus nephritis and spontaneous LE-like skin lesions beginning at age 3 months, even under pathogen-free conditions (Furukawa et al. 1984, Kanauchi et al. 1991, Murphy and Roths 1978). The congenic MRL/n mouse strain is more than 99.6% homozygous to MRL/lpr mice but lacks the *lpr* mutation and is almost normal during the first 6 months of life (Murphy and Roths 1978).

The MRL/lpr Mouse as a Good Model of Cutaneous Lupus Erythematosus

The MRL/lpr mouse is a good model for the spontaneous development of skin lesions similar to those seen in human LE (Furukawa et al. 1984, Horiguchi et al. 1986a,b, Provost and Watson 1993). Macroscopically, these skin lesions have been described as showing "alopecia and scab formation" by Murphy and Roths (Murphy and Roths 1978). Such skin lesions are not observed in NZB, B/W F1, or BXSB mice. Our immunopathologic studies have revealed liquefaction-like changes in basal keratinocytes, dermal T-cell infiltration, and vasodilatation (Furukawa et al. 1984), as well as ultrastructural changes very similar to those seen in human LE skin lesions (Horiguchi et al. 1984, 1986b). The incidence of IgG deposition at the DEJ of MRL/lpr mice increases with age and reaches more than 80% after age 5 months (Furukawa et al. 1984, Horiguchi et al. 1986a). Subepithelial immunoglobulin deposits are also found in the esophagus and uterus (Furukawa et al. 1986a, Horiguchi 1987a). These subepidermal immounglobulin deposits are eliminated by neonatal thymectomy (Furukawa et al. 1986bc). CD4$^+$ cells are predominant, and the CD4/CD8 ratio is high in dermal infiltrates with increased expression of *c-myb* and *c-myc* protooncogenes (Kanauchi et al. 1991, Kitajima et al. 1992). The number of Ia+-Langerhans' cells (LC) is increased significantly in the central portion of these lesions at an early stage and in the peripheral portions of the lesions later on. In contrast, Ia$^+$-LC and Thy-1$^+$-dendritic epidermal cells are markedly decreased in the skin lesions at a later stage. Therefore, there is a good deal of information that strongly suggests that this mouse model develops cutaneous lesions that are pathologically similar to human CLE lesions (Furukawa 1994, Furukawa 1999, Provost and Watson 1993).

Similarities and Differences in Skin Lesions of MRL/n vs MRL/lpr Mice

It is believed that the *lpr* mutation causes an acceleration of the subclinical autoimmune-prone background of MRL/n mice (Theofilopoulos 1995). Although the *lpr* mutation has also been reproduced in several other mouse strains, such as the C3H, C57BL/6J, and AKR mouse, these strains do not show the same severity of lupus nephritis, vasculitis, or arthritis as the MRL/lpr mouse, except for the appearance of lymphoproliferation, the presence of rheumatoid factor, and a decrease in interleukin (IL) 2 production (Berney et al. 1992, Izui 1994, Takahashi et al. 1991, Theofilopoulos 1981). Therefore, the autoimmune disease–prone genetic background of the MRL mice is important for the investigation of autoimmune phenomena in MRL/lpr mice.

The skin manifestations of aged MRL/n mice are found on the upper dorsal surface, and a few mice also show necrotic skin lesions on the ears (Fig. 16.1) (Furukawa et al. 1996). One-third of MRL/lpr mice have spontaneous LE-like eruptions at 3 months of age, and the incidence rises to 80% at 5 months of age. In MRL/n mice, at 12 months of age, almost half have skin lesions similar to MRL/lpr mice, and 75% of 21-month-old MRL/n mice have such skin lesions. The histology of these MRL/n mice includes hyperkeratosis, acanthosis, mononuclear cell infiltration into the dermis, an increased number of collagen bundles, and fibrosis. Vasodilatation, bleeding, or liquefaction-like changes, which are common in MRL/lpr mice, are not observed in MRL/n mice. The mononuclear cell infiltration seen in the MRL/n mice is also milder than in the MRL/lpr mice (Furukawa et al. 1996).

In MRL/n mice, immunoglobulin deposits are also found at the DEJ in aged mice, but the incidence is very low compared with that in MRL/lpr mice. A more characteristic finding in aged MRL/n mice is epidermal cell nuclear staining on direct immunofluorescence with a homogeneous pattern (Furukawa et al. 1996). In humans, such unique immunofluorescence results are often observed in patients with mixed

Fig. 16.1. Macroscopic and immuno-pathologic characteristics of the aged MRL/n mouse. Nuclear stainings are shown in the skin (*bottom left*) and the kidney (*bottom right*)

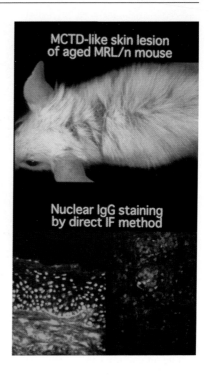

MCTD-like skin lesion of aged MRL/n mouse

Nuclear IgG staining by direct IF method

connective tissue diseases and in one third of patients with SLE with a slightly different staining pattern (Burrows et al. 1993, Velthuis et al. 1990). At 21 months of age, 50% of the MRL/n mice show epidermal cell nuclear staining, which is not observed in any of the MRL/lpr mice. The epidermal cell nuclear staining is always associated with nuclear staining in the kidney, lung, and spleen. In addition, sera from aged MRL/n mice show homogeneously positive binding to the nuclei of keratinocytes cultured from newborn MRL/n mice. This in vitro binding to the keratinocytes also correlates with epidermal cell nuclear staining using direct immunofluorescence.

From these studies, we can conclude that the *lpr* mutation accelerates the progression of a mild type of systemic and cutaneous connective tissue disease into a more severe type, such as SLE (Fig. 16.2). Furthermore, skin lesions from aged MRL/n mice can provide new insights into the long-standing controversy over whether epidermal cell nuclear staining occurs in vivo. Based on the little evidence of the cellular penetration of anti-RNP IgGs through Fc receptors (Alarcon-Segovia et al. 1978), and the in vivo binding of antiribonucleoprotein and anti-DNA antibodies to a cell suspension of live keratinocytes (Galoppin and Saurat 1981), epidermal nuclear staining may indeed be an in vivo immunologic event.

Lessons from MRL Mice for Human Cutaneous Lupus Erythematosus

Because the MRL/lpr mouse is a macroscopic and immunohistologic model for CLE, it is possible to elucidate the role of the *lpr* mutation in the development of LE-like

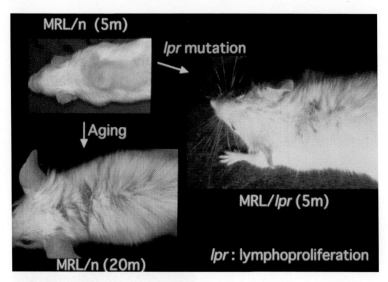

Fig. 16.2. Association between the MRL/n mouse and the Fas-defect MRL/Mp-lpr/lpr mouse

skin lesions in MRL mice. The basic analysis was conducted according to our previous genetic studies in NZ mice (Furukawa 1985b, Maruyama et al. 1983, Shirai et al. 1986). The results from the F1 hybrids (MRL/lpr×MRL/n) and F2 (F1×F1) hybrid mice indicated that the *lpr* mutation regulated lymphoproliferation and subepidermal immunoglobulin deposition at the DEJ. Interestingly, the appearance of macroscopic skin lesions was not regulated by the *lpr* mutation alone (Furukawa 1997, Furukawa et al. 1996). Previously, we demonstrated that subepidermal immunoglobulin deposits are completely eliminated by neonatal thymectomy but that macroscopic LE-like lesions are not (Furukawa et al. 1986b, c). In addition, the transfer of proliferative double-negative T cells from MRL/lpr mice to MRL/n mice can induce perivascular lymphocyte infiltration in the dermis, and additional treatment with polyclonal B-cell activators can successfully reproduce the subepidermal immunoglobulin deposits, in which macroscopic skin lesions do not develop (Furukawa et al. 1993b). Rheumatoid factors of the cryoprecipitable IgG3 subclass derived from MRL/lpr mice can also induce skin leukocytoclastic vasculitis (Berney et al. 1992). Based on these results, the appearance of macroscopic LE-like skin lesions can therefore be speculated to be due to the *lpr* mutation plus an additional factor, which probably affects the induction of these macroscopic skin lesions in an autosomal dominant fashion (Fig. 16.3). Candidates for such an additional factor may include environmental stimuli such as changes in temperature, UV light, and biological stress (Furukawa et al. 1993a, Horiguchi et al. 1987b).

Fig. 16.3. Association between the *lpr* mutation and lupus dermatoses in the MRL/Mp-lpr/lpr mouse. Subepidermal IgG deposition, written as LBT(+), is regulated by the *lpr* mutation in an autosomal recessive manner. Spontaneous lupus erythematosus-like skin lesions, written as lupus dermatoses, are speculated to be regulated by the *lpr* mutation in a recessive manner plus an additional factor in a dominant manner

Role of responsible genes

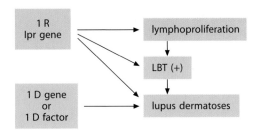

NZ Mouse

Genetic Basis of Subepidermal Immunoglobulin Deposits in NZB and B/W F1 Mice

Bielschowsky et al. (Bielschowsky et al. 1959) first reported the development of autoimmune disease in the inbred NZB mouse strain. The NZB mouse is characterized by many SLE-like symptoms, such as autoimmune hemolytic anemia, hyper-γ-globulinemia, hypocomplementemia, occasional lymphoproliferative disorders, and immune complex–type glomerulonephritis. More interesting is the F1 progeny from the NZB and the nonautoimmune NZW strain (B/W F1), which has an earlier onset and a higher incidence of lupus nephritis (Table 16.1) than the parental NZB strain as well as the renal disease associated with higher titers of antinuclear antibodies (Howie and Helyer 1968). This augmented presentation of autoimmune disease has been explained by the involvement of one or more NZW genes, which act to modify the expression of the major autoimmune NZB gene(s) (Shirai 1982, Wandstract and Wakeland 2002). Conventional genetic studies indicate that each parental strain contributes at least one or two genes, one of which is linked to the MHC locus, with heterozygosity (H-2d/z) conferring the maximal susceptibility. Furthermore, molecular technology has enabled us to determine the lupus susceptibility locus (Kono et al. 1994) and to speculate a relationship between this locus and the gene-encoding receptors for tumor necrosis factor (Drake et al. 1994).

NZ mice rarely show macroscopic skin lesions. However, subepidermal immunoglobulin deposition in B/W F1 mice has been reported by Gilliam and associates (Gilliam et al. 1975) and is equivalent to human skin lupus band test (LBT) in patients with SLE. The immunoglobulin deposits are highest in the keratinizing lip (Sontheimer and Gilliam 1979) or tail skin (Furukawa and Hamashima 1982) (Fig. 16.4), which suggests a correlation with epidermal DNA synthesis (Sontheimer and Gilliam 1979). Our previous genetic studies on the LBT showed that the incidence in female NZB, NZW, B/W F1, and B/W F1×NZW backcross mice was 60%, 0%, 100%, and 42% at 12 months of age, respectively (Furukawa et al. 1985b). B/W F1 mice have not only a higher incidence but also an earlier onset of LBT positivity than the parental NZB mice. Thus, a single dominant locus in the NZB strain determines the appearance of a positive LBT result, and this trait is intensified to a great degree by the involvement

Fig. 16.4. Immunoglobulin deposition at the dermoepidermal junction of the tail skin of the F1 progeny from the New Zealand Black and the nonautoimmune New Zealand White strain (B/W F1)

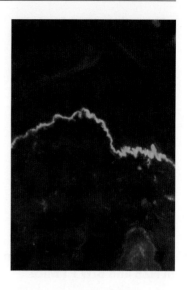

of the NZW gene(s) in B/W F1 mice. Linkage studies reveal that the NZB gene is linked to some extent to the H-2 complex and that there is a significant association between LBT positivity and the appearance of anti-double-stranded DNA antibodies and renal disease in B/W F1×NZW backcross mice. Therefore, it is postulated that the NZB-LBT gene (provisionally designated *Lbt-1*), if present on chromosome 17, is closely linked to the occurrence of anti-DNA antibodies and renal disease. There is a lack of retroviral gp70 deposition at the DEJ of NZB and B/W F1 mice, especially given the fact that gp70 is the predominant antigen in the immune complexes of diseased renal glomeruli (Maruyama et al. 1983). It is thus possible that there is a difference in the pathogenesis between lupus dermatoses and lupus nephritis (Furukawa 1997).

NZB/KN Mice as a Model of Autoimmune Alopecia

The NZB/KN mouse was established by Nakamura et al. (Nakamura et al. 1991). This strain is characterized by degenerative polyarthritis in the joints of the forepaw and hindpaw, beginning at age 2 months, which is more frequently observed in male mice than in female mice. NZB/KN is considered to be a model of rheumatoid arthritis. An additional interesting finding is the presence of alopecia over the tail to the lower back regions (Hiroi et al. 2001). Alopecia starts at 3 months of age and appears in 80% of 9-month-old NZB/KN mice (Fig. 16.5). Macroscopically, the alopecia lesion shows no scab formation or erythematous changes, and immunohistologically subepidermal IgM deposits are frequently demonstrated. These unique points raise the possibility that the NZB/KN mouse is a model of autoimmune alopecia.

There have been no good models of murine autoimmune alopecia. One exception was the NC mouse investigated by Tamada et al. (Tamada et al. 1976). The NC mouse was developed by Japanese investigators (Kondo et al. 1969) and has been considered to be a useful model of a certain type of autoimmune anemia, glomerulonephritis,

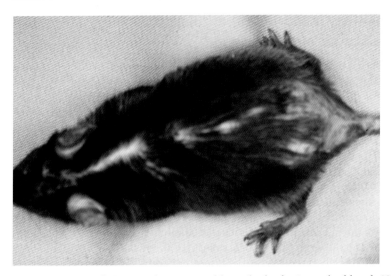

Fig. 16.5. Alopecia lesions on the upper and lower back of a 9-month-old male New Zealand Black/KN mouse

and amyloidosis. Erythema and diffuse alopecia appears on the face and ears, and alopecia without erythema occurs on the back. Such skin lesions start at age 3 months and appear cumulatively in more than 80% of the mice. However, subepidermal immunoglobulins are not deposited. In this sense, it remains unclear whether the NC mouse is a model of autoimmune alopecia. Interestingly, this inbred strain is now being investigated as a model of atopic dermatitis because of the hyper-IgE in the sera (Matsuda et al. 1997).

As described previously in this review, the MRL mice also show alopecia lesions with erythematous changes, in which histologic changes in the epidermis, vasodilatation, and bleeding are all observed. These changes are similar to the alopecia lesions seen in patients with discoid LE.

Autoimmune Diseases in Hybrid Mouse

Several F1 hybrid mice have been used for the investigation of autoimmunity. The (NZW×BXSB)F1 mouse, which develops lupus nephritis with myocardial infarctions, is a model of idiopathic thrombocytopenic purpura (Oyaizuet al. 1988), and also shows serologic features resembling human antiphospholipid syndrome (Monestier et al. 1996). The (NZB×BXSB)F1 mouse is also a model of lupus nephritis (Merino et al. 1994). These studies gave new insights and a better understanding into the role of the *Yaa* gene in lupus development (Table 16.2). Although several other hybrid strains, including the (SWR×SJL)F1 mouse, in which both parental strains show lymphadenopathy, splenomegaly, and hyper-γ-globulinemia (Vidal et al. 1994), have been proposed as models of SLE, there is little information available on lupus dermatoses.

Photosensitivity in Murine Experimental and Inbred Lupus Models

Photosensitivity is one of the major symptoms of SLE and related diseases, including subacute CLE and neonatal LE. Although it remains unclear how "photosensitivity" can be examined using laboratory tests, experimental models have been developed and inbred SLE-prone mice have been investigated for a better understanding of the "photosensitivity" phenomenon in relation to autoimmunity (reviewed by Sontheimer 1996).

Natali and Tan (Natali and Tan 1973) first reported experimental skin lesions in mice that resembled SLE. In their experiment, the mice were immunized with UVC-irradiated DNA to produce high titers of circulating antibodies against a DNA photoproduct, the thymic dimer. After these mice were whole-body irradiated with UVC, subepidermal immunoglobulin and complement deposition were produced. This result supports the importance of DNA-anti-DNA antibody complexes in the pathogenesis of CLE and the significant influence of UV. However, the role of UVA and UVB irradiation remains obscure because UVC does not reach the earth. The transient occurrence of subepidermal immunoglobulin deposits and macroscopic LE-like lesions was successfully induced in UVB-irradiated rabbits that were previously immunized with heat-denatured DNA (Imamura 1981).

It is well known that patients with LE show hypersensitivity to UVB light (Epstein et al. 1965, Kochevar 1985). In NZB mice, the relationships between autoimmunity, chromosomal abnormalities, and clastogenic factors have been discussed by a few investigators (Emerit 1982, Halpern et al. 1972, Reddy et al. 1978), and the UV sensitivity of NZB cell lines has also been reported (Zamanski et al. 1980). The clastogenic factors were reported to be sensitive to near-UV light (360–400 nm) (Emerit 1982), but the significance of this finding has not been completely understood. B/W F1 mice, which have manifestations more similar to human SLE than NZB mice, produce high serum titers of antinuclear antibodies and anti-DNA antibodies following whole-body irradiation with UVC light (Natali et al. 1978). However, this UV-induced acceleration of autoimmune traits in B/W F1 mice is still controversial (Davis and Percy 1978).

MRL/lpr mice, which have LE-like skin lesions and subepidermal immunoglobulin deposits, have yielded us more informative insights into the pathogenesis of UV-related dermatoses than either NZ or BXSB mice, both of which lack macroscopic skin lesions. Long-term exposure to a low dose of UVB radiation accelerates the development of LE-like skin lesions and enhances the intensity of subepidermal immunoglobulin deposits (Horiguchi et al. 1987b). In contrast, UVB irradiation has no effect on the anti-DNA antibody titer of the sera, the incidence of subepidermal immunoglobulin deposits, and the extent of glomerulonephritis (Ansel et al. 1985, Horiguchi et al. 1987b). When subepithelial immunoglobulin deposits in the uteri of MRL/lpr mice are examined after whole-body UVB irradiation, the intensity and incidence of such deposits are not changed, whereas the intensity of these deposits in the skin is enhanced (Furukawa et al. 1986a). Therefore, the promotion of skin lesions in MRL/lpr mice by UVB exposure may not be associated with the acceleration of intrinsic SLE phenomena but rather with reactive changes of the skin against environmental stimuli.

Similar to the susceptible UV-induced cytotoxicity from fibrocytes of NZB mice (Zamanski et al. 1980), fibrocytes and keratinocytes cultured from MRL/lpr mice are susceptible to UVB-induced cytotoxicity (Furukawa et al. 1989). Fibroblasts cultured from newborn MRL/lpr mice show a higher susceptibility to a single UVB light irradiation than MRL/n, F1 hybrids of (MRL/lpr × MRL/n mice) or BALB/c mice. Such susceptibility to UVB irradiation is not observed in young or adult MRL/lpr mice. UVA light irradiation is not cytotoxic. Keratinocytes cultured from MRL mice have a lower cytotoxicity to UVB irradiation than fibroblasts cultured. However, keratinocytes from newborn MRL/lpr mice show higher cytotoxicity to relatively low doses of UVB light irradiation than cells from MRL/n mice. Furthermore, syngeneic or allogeneic sera augment the UVB-induced cytotoxicity seen in cultured fibroblasts. However, UVB irradiation of spleen cells results in no significant difference in cytotoxicity between MRL/lpr mice and MRL/n mice. Unlike the in vivo whole-body irradiation with UVB, susceptibility to UVB light cytotoxicity in vitro may be associated with intrinsic SLE phenomena and may be regulated by the individual's genetic background.

Ansel et al. (Ansel et al. 1985) described the unique effects of broad-spectrum UV irradiation on BXSB mice. UV irradiation increases mortality in BXSB male mice and accelerates autoimmune traits, including anti-DNA antibody production, splenic polyclonal B-cell activity, and glomerulonephritis. These UVB-induced changes in serology and renal function are not observed in MRL/lpr mice (Horiguchi et al. 1987b). In contrast, the macroscopic changes found in MRL/lpr mice are not induced in UVB-irradiated BXSB mice. Therefore, the strain difference between SLE-prone mice irradiated with UV light may serve as useful clues for the investigation of multiple manifestations of photosensitivity in CLE. All SLE-prone mouse strains, in contrast to all non-SLE-prone mouse strains, show increased susceptibility to the induction of DNA damage by UVA and increased DNA synthesis and release after UVA exposure (Golan et al. 1984). Regarding the effects of UVA on SLE symptoms, it is interesting that UVA1 light irradiation decreases clinical disease activity and autoantibodies in patients with human SLE (McGrath 1994).

Graft-vs-Host Disease as a Model of Systemic Lupus Erythematosus

It is well known that chronic graft-vs-host (GVH) disease in mice has similarities to human SLE, and several models have been used for these investigations. The GVH model offers significant advantages over the existing, spontaneous SLE-prone mice in that it can be reliably induced and it follows a predictable, relatively short time course. Gleichmann and associates successfully induced a syndrome strongly resembling SLE in a suitable chronic GVH disease made in nonirradiated, H-2-incompatible (C57BL/10 × DBA/2)F1 mice injected intravenously with DBA/2 spleen cells and lymph node cells (Gleichmann et al. 1982, Van Rappard-Van Der Veen et al. 1983). Their model develops subepidermal immunoglobulin deposits like inbred SLE-prone mice. (BALB/c × A/J)F1 mice inoculated with A/J lymphocytes show mixed connective tissue disease-like symptoms, including finger swelling, alopecia, and proteinuria (Gelpi et al. 1988). Because chronic GVH models for SLE are useful for investigating cellular-level immune abnormalities, it is likely that the effects and mechanisms of immunosuppressive drugs or therapy can be investigated more precisely in GVH models than in inbred mouse models (Appleby et al. 1989). The 8-methoxypsoralen and UVA light treatment of DBA/2 cells can vaccinate recipient mice against the progression of GVH reaction-initiated SLE-like disease by using the same GVH disease system (Girardi et al. 1995). Anti-αβTCR monoclonal antibody is also effective as a therapeutic agent (Maeda and Nomoto 1995).

SCID Mouse as a Model of Systemic Lupus Erythematosus

The SCID mouse is a mutant of the mouse strain C.B-17, an IgHb congenic partner of the BALB/c (H-2d) mouse. The mutation in the SCID mouse is autosomal recessive and is mapped to the centromeric region of chromosomes (Vladutiu 1993). The effect of the SCID mutation is manifested in lymphoid cells. Myeloid, erythroid, antigen-presenting cells, splenic colony stem cells, and NK cell development and function are not influenced by the SCID mutation. There is a defect in a DNA break repair enzyme; this V(D)J recombinase–associated defect affects somatic rearrangement of TCR genes and immunoglobulin genes in B lymphocytes. The development of T lymphocytes is stopped at the CD4$^-$, CD8 immature thymocyte stage, and the maturation of B lymphocytes is arrested at the pro-B lymphocytes (from the review of Vladutiu 1993).

Because the SCID mouse is deficient in active T and B lymphocytes, this mutant can be reconstituted with different allogeneic as well as xenogeneic hematopoietic and lymphoid cells. Indeed, studies using SCID mice as the recipients of peripheral blood lymphocytes from patients with SLE or experimental SLE mice have been reported (Duchosal et al. 1990, Reininger et al. 1992, Segal et al. 1992, Vladutiu 1993). Dixon and associates reported that SCID mice reconstituted with peripheral blood lymphocytes from patients with SLE showed the long-term presence of donor-type autoantibodies in their sera, as well as human immunoglobulin deposits in their renal glomeruli (Duchosal et al. 1990). The development of autoimmune disease can also be induced in SCID mice populated with long-term in vitro proliferating B/W F1 pre-B cells (Reininger et al. 1992). This SCID model for SLE allows us to directly evaluate the effects of cellular and humoral function in the progression of SLE and enables us to compare various potential therapies (e. g., the use of antisense oligonucleotides, anti-TCR antibodies) simultaneously on the disease-producing cells of a single human patient.

Lupus-like Syndromes Related to Drugs and Environmental Factors

Autoimmunity develops in relation to many environmental agents, including drugs, chemical agents, dietary factors, and infectious agents (Mongey and Hess 1996). Until now, more than 70 drugs have been related to the onset of drug-related lupus. In general, skin manifestation is not frequently observed in patients with drug-related lupus, although there are no specific diagnostic criteria. Approximately 25% of patients with hydralazine-induced lupus develop skin manifestations. In contrast, skin lesions in procainamide-induced lupus are said to absent. Some anticancer agents are well known to induce photosensitivity and lupus-like lesions (Ghate JV et al. 2001, Yoshimasu et al. 2001b). Among anticancer agents, a mixture of uracil and tegafur is common in Japan. The review of 17 Japanese cases of discoid LE-like lesions induced by fluorouracil agents enabled us to establish the mouse model (Yoshimasu et al. 2001a, 2004), which provides new insights for better understanding the discoid lupus lesions because experimental studies in induced models have the advantage over those in spontaneous models in that the onset and progression of disease can be controlled (Taneja and David 2001). Paraffin, silicone, and pristen also have the possibility of introducing the new aspects in drug-induced CLE (Satoh et al. 1999).

Summary and Conclusion

During the past decade, the most exciting and important finding in SLE-prone mice has been the discovery of Fas/Fas ligand systems in the pathogenesis of autoimmune phenomena. A human model for murine lpr/gld disease has also been reported (Sneller et al. 1992). Furthermore, as shown in Table 16.2, studies on immunoglobulin variable region genes, TCR genes, and MHC class II genes have given us much information concerning human and murine SLE. With respect to cytokines, IL-2 deficiency (Dauphinee et al. 1981) and the key role of IL-6 (Finck et al. 1994, Tang et al. 1991) have been found in SLE-prone mouse strains, and Th2 cytokine production has been demonstrated to play a more pathogenic role than Th1 cytokine production in human and murine SLE (Klinman and Steinberg 1995), except in MRL/lpr mice (Takahashi et al. 1996.). Transforming growth factor is also intriguing because transforming growth factor β-knockout mice show SLE-like autoantibodies and Sjögren's syndrome-like lymphoproliferation (Dang et al. 1995). Apart from these basic scientific investigations, there are also many promising and practical therapeutic approaches (Shoenfeld 1994). In particular, treatments with anti-CD4 antibody (Gilkeson et al. 1992) and murine CTLA4Ig, which bound B7 and blocked binding of CD28 to B7 (Finck et al. 1994), are outstanding. Recently, vaccine therapy has been attempted (Rook et al. 2000). However, it remains obscure whether such new approaches are effective for the skin lesions of SLE-prone mice, although some immunosuppressive agents, such as FK506, cyclosporine, and Chinese herbal medicines, have been evaluated to determine their selective effects on the skin lesions of MRL/lpr mice (Furukawa et al. 1995, Ito et al. 2002, Kanauchi et al. 1994a, b).

Needless to say, mouse models are not identical, but are similar, to human diseases. However, they are important in the search for the underlying pathogenesis of autoimmune diseases on the basis of careful evaluation of the similarities and differences between human diseases and these models. If such studies are steadily performed, then inbred or experimental models will become more promising tools for the investigation of CLE.

Acknowledgements. The author is grateful to T. Shirai of Juntendo University, M. Takigawa of Hamamatsu University, S. Imamura and Y. Hamashima of Kyoto University, Japan, and D. A. Norris of the University of Colorado, USA, for their scientific support. This work was also supported by grants from the Japanese Ministry of Education, Science, Culture, and Sports and from the Japanese Ministry of Health and Welfare. This review article is a minor modified version of our previous report (Furukawa 1997).

References

Alarcon-Segovia D, Ruiz-Arguelles A, Fishbein E (1978) Antibody to nuclear ribonucleoprotein penetrates live human mononuclear cells through Fc receptors. Nature 271:67–69

Andrews BS, Eisenberg RA, Theofilopoulos AN, Izui S, Wilson CB, McConahey PJ, Murphy ED, Roths JB, Dixon FJ (1978) Spontaneous murine lupus-like syndrome. Clinical and immunopathological manifestations in several strains. J Exp Med 148:1198–1215

Ansel JC, Mountz J, Steinberg AD, DeFabo E, Green J (1985) Effects of UV radiation on autoimmune strains of mice: increased mortality and accelerated autoimmunity in BXSB mice. J Invest Dermatol 85:181–186

Appleby P, Webber DG, Bowen JG (1989) Murine chronic graft-versus-host disease as a model of systemic lupus erythematosus: effect of immunosuppressive drugs on disease development. Clin Exp Immunol 78:449–453

Berney T, Fulpius T, Shibata T, Reininger L, Van Snick J, Shan H, Weigert M, Marshak-Rothstein A, Izui S (1992) Selective pathogenicity of murine rheumatoid factors of the cryoprecipitable IgG3 subclass. Int Immunol 4:93–99

Bielschowsky M, Helyer BJ, Howie JB (1959) Spontaneous anemia in mice of the NZB/BL strain. Proc Univ Otago Med Sch 37:9–11

Burrows NP, Bhogal BS, Jones RR, Black MM (1993) Clinicopathological significance of cutaneous epidermal nuclear staining by direct immunofluorescence. J Cutan Pathol 20: 159–162

Dang H, Geiser AG, Letterio JJ, Nakabayashi T, Kong L, Fernandes G, Talal N (1995) SLE-like autoantibodies and Sjogren's syndrome-like lymphoproliferation in TGF-γ-knockout mice. J Immunol 155:3205–3212

Dauphinee MJ, Kipper SB, Wofsy D, Talal N (1981) Interleukin 2 deficiency is a common feature of autoimmune mice. J Immunol 127:2483–2487

Davis P, Percy JS (1978) Effect of ultraviolet light on disease characteristics of NZB/W mice. J Rheumatol 5:125–128

Drake CG, Babcock SK, Palmer E, Kotzin BL (1994) Genetic analysis of the NZB contribution to lupus-like autoimmune disease in (NZB×NZW)F1 mice. Proc Natl Acad Sci USA 91:4062–4066

Duchosal MA, McConahey PJ, Robinson CA, Dixon FJ (1990) Transfer of human systemic lupus erythematosus in severe combined immunodeficient (SCID) mice. J Exp Med 172:985–988

Emerit I (1982) Chromosome breakage factors: origin and possible significance. Proc Muta Res 4:61–74

Epstein JH, Tuffanelli DL, Dubois EL (1965) Light sensitivity and lupus erythematosus. Arch Dermatol 91:483–485

Finck BK, Chan B, Wofsy D (1994) Interleukin 6 promotes murine lupus in NZB/NZW F1 mice. J Clin Invest 94:585–591

Finck BK, Linsley PS, Wofsy D (1994) Treatment of murine lupus with CTLA4Ig. Science 265: 1225–1227

Furukawa F (1997) Animal models of cutaneous lupus erythematosus and lupus erythematosus photosensitivity. Lupus 6:193–202

Furukawa F (1999) Anti-nuclear antibody-keratinocyte interaction in photosensitive cutaneous lupus erythematosus. Histol Histopathol 14:627–63

Furukawa F, Hamashima Y (1982) Lupus band test in New Zealand mice and MRL mice. J Dermatol 9:467–471

Furukawa F, Tanaka H, Sekita K, Nakamura T, Horiguchi Y, Hamashima Y (1984) Dermato-pathological studies on skin lesions of MRL mice. Arch Dermatol Res 276:186–194

Furukawa F, Kohno A, Ohshio G, Suzuki K, Hamashima Y (1985a) Pathogenesis of lupus der-matoses in autoimmune mice. IV. Association between cutaneous immunoglobulin deposi-tion and anti-single-stranded DNA antibodies in sera. Arch Dermatol Res 277:79–83

Furukawa F, Maruyama N, Yoshida H, Hamashima Y, Hirose S (1985b) Genetic studies on the skin lupus band test in New Zealand mice. Clin Exp Immunol 59:146–152

Furukawa F, Horiguchi Y, Kanauchi Y, Hamashima Y, Imamura S (1986a) The uterus lupus band test and its correlation with the skin lupus band test in autoimmune mice. Microbiol Immunol 30:395–400

Furukawa F, Imamura S, Horiguchi Y et al (1986b) New horizons in murine lupus dermatoses. Proc Jpn Soc Invest Dermatol 10:57–62

Furukawa F, Ohshio G, Tanaka H, Nakamura T, Ikehara S, Imamura S, Hamashima Y (1986c) Pathogenesis of lupus dermatoses in autoimmune mice. VI. Correlation between positivity of lupus band test and lupus nephritis. Arch Dermatol Res 278:343–346

Furukawa F, Lyons MB, Norris DA (1989) Susceptible cytotoxicity to ultraviolet B light in fibro-blasts and keratinocytes cultured from autoimmune-prone MRL/Mp-lpr/lpr mice. Clin Immunol Immunopathol 52:460–472

Furukawa F, Ikai K, Matsuyoshi N, Shimizu K, Imamura S (1993a) Relationship between heat shock protein induction and the binding of antibodies to the extractable nuclear antigens on cultured human keratinocytes. J Invest Dermatol 101:191–195

Furukawa F, Ohshio G, Imamura S (1993b) Pathogenesis of lupus dermatoses in autoimmune mice. XIX. Attempts to induce subepidermal immunoglobulin deposition in MRL/Mp-+/+mice. Arch Dermatol Res 285:20–26

Furukawa F, Kanauchi H, Imamura S (1994) Susceptibility to UVB light in cultured kera-tinocytes of cutaneous lupus erythematosus. Dermatology 189 (Suppl 1):18–23

Furukawa F, Imamura S, Takigawa M (1995) FK506: therapeutic effects on lupus dermatoses in autoimmune-prone MRL/Mp-lpr/lpr mice. Arch Dermatol Res 287:558–563

Furukawa F, Kanauchi H, Wakita H, Tokura Y, Tachibana T, Horiguchi Y, Imamura S, Ozaki S, Taki-gawa M (1996) Spontaneous autoimmune skin lesions of MRL/n mice – autoimmune disease-prone genetic background in relation to Fas-defect MRL/lpr mice. J Invest Dermatol 107: 95–100

Galoppin L, Saurat JH (1981) In vitro study of the binding of antiribonucleoprotein antibodies to the nucleus of isolated living keratinocytes. J Invest Dermatol 76:264–267

Gelpi C, Rodriguez-Sanchez JL, Martinez MA, Craft J, Hardin JA (1988) Murine graft vs host dis-ease. A model for study of mechanisms that generate autoantibodies to ribonucleoproteins. J Immunol 140:4160–4166

Ghate JV, Turner ML, Rudek MA , Figg WD, Dahut W, Dyer V, Pluda JM, Reed E (2001) Drug-induced lupus associated with COL-3. J Am Acad Dermatol 137:471–474

Gilkeson GS, Spurney R, Coffman TM, Kurlander R, Ruiz P, Piestsky DS (1992) Effect of anti-CD4 antibody treatment on inflammatory arthritis in MRL-lpr/lpr mice. Clin Immunol Immuno-pathol 64:166–172

Gilliam JN, Hurd ER, Ziff M (1975) Subepidermal deposition of immunoglobulin in NZB/NZW F1 hybrid mice. J Immunol 114:33–137

Girardi M, Herreid P, Tigelaar RE (1995) Specific suppression of lupus-like graft-versus-host dis-ease using extracorporeal photochemical attenuation of effector lymphocytes. J Invest Der-matol 104:177–182

Gleichmann E, Van Elven EH, Van der Veen JPW (1982) A systemic lupus erythematosus (SLE)-like disease in mice induced by abnormal T-B cell cooperation: preferential formation of autoantibodies characteristic of SLE. Eur J Immunol 12:152–159

Golan DT, Borel Y (1984) Increased phtosensitivity to near-ultraviolet light in murine SLE. J Immunol 132:705–710

Halpern B, Emerit I, Housset E (1972) Possible autoimmune processes related to chromosomal abnormalities (breakage) in NZB mice. Nature 235:214–215

Hiroi A, Ito T, Furukawa F (2001) Immunopathological study on alopecia of the NZB/KN mouse. J Wakayama Med Soc 52:377–383

Horiguchi Y, Furukawa F, Hamashima Y, Imamura S (1984) Ultrastructural observations of skin lesions in MRL mice – dermoepidermal junction. Arch Dermatol Res 276:229–234

Horiguchi Y, Furukawa F, Imamura S (1986a) Ultrastructural observations of skin lesions in MRL mice – dermal infiltrations and capillary changes. J Dermatol 6:440–447

Horiguchi Y, Furukawa F, Hamashima Y, Imamura S (1986b) Ultrastructural lupus band test in skin of MRL/l mice. Arch Dermatol Res 278:474–480

Horiguchi Y, Furukawa F, Kanauchi H, Imamura S (1987a) Comparative electron and immuno-electron microscopic studies on immunoglobulin deposits in the glomeruli of the kidney, skin, esophagus and uterus of MRL/l mice. Acta Histochem Cytochem 20: 217–227

Horiguchi Y, Furukawa F, Ohshio G, Horio T, Imamura S (1987b) Effects of ultraviolet light irradiation on the skin of MRL/l mice. Arch Dermatol Res 279:478–483

Howie JB, Helyer BJ (1968) The immunology and pathology of NZB mice. Adv Immunol 9:215–266

Imamura S (1981) Skin lesion of SLE and its pathomechanisms. Nishinihon J Dermatol 43:1119–1125 (in Japanese)

Ito T, Seo N, Yagi H, Ohtani T, Tokura Y, Takigawa M, Furukawa F (2002) Unique therapeutic effects of the Japanese-Chinese herbal medicine, Sairei-to, on Th1/Th2 balance of the autoimmunity of MRL/lpr mice. J Dermatol Sci 28:198–210

Izui S, Merino R, Iwamoto M, Fossati L (1994) Mechanisms of genetic control of murine systemic lupus erythematosus. Springer Semin Immunopathol 16:133–152

Kanauchi H, Furukawa F, Imamura S (1991) Characterization of cutaneous infiltrates in MRL/lpr mice monitored from onset to the full development of lupus erythematosus-like skin lesions. J Invest Dermatol 96:478–483

Kanauchi H, Imamura S, Takigawa M, Furukawa F (1994a) Effects of cyclosporin A on lupus dermatoses in autoimmune-prone MRL/Mp-lpr/lpr mice. J Dermatol Treat 5:187–191

Kanauchi H, Imamura S, Takigawa M, Furukawa F (1994b) Evaluation of the Japanese-Chinese herbal medicine, Kampo, for the treatment of lupus dermatoses in autoimmune prone MRL/Mp-lpr/lpr mice. J Dermatol 21:935–939

Kitajima T, Furukawa F, Kanauchi H, Imamura S, Ogawa K, Sugiyama T (1992) Histological detection of c-myb and c-myc proto-oncogene expression in infiltrating cells in cutaneous lupus erythematosus-like lesions of MRL/l mice by in situ hybridization. Clin Immunol Immunopathol 62:119–123

Klinman DM, Steinberg AD (1995) Inquiry into murine and human lupus. Immunol Rev 144:157–193

Kochevar IE (1985) Action spectrum and mechanisms of UV radiation-induced injury in lupus erythematosus. J Invest Dermatol 85:140S-143S

Kondo K, Nagami T, Teramoto S (1969) Differences in hematopoietic death among inbred strains of mice. In: Bond PV, Sugahara T (eds) Comparative cellular and species radiosensitivity. Igakushoin, Tokyo, pp 20–29

Kono DH, Burlingame RW, Owens DG, Kuramochi A, Balderas RS, Balomenos D, Theofilopoulos AN (1994) Lupus susceptibility loci in New Zealand mice. Proc Natl Acad Sci USA 91: 10168–10172

Maeda T, Nomoto K (1995) Anti-T cell receptor antibody treatment of mice with lupus-like graft versus host disease: suppression of glomerulonephritis without reduction in anti-DNA antibody levels. J Rheumatol 22:2259–2265

Maruyama N, Furukawa F, Nakai Y, Sasaki Y, Ohta K, Ozaki S, Hirose S, Shirai T (1983) Genetic studies of autoimmunity in New Zealand mice. IV. Contribution of NZB and NZW genes to the spontaneous occurrence of retroviral gp70 immune complexes in (NZB×NZW) F1 hybrid and the correlation to renal disease. J Immunol 130:740–746

Matsuda H, Watanabe N, Geba GP, Sperl J, Tsudzuki M, Hiroi J, Matsumoto M, Ushio H, Saito S, Askenase PW, Ra C (1997) Development of atopic dermatitis-like skin lesion with IgE hyper-production in NC/Nga mice. Int Immunol 9:461–466

Merino R, Iwamoto M, Gershwin ME, Izui S (1994) The *Yaa* gene abrogates the major histocompatibility complex association of murine lupus in (NZB×BXSB)F1 hybrid mice. J Clin Invest 94:521–525

Mongey AB, Hess EV (1996) Lupus-like syndrome related to drugs and environmental factors. In: Schur PH (ed) the clinical management of systemic lupus erythematosus. Lippincott Raven, Philadelphia, pp 183–193

Murphy ED, Roths JB (1978) Autoimmunity and lymphoproliferation. Induction by mutant gene lpr, and acceleration by a male-associated factor in strain BXSB mice. In: Bigazzi PE, Warner NL (eds) Genetic control of autoimmune disease. Elsevier, New York, pp 207–221

Nakamura K, Kashiwazaki S, Takagishi K, Tsukamoto Y, Morohoshi Y, Nakano T, Kimura M (1991) Spontaneous degenerative polyarthritis in male New Zealand Black/KN mice. Arthritis Rheum 34:171–179

Natali PG, Mottolese M, Nicotra M (1978) Immune complex formation in NZB/W mice after ultraviolet radiation. Clin Immunol Immunopathol 10:414–419

Natali PG, Tan EM (1973) Experimental skin lesions in mice resembling systemic lupus erythematosus. Arthritis Rheum 16:579–589

Oyaizu N, Yasumizu R, Miyama-Inaba M, Nomura S, Yoshida H, Miyawaki S, Shibata Y, Mitsuoka S, Yasunaga K, Morii S et al (1988) (NZW×BXSB) F1 mouse. a new animal model of idiopathic thrombocytopenic purpura. J Exp Med 167:2017–2022

McGrath H Jr (1994) Ultraviolet-A1 irradiation decreases clinical disease activity and autoantibodies in patients with systemic lupus erythematosus. Clin Exp Rheumatol 12:129–135

Monestier M, Kandiah DA, Kouts S, Novick KE, Ong GL, Radic MZ, Krilis SA (1996) Monoclonal antibodies from NZW×BXSB F1 mice to β2-glycoprotein I and cardiolipin. J Immunol 156:2631–2641

Nishimura H, Honjo T (2001) PD-1: an inhibitory immunoreceptor involved in peripheral tolerance. Trends Immunol 22:265–268

Provost TT, Watson R (1993) The MRL/lpr mouse model of cutaneous lupus. In: Wallace DJ, Hahn BH (eds) Dubois' lupus erythematosus, 4th ed. Lea & Febiger, Baltimore, p 282

Reddy AL, Fialkow PJ, Salo A (1978) Ultraviolet radiation-induced chromosomal abnormalities in fetal fibroblasts from New Zealand black mice. Science 201:920–922

Reininger L, Radaszkiewicz T, Kosco M, Melchers F, Rolink AG (1992) Development of autoimmune disease in SCID mice populated with long-term "in vitro" proliferating (NZB×NZW)F1 pre-B cells. J Exp Med 176:1343–1353

Rook GAW, Ristori G, Salvetti M, Giovannoni G, Thompson EJ, Standford JL (2000) Bacterial vaccines for the treatment of multiple sclerosis and other autoimmune diseases. Immunol Today 21:503–507

Satoh M, Richards HB, Reeves WH (1999) Pathogenesis of autoantibody production and glomerulonephritis in pristane-treated mice. In: Kammer GM, Tsokos GC (eds) Lupus molecular and cellular pathogenesis. Humana Press, Totowa, NJ, pp 399–416

Segal R, Globerson A, Zinger H, Mozes E (1992) Induction of experimental systemic lupus erythematosus (SLE) in mice with severe combined immunodeficiency (SCID). Clin Exp Immunol 89:239–243

Shimizu J, Yamazaki S, Takahashi T, Ishida Y, Sakaguchi S (2002) Stimulation of CD25⁺CD4⁺ regulatory T cells through GITR breaks immunological self-tolerance. Nature Immunol 3:135–142

Shirai T (1982) The genetic basis of autoimmunity in murine lupus. Immunol Today 7:187–194

Shirai T, Ohta K, Kohno A, Furukawa F, Yoshida H, Maruyama N, Hirose S (1986) Naturally occurring antibody response to DNA is associated with the response to retroviral gp70 in autoimmune New Zealand mice. Arthritis Rheum 29:242–250

Shoenfeld Y (1994) Immunosuppression of experimental systemic lupus erythematosus and antiphospholipid syndrome. Transplant Proc 26:3211–3213

Sneller MC, Straus SE, Jaffe ES, Fleisher TA, Stetler-Stevenson M, Strober W (1992) A novel lymphoproliferative/autoimmune syndrome resembling murine lpr/gld disease. J Clin Invest 90:334–341

Sontheimer RD (1996) Photoimmunology of lupus erythematosus and dermatomyositis: a spec-
    ulative review. Photochem Photobiol 63:583–594
Sontheimer RD, Gilliam JN (1979) Regional variation in the deposition of subepidermal
    immunoglobulin in NZB/W F1 mice: association with epidermal DNA synthesis. J Invest
    Dermatol 72:25–28
Steinberg AD (1995) Insights into the basis of systemic lupus. J Autoimmunity 8:771–785
Takahashi S, Fossati L, Iwamoto M, Merino R, Motta R, Kobayakawa T, Izui S (1996) Imbalance
    towards Th1 predominance is associated with acceleration of lupus-like autoimmune syn-
    drome in MRL mice. J Clin Invest 97:1597–1604
Takahashi S, Nose M, Sasaki J, Yamamoto T, Kyogoku M (1991) IgG3 production in MRL/lpr mice
    is responsible for development of lupus nephritis. J Immunol 147:515–519
Tamada Y, Ohhashi M, Kobayashi T et al (1976) Pathological studies on NC mouse with ery-
    thema and alopecia. Jpn J Allergol 25:829–836
Taneja V, David CS (2001) Lessons from animal models for human autoimmune diseases. Nature
    Immunol 2:781–784
Tang B, Matsuda M, Akira S, Nagata N, Ikehara S, Hirano T, Kishimoto T (1991) Age-associated
    increase in interleukin 6 in MRL/lpr mice. Int Immunol 3:273–278
Theofilopoulos AN (1995) The basis of autoimmunity. 2. Genetic predisposition. Immunol
    Today 6:150–159
Theofilopoulos AN, Dixon FJ (1981) Etiopathogenesis of murine SLE. Immunol Rev 55:179–216
Van Rappard-Van Der Veen FM, Radaszkiewicz R, Terraneo L, Gleichmann E (1983) Attempts at
    standardization of lupus-like graft-vs-host disease: inadvertent repopulation by DBA/2
    spleen cells of H-2-different nonirradiated F1 mice. J Immunol 130:2693–2701
Vladutiu AO (1993) The severe combined immunodeficient (SCID) mouse as a model for the
    study of autoimmune diseases. Clin Exp Immunol 93:1–8
Velthuis PJ, Kater L, van der Tweel I, Meyling FG, Derksen RH, Hene RJ, van Geutselaar JA, Baart
    de la Faille H (1990) In vivo antinuclear antibody of the skin: diagnostic significance and
    association with selective antinuclear antibodies. Ann Rheum Dis 49:163–167
Vidal S, Gelpi C, Rodriguez-Sanchez JL (1994) (SWR×SJL)F1 mice: a new model of lupus-like
    disease. J Exp Med 179:1429–1435
Wandstract A, Wakeland E (2001) The genetics of complex autoimmune diseases: non-MHC sus-
    ceptibility genes. Nature Immunol 2:802–809
Watanabe-Fukunaga R, Brannan CI, Copeland NG, Jenkins NA, Nagata S (1992) Lymphoprolif-
    eration disorder in mice explained by defects in Fas antigen that mediates apoptosis. Nature
    356:314–317
Yoshimasu T, Hiroi A, Ohtani T, Furukawa F (2001a) Establishment of a model for drug induced
    discoid lupus erythematosus in TCR alpha chain knockout mouse. Exp Dermatol 10:213
Yoshimasu T, Hiroi A, Uede K, Furukawa F (2001b) Discoid lupus erythematosus(DLE)-like
    lesion induced by uracil-tegafur(UFT). Eur J Dermatol 11:54–57
Yoshimasu T, Nishide T, Seo N, Hiroi A, Ohtani T, Uede K, Furukawa F (2004) Susceptibility of T
    cell receptor-alpha chain knock-out mice to ultraviolet B light and fluorouracil: a novel
    model for drug-induced cutaneous lupus erythematosus. Clin Exp Immunol 136:245–254
Zamanski GB, Kleinman LF, Kaplan JC, Black PH (1980) Effect of ultraviolet light irradiation on
    the survival of New Zealand black mouse cells. Arthritis Rheum 23:866–867

CHAPTER 17

Apoptosis in Lupus Erythematosus 17

FELIPE ANDRADE, ANTONY ROSEN, LIVIA CASCIOLA-ROSEN

Systemic lupus erythematosus (SLE) is a multisystem autoimmune disease of unknown etiology characterized by chronic, inflammatory damage of numerous tissues. The highly specific clinical phenotypes of SLE, the unique pathology, and the very specific autoantibody response associated with these phenotypes have provided critical insights into the pathogenesis of lupus. In this regard, photosensitive lupus skin disease and neonatal lupus have been particularly instructive, providing both common and unique insights into disease mechanisms (Buyon 1996, Orteu et al. 2001, Sontheimer 1989). For example, the skin is a prominent target tissue in both phenotypes, and there is a characteristic exacerbation of cutaneous disease after exposure to sunlight or to artificial sources of ultraviolet (UV) radiation (Buyon 1996, Orteu et al. 2001, Simmons-O'Brian et al. 1995, Sontheimer 1989). Similarly, both phenotypes are associated with the production of autoantibodies to highly specific targets, for example, Ro/SSA and La/SSB (Lee et al. 1994a, b, Provost and Reichlin 1988). The neonatal lupus phenotype is particularly instructive in this regard, as it demonstrates that passive transfer of autoantibodies plays a critical role in lesion generation. Such lesion induction by an environmental exposure in the setting of specific autoantibodies strongly suggests that the stimulus alters the tissue to render it sensitive to autoamplifying damage by inflammatory pathways. Recent data have defined an important role for apoptotic death of cells in generating this ongoing tissue damage (Casciola-Rosen et al. 1994, Casiola-Rosen and Rosen 1997, 1999, Miranda et al. 1998, 2000, Tran et al. 2002). This review focuses on the roles of apoptosis in SLE, with particular emphasis on its relevance to skin disease. Although some aspects of the model presented have yet to be proven in vivo, recognition that apoptotic death is an important source of the ongoing antigenic drive in SLE has significant implications for rational therapy and for prevention of complications in this group of diseases.

The Relationship of Cutaneous Lupus Erythematosus Lesions and UV Light: Implications for Pathogenesis

In numerous studies, a striking relationship has emerged between sunlight exposure and the lesions of cutaneous LE (reviewed in Orteu et al. 2001). For example, disease sometimes manifests de novo after extended sunlight exposure, and ongoing skin disease is frequently exacerbated by such exposure. Furthermore, skin lesions are most frequently found in sun-exposed skin, and lesions can be induced experimentally by exposure to artificial sources of UV radiation (reviewed in Orteu et al. 2001).

The description of the markedly photosensitive subset of subacute cutaneous LE further clarified this relationship between UV irradiation and lesion development (Sontheimer 1989). UV irradiation of skin is associated with the generation of increased numbers of apoptotic keratinocytes ("sunburn cells"), and UV irradiation of keratinocytes in vitro induces apoptotic death (Casiola-Rosen et al. 1994, Young 1987). It is therefore of particular interest that the pathology of cutaneous lupus is predominantly a lichenoid reaction in which apoptotic keratinocytes are enriched (Chung et al. 1998, Pablos et al. 1999). The association of photosensitivity with a unique autoantibody response to Ro and La in both adult and neonatal forms of LE has suggested that skin lesions result from an interplay between UV-induced skin changes and preexistent, specific immune effector pathways. Significant evidence in support of such a model has accumulated in recent years.

The Specific Autoantibody Response as a Probe of Disease Mechanisms in Systemic Lupus Erythematosus

There is a growing consensus that the highly specific humoral immune response to autoantigens in systemic autoimmune diseases is T-cell dependent and that flares of disease result when this primed immune system is rechallenged with self-antigen (Diamond et al. 1992, Radic and Weigert 1994). The molecules targeted in SLE are ubiquitously expressed in most nucleated cells but seem to share nothing in common in terms of structure, function, or subcellular distribution in control cells (Casciola-Rosen et al. 1995, Rosen and Casciola-Rosen 1999). The mechanisms responsible for initiation and propagation of the immune response to this highly specific group of autoantigens remain unclear (Bach and Koutouzov 1997). Several years ago, we postulated that although these autoantigens have no apparent unifying characteristics, they likely satisfied the stringent criteria for initiation of a primary immune response at the onset of disease (e. g., presentation in a proimmune context of suprathreshold concentrations of molecules with structure not tolerized during development of the immune system) (Casciola-Rosen and Rosen 1997, Rosen and Casciola-Rosen 1999, Casciola-Rosen et al. 1994, 1995). The corollary of this proposal is that if the perturbed state can be re-created in vitro, these common features of autoantigens (i.e., similar alterations in concentration, distribution, and structure) can be observed. The photosensitivity observed in adult and neonatal forms of SLE and the unique cardiac conduction defects observed in the neonatal lupus syndrome have provided a unique opportunity to search for such unifying mechanisms by studying the cell biology and biochemistry of lupus autoantigens after UV irradiation (Casciola-Rosen et al. 1994, Golan et al. 1992, LeFeber et al. 1984) or during cardiac development (Miranda et al. 1998, Miranda-Carus et al. 2000, Tran et al. 2002). These studies have highlighted apoptosis as the potential perturbed state underlying the initiation and propagation of SLE and focus attention on the alterations in the cell biology and biochemistry that unify autoantigens during this form of cell death as important mechanistic principles in this disease.

UV Irradiation Induces Apoptosis of Keratinocytes and Clustering of Lupus Autoantigens in Apoptotic Surface Blebs

Because the epidermis is one of the physiologic targets of the immunopathologic response in lupus, several groups have established an in vitro epidermal model to address the fate of autoantigens in keratinocytes after irradiation with UVB (Casciola-Rosen et al. 1994, Furukawa et al. 1990, Golan et al. 1992, LeFeber et al. 1984, Natali and Tan 1973). One of the striking observations made was that several lupus autoantigens (including Ro/SSA, La/SSB, snRNP, and Sm) that are normally intracellular could be stained extracellularly in monolayers of human keratinocytes incubated for 20–24 hours after UV irradiation (Furukawa et al. 1990, Golan et al. 1992, LeFeber et al. 1984). Using a similar in vitro system, we demonstrated that keratinocytes become apoptotic within a few hours of irradiation (Casciola-Rosen et al. 1994). Further studies showed that the lupus autoantigens are strikingly redistributed in apoptotic cells, and they become clustered into two populations of structure at the surface of apoptotic cells: small blebs and apoptotic bodies (Fig. 17.1). Small surface blebs arise from fragmented rough endoplasmic reticulum and are highly enriched in Ro/SSA (52 kDa), ribosomal autoantigens, as well as those autoantigens found within the endoplasmic reticulum lumen (e. g., calreticulin). This marked enrichment in autoantigens in small surface blebs was accompanied by a concomitant depletion of these molecules from the cytosol. Apoptotic bodies contain nuclear autoantigens, which also undergo a striking redistribution and concentration during apoptosis. Thus,

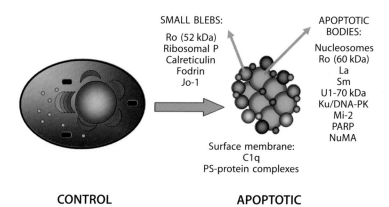

Fig. 17.1. Autoantigens cluster in unique apoptotic subcellular structures. Lupus autoantigens are not restricted to any specific subcellular compartment in normal cells. However, in cells dying by apoptosis induced by numerous different apoptotic stimuli, they become clustered and concentrated within small surface blebs and apoptotic bodies. In addition, phosphatidylserine, which is normally restricted to the inner surface of the plasma membrane bilayer, becomes rapidly redistributed early in apoptosis and appears at the external membrane surface. Interestingly, surface blebs of apoptotic keratinocytes bind C1q, whose collagen-like domains are the frequent (~47%) target of a high titer antibody response in patients with systemic lupus erythematosus. PS, phosphatidylserine

Ro/SSA (60 kDa), La/SSB, snRNPs, Ku, and poly(ADP-ribose)polymerase (normally diffusely distributed throughout the nucleus) became concentrated as a rim around the condensing chromatin and apoptotic bodies. In addition to the enrichment of lupus autoantigens within apoptotic surface blebs, anionic phospholipids, particularly phosphatidylserine (PS), are also found concentrated at the surface of these structures (Casciola-Rosen et al. 1996, Fadok et al. 1992, Price et al. 1996). The humoral response to anionic phospholipids in lupus seems to recognize complexes of the phospholipid and one of several PS-binding proteins, for example, β2-glycoprotein 1 or annexin V. Recent studies have also demonstrated that anti-DNA antibodies recognize their cognate antigens at the surface of apoptotic cells (Cocca et al. 2001).

Clustering of Autoantigens on Apoptotic Cells: Insights from Phenotype Development in Neonatal Systemic Lupus Erythematosus

The striking clustering of autoantigens at the surface of apoptotic cells, the unique phenotypes of neonatal SLE, and the association of phenotype development with specific autoantibodies provide important mechanistic insights into the role of apoptosis in terms of phenotype development in neonatal SLE. It is important to note that this phenotype occurs in the presence of preformed maternal autoantibodies and likely reports on disease propagation mechanisms also relevant in established adult disease. The role of apoptosis in disease initiation (i.e., induction of a specific autoantibody response) is dealt with in more detail in the next section.

Several recent studies have demonstrated that although apoptotic cells are actively anti-inflammatory and tolerance inducing (Fadok et al. 1998, Gallucci et al. 1999, Huyn et al. 2002, Voll et al. 1997, Sauter et al. 2000), binding of antibodies to the cell surface abrogates these anti-inflammatory properties and renders apoptotic cells proinflammatory (Manfredi et al. 1998). Thus, apoptotic cells opsonized with autoantibodies that recognize antigens at the apoptotic cell surface are efficiently phagocytosed by macrophages, and their phagocytosis is accompanied by the secretion of tumor necrosis factor α. The presence of autoantibodies recognizing the apoptotic cell surface can therefore render normally quiet forms of apoptotic death occurring during development or homeostasis markedly proinflammatory. Buyon and colleagues recently demonstrated that in the developing conduction system of the heart, for example, apoptotic death of myocardial cells is associated with autoantigen accessibility and autoantibody binding at the cell surface (Miranda-Carus et al. 2000). They further demonstrate in vitro that antibodies to Ro and La bind to the surface of apoptotic cardiomyocytes and induce the secretion of tumor necrosis factor α on co-culture with macrophages. This was not a feature of nonapoptotic cardiomyocytes or apoptotic myocytes not opsonized with autoantibodies. Buyon and colleagues propose that damage to additional cells in the developing conducting system may thus represent damage to healthy bystander cells through these recruited inflammatory mechanisms (Miranda-Carus et al. 2000). A similar mechanism might account for the photosensitive skin lesions that develop in neonates and adults, where UV exposure induces keratinocyte apoptosis, exposure of relevant autoantigens to autoantibody binding, and activation of a proinflammatory pathway of apoptotic cell clearance.

Induction of a Specific Autoantibody Response: Critical Component of Pathogenesis

Recent studies have demonstrated that apoptotic cells are a dominant toleragen for the immune system (Henson et al. 2001, Savill and Fadok 2000), with apoptosis occurring universally during development, homeostasis, and lymphocyte selection and actively inducing anti-inflammatory cytokine secretion on phagocytosis by macrophages (Hengartner 2000). Abnormalities in (a) the efficient, noninflammatory clearance of apoptotic cells or (b) the occurrence of unusual forms of apoptotic death that generate unique structures of autoantigens not generated during "tolerizing" apoptosis may render an individual susceptible to immunization with apoptotic cells. Examples of both mechanisms are dealt with in the following subsections.

Abnormal Clearance of Apoptotic Cells Renders Individuals Susceptible to Initiation of Systemic Autoimmunity

Apoptotic cell clearance is a complex process that actively inhibits the initiation of inflammation and immune responses, in part through the release of anti-inflammatory cytokines (Henson et al. 2001, Savill and Fadok 2000). Clearance involves numerous components on both the phagocytic cell (including CD14, the PS receptor, CD36, and scavenger receptor class A) and the cell being engulfed (e. g., PS). Although numerous cell surface receptors on macrophages seem to be responsible for binding of the apoptotic cell, recent studies have demonstrated that ligation of the PS receptor by surface PS on the apoptotic cell is responsible for inducing the rapid and efficient uptake of the bound cell through stimulated macropinocytosis (Fadok et al. 2001, Hoffmann et al. 2001, Somersan et al. 2001). Recent studies have also implicated soluble components of the innate immune system in the efficient clearance of, and the induction of immune tolerance to, apoptotic material (Botto et al. 1998, Carroll 1998). For example, mice deficient in C1q or SAP develop autoantibodies to DNA and immune complex-mediated renal disease, and C1q-deficient animals show delayed clearance of apoptotic cells (Taylor et al. 2000). A central mechanism for accessing anti-inflammatory pathways of macrophages seems to involve the interactions of early components of the classic complement cascade with C-reactive protein (Botto et al. 1998, Gershov et al. 2000). The recent observation that deficiency of members of the Mer family of tyrosine kinases (which are required for both efficient clearance of apoptotic cells and induction of anti-inflammatory consequences) renders animals susceptible to initiation of systemic autoimmunity further underscores the importance of this mechanism (Lu and Homeostatic 2001, Scott et al. 2001). It is likely that initiation of an immune response to components clustered at the surface of apoptotic cells results from susceptibility defects along this pathway.

The milieu surrounding the engulfed apoptotic cell might also determine the fate of this material. Interestingly, transgenic mice expressing interferon (IFN)-γ in the epidermis develop inflammatory skin disease and features of SLE such as antinuclear antibodies and lupus nephritis resembling the human condition (Seery et al. 1997). Although the mechanisms involved have not been well defined, the authors suggest that apoptotic keratinocytes provide the source of self-antigens, which are likely processed by professional antigen-presenting cells that migrate from the epidermis to the dermis (likely attracted by IFN-γ) and the draining lymph nodes.

Occurrence of Unusual Forms of Apoptotic Death that Generate Unique Autoantigen Structures Not Generated During "Tolerizing" Apoptosis

The noninflammatory, tolerance-inducing forms of apoptosis that typify developmental and homeostatic situations generate a highly stereotyped form of death, both morphologically and biochemically (Hengartner 2000). This final common death pathway in this form of tolerance-inducing death is mediated by a family of highly specific death proteases (caspases), which operate in an autoamplifying cascade that can be activated by numerous upstream signals (Thornberry and Lazebnik 1998). Recent studies have stressed that distinct autoantigen structures can be generated when this default caspase-dependent pathway is inhibited or bypassed (Andrade et al. 1998, Casciola-Rosen et al. 1999, Odin et al. 2001). Numerous factors have now been demonstrated to be relevant in the inhibition of caspase-mediated death of keratinocytes, including expression of antiapoptotic Bcl-2 family members, expression of high levels of heat shock proteins, and potentially direct endogenous or viral protease inhibitors of the caspases. Several alternate pathways that are of particular relevance in the skin are discussed below.

Generation of Unique Autoantigen Cleavage Fragments During Cytotoxic Lymphocyte Granule-Induced Death

The cytotoxic lymphocyte granule pathway is expressed in cytotoxic T lymphocytes and natural killer cells, which are active in target cell killing of infected, stressed, transformed, or antibody-coated cells. Recent studies from our laboratory have demonstrated that numerous SLE ribonucleoprotein autoantigens (e. g., U1-70 kDa, La/SSB) are directly and efficiently cleaved by the cytotoxic lymphocyte granule protease granzyme B (Andrade et al. 1998, Casciola-Rosen et al. 1999). The fragments generated by such cleavage are distinct from those generated by caspases in other forms of cell death. We proposed that such unique autoantigen fragments may expose cryptic epitopes in these self-antigens, which have not previously been tolerized, and activate autoreactive T cells. Exposure to altered forms of self-antigens may play an important role in the initiation of immune responses to the highly select group of autoantigens targeted in this group of diseases. Because the granule pathway may also play an important role in inducing cytotoxicity of antibody-coated target cells, it may also be involved in the propagation/amplification phases of disease. It is of interest that granzyme B expression in inflamed epidermis has previously been demonstrated (Berthou et al. 1997).

Generation of Unique UV-Induced Photoproducts
During Irradiation of the Skin

Although many autoantigens targeted in SLE are redistributed in cells dying by apoptosis, only ribonucleoprotein complexes containing La/SSB, Ro/SSA, Sm, and U1-70 kDa have been implicated in the pathogenesis of experimental photo-induced epidermal damage. It has been proposed that a pathologic immune response develops in patients with lupus against one or more of the photoproducts found in normal skin after UV irradiation, raising the possibility that these ribonucleoprotein complexes themselves (unlike other autoantigens) might be lupus chromophores. It is also possible that photoproducts that present in normal skin after UV irradiation might be metabolized abnormally in patients with lupus owing to genetic polymorphisms, predisposing to an exaggerated autoimmune response against these photoproducts. The resulting immune response is directed against the UVB-induced complexes and subsequently spreads to individual component molecules (RNA and protein), generating an autoamplifying injury characteristic of these self-sustaining diseases (Fig. 17.2). Our laboratory recently demonstrated that such covalent RNA-

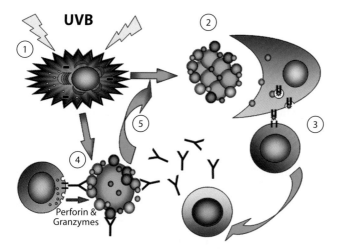

Fig. 17.2. Model of photo-induced epidermal damage (Buyon 1996). UVB irradiation generates novel autoantigen photoproducts by inducing RNA/protein cross-linked complexes (Sontheimer 1989). In the irradiated cells dying by apoptosis, these novel photoproducts are concentrated in apoptotic surface blebs (Orteu et al. 2001). In genetically susceptible individuals, an exaggerated autoimmune response against these photoproducts might result in an immune response initially directed against the UVB-induced complexes and could subsequently spread to monomeric molecules (RNA and protein) (Simmons-O'Brian et al. 1995). Autoantibody binding to UV-exposed antigens might induce lysis of keratinocytes by antibody-dependent cellular cytotoxicity and subsequent epidermal damage. The initial antibody-dependent cellular cytotoxicity against keratinocytes might spread the immune response to other autoantigens (via granzyme B autoantigen cleavage), resulting in systemic disease flares (Provost and Reichlin 1988). Autoantibody binding to apoptotic surface blebs might also enhance their capture and presentation by Fc receptor-expressing antigen-presenting cells, favoring spreading of the immune response to other modified autoantigens in the blebs

autoantigen complexes are indeed generated in keratinocytes after UV irradiation (Andrade et al. 2001). Studies to define the immune response to the biochemically unique antigen forms and the clearance of such complexes in patients with SLE are currently under way.

The generation of these autoantibodies might have important consequences in the propagation and amplification of the autoimmune response to apoptotic cells in several ways: (a) antibody binding to UV-exposed autoantigens might induce keratinocyte lysis by antibody-dependent cellular cytotoxicity; (b) antibody binding to apoptotic keratinocytes might enhance the capture and presentation of apoptotic surface blebs by B cells, favoring spreading of the immune response to other modified autoantigens in the blebs; (c) antibodies are likely to change the nature of the response upon phagocytosis from noninflamatory to inflammatory; and (d) antibodies might themselves induce cell damage and death and thereby autoamplify any injury.

Conclusion

Although the studies discussed herein focused attention on unique forms of apoptosis (e. g., UV radiation and antibody-dependent cellular cytotoxicity) as candidate processes associated with the initiation and propagation of cutaneous and systemic lupus, other cellular stress factors (e. g., infectious agents or drugs) might contribute to the pathogenic process. In the genetically susceptible individual (e. g., someone who has a defect in the ability to efficiently phagocytose and degrade apoptotic cells and debris, or to mount an adequate anti-inflammatory response after ingestion of apoptotic material), the confluence of several forces allows the generation of suprathreshold concentrations of nontolerized structure. If such material accesses the major histocompatibility complex class II antigen-presenting pathway in the presence of appropriate co-stimulatory signals, a primary T-cell response directed at modified antigens will be efficiently initiated and will drive the production of autoantibodies to these antigens. The low frequency of this form of autoimmunity in the population is likely to reflect this need to simultaneously satisfy several stringent criteria to initiate the primary immune response. The molecules targeted are unified by their susceptibility to modification (e. g., cleavage by caspases and/or granzyme B; oxidation) during the perturbing process, likely revealing a previously cryptic structure. Such modifications could include novel UVB-induced RNA/protein cross-linked structures that are generated in cells undergoing UVB-induced apoptosis. Once primary immunization has occurred, the repeated generation of apoptotic material (e. g., during sun exposure, viral infection, or drug exposure) might efficiently rechallenge the primed immune system (the stringency of this secondary response being significantly lower than that of the primary response). The effector pathways activated by the primed immune system include several that generate loads of apoptotic material (e. g., cellular cytotoxicity and inflammatory cell apoptosis). The opsonization of apoptotic material by antibodies against ribonucleoprotein complexes (specifically in photosensitive lupus) may increase the efficiency of apoptotic antigen capture and induce the production of proinflammatory rather than anti-inflammatory cytokines, potentially further driving the immune response. This capacity for immune-driven autoamplification may be one of the critical principles underlying severe systemic autoimmune disease. An important target of future therapeutic intervention may include interrupting the autoamplifying loop by decreasing apoptosis during flares. Identifying the factors that have an impact on the production of unique forms and proper clearance of apoptotic cells may suggest other novel pathways for intervention.

Acknowledgements. These studies were supported by National Institutes of Health grants AR44684 and DE 12354 and the SLE Foundation. A. Rosen is supported by a Burroughs Wellcome Fund Translational Research Award. L. Casciola-Rosen is a recipient of a research grant from the Arthritis Foundation, MD Chapter, MARRC Program.

References

Andrade F, Roy S, Nicholson D, Thornberry N, Rosen A, Casciola-Rosen L (1998) Granzyme B directly and efficiently cleaves several downstream caspase substrates: Implications for CTL-induced apoptosis. Immunity 8:451–460

Andrade F, Casciola-Rosen L, Rosen A (2001) Novel covalent U1RNA-protein complexes are generated in cells by ultraviolet B (UVB) irradiation: implications for autoimmunity. Arthritis Rheum 44:S304

Bach JF, Koutouzov S (1997) Immunology. New clues to systemic lupus. Lancet 350(Suppl 3):11

Berthou C, Michel L, Soulié A, Jean-Louis F, Flageul B, Dubertret L, Sigaux F, Zhang Y, Sasportes M (1997) Acquisition of granzyme B and Fas ligand proteins by human keratinocytes contributes to epidermal cell defense. J Immunol 159:5293–5300

Botto M, Dell'Agnola C, Bygrave AE, Thompson EM, Cook HT, Petry F, Loos M, Pandolfi PP, Walport MJ (1998) Homozygous C1q deficiency causes glomerulonephritis associated with multiple apoptotic bodies. Nat Genet 19:56–59

Buyon JP (1996) Neonatal lupus: bedside to bench and back. Scand J Rheumatol 25:271–276

Carroll MC (1998) The lupus paradox. Nat Genet 19:3–4

Casciola-Rosen LA, Rosen A (1997) Ultraviolet light-induced keratinocyte apoptosis: a potential mechanism for the induction of skin lesions and autoantibody production in LE. Lupus 6:175–180

Casciola-Rosen LA, Anhalt G, Rosen A (1994) Autoantigens targeted in systemic lupus erythematosus are clustered in two populations of surface structures on apoptotic keratinocytes. J Exp Med 179:1317–1330

Casciola-Rosen LA, Anhalt GJ, Rosen A (1995) DNA-dependent protein kinase is one of a subset of autoantigens specifically cleaved early during apoptosis. J Exp Med 182:1625–1634

Casciola-Rosen LA, Rosen A, Petri M, Schlissel M (1996) Surface blebs on apoptotic cells are sites of enhanced procoagulant activity: implications for coagulation events and antigenic spread in systemic lupus erythematosus. Proc Natl Acad Sci USA 93:1624–1629

Casciola-Rosen LA, Andrade F, Ulanet D, Wong WB, Rosen A (1999) Cleavage by granzyme B is strongly predictive of autoantigen status: implications for initiation of autoimmunity. J Exp Med 190:815–825

Chung JH, Kwon OS, Eun HC, Youn JI, Song YW, Kim JG, Cho KH (1998) Apoptosis in the pathogenesis of cutaneous lupus erythematosus. Am J Dermatopathol 20:233–241

Cocca BA, Seal SN, D'Agnillo P, Mueller YM, Katsikis PD, Rauch J, Weigert M, Radic MZ (2001) Structural basis for autoantibody recognition of phosphatidylserine-beta 2 glycoprotein I and apoptotic cells. Proc Natl Acad Sci U S A 98:13826–13831

Diamond B, Katz JB, Paul E, Aranow C, Lustgarten D, Scharff MD (1992) The role of somatic mutation in the pathogenic anti-DNA response. Ann Rev Immunol 10:731–757

Fadok VA, Voelker DR, Campbell PA, Cohen JJ, Bratton DL, Henson PM (1992) Exposure of phosphatidylserine on the surface of apoptotic lymphocytes triggers specific recognition and removal by macrophages. J Immunol 148:2207–2216

Fadok VA, Bratton DL, Konowal A, Freed PW, Westcott JY, Henson PM (1998) Macrophages that have ingested apoptotic cells in vitro inhibit proinflammatory cytokine production through autocrine/paracrine mechanisms involving TGF-β, PGE2, and PAF. J Clin Invest 101:890–898

Fadok VA, Bratton DL, Henson PM (2001) Phagocyte receptors for apoptotic cells: recognition, uptake, and consequences. J Clin Invest 108:957–962

Furukawa F, Kashihara-Sawami M, Lyons MB, Norris DA (1990) Binding of antibodies to the extractable nuclear antigens of SS-A/Ro and SS-B/La is induced on the surface of human keratinocytes by ultraviolet light (UVL): implications for the pathogenesis of photosensitive cutaneous lupus. J Invest Dermatol 94:77–85

Gallucci S, Lolkema M, Matzinger P (1999) Natural adjuvants: endogenous activators of dendritic cells. Nat Med 5:1249–1255

Gershov D, Kim S, Brot N, Elkon KB (2000) C-Reactive protein binds to apoptotic cells, protects the cells from assembly of the terminal complement components, and sustains an antiinflammatory innate immune response: implications for systemic autoimmunity. J Exp Med 192:1353–1364

Golan TD, Elkon KB, Gharavi AE, Krueger JG (1992) Enhanced membrane binding of autoantibodies to cultured keratinocytes of systemic lupus erythematosus patients after ultraviolet B/ultraviolet A irradiation. J Clin Invest 90:1067–1076

Hengartner MO (2000) The biochemistry of apoptosis. Nature 407:770–776

Henson PM, Bratton DL, Fadok VA (2001) Apoptotic cell removal. Curr Biol 11:R795–805

Hoffmann PR, deCathelineau AM, Ogden CA, Leverrier Y, Bratton DL, Daleke DL, Ridley AJ, Fadok VA, Henson PM (2001) Phosphatidylserine (PS) induces PS receptor-mediated macropinocytosis and promotes clearance of apoptotic cells. J Cell Biol 155:649–659

Huynh ML, Fadok VA, Henson PM (2002) Phosphatidylserine-dependent ingestion of apoptotic cells promotes TGF-beta1 secretion and the resolution of inflammation. J Clin Invest 109:41–50

Lee LA, Frank MB, McCubbin VR, Reichlin M (1994a) Autoantibodies of neonatal lupus erythematosus. J Invest Dermatol 102:963–966

Lee LA, Roberts CM, Frank MB, McCubbin VR, Reichlin M (1994b) The autoantibody response to Ro/SSA in cutaneous lupus erythematosus. Arch Dermatol 130:1262–1268

LeFeber WP, Norris DA, Ryan SR, Huff JC, Lee LA, Kubo M, Boyce ST, Kotzin BL, Weston WL (1984) Ultraviolet light induces binding of antibodies to selected nuclear antigens on cultured human keratinocytes. J Clin Invest 74:1545–1551

Lu Q, Lemke G (2001) Homeostatic regulation of the immune system by receptor tyrosine kinases of the Tyro 3 family. Science 293:306–311

Manfredi AA, Rovere P, Galati G, Heltai S, Bozzolo E, Soldini L, Davoust J, Balestrieri G, Tincani A, Sabbadini MG (1998) Apoptotic cell clearance in systemic lupus erythematosus. 1. Opsonization by antiphospholipid antibodies. Arthritis Rheum 41:205–214

Miranda ME, Tseng CE, Rashbaum W, Ochs RL, Casiano CA, Di Donato F, Chan EK, Buyon JP (1998) Accessibility of SSA/Ro and SSB/La antigens to maternal autoantibodies in apoptotic human fetal cardiac myocytes. J Immunol 161:5061–5069

Miranda-Carus ME, Askanase AD, Clancy RM, Di Donato F, Chou TM, Libera MR, Chan EK, Buyon JP (2000) Anti-SSA/Ro and anti-SSB/La autoantibodies bind the surface of apoptotic fetal cardiocytes and promote secretion of TNF-alpha by macrophages. J Immunol 165:5345–5351

Natali PG, Tan EM (1973) Experimental skin lesions in mice resembling systemic lupus erythematosus. Arthritis Rheum 16:579–589

Odin JA, Huebert RC, Casciola-Rosen L, LaRusso NF, Rosen A (2001) Bcl-2-dependent oxidation of pyruvate dehydrogenase-E2, a primary biliary cirrhosis autoantigen, during apoptosis. J Clin Invest 108:223–232

Orteu CH, Sontheimer RD, Dutz JP (2001) The pathophysiology of photosensitivity in lupus erythematosus. Photodermatol Photoimmunol Photomed 17:95–113

Pablos JL, Santiago B, Galindo M, Carreira PE, Ballestin C, Gomez-Reino JJ (1999) Keratinocyte apoptosis and p53 expression in cutaneous lupus and dermatomyositis. J Pathol 188:63–68

Price BE, Rauch J, Shia MA, Walsh MT, Lieberthal W, Gilligan HM, O'Laughlin T, Koh JS, Levine JS (1996) Anti-phospholipid autoantibodies bind to apoptotic, but not viable, thymocytes in a β_2-glycoprotein I-dependent manner. J Immunol 157:2201–2208

Provost TT, Reichlin M (1988) Immunopathologic studies of cutaneous lupus erythematosus. J Clin Invest 8:223–232

Radic MZ, Weigert M (1994) Genetic and structural evidence for antigen selection of anti-DNA antibodies. Ann Rev Immunol 12:487–520

Rosen A, Casciola-Rosen L (1999) Autoantigens as substrates for apoptotic proteases: Implications for the pathogenesis of systemic autoimmune disease. Cell Death Differ 6:6–12

Sauter B, Albert ML, Francisco L, Larsson M, Somersan S, Bhardwaj N (2000) Consequences of cell death: exposure to necrotic tumor cells, but not primary tissue cells or apoptotic cells, induces the maturation of immunostimulatory dendritic cells. J Exp Med 191:423–434

Savill J, Fadok V (2000) Corpse clearance defines the meaning of cell death. Nature 407:784–788

Scott RS, McMahon EJ, Pop SM, Reap EA, Caricchio R, Cohen PL, Earp HS, Matsushima GK (2001) Phagocytosis and clearance of apoptotic cells is mediated by MER. Nature 411:207–211

Seery JP, Carroll JM, Cattell V, Watt FM (1997) Antinuclear autoantibodies and lupus nephritis in transgenic mice expressing interferon gamma in the epidermis. J Exp Med 186:1451–1459

Simmons-O'Brien E, Chen S, Watson R, Antoni C, Petri M, Hochberg M, Stevens MB, Provost TT (1995) One hundred anti-Ro (SS-A) antibody positive patients: a 10-year follow-up. Medicine (Baltimore) 74:109–130

Somersan S, Bhardwaj N (2001) Tethering and tickling: a new role for the phosphatidylserine receptor. J Cell Biol 155:501–504

Sontheimer RD (1989) Subacute cutaneous lupus erythematosus: a decade's perspective. Med Clin North Am 73:1073–1090

Taylor PR, Carugati A, Fadok VA, Cook HT, Andrews M, Carroll MC, Savill JS, Henson PM, Botto M, Walport MJ (2000) A hierarchical role for classical pathway complement proteins in the clearance of apoptotic cells in vivo. J Exp Med 192:359–366

Thornberry NA, Lazebnik Y (1998) Caspases: enemies within. Science 281:1312–1316

Tran HB, Ohlsson M, Beroukas D, Hiscock J, Bradley J, Buyon JP, Gordon TP (2002) Subcellular redistribution of la/SSB autoantigen during physiologic apoptosis in the fetal mouse heart and conduction system: a clue to the pathogenesis of congenital heart block. Arthritis Rheum 46:202–208

Voll RE, Herrmann M, Roth EA, Stach C, Kalden JR, Girkontaite I (1997) Immunosuppressive effects of apoptotic cells. Nature 390:350–351

Young AR (1987) The sunburn cell. Photoderm 4:127–134

CHAPTER 18

Pathogenesis of Cutaneous Lupus Erythematosus: The Role of Ultraviolet Light

18

MICHELE L. ROSENBAUM, VICTORIA P. WERTH

Cutaneous lupus erythematosus (CLE) defines a spectrum of diseases, including subacute CLE (SCLE), LE tumidus (LET), discoid LE (DLE), and systemic LE (SLE). Of these, the most photosensitive are SCLE and LET. The anti-Ro/SSA antibody and the human leukocyte antigen (HLA) DR3 genotype are strongly correlated with SCLE but are rarely present in DLE (Lee and Farris 1999) or LET (Alexiades-Armenakas et al. 2003).

Photosensitivity defines a predisposition to developing lesions from the sun, as these patients have a normal range of minimal erythema dose compared with the general population (Sanders et al. 2003). Photoprovocation studies clearly demonstrate that ultraviolet (UV) light (UVA, UVB) (Kuhn et al. 2001a, b, Lehmann et al. 1990, Walchner et al. 1997), and visible light (Sanders et al. 2003) can provoke lesions in all photosensitive forms of LE (Cheong et al. 1994).

UV Light, Apoptosis, and Autoimmunity

The link between photosensitivity and the induction of autoimmune disease can be understood through a model centered on the apoptotic cell. Apoptosis is a process of programmed cell death during which intracellular antigens are translocated to the cell surface, allowing for detection by the immune system (Casciola-Rosen and Rosen 1997, Casciola-Rosen et al. 1994, 1995, 1999, Schultz and Harrington 2003). Because apoptosis is required for the development and maintenance of tissue homeostasis in multicellular organisms, the immune system has developed mechanisms to cope with the removal of apoptotic debris. Under noninflammatory conditions, immature dendritic cells (DCs) or local macrophages phagocytose apoptotic cells and prevent the development of autoantibodies in a process of tolerance (White and Rosen 2003). If the balance is distorted by an increase in the production of apoptotic cells, by an increase in the amount of inflammatory cytokines, or by a deficiency in the proteins involved in clearance, apoptotic debris may be processed by antigen-presenting cells (APCs) and may gain access to major histocompatibility complex (MHC) class I and II pathways to efficiently stimulate $CD4^+$ and $CD8^+$ cells (Rovere-Querini and Dumitriu 2003). This would promote the development of autoantibodies, possibly leading to the development of autoimmunity (Fig. 18.1).

It is unlikely that the development of autoimmunity relies solely on the inability of the immune system to cope with apoptotic debris. Rather, it is likely a combination of factors relating to the inefficient killing and removal of T and B cells in the setting of

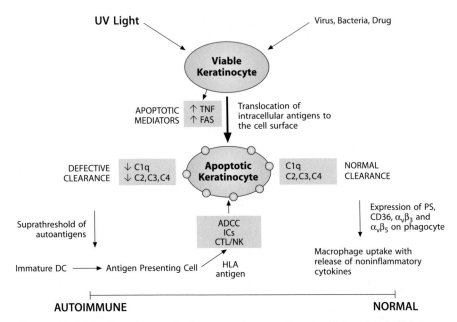

Fig. 18.1. Model for the pathogenesis of cutaneous lupus erythematosus. Apoptotic cells are usually cleared by noninflammatory pathways that involve macrophages. If this system is overloaded, by either an increase in proapoptotic signals or a decrease in clearance mechanisms, apoptotic debris can be taken up by DCs to initiate an immune response. ADCC, antibody-dependent cellular cytotoxicity; DC, dendritic cell; PS, phosphatidylserine; TNF, tumor necrosis factor; UV, ultraviolet

specific autoantigen triggers, leading to the development of autoreactive T cells (Kretz-Rommel and Rubin 1999, Takeuchi et al. 1995). The importance of eliminating autoreactive T and B cells has been demonstrated by the presence of autoimmunity in Fas-deficient mice and humans and in mice overexpressing the anti-apoptotic protein Bcl-2 in B cells (Mevorach 2003, Watanabe-Fukunaga et al. 1992).

Ultraviolet Radiation Induces Apoptosis

SCLE and DLE are characterized by increased numbers of apoptotic cells in lesional skin (Baima and Sticherling 2001, Pablos et al. 1999). Both UVA (320–400 nm) and UVB (290–320 nm) are potent inducers of apoptosis in the epidermis, as evidenced by the presence of the sunburned cell (SBC) (morphologically distinguished by the presence of pyknotic nuclei and a shrunken and eosinophilic cytoplasm) or by DNA fragmentation detection assays (Murphy et al. 2001). Although the final product is similar, the mechanism and timeframe related to apoptosis induction differ between UVA and UVB (Godar 1999, Nghiem et al. 2002).

UVR Light Causes Exposure of Autoantigens to the Immune System

SCLE and neonatal LE are associated with the presence of antibodies to Ro/SSA and La/SSB (Mond et al. 1989, Sontheimer et al. 1982). The importance of anti-Ro/SSA antibody in the pathogenesis of SCLE is demonstrated by the fact that the lesions of neonatal LE resolve within a few months of onset, likely with the degradation of maternal antibodies (Lee and Farris 1999). These antibodies are necessary but insufficient for the development of SCLE, demonstrating that there are multiple factors required for the development of autoimmunity.

The link between apoptotic cells and the development of autoantibodies was eloquently shown in vitro by demonstrating that during UVB-induced keratinocyte apoptosis, intracellular antigens, including 52-kDa Ro/SSA, ribosomes, calreticulin, and phospholipid complexes, were translocated to two distinct blebs on the cell surface (Casciola-Rosen et al. 1994). Interestingly, during apoptosis, these antigens could be structurally modified by granzyme B, ICE-like proteases, and reactive oxygen intermediates to produce cryptic epitopes that can bind to MHC II molecules and produce an antibody response (Casciola-Rosen and Rosen 1997, Casciola-Rosen et al. 1995, 1999).

Studies demonstrate a clonal expansion of T cells from CLE blood and skin, suggesting that lesions may be secondary to antibody-dependent cellular cytotoxicity (ADCC) (Furukawa et al. 1996, Kita et al. 1998). In vitro and in vivo studies show that antibodies from the serum of patients with LE bind to the surface of UVB-irradiated keratinocytes (Furukawa et al. 1990, LeFeber et al. 1984) and that this binding, along with UVB cytotoxicity, increases when using keratinocytes from patients with LE, DLE, or SCLE compared with controls (Furukawa et al. 1999). This increased binding is likely responsible for ADCC to keratinocytes (Furukawa et al. 1994, 1999). Other studies demonstrate that IgG1 anti-Ro/SSA autoantibody can activate complement and ADCC (Bennion et al. 1990). Interestingly, estradiol augments the binding of anti-Ro/SSA and anti-La/SSB antibodies to irradiated keratinocytes, suggesting a link between increased prevalence of SCLE and LE in females (Furukawa et al. 1988). Estrogen likely has a direct effect on the development of autoantibodies, as studies treating lupus-prone mice with tamoxifen have demonstrated a decrease in IgG3 antibodies against DNA and nuclear proteins along with a clinical reduction in proteinuria and a decrease in mortality (Sthoeger et al. 2003).

The exact function of Ro/SSA is unknown, but a recent study demonstrated that it may have a role in cytokine production by activated T cells (Ishii et al. 2003). Recently, a Ro/SSA knockout mouse was developed that was characterized by the development of an autoimmune syndrome with increased sensitivity to light. This suggests that Ro/SSA antibodies may actually contribute to the development of the autoimmune response by allowing cryptic epitopes to be presented to the immune system in response to UV apoptosis (Xue et al. 2003).

UVR Is an Important Immunomodulator

UVA and UVB induce distinct sets of inflammatory mediators and, therefore, have different impacts on the immune and inflammatory responses (O'Garra and Murphy 1993). First, UVA and UVB increase levels of both interleukin (IL)-10 and IL-12, but the levels induced differ, with UVB producing more IL-10 than UVA and UVA1 producing more IL-12 than UVB (Kondo and Jimbow 1998, Skov et al. 1997, Werth et al. 2003). IL-10 produced from irradiated keratinocytes induces systemic immunosuppression and tolerance by promoting the Th2 response (Rivas and Ullrich 1992), whereas IL-12 seems to promote a Th1 response (Adorini 1999). IL-12 can reverse UV-induced IL-10 immunosuppression and tolerance (Schmitt et al. 1995, Schwarz et al. 1996), either by inhibiting Th2 cells from secretion of IL-4 and IL-10 (Schmitt et al. 1995) or by blocking IL-10 and tumor necrosis factor (TNF)-α release at the level of the keratinocyte (Schmitt et al. 2000, Werth et al. 2003). IL-10 and TNF-α likely have different roles in UV-induced immunosuppression and tolerance, with TNF-α involved in the induction of immune suppression and IL-10 involved in tolerance (Niizeki and Streilein 1997).

Second, UV induces IL-1α and TNF-α, which leads to increased expression of adhesion molecules on keratinocytes and endothelial cells, which causes local recruitment of inflammatory cells (Bennion et al. 1995, Dorner et al. 1995b, Heckmann et al. 1994). The importance of adhesion molecules in the pathogenesis of photosensitive disease is demonstrated by the fact that there is increased expression of intercellular adhesion molecule-1 (ICAM-1), histocompatibility class II molecules (HLA-DR), E-selectin, and vascular cell adhesion molecule-1 (VCAM-1) in lesional skin of patients with SCLE, DLE, or LET compared with controls (Hausmann et al. 1996, Kuhn et al. 2002). Soluble E-selectin is increased in CLE (Kubo et al. 2000), as is soluble ICAM-1 (Kumamoto et al. 1997) and soluble VCAM-1. Finally, MRL/lpr mice have an exaggerated ICAM-1-dependent leukocyte endothelial interaction, which may contribute to increased inflammation in this murine model of LE (Marshall et al. 2003).

Third, UVB modifies the production of the chemokines CXCL1 and CXCL2 (Kondo et al. 2000), whereas UVA inhibits chemokine CCL17 production from keratinocytes (Zheng et al. 2003). CXCR3-activating chemokines (CXCL9, CXCL10, and CXCL11), as well as HLA-DR3 and ICAM-1, are preferentially expressed at the dermal-epidermal junction and periadnexal areas in DLE lesional skin. CD4[+] and CD8[+] dermal T cells are located in the same areas that express the CXCR3 receptor, suggesting that these chemokines may have an effect on leukocyte recruitment. Interferon (IFN)-γ induces keratinocyte and macrophage expression of chemokines, HLA-DR3, and ICAM-1, suggesting that IFN-γ has an important immunomodulatory role in DLE (Flier et al. 2001). Low levels of IFN-γ are associated with a reduced autoantibody response in murine lupus models (Pollard 2002).

UVR Induces the Release of Pro-apoptotic Cytokines

UVR alters the expression of cytokines and adhesion molecules in the skin to cause apoptosis and inflammation. Primary cytokines released by keratinocyte cells in response to UVB are IL-1 and TNF-α (Norris et al. 1997). TNF-α and IL-1α have been demonstrated to cause increased production of TNF-α by keratinocytes in an autocrine manner (Lisby and Hauser 2002). Interestingly, TNF-α induces apoptosis and the translocation of intracellular Ro and La antigens to surface blebs on cultured keratinocyte cells (Dorner et al. 1995a). Early studies searching for candidate genes involved in SLE demonstrated that a polymorphism in the promoter region of TNF-

Table 18.1. Prevalence of the −308A polymorphism in cutaneous lupus erythematosus (CLE)

	DLE	SCLE	Control
GG	48	25	133
GA	15	33	48
AA	2	8	2
Total	65	66	183
−308A frequency	0.15	0.37	0.142

DLE, discoid LE; SCLE, subacute CLE.

α, termed "TNF2", was strongly linked to HLA-A1, -B8, and -DR3 (Wilson et al. 1993). Subsequent studies showed that this promoter polymorphism, which consisted of a substitution of guanine by adenosine at the −308 base pair in the promoter region of TNF-α, was more common in patients with SLE than in controls, but the linkage was not independent of the DR3 haplotype (Wilson et al. 1994). HLA-DR3 but not the −308A polymorphism is strongly linked to the presence of anti-Ro/SSA and anti-La/SSB autoantibodies (Wilson et al. 1994).

The TNF2 polymorphism has subsequently been demonstrated to act as an independent susceptibility factor from the DR3 locus for SLE in two separate cohorts of African American (Sullivan and Furst 1997) and Caucasian (Rood et al. 2000) patients with SLE. Studies on human B cells transfected with the CAT reporter gene under the control of the TNF2 promoter have an increase in transcription compared with TNF1 promoter, demonstrating that the polymorphism may impact autoimmunity via production of increased TNF-α (Wilson et al. 1997). TNF-α levels do not differ between patients with active or clinical remission (Wais et al. 2003).

The TNF2 promoter is also linked to photosensitive cutaneous autoimmune disease. Patients with SCLE have an increased prevalence of the −308A promoter vs controls, and the −308A polymorphism is linked to DR3 in patients with SCLE but not with DM (Millard et al. 2001, Pachman et al. 2000, Werth et al. 2000, 2002) (Table 18.1). Patients with DLE do not have a statistically significant increase in TNF2 (Millard et al. 2001, Werth et al. 2000). In vitro assays using the CAT-construct under control of the full-length TNF1 promoter demonstrate that KCs produce TNF-α in response to IL-1α and TNF-α (Lisby and Hauser 2002). Further studies demonstrated that −308A is a much stronger transcriptional activator than the −308G wild-type promoter in UVB- but not UVA-irradiated KCS (Silverberg et al. 1999) and fibroblasts in the presence of IL-1α (Werth et al. 2000).

The functional link between photosensitive disease and the TNF2 promoter is still unclear, but it may be that increased production of TNF-α in response to UV light leads to an increase in apoptotic cells and inflammatory mediators. In the right MHC background, this increase in apoptotic cells may overwhelm the noninflammatory clearance of apoptotic debris and may lead to the development of autoantibodies.

IL-12 may also have a role in controlling UV-mediated apoptosis. Both UVA and UVB induce IL-12, and IL-12 causes suppression of TNF-α at the level of the promoter (Werth et al. 2003). Interestingly, IL-12 was found to promote survival of UV-irradiated keratinocytes in vivo, likely by increasing the activity of DNA repair enzymes (Schwarz et al. 2002). It is tempting to speculate that UVA1-induced IL-12 may be responsible for inhibition of TNF-α, possibly working through DNA repair enzymes, and thus accounting for the therapeutic effects of UVA1 seen in particular with anti-Ro/SSA-positive photosensitive LE patients (McGrath 1994).

Decreased Clearance of Apoptotic Cells

There is growing evidence in patients with SLE and autoimmune mouse models that defects in the clearance of apoptotic cells may be important in triggering the immune response. First, in the absence of apoptotic cell uptake, multiple apoptotic bodies can be found in tissues, and these remnants are often associated with the presence of autoimmune disease (Botto et al. 1998, Potter et al. 2003, Scott et al. 2001). Second, deficiencies in the receptor tyrosine kinases Tyro 3, Axl, and Mer lead to autoimmunity (Cohen et al. 2002, Lu and Lemke 2001), and Mer knockout mice have impaired phagocytosis and clearance of apoptotic cells, leading to increased numbers of nuclear autoantibodies (Scott et al. 2001). Third, there is abnormal clearance of apoptotic lymphocytes and fragments by macrophages in SLE (Hermann et al. 1998). Finally, there is impaired uptake of apoptotic cells and macrophages in germinal centers in some patients with SLE (Baumann et al. 2002), and uptake of apoptotic polymorphonuclear leukocytes and macrophages was increased by the addition of serum from healthy patients (Ren et al. 2003).

Apoptotic cells display an array of surface ligands to provide uptake signals to local and circulating phagocytic cells. These ligands cause a "tether and tickle" response in the phagocyte to induce macropinocytosis and the secretion of noninflammatory cytokines. The "tether" signal is thought to be mediated through phosphatidylserine (PS), which is flipped to the outer cell membrane early in the apoptotic process (Hoffmann et al. 2001). PS likely causes attachment of the phagocyte to the apoptotic cell, whereby other receptors are needed to mediate the "tickle" response or change in actin skeleton in the phagocyte to mediate macropinocytosis (Somersan and Bhardwaj 2001). Other receptors that are likely to be important in uptake include CD36, αvβ3 and αVβ5 integrins, and CD68 (Hoffmann et al. 2001). Engagement of these receptors in the right inflammatory setting causes the phagocyte to suppress the immune response through production of IL-10, transforming growth factor (TGF) β, platelet activating factor, and prostaglandin E (Gaipl et al. 2003, Huynh et al. 2002, Somersan and Bhardwaj 2001). Uptake of apoptotic cells also decreases the amount of IL-12 secreted by the macrophage (Kim et al. 2003). The amount of PS displayed on the cell surface may be important for macrophage uptake (Borisenko et al. 2003), as may timing, as uptake by macrophages of very early apoptotic cells expressing low levels of PS did not result in any cytokine production, suggesting that early uptake was not associated with inflammation (Kurosaka et al. 2003).

In the absence of PS, or in the presence of inflammatory mediators, other signals may dominate. Annexin I, which colocalizes with PS on the cell membrane, is also important for uptake (Arur et al. 2003), but phagocytosis through this ligand induces the humoral immune response (Gaipl et al. 2003). Collectins, complement, and pentraxins are also important in the uptake of apoptotic cells by macrophages, and deficiencies in these proteins are a strong predictor of autoimmunity (Nauta et al. 2003).

C1q is a component of the classical complement pathway. It is structurally homologous to the collectin family of proteins and contains a collagen-like tail and globular head with binding domains. Early complement deficiency is a strong predictor for the development of SLE (Pickering et al. 2001). Individuals with homozygous C1q deficiency have a 98% likelihood of developing a lupus syndrome (Walport et al. 1998) and develop photosensitive eruptions (Bowness et al. 1994). C1q knockout mice develop high titers of autoantibodies and glomerulonephritis characterized histologically by immune deposits and multiple apoptotic bodies (Botto et al. 1998). Complement components are necessary for the uptake of apoptotic cells (Mevorach et al. 1998, Taylor et al. 2000), and C1q has been demonstrated to bind to apoptotic cells and to induce complement activation (Nauta et al. 2002) as well as uptake by macrophage via the CD91 and calreticulin receptor (CRT) (Ogden et al. 2001).

There is evidence that suggests that C1q may be important in the pathogenesis of photosensitive LE. First, in vitro studies demonstrate that C1q binds directly and specifically to surface blebs of apoptotic human keratinocytes (Korb and Ahearn 1997). Second, SCLE has been linked to a low-producing variant of the C1q gene (Racila et al. 2003). Interestingly, UV-irradiated C1q knockout mice do not demonstrate an alteration in the rate of clearance of SBCs after UV exposure, and chronic UV exposure does not alter systemic disease (Pickering et al. 2001). However, this was done on a C57BL/6 background, and there is evidence that the manifestations of C1q deficiency depend on genetic background, with acceleration of the presence of the production of autoantibodies and severity of renal disease in the MRL/MpJ background (Mitchell et al. 2002). UV irradiation studies have not been reported in these mice. It is likely that persistence of apoptotic and necrotic keratinocyte cells leads to phagocytosis by immature DCs, which can then gain access to the MHC class I and II pathway and initiate a primary response (Rovere et al. 2000b).

Other collectins and complement components may also play a role in the clearance of apoptotic cells. C3 has been shown on sunburn cells in C1q-deficient mice, and it is likely that C3 opsonic fragments play a role in the recognition and removal of sunburn cells in skin (Pickering et al. 2001). It is likely that C2, C3, and C4 complement deficiencies, also associated with SCLE, play a role in decreased clearance of apoptotic cells. There is redundancy in the clearance mechanism, demonstrating the importance of presenting apoptotic debris to the immune system. Clearly, defects in different clearance mechanisms may be important for different diseases.

Antigen Presentation and Inflammatory Responses

Cross-Presentation of Apoptotic Antigens

After uptake of apoptotic cells by phagocytes, the cellular components are processed and either incorporated by the phagocyte or, provided that the apoptotic protein fragments can fit into the MHC binding groove, presented to CD4$^+$ T cells by MHC class II or to CD8$^+$ T cells by MHC class I molecules in a process called "cross-presentation." Cross-presentation of apoptotic debris to MHC class I–restricted T cells is surprising because MHC class I–associated proteins are usually cytosolic proteins that are processed through proteosomes and subsequently enter the ER by a transporter associated with antigen processing. Further attachment to the MHC class I complex is mediated through the proteins tapasin, calnexin, and Erp57. The pathway by which the epitopes from apoptotic cells gain access to MHC class I proteins has not been fully elucidated, and it is unclear whether there is a direct phagosome to cytosol pathway, direct access to the cytosol of apoptotic antigens, or a separate phagosome that contains the MHC class I loading machinery. MHC class II presentation of apoptotic debris is more direct, as phagocytic uptake of apoptotic debris is processed through the lysosome and endoplasmic reticulum (ER), where it can attach to MHC class II molecules (Rovere-Querini and Dumitriu 2003).

Dendritic Cells and Photosensitive Autoimmune Disease

Despite the ability of macrophages to cross-present antigens, in vivo studies have demonstrated that they are not efficient in initiating immune responses (Rovere-Querini and Dumitriu 2003). DCs, on the other hand, have been demonstrated to be strong inducers of the immune response (Bondanza et al. 2003, Jung et al. 2002), and there is reason to believe that they are involved in the pathogenesis of SLE and photosensitive LE.

Immature DCs are responsible for maintenance of peripheral tolerance to self-antigens, whereas mature DCs are responsible for the induction of immunity. IFN-γ causes maturation of immature DCs into efficient APCs, and IFN-γ can then act in an autocrine manner to activate DCs (Montoya et al. 2002). In patients with SLE, increased levels of IFN-γ lead to DC activation and may be responsible for a break in tolerance to self-antigens and an activation of the immune system (Pascual et al. 2003). Interestingly, IFN-γ serum levels closely mirror disease activity in patients with lupus, and gene signatures of peripheral bone marrow cells from patients with SLE match those of IFN-γ-regulated genes (Pascual et al. 2003). Further evidence that IFN-γ drives DC differentiation in SLE is generated by the fact that antibodies to IFN-γ block the ability of SLE serum to induce differentiation of immature DCs, and addition of IFN-γ to normal serum reproduces DC maturation (Blanco et al. 2001).

Plasmacytoid DCs (PDCs) are efficient producers of IFN-γ, IL-10, or IL-12 depending on the stimulus (Pascual et al. 2003), and increased pDCs and IFN-γ-producing cells are found in the skin of patients with CLE (Blomberg et al. 2001, Farkas et al. 2001, Wollenberg et al. 2002). The amount of PDCs in the lesions correlates with the amount of IFN-γ target protein expression and with the amount of L-selectin ligand in peripheral lymph node endothelial cells (Farkas et al. 2001). With the proper trigger, PDCs can produce IFN-α/β in large amounts. IFN-α favors a type 1 cytokine response, suggesting that SLE may be mediated by type 1 cytokines. Increased type 1 cytokines, IFN-α and IL-2, have been detected in lesional skin of DLE, supporting that a Th1 response is involved in mediating inflammation in CLE (Toro et al. 2000).

The function of PDCs likely depends on the local environment (Kadowaki et al. 2000). In the presence of IL-3 and CD40L, PDCs can become mature DCs and initiate a Th2 immune response. IL-1α and TNF-α, stimulated by UVB irradiation of keratinocytes, promote DC maturation and efficient antigen presentation (Cumberbatch et al. 2002), whereas IL-10 prevents DC maturation (Moore et al. 2001). It is therefore likely that in times of massive apoptosis and lack of clearance, DCs are recruited and, in the proper inflammatory setting, mature to efficient APCs initiating an immune response (Rovere et al. 1999). Mature DCs express high levels of MHC but clearly need another signal to generate immunity vs tolerance (Albert et al. 2001). This signal may be TNF-α, as, in conjunction with anti-CD40 ligand, TNF-α induces maturation of DCs (Menges et al. 2002).

Proteins important in the clearance of apoptotic cells are also important signals to DC maturation. Immature and mature DCs express different amounts of receptor for C1q (Vegh et al. 2003). PTX3 prevents uptake of apoptotic cells by DCs (Rovere et al. 2000a). Other components that prevent maturation of immature DCs include αvβ3 and αvβ5 integrins, CD36, and C3b (Verbovetski et al. 2002).

Effect of Genetic Background on Antigen Presentation

The presence of anti-Ro/SSA antibody is influenced by the presence of specific HLA class II genes (Provost and Watson 1993, Sontheimer et al. 1982). HLA class II genes are important in the mode of T-cell response to antigens. Mice transgenic for DR2, DR3, and DQ8 showed stronger T- and B-cell responses to human Ro antigen than did DQ6 mice (Paisansinsup et al. 2002). In addition, HLA class II genes influence epitope spreading from activated T and/or B lymphocytes (Paisansinsup et al. 2002).

The association of HLA-DR3 with SCLE likely has a strong influence on antigen presentation. The linkage disequilibrium of the –308A TNF promoter polymorphism with DR3 seen in SCLE is likely to be important in determining immune response (Werth et al. 2002). One could imagine that increased TNF-α production from the –308A polymorphism leads to increased apoptosis and Ro antigen presentation. In the context of HLA-DR3, this could stimulate an autoantibody response and trigger the development of autoimmunity.

Inflammatory Cells in Photosensitive Autoimmune Disease: The Link to Antigen Presentation

We explained how during the physiologic turnover of apoptotic cells, autoantigens are displayed to the immune system for the maintenance of tolerance or, when there is an imbalance in the system, the production of autoimmunity. Furthermore, during the normal uptake of apoptotic debris, antigens can be processed to bind to MHC I or MHC II molecules to activate CD4[+] or CD8[+] T cells. It is still unclear how the inflammatory response in CLE is initiated and maintained, but there is evidence to support that it is an antigen-driven response. First, cutaneous lesions contain a patchy infiltrate of activated T cells that are predominantly CD4[+] (David-Bajar 1993). Second, there is a selective expansion of Vβ8.1 CD3[+] cells in the skin of patients with CLE (Furukawa et al. 1996). Third, sequencing of T-cell receptor clonotypes from skin suggests an antigen-driven response (Kita et al. 1998). Fourth, APCs in skin from DLE, SCLE, and CLE express B7-1 and B7-2 surface molecules that bind to CD28[+], suggesting that these cells can activate a T-cell response (Denfeld et al. 1997).

CD3[+] cells are present in the lesions of CLE, with more CD4[+] cells than CD8[+] cells. Evidence supporting that a Th1 response may be responsible for cutaneous autoimmunity includes the following: increased type 1 cytokines, IFN-γ and IL-2, are detected in lesional skin of DLE (Toro et al. 2000); high levels of IL-10, which suppresses the Th1 response and activates a Th2 response, do not correlate with the occurrence of CLE (van der Linden et al. 2000); and type 2 cytokine IL-4 is decreased in monocytes from patients with SLE (Horwitz et al. 1994).

It is likely that combinations of genetic polymorphisms are at least in part responsible for most CLE. In SCLE, individuals who are homozygous for the –308A TNF promoter polymorphism may have enough residual antigens from apoptotic cells to trigger an immunologic response, whereas patients who are heterozygous for the polymorphism may have to also have a deficiency in the genes responsible for clearance, such as C1q. Clearly, in the proper HLA background, the presence of pro-apoptotic and anti-clearance polymorphisms will play a role in antigen presentation, autoantibody production, and the subsequent immune response to nontolerized apoptotic antigens.

References

Adorini L (1999) Interleukin-12, a key cytokine in Th1-mediated autoimmune diseases. Cell Mol Life Sci 55:1610–1625

Albert ML, Jegathesan M, Darnell RB (2001) Dendritic cell maturation is required for the cross-tolerization of CD8+ T cells. Nat Immunol 2:1010–1017

Alexiades-Armenakas MR, Baldassano M, Bince B, Werth V, Bystryn JC, Kamino H, Soter NA, Franks AG, Jr. (2003) Tumid lupus erythematosus: criteria for classification with immunohistochemical analysis. Arthritis Rheum 49:494–500

Arur S, Uche UE, Rezaul K, Fong M, Scranton V, Cowan AE, Mohler W, Han DK (2003) Annexin I is an endogenous ligand that mediates apoptotic cell engulfment. Dev Cell 4:587–598

Baima B, Sticherling M (2001) Apoptosis in different cutaneous manifestations of lupus erythematosus. Br J Dermatol 144:958–966

Baumann I, Kolowos W, Voll RE, Manger B, Gaipl U, Neuhuber WL, Kirchner T, Kalden JR, Herrmann M (2002) Impaired uptake of apoptotic cells into tingible body macrophages in germinal centers of patients with systemic lupus erythematosus. Arthritis Rheum 46:191–201

Bennion SD, Ferris C, Lieu TS, Reimer CB, Lee LA (1990) IgG subclasses in the serum and skin in subacute cutaneous lupus erythematosus and neonatal lupus erythematosus. J Invest Dermatol 95:643–646

Bennion SD, Middleton MH, David-Bajar KM, Brice S, Norris DA (1995) In three types of interface dermatitis, different patterns of expression of intercellular adhesion molecule-1 (ICAM-1) indicate different triggers of disease. J Invest Dermatol 105:71S-79S

Blanco P, Palucka AK, Gill M, Pascual V, Banchereau J (2001) Induction of dendritic cell differentiation by IFN-alpha in systemic lupus erythematosus. Science 294:1540–1543

Blomberg S, Eloranta ML, Cederblad B, Nordlin K, Alm GV, Ronnblom L (2001) Presence of cutaneous interferon-alpha producing cells in patients with systemic lupus erythematosus. Lupus 10:484–490

Bondanza A, Zimmermann VS, Dell'Antonio G, Dal Cin E, Capobianco A, Sabbadini MG, Manfredi AA, Rovere-Querini P (2003) Cutting edge: dissociation between autoimmune response and clinical disease after vaccination with dendritic cells. J Immunol 170:24–27

Borisenko GG, Matsura T, Liu SX, Tyurin VA, Jianfei J, Serinkan FB, Kagan VE (2003) Macrophage recognition of externalized phosphatidylserine and phagocytosis of apoptotic Jurkat cells–existence of a threshold. Arch Biochem Biophys 413:41–52

Botto M, Dell'Agnola C, Bygrave AE, Thompson EM, Cook HT, Petry F, Loos M, Pandolfi PP, Walport MJ (1998) Homozygous C1q deficiency causes glomerulonephritis associated with multiple apoptotic bodies. Nat Genet 19:56–59

Bowness P, Davies KA, Norsworthy PJ, Athanassiou P, Taylor-Wiedeman J, Borysiewicz LK, Meyer PA, Walport MJ (1994) Hereditary C1q deficiency and systemic lupus erythematosus. QJM 87:455–464

Casciola-Rosen LA, Rosen, A (1997) Ultraviolet light-induced keratinocyte apoptosis: a potential mechanism for the induction of skin lesions and autoantibody production in LE. Lupus 6:175–180

Casciola-Rosen LA, Anhalt G, Rosen A (1994) Autoantigens targeted in systemic lupus erythematosus are clustered in two populations of surface structures on apoptotic keratinocytes. J Exp Med 179:1317–1330

Casciola-Rosen LA, Anhalt GJ, Rosen A (1995) DNA-dependent protein kinase is one of a subset of autoantigens specifically cleaved early during apoptosis. J Exp Med 182:1625–1634

Casciola-Rosen LA, Andrade F, Ulanet D, Wong WB, Rosen A (1999) Cleavage by granzyme B is strongly predictive of autoantigen status: implications for initiation of autoimmunity. J Exp Med 190:815–826

Cheong WK, Hughes GR, Norris PG, Hawk JL (1994) Cutaneous photosensitivity in dermatomyositis. Br J Dermatol 131:205–208

Cohen PL, Caricchio R, Abraham V, Camenisch TD, Jennette JC, Roubey RA, Earp HS, Matsushima G, Reap EA (2002) Delayed apoptotic cell clearance and lupus-like autoimmunity in mice lacking the c-mer membrane tyrosine kinase. J Exp Med 196:135–140

Cumberbatch M, Dearman RJ, Groves RW, Antonopoulos C, Kimber I (2002) Differential regulation of epidermal Langerhans cell migration by interleukins (IL)-1α and IL-1β during irritant- and allergen-induced cutaneous immune responses. Toxicol Appl Pharmacol 182:126–135

David-Bajar KM (1993) Subacute cutaneous lupus erythematosus. J Invest Dermatol 100:2S–8S

Denfeld RW, Kind P, Sontheimer RD, Schopf E, Simon JC (1997) In situ expression of B7 and CD28 receptor families in skin lesions of patients with lupus erythematosus. Arthritis Rheum 40:814–821

Dorner T, Hucko M, Mayet WJ, Trefzer U, Burmester GR, Hiepe F (1995b) Enhanced membrane expression of the 52 kDa Ro(SS-A) and La(SS-B) antigens by human keratinocytes induced by TNF alpha. Ann Rheum Dis 54:904–909

Dorner T, Hucko M, Mayet WJ, Trefzer U, Burmester GR, Hiepe F (1995a) Enhanced membrane expression of the 52 kDa Ro(SS-A) and La(SS-B) antigens by human keratinocytes induced by TNF alpha. Ann Rheum Dis 54:904–909

Farkas L, Beiske K, Lund-Johansen F, Brandtzaeg P, Jahnsen FL (2001) Plasmacytoid dendritic cells (natural interferon- alpha/beta-producing cells) accumulate in cutaneous lupus erythematosus lesions. Am J Pathol 159:237–243

Flier J, Boorsma DM, van Beek PJ, Nieboer C, Stoof TJ, Willemze R, Tensen CP (2001) Differential expression of CXCR3 targeting chemokines CXCL10, CXCL9, and CXCL11 in different types of skin inflammation. J Pathol 194:398–405

Furukawa F, Lyons MB, Lee LA, Coulter SN, Norris DA (1988) Estradiol enhances binding to cultured human keratinocytes of antibodies specific for SS-A/Ro and SS-B/La. Another possible mechanism for estradiol influence of lupus erythematosus. J Immunol 141:1480–1488

Furukawa F, Kashihara-Sawami M, Lyons MB, Norris DA (1990) Binding of antibodies to the extractable nuclear antigens SS-A/Ro and SS-B/La is induced on the surface of human keratinocytes by ultraviolet light (UVL): implications for the pathogenesis of photosensitive cutaneous lupus. J Invest Dermatol 94:77–85

Furukawa F, Kanauchi H, Imamura S (1994) Susceptibility to UVB light in cultured keratinocytes of cutaneous lupus erythematosus. Dermatology 189 (Suppl 1):18–23

Furukawa F, Tokura Y, Matsushita K, Iwasaki-Inuzuka K, Onagi-Suzuki K, Yagi H, Wakita H, Takigawa M (1996) Selective expansions of T cells expressing V beta 8 and V beta 13 in skin lesions of patients with chronic cutaneous lupus erythematosus. J Dermatol 23:670–676

Furukawa F, Itoh T, Wakita H, Yagi H, Tokura Y, Norris DA, Takigawa M (1999) Keratinocytes from patients with lupus erythematosus show enhanced cytotoxicity to ultraviolet radiation and to antibody-mediated cytotoxicity. Clin Exp Immunol 118:164–170

Gaipl US, Beyer TD, Baumann I, Voll RE, Stach CM, Heyder P, Kalden JR, Manfredi A, Herrmann M (2003) Exposure of anionic phospholipids serves as anti-inflammatory and immunosuppressive signal–implications for antiphospholipid syndrome and systemic lupus erythematosus. Immunobiology 207:73–81

Godar DE (1999) Light and death: photons and apoptosis. J Investig Dermatol Symp Proc 4:17–23

Hausmann G, Mascaro JM Jr, Herrero C, Cid MC, Palou J, Mascaro JM (1996) Cell adhesion molecule expression in cutaneous lesions of dermatomyositis. Acta Derm Venereol 76:222–225

Heckmann M, Eberlein-Konig B, Wollenberg A, Przybilla B, Plewig G (1994) Ultraviolet-A radiation induces adhesion molecule expression on human dermal microvascular endothelial cells. Br J Dermatol 131:311–318

Hermann M, Niemitz C, Marafioti T, Schriever F (1998) Reduced phagocytosis of apoptotic cells in malignant lymphoma. Int J Cancer 75:675–679

Hoffmann PR, deCathelineau AM, Ogden CA, Leverrier Y, Bratton DL, Daleke DL, Ridley AJ, Fadok VA, Henson PM (2001) Phosphatidylserine (PS) induces PS receptor-mediated macropinocytosis and promotes clearance of apoptotic cells. J Cell Biol 155:649–659

Horwitz DA, Wang H, Gray JD (1994) Cytokine gene profile in circulating blood mononuclear cells from patients with systemic lupus erythematosus: increased interleukin-2 but not interleukin-4 mRNA. Lupus 3:423–428

Huynh ML, Fadok VA, Henson PM (2002) Phosphatidylserine-dependent ingestion of apoptotic cells promotes TGF-beta1 secretion and the resolution of inflammation. J Clin Invest 109: 41–50

Ishii T, Ohnuma K, Murakami A, Takasawa N, Yamochi T, Iwata S, Uchiyama M, Dang NH, Tanaka H, Morimoto C (2003) SS-A/Ro52, an autoantigen involved in CD28-mediated IL-2 production. J Immunol 170:3653–3661

Jung S, Unutmaz D, Wong P, Sano G, De los Santos K, Sparwasser T, Wu S, Vuthoori S, Ko K, Zavala F, Pamer EG, Littman DR, Lang RA (2002) In vivo depletion of CD11 c(+) dendritic cells abrogates priming of CD8(+) T cells by exogenous cell-associated antigens. Immunity 17:211–220

Kadowaki N, Antonenko S, Lau JY, Liu YJ (2000) Natural interferon alpha/beta-producing cells link innate and adaptive immunity. J Exp Med 192:219–226

Kim SJ, Gershov D, Ma X, Brot N, Elkon KB (2003) Opsonization of apoptotic cells and its effect on macrophage and T cell immune responses. Ann N Y Acad Sci 987:68–78

Kita Y, Kuroda K, Mimori T, Hashimoto T, Yamamoto K, Saito Y, Iwamoto I, Sumida T (1998) T cell receptor clonotypes in skin lesions from patients with systemic lupus erythematosus. J Invest Dermatol 110:41–46

Kondo S, Jimbow K (1998) Dose-dependent induction of IL-12 but not IL-10 from human keratinocytes after exposure to ultraviolet light A. J Cell Physiol 177:493–498

Kondo S, Yoneta A, Yazawa H, Kamada A, Jimbow K (2000) Downregulation of CXCR-2 but not CXCR-1 expression by human keratinocytes by UVB. J Cell Physiol 182:366–370

Korb LC, Ahearn JM (1997) C1q binds directly and specifically to surface blebs of apoptotic human keratinocytes: complement deficiency and systemic lupus erythematosus revisited. J Immunol 158:4525–4528

Kretz-Rommel A, Rubin RL (1999) Persistence of autoreactive T cell drive is required to elicit antichromatin antibodies in a murine model of drug-induced lupus. J Immunol 162: 813–820

Kubo M, Ihn H, Yamane K, Yazawa N, Kikuchi K, Soma Y, Tamaki K. (2000) Increased serum levels of soluble vascular cell adhesion molecule-1 and soluble E-selectin in patients with polymyositis/dermatomyositis. Br J Dermatol 143:392–398

Kuhn A, Sonntag M, Richter-Hintz D, Oslislo C, Megahed M, Ruzicka T, Lehmann P (2001a) Phototesting in lupus erythematosus tumidus: review of 60 patients. Photochem Photobiol 73:532–536

Kuhn A, Sonntag M, Richter-Hintz D, Oslislo C, Megahed M, Ruzicka T, Lehmann P (2001b) Phototesting in lupus erythematosus: a 15-year experience. J Am Acad Dermatol 45:86–95

Kuhn A, Sonntag M, Sunderkotter C, Lehmann P, Vestweber D, Ruzicka T (2002) Upregulation of epidermal surface molecule expression in primary and ultraviolet-induced lesions of lupus erythematosus tumidus. Br J Dermatol 146:801–809

Kumamoto T, Abe T, Ueyama H, Sugihara R, Shigenaga T, Tsuda T (1997) Elevated soluble intercellular adhesion molecules-1 in inflammatory myopathy. Acta Neurol Scand 95:34–37

Kurosaka K, Takahashi M, Watanabe N, Kobayashi Y (2003) Silent cleanup of very early apoptotic cells by macrophages. J Immunol 171:4672–4679

Lee LA, Farris AD (1999) Photosensitivity diseases: cutaneous lupus erythematosus. J Investig Dermatol Symp Proc 4:73–78

LeFeber WP, Norris DA, Ryan SR, Huff JC, Lee LA, Kubo M, Boyce ST, Kotzin BL, Weston WL (1984) Ultraviolet light induces binding of antibodies to selected nuclear antigens on cultured human keratinocytes. J Clin Invest 74:1545–1551

Lehmann P, Holzle E, Kind P, Goerz, G, Plewig G (1990) Experimental reproduction of skin lesions in lupus erythematosus by UVA and UVB radiation. J Am Acad Dermatol 22:181–187

Lisby S, Hauser C (2002) Transcriptional regulation of tumor necrosis factor-alpha in keratinocytes mediated by interleukin-1beta and tumor necrosis factor-alpha. Exp Dermatol 11:592–598

Lu Q, Lemke G (2001) Homeostatic regulation of the immune system by receptor tyrosine kinases of the Tyro 3 family. Science 293:306–311

Marshall D, Dangerfield JP, Bhatia VK, Larbi KY, Nourshargh S, Haskard DO (2003) MRL/lpr lupus-prone mice show exaggerated ICAM-1-dependent leucocyte adhesion and transendothelial migration in response to TNF-alpha. Rheumatology (Oxford) 42:929–934

McGrath H Jr (1994) Ultraviolet-A1 irradiation decreases clinical disease activity and autoantibodies in patients with systemic lupus erythematosus. Clin Exp Rheumatol 12:129–135

Menges M, Rossner S, Voigtlander C, Schindler H, Kukutsch NA, Bogdan C, Erb K, Schuler G, Lutz MB (2002) Repetitive injections of dendritic cells matured with tumor necrosis factor alpha induce antigen-specific protection of mice from autoimmunity. J Exp Med 195:15–21

Mevorach D (2003) Systemic lupus erythematosus and apoptosis: a question of balance. Clin Rev Allergy Immunol 25:49–60

Mevorach D, Zhou JL, Song X, Elkon KB (1998) Systemic exposure to irradiated apoptotic cells induces autoantibody production. J Exp Med 188:387–392

Millard TP, Kondeatis E, Cox A, Wilson AG, Grabczynska SA, Carey BS, Lewis CM, Khamashta MA, Duff GW, Hughes GR, Hawk JL, Vaughan RW, McGregor JM (2001) A candidate gene analysis of three related photosensitivity disorders: cutaneous lupus erythematosus, polymorphic light eruption and actinic prurigo. Br J Dermatol 145:229–236

Mitchell DA, Pickering MC, Warren J, Fossati-Jimack L, Cortes-Hernandez J, Cook HT, Botto M, Walport MJ (2002) C1q deficiency and autoimmunity: the effects of genetic background on disease expression. J Immunol 168:2538–2543

Mond CB, Peterson MG, Rothfield NF (1989) Correlation of anti-Ro antibody with photosensitivity rash in systemic lupus erythematosus patients. Arthritis Rheum 32:202–204

Montoya M, Schiavoni G, Mattei F, Gresser I, Belardelli F, Borrow P, Tough DF (2002) Type I interferons produced by dendritic cells promote their phenotypic and functional activation. Blood 99:3263–3271

Moore KW, de Waal Malefyt R, Coffman RL, O'Garra A (2001) Interleukin-10 and the interleukin-10 receptor. Annu Rev Immunol 19:683–765

Murphy G, Young AR, Wulf HC, Kulms D, Schwarz T (2001) The molecular determinants of sunburn cell formation. Exp Dermatol 10:155–160

Nauta AJ, Daha MR, van Kooten C, Roos A (2003) Recognition and clearance of apoptotic cells: a role for complement and pentraxins. Trends Immunol 24:148–154

Nauta AJ, Trouw LA, Daha MR, Tijsma O, Nieuwland R, Schwaeble WJ, Gingras AR, Mantovani A, Hack EC, Roos A (2002) Direct binding of C1q to apoptotic cells and cell blebs induces complement activation. Eur J Immunol 32:1726–1736

Nghiem DX, Kazimi N, Mitchell DL, Vink AA, Ananthaswamy HN, Kripke ML, Ullrich SE (2002) Mechanisms underlying the suppression of established immune responses by ultraviolet radiation. J Invest Dermatol 119:600–608

Niizeki H, Streilein JW (1997) Hapten-specific tolerance induced by acute, low-dose ultraviolet B radiation of skin is mediated via interleukin-10. J Invest Dermatol 109:25–30

Norris DA, Whang K, David-Bajar K, Bennion SD (1997) The influence of ultraviolet light on immunological cytotoxicity in the skin. Photochem Photobiol 65:636–646

O'Garra A, Murphy K (1993) T-cell subsets in autoimmunity. Curr Opin Immunol 5:880–886

Ogden CA, deCathelineau A, Hoffmann PR, Bratton D, Ghebrehiwet B, Fadok VA, Henson PM (2001) C1q and mannose binding lectin engagement of cell surface calreticulin and CD91 initiates macropinocytosis and uptake of apoptotic cells. J Exp Med 194:781–795

Pablos JL, Santiago B, Galindo M, Carreira PE, Ballcstin C, Gomez-Reino JJ (1999) Keratinocyte apoptosis and p53 expression in cutaneous lupus and dermatomyositis. J Pathol 188:63–68

Pachman LM, Liotta-Davis MR, Hong DK, Kinsella TR, Mendez EP, Kinder JM, Chen EH (2000) TNFα-308A allele in juvenile dermatomyositis: association with increased production of tumor necrosis factor alpha, disease duration, and pathologic calcifications. Arthritis Rheum 43:2368–2377

Paisansinsup T, Deshmukh US, Chowdhary VR, Luthra HS, Fu SM, David CS (2002) HLA class II influences the immune response and antibody diversification to Ro60/Sjogren's syndrome-A: heightened antibody responses and epitope spreading in mice expressing HLA-DR molecules. J Immunol 168:5876–5884

Pascual V, Banchereau J, Palucka AK (2003) The central role of dendritic cells and interferon-alpha in SLE. Curr Opin Rheumatol 15:548–556

Pickering MC, Fischer S, Lewis MR, Walport MJ, Botto M, Cook HT (2001) Ultraviolet-radiation-induced keratinocyte apoptosis in C1q-deficient mice. J Invest Dermatol 117:52–58

Pollard KM (2002) Cell death, autoantigen cleavage, and autoimmunity. Arthritis Rheum 46:1699–1702

Potter PK, Cortes-Hernandez J, Quartier P, Botto M, Walport MJ (2003) Lupus-prone mice have an abnormal response to thioglycolate and an impaired clearance of apoptotic cells. J Immunol 170:3223–3232

Provost TT, Watson R (1993) Anti-Ro(SS-A) HLA-DR3-positive women: the interrelationship between some ANA negative, SS, SCLE, and NLE mothers and SS/LE overlap female patients. J Invest Dermatol 100:14S-20S

Racila DM, Sontheimer CJ, Sheffield A, Wisnieski JJ, Racila E, Sontheimer RD (2003) Homozygous single nucleotide polymorphism of the complement C1QA gene is associated with decreased levels of C1q in patients with subacute cutaneous lupus erythematosus. Lupus 12:124–132

Ren Y, Tang J, Mok MY, Chan AW, Wu A, Lau CS (2003) Increased apoptotic neutrophils and macrophages and impaired macrophage phagocytic clearance of apoptotic neutrophils in systemic lupus erythematosus. Arthritis Rheum 48:2888–2897

Rivas JM, Ullrich SE (1992) Systemic suppression of delayed-type hypersensitivity by supernatants from UV-irradiated keratinocytes. An essential role for keratinocyte-derived IL-10. J Immunol 149:3865–3871

Rood MJ, van Krugten MV, Zanelli E, van der Linden MW, Keijsers V, Schreuder GM, Verduyn W, Westendorp RG, de Vries RR, Breedveld FC, Verweij CL, Huizinga TW (2000) TNF-308A and HLA-DR3 alleles contribute independently to susceptibility to systemic lupus erythematosus. Arthritis Rheum 43:129–134

Rovere P, Sabbadini MG, Vallinoto C, Fascio U, Zimmermann VS, Bondanza A, Ricciardi-Castagnoli P, Manfredi AA (1999) Delayed clearance of apoptotic lymphoma cells allows cross-presentation of intracellular antigens by mature dendritic cells. J Leukoc Biol 66:345–349

Rovere P, Peri G, Fazzini F, Bottazzi B, Doni A, Bondanza A, Zimmermann VS, Garlanda C, Fascio U, Sabbadini MG, Rugarli C, Mantovani A, Manfredi AA (2000a) The long pentraxin PTX3 binds to apoptotic cells and regulates their clearance by antigen-presenting dendritic cells. Blood 96:4300–4306

Rovere P, Sabbadini MG, Fazzini F, Bondanza A, Zimmermann VS, Rugarli C, Manfredi AA (2000b) Remnants of suicidal cells fostering systemic autoaggression. Apoptosis in the origin and maintenance of autoimmunity. Arthritis Rheum 43:1663–1672

Rovere-Querini P, Dumitriu IE (2003) Corpse disposal after apoptosis. Apoptosis 8:469–479

Sanders CJ, Van Weelden H, Kazzaz GA, Sigurdsson V, Toonstra J, Bruijnzeel-Koomen C A (2003) Photosensitivity in patients with lupus erythematosus: a clinical and photobiological study of 100 patients using a prolonged phototest protocol. Br J Dermatol 149:131–137

Schmitt DA, Owen-Schaub L, Ullrich SE (1995) Effect of IL-12 on immune suppression and suppressor cell induction by ultraviolet radiation. J Immunol 154:5114–5120

Schmitt DA, Walterscheid JP, Ullrich SE (2000) Reversal of ultraviolet radiation-induced immune suppression by recombinant interleukin-12: suppression of cytokine production. Immunology 101:90–96

Schultz DR, Harrington WJ (2003) Apoptosis: programmed cell death at a molecular level. Semin Arthritis Rheum 32:345–369

Schwarz A, Grabbe S, Aragane Y, Sandkuhl K, Riemann H, Luger TA, Kubin M, Trinchieri G, Schwarz T (1996) Interleukin-12 prevents ultraviolet B-induced local immunosuppression and overcomes UVB-induced tolerance. J Invest Dermatol 106:1187–1191

Schwarz A, Stander S, Berneburg M, Bohm M, Kulms D, van Steeg H, Grosse-Heitmeyer K, Krutmann J, Schwarz T (2002) Interleukin-12 suppresses ultraviolet radiation-induced apoptosis by inducing DNA repair. Nat Cell Biol 4:26–31

Scott RS, McMahon EJ, Pop SM, Reap EA, Caricchio R, Cohen PL, Earp HS, Matsushima GK (2001) Phagocytosis and clearance of apoptotic cells is mediated by MER. Nature 411:207–211

Skov L, Hansen H, Barker JN, Simon JC, Baadsgaard O (1997) Contrasting effects of ultraviolet-A and ultraviolet-B exposure on induction of contact sensitivity in human skin. Clin Exp Immunol 107:585–588

Somersan S, Bhardwaj N (2001) Tethering and tickling: a new role for the phosphatidylserine receptor. J Cell Biol 155:501–504

Sontheimer RD, Maddison PJ, Reichlin M, Jordon RE, Stastny P, Gilliam JN (1982) Serologic and HLA associations in subacute cutaneous lupus erythematosus, a clinical subset of lupus erythematosus. Ann Intern Med 97:664–671

Sthoeger ZM, Zinger H, Mozes E (2003) Beneficial effects of the anti-oestrogen tamoxifen on systemic lupus erythematosus of (NZB×NZW)F1 female mice are associated with specific reduction of IgG3 autoantibodies. Ann Rheum Dis 62:341–346

Sullivan KM, Furst DE (1997) The evolving role of blood and marrow transplantation for the treatment of autoimmune diseases. J Rheumatol Suppl 48:1–4

Takeuchi K, Turley SJ, Tan EM, Pollard KM (1995) Analysis of the autoantibody response to fibrillarin in human disease and murine models of autoimmunity. J Immunol 154: 961–971

Taylor PR, Carugati A, Fadok VA, Cook HT, Andrews M, Carroll MC, Savill JS, Henson PM, Botto M, Walport MJ (2000) A hierarchical role for classical pathway complement proteins in the clearance of apoptotic cells in vivo. J Exp Med 192:359–366

Toro JR, Finlay D, Dou X, Zheng SC, LeBoit PE, Connolly MK (2000) Detection of type 1 cytokines in discoid lupus erythematosus. Arch Dermatol 136:1497–1501

van der Linden MW, Westendorp RG, Sturk A, Bergman W, Huizinga TW (2000) High interleukin-10 production in first-degree relatives of patients with generalized but not cutaneous lupus erythematosus. J Investig Med 48:327–334

Vegh Z, Goyarts EC, Rozengarten K, Mazumder A, Ghebrehiwet B (2003) Maturation-dependent expression of C1q-binding proteins on the cell surface of human monocyte-derived dendritic cells. Int Immunopharmacol 3:345–357

Verbovetski I, Bychkov H, Trahtemberg U, Shapira I, Hareuveni M, Ben Tal O, Kutikov I, Gill O, Mevorach D (2002) Opsonization of apoptotic cells by autologous iC3b facilitates clearance by immature dendritic cells, down-regulates DR and CD86, and up-regulates CC chemokine receptor 7. J Exp Med 196:1553–1561

Wais T, Fierz W, Stoll T, Villiger PM (2003) Subclinical disease activity in systemic lupus erythematosus: immunoinflammatory markers do not normalize in clinical remission. J Rheumatol 30:2133–2139

Walchner M, Messer G, Kind P (1997) Phototesting and photoprotection in LE. Lupus 6: 167–174

Walport MJ, Davies KA, Botto M (1998) C1q and systemic lupus erythematosus. Immunobiology 199:265–285

Watanabe-Fukunaga R, Brannan CI, Copeland NG, Jenkins NA, Nagata S (1992) Lymphoproliferation disorder in mice explained by defects in Fas antigen that mediates apoptosis. Nature 356:314–317

Werth VP, Callen JP, Ang G, Sullivan KE (2002) Associations of tumor necrosis factor alpha and HLA polymorphisms with adult dermatomyositis: implications for a unique pathogenesis. J Invest Dermatol 119:617–620

Werth VP, Bashir MM, Zhang W (2003) IL-12 completely blocks ultraviolet-induced secretion of tumor necrosis factor alpha from cultured skin fibroblasts and keratinocytes. J Invest Dermatol 120:116–122

Werth VP, Zhang W, Dortzbach K, Sullivan K (2000) Association of a promoter polymorphism of tumor necrosis factor-alpha with subacute cutaneous lupus erythematosus and distinct photoregulation of transcription. J Invest Dermatol 115:726–730

White S, Rosen A (2003) Apoptosis in systemic lupus erythematosus. Curr Opin Rheumatol 15:557–562

Wilson AG, de Vries N, Pociot F, di Giovine FS, van der Putte LB, Duff GW (1993) An allelic polymorphism within the human tumor necrosis factor alpha promoter region is strongly associated with HLA A1, B8, and DR3 alleles. J Exp Med 177:557–560

Wilson AG, Gordon C, di Giovine FS, de Vries N, van de Putte LB, Emery P, Duff GW (1994) A genetic association between systemic lupus erythematosus and tumor necrosis factor alpha. Eur J Immunol 24:191–195

Wilson AG, Symons JA, McDowell TL, McDevitt HO, Duff GW (1997) Effects of a polymorphism in the human tumor necrosis factor alpha promoter on transcriptional activation. Proc Natl Acad Sci U S A 94:3195–3199

Wollenberg A, Wagner M, Gunther S, Towarowski A, Tuma E, Moderer M, Rothenfusser S, Wetzel S, Endres S, Hartmann G (2002) Plasmacytoid dendritic cells: a new cutaneous dendritic cell subset with distinct role in inflammatory skin diseases. J Invest Dermatol 119:1096–1102

Xue D, Shi H, Smith JD, Chen X, Noe DA, Cedervall T, Yang DD, Eynon E, Brash DE, Kashgarian M, Flavell RA, Wolin SL (2003) A lupus-like syndrome develops in mice lacking the Ro 60-kDa protein, a major lupus autoantigen. Proc Natl Acad Sci U S A 100:7503–7508

Zheng X, Nakamura K, Tojo M, Akiba H, Oyama N, Nishibu A, Kaneko F, Tsunemi Y, Kakinuma T, Saeki H, Tamaki K (2003) Ultraviolet A irradiation inhibits thymus and activation-regulated chemokine (TARC/CCL17) production by a human keratinocyte HaCaT cell line. Eur J Dermatol 13:348–353

CHAPTER 19

The Role of T Cells and Adhesion Molecules in Cutaneous Lupus Erythematosus

19

FILIPPA NYBERG, EIJA STEPHANSSON

E. Stephansson has also published articles under the author name E.A. Johansson

Immune response to skin antigens modified by ultraviolet (UV) radiation is currently proposed as the pathomechanism for skin lesions in lupus erythematosus (LE) (Casciola-Rosen and Rosen 1997, Norris 1993, 1995, Norris et al. 1997). Cellular apoptosis brought about by UV radiation is believed to have an important role in inducing and perpetuating the disease, but the in vivo role for apoptosis in cutaneous LE (CLE) remains unclear (Orteu et al. 2001). A multistep model has been proposed in which the first step is the release of soluble proinflammatory epidermal and dermal mediators, which may be genetically regulated. A particular allele of interleukin (IL) 1 has been associated with systemic LE (SLE) severity and photosensitivity (Blakemore et al. 1994), and a high tumor necrosis factor (TNF)-α response is linked to the HLA-DR3 gene (Wilson and Duff 1995, Wilson et al. 1993). The HLA-DR3 gene is reported to associate with the most photosensitive variant of CLE, subacute CLE (SCLE) (Callen and Klein 1988, Sontheimer et al. 1982), also in Scandinavia (Johansson-Stephansson et al. 1989). The second step is increased expression of cellular adhesion molecules (CAMs) on keratinocytes and on subepidermal endothelial cells. The increases in cytokine and CAM expression direct cytotoxic T cells to the skin. Nuclear antigens such as Ro/SSA, translocated to the keratinocyte surfaces, possibly involving the heat-shock proteins, are then targeted by circulating anti-Ro/SSA antibodies and cytotoxic T cells (Bennion and Norris 1997, Norris 1993, 1995, Norris et al. 1997).

T Lymphocytes

Antigen-stimulated, so-called armed T cells are generally of CD8 (mainly "killer" T cells) or CD4 (T helper [Th]) type. CD8 cells recognize peptides bound to major histocompatibility complex (MHC) class I molecules. The membrane-bound receptor on these cells is a ligand for Fas and is involved in apoptosis. CD4 cells recognize the antigen-MHC class II complex. They are further subdivided into two groups by the cytokine profile they produce. Type 1 T-helper (Th1) cells secrete IL-2, IL-12, and interferon (IFN)-γ. They are involved in cell-mediated immune reactions and stimulate B cells to produce complement-fixing antibodies. Type 2 T-helper (Th2) cells secrete IL-4, IL-5, IL-6, and IL-10 and are involved in IgE-mediated allergic reactions and the production of non-complement-fixing antibodies (Janeway and Travers 1994). In addition, there are also so-called Th0 cells producing IL-4 and IFN-γ. Also, IL-10, a cytokine that has down-regulating properties, is produced by both Th1 and Th2 cells (Stevens and Bergstresser 1998). In normal human skin, some T cells are found, mostly around dermal postcapillary venules and appendages. Most of them express the αβ T-cell antigen receptor, and vβs 1, 7, 14, and 16 are enriched compared with circulating T cells (Sugerman and Bigby 2000). γδ T cells have cytotoxic potential and are present in murine epithelia with a possible role in immunosurveillance of epithelia but are not found in normal human skin (Alaibac et al. 1992, Bos et al. 1990).

Based on CD45 isoforms, T cells can be divided into CD45RA[+] (suppressor inducer) cells, with functional characteristics of naive T lymphocytes, and CD45RO[+] (helper inducer) cells, with functional characteristics of memory T cells, responding to recall antigens (Kristensson et al. 1992, Morimoto et al. 1985a, b). Also, CD31 cell surface antigen (platelet endothelial adhesion molecule-1) has been shown to define naive T cells (Morimoto and Schlossman 1993, Torimoto et al. 1992). UVB irradiation has been shown to recruit nonactivated CD4[+]CD45RO[+] T cells into both the epidermis and the dermis. Antigen presentation to these cells is thought to result in activation of the suppressor pathway (Di Nuzzo et al. 1998). Contrary to this, UVA irradiation has been shown to deplete skin-infiltrating T cells via apoptosis (Morita et al. 1997).

T Lymphocytes in Cutaneous Lupus Erythematosus

The model of antibody-dependent cellular cytotoxicity fits well with Ro/SSA antibody-associated forms of LE, such as SCLE, neonatal LE, and possibly SLE. However, non-antibody-associated forms of CLE, such as chronic CLE (CCLE), fit less well, although low levels of anti-Ro/SSA antibody production have been noted in patients with CCLE (Lee et al. 1993). Furthermore, polyclonal B-cell activation was detected in serum from patients with discoid LE (DLE) compared with healthy controls (Wangel et al. 1984). Instead, it has been suggested that autoantigen-specific lymphocytes are involved in the pathogenesis of skin lesions of CCLE with a delayed-type hypersensitivity reaction (Sontheimer 1996, Volc-Platzer et al. 1993). Several authors have found higher numbers of CD4 than CD8 cells in the dermal inflammatory infiltrate in CLE (Hasan et al. 1999, Jerdan et al. 1990, Tebbe et al. 1994, Velthuis et al. 1990, Viljaranta et al. 1987). Monoclonal CD4 antibodies have been successfully used to treat severe CLE (Prinz et al. 1996).

A mixed cytokine pattern with IFN-γ-induced intercellular adhesion molecule-1 (ICAM-1) expression, as in Th1-type response, and a Th2-type response with significant IL-5 production and detectable IL-10 production was found in LE lesions (Stein et al. 1997). The authors found no differences in cytokine profiles between LE subgroups.

Recent reports indicate a central role for the T-cell receptor on autoreactive T cells in SLE, and a genetic background was proposed (Tsokos and Liossis 1998). The significance of these findings to CLE is not known at present. Vβ8.1 CD3[+] cells were elevated in skin lesions from CCLE and acute CLE (ACLE) compared with psoriasis and atopic dermatitis, with a higher percentage of vβ8.1 and vβ13.3 in skin lesions from CCLE than from ACLE. There was also a skew toward these vβ types in the peripheral blood (Furukawa et al. 1996, Werth et al. 1997). This is consistent with an antigen-driven response. Sequencing of T-cell receptor clones from infiltrates in skin of patients with SLE further supports antigen-induced clonal accumulation (Kita et al.

1998). The chemokine receptor CXCR3 is expressed by CD45RO$^+$ (helper inducer) cells, preferentially by the Th1 subset and by natural killer cells. In a recent study, CXCR3 was expressed by both CD4$^+$ and CD8$^+$ dermal T cells in various inflammatory skin conditions, including CLE. CXCR3-activating chemokines CXL9, CXL10, and CXL11 were expressed at the dermoepidermal junction at sites where macrophages and lymphocytes were in close contact with the epidermis. The distribution patterns were different, with a patchy pattern and distribution around hair follicles in CLE. A strong correlation with ICAM-1 and HLA-DR expression was seen. IFN-γ induces CXR3-activating chemokines, ICAM-1, and HLA-DR (Flier et al. 2001).

A specific subset of γδ T cells has been observed in the epidermis of CCLE lesions but not in the blood, and the authors proposed that these cells were preferentially expanded within the epidermis (Volc-Platzer et al. 1993). γδ T cells recognize heat-shock proteins, and response by these cells to heat-shock proteins released from UV-injured keratinocytes has been suggested as a mechanism in UV-induced LE (Sontheimer 1996). In SLE, numbers of γδ T cells were lower in peripheral blood than in healthy controls, but the percentage of γδ T cells in clinically healthy skin of patients with SLE was twice as high as in healthy persons. A correlation with SLE activity was found (Robak et al. 2001). However, other authors did not find γδ T cells in the epidermis of patients with CLE (Fivensson et al. 1991), and all our biopsies from lesional skin were negative (F. Nyberg, E. Stephansson, unpublished observation).

A decreased number of epidermal Langerhans' cells is found in human CLE lesions (Andrews et al. 1986, Sontheimer and Bergstresser 1982) and during the induction of cell-mediated hypersensitivity reaction (Mommaas et al. 1993). Dermal dendritic macrophages (CD36$^+$), which infiltrate the human dermis after UVB irradiation (Meunier et al. 1995), associate with CD4$^+$ cells and are suggested to be pathogenically important in CLE lesions (Mori et al. 1994). They also activate human CD45RA$^+$ (suppressor inducer) cells (Baadsgard et al. 1988). A major proportion of inflammatory cells were CD45RA$^+$ cells in photo-provoked and spontaneous CLE lesions, but not in polymorphous light eruption (PLE); in serial biopsies, CD45RO$^+$ (helper inducer) cells tended to infiltrate the epidermis and subepidermal area earlier than CD45RA$^+$ and CD31$^+$ cells (Hasan et al. 1999). The authors concluded that CD45RA$^+$ cells may have a role in maintaining the CLE skin lesions by their ability to induce CD8$^+$ cells. CD8$^+$ cells have been found to mediate delayed-type hypersensitivity reactions (Kalish and Askenase 1999).

The binding of co-stimulatory molecules (B7 family) on antigen-presenting cells to their counterreceptors CD28 and CTLA-4 on T cells results in activated Th or cytotoxic T cells, which is required to optimally activate T cells and prevent antigen-specific tolerance (June et al. 1994, Werth et al. 1997). In situ expression of B7 and CD28 was examined in active skin lesions of patients with SLE, SCLE, and CCLE by immunohistochemical analysis and reverse transcription polymerase chain reaction. B7–1(CD80) and B7–2(CD86) were expressed on dermal and minimally on epidermal antigen-presenting cells and T cells but not on keratinocytes. These cells were able to bind CTLA-4 immunoglobulin in situ. CD28 was expressed by most T cells infiltrating the dermis and epidermis and was reduced during treatment (Denfeld et al. 1997). Plasmacytoid dendritic cell (PDC) precursors in peripheral blood produce large amounts of IFN-α/β when triggered by viruses. On stimulation with IL-3 and CD40 ligand, the same precursors differentiate into mature DCs that stimulate naive

CD4[+] T cells to produce Th2 cytokines. In a recent study, PDCs were present in human CLE lesions but not in normal skin, and the density of PDCs in affected skin correlated with the number of cells expressing the IFN-α/β-inducible protein MxA. This could suggest that PDCs produce IFN-α/β locally. Accumulation of PDCs coincided also with the expression of L-selectin on dermal vascular endothelium (Farkas et al. 2001).

A recent study showed dissociation of target organ disease in beta(2)-microglobulin–deficient MRL-Fas(lpr) mice: lupus skin lesions were accelerated, whereas nephritis was ameliorated. Beta(2)-microglobulin affects the expression of classic and nonclassic MHC molecules and thus prevents the normal development of CD8[−] as well as CD1-dependent NK1[+] T cells. The finding was not reproduced in CD1-deficient mice, excluding CD1[−] or NK1[+] T-cell-dependent mechanism. The authors conclude that regulation of autoimmunity can also occur at the target organ level (Chan et al. 2001).

Adhesion Molecules

A necessary step for lymphocytes to leave the blood vessel and migrate to the target organ, in this case the skin, is the expression of CAMs. CAMs are necessary for cell-cell and cell-matrix contact in inflammatory reactions (Chapman and Haskard 1995, McMurray 1996, Shiohara et al. 1992, Springer 1990).

ICAM-1 and vascular adhesion molecule-1 (VCAM-1) are members of the immunoglobulin gene superfamily and are induced or up-regulated on several cell types in the skin during inflammation. E-selectin is exclusively expressed by activated endothelial cells (Frenette and Wagner 1996). Soluble forms of these CAMs have been reported and are possibly related to disease activity in LE as well as many other neoplastic and inflammatory conditions (Gearing and Newman 1993).

CAMs in the Skin

ICAM-1 is an 85- to 110-kDa transmembrane glycoprotein mapped to human chromosome 19 and constitutively expressed by a variety of cells. Binding of ICAM-1 to its ligand, lymphocyte function-associated antigen 1, is the major pathway for keratinocytes and Langerhans' cells to interact with leukocytes and mediates both antigen-independent and antigen-dependent adhesion (Trefzer and Krutmann 1995). In addition, ICAM-1 has been shown to function as a receptor for human rhinoviruses ("common cold") (Greve et al. 1989, Staunton et al. 1989) and as an endothelial cell receptor for *Plasmodium falciparum* in malaria (Behrendt et al. 1989).

Keratinocytes normally express no or minimal ICAM-1, and this is regulated at the transcriptional level (Norris 1995). ICAM-1 can be induced or up-regulated by cytokines such as TNF-α, IL-1, and IFN-γ (Dustin et al., 1986) and by TNF-β (Krutmann et al. 1990, 1991). The responsiveness to cytokines that induce ICAM-1 transcription differs between tissues (Cornelius et al. 1993, 1994). An example of this different responsiveness is that IL-1 induces ICAM-1 on endothelial cells but, although debated, probably not on keratinocytes (Norris 1995, Trefzer and Krutmann 1995). ICAM-1 expression induced by TNF-α and IFN-γ is maximal in basal, undifferentiated keratinocytes. IFN-γ from dermal inflammatory cells and histamine from dermal mast cells are thought to influence basal ICAM-1 expression (Norris 1995).

Expression of CAMs on endothelial cells is essential for leukocyte margination, rolling, adhesion, and emigration from the bloodstream into tissue (Butcher 1991, Butcher et al. 1986, Shimizu et al. 1992).

VCAM-1 is minimally expressed on resting endothelial cells, but it is expressed by various cell types on activation. IL-1 and TNF-α but not UV light induces VCAM-1 on endothelial cells. The receptor for VCAM-1 is VLA-4 on monocytes and lymphocytes (Norris 1993).

E-selectin (115 kDa) is one of three proteins in the selectin family encoded on the long arm of human chromosome 1. E-selectin is only expressed by activated postcapillary venules (Rodhe et al. 1992) and shows specificity for skin homing T cells (Picker et al. 1991, Zimmerman et al. 1992).

Effects of UV Irradiation on CAMs

In the past decade, many researchers have studied the effect of UV irradiation on adhesion molecule expression, with possible clinical implications for photosensitive disorders such as CLE. A nuclear factor (NFκB) has been implicated by DNA sequencing as potential transcriptional activator for ICAM-1 (Muller et al. 1995), and it has been shown in vitro that UVB activates the NFκB in the cytosol of epidermal cells (Simon et al. 1994). A direct effect of UVA on transcription of the ICAM-1 gene has been shown via a singlet-oxygen-dependent mechanism (Grether-Beck et al. 1996). After UVB irradiation of cultured keratinocytes, a biphasic effect is seen on ICAM-1 expression, with suppression in the first 24 h and then up-regulation (Norris 1995). DNA photoproducts such as pyrimidine-dimers are directly involved in the UV-induced suppression of IFN-γ-induced ICAM-1 expression on keratinocytes (Krutmann et al. 1994).

In vitro studies have shown direct induction of ICAM-1 but not of VCAM-1 or E-selectin by UVB irradiation of cultured human dermal endothelial cells (Cornelius et al. 1994, Rhodes et al. 1996). Anti-double-stranded DNA has been shown to induce ICAM-1 and VCAM-1 but not E-selectin on cultured human umbilical vein endothelial cells, and increased levels of soluble ICAM-1 and VCAM-1 were also found in supernatants from the cell cultures (Lai et al. 1996).

PA Norris and coworkers reported in vivo sequential expression of CAMs in UVB-induced erythema compared with intracutaneous injection of purified protein derivative (PPD). E-selectin expression on endothelial cells was seen after 6 h in both reactions, with a prolonged expression (1 week) in the PPD reaction. PPD but not UVB induced basal keratinocyte ICAM-1 expression and VCAM-1 expression on stellate-shaped cells in the upper dermis, first seen at 24 h (Norris et al. 1991). In PLE, similar findings regarding CAM expression were found as after PPD injection, but keratinocyte ICAM-1 expression was strong already after 5 h, and VCAM-1 was expressed on perivascular cells (Norris et al. 1992). UVA irradiation in vivo on healthy skin increased endothelial ICAM-1 after 24 h, whereas ICAM-1 expression on cultured keratinocytes decreased after UVA but increased on cultured fibroblasts 6–48 h after irradiation. These authors also reported constitutive keratinocyte ICAM-1 expression (Treina et al. 1996), whereas most authors claim that keratinocytes normally do not express ICAM-1 in vivo (Trefzer and Krutmann 1995). In another study, both UVA and UVB induced endothelial ICAM-1 and E-selectin expression in vivo, but only UVA induced these molecules on cultured human dermal endothelial cells. The induction was dose dependent, peaking at 20 J/cm^2 for both molecules, and time dependent, peaking at 6 h for E-selectin and 24 h for ICAM-1 (Heckmann et al. 1994).

CAMs in Cutaneous Lupus Erythematosus

Different patterns of ICAM-1 expression in the epidermis have been documented in LE vs other cutaneous inflammation and also between subsets of LE. In experimentally UVA- and UVB-induced lesions in patients with LE and PLE, those with SCLE showed ICAM-1 expression throughout the epidermis, those with DLE showed basal ICAM-1 staining, and those with PLE showed focal basal ICAM-1 staining associated with lymphocyte infiltrates (Stephansson and Ros 1993). SCLE, erythema multiforme, and lichen planus showed diffuse ICAM-1 expression throughout the epidermis in SCLE, basal and focal suprabasal ICAM-1 expression in erythema multiforme, and ICAM-1 expression on basal keratinocytes in lichen planus. Virus, UVB, and perhaps other triggers of cytokine release or possibly of ICAM-1 directly were suggested to explain these different ICAM-1 expression patterns (Bennion et al. 1995). Another group found no significant differences in CAM expression patterns in biopsy samples from spontaneous CCLE and SCLE lesions; they found ICAM-1 expression on keratinocytes, dermal inflammatory cells, and endothelial cells in the LE lesions (Tebbe et al. 1994).

Endothelial VCAM-1 staining was increased in biopsy samples from LE lesions compared with scleroderma and morphea (Jones et al. 1996), and increased expression of VCAM-1 has been found in nonlesional skin in patients with SLE and correlated to disease activity (Belmont et al. 1994). Activated endothelium, perhaps associated with increased endothelial expression of nitric oxide synthase, has been proposed as a unifying hypothesis for the diverse nature of SLE vascular lesions (Belmont and Abramson 1997). Patients with LE display aberrant kinetics and a prolonged time course of the epidermal expression of inducible nitric oxide synthase after UV provocation (Kuhn et al. 1998).

To study possible differences in CAM expression in PLE vs different subsets of CLE, photoprovocation and serial biopsy samples were studied (Hasan et al. 1997, Nyberg et al. 1997, Nyberg et al. 1999). We found different expression patterns of ICAM-1, VCAM-1, and E-selectin in patients with SLE and SCLE compared with patients with DLE and patients with PLE in our serial biopsy samples from evolving UV-induced reactions (Figs. 19.1–19.5). Transient vs persistent skin reactions revealed differences especially regarding ICAM-1 expression by day 7. It is possible that these early differences indicate different control mechanisms in different UV radiation-induced skin lesions. Negative control of ICAM-1 is associated with the f-actin cytoskeleton network, and disruption of f-actin enhances cytokine-induced ICAM-1 transcription (Trefzer and Krutmann 1995). A possible interpretation of the findings that patients with SLE and SCLE show linear expression of ICAM-1 in the whole epidermis whereas patients with DLE show mostly focal, basal staining is that UV irradiation plays a more direct role in the induction of ICAM-1 in SLE and SCLE. In DLE, cytokines such as IFN-γ and TNF-α released from the dermal infiltrate on UV irradiation are more likely to

Figs. 19.1–19.5. Examples of expression patterns of cellular adhesion molecules (CAMs) in UV-induced skin lesions in patients with cutaneous lupus erythematosus (CLE). Cryostat sections, mouse monoclonal antibodies against intercellular adhesion molecule-1 (ICAM-1), E-selectin, and vascular adhesion molecule-1 (VCAM-1) (Vectastain Elite ABC)

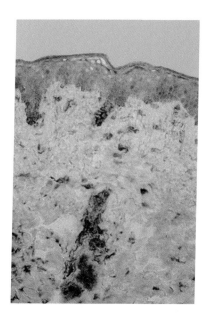

Fig. 19.1. Basal expression of ICAM-1 on keratinocytes and increased expression in the follicular epithelium. Endothelial cells and scattered inflammatory cells in the upper dermis express ICAM-1. UV-induced CLE lesion in a patient with chronic CLE (×250)

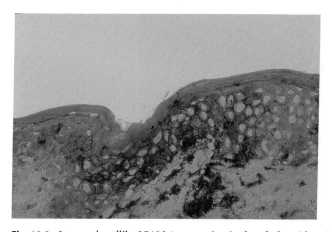

Fig. 19.2. Intense, bandlike ICAM-1 expression in the whole epidermis. UV-induced lesion in subacute CLE (×250)

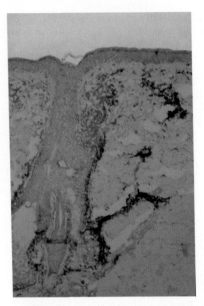

Fig. 19.3. Lymphocyte function-associated antigen 1-positive lymphocytes accumulating around hair follicle. UV-induced lesion in a patient with chronic CLE (×250)

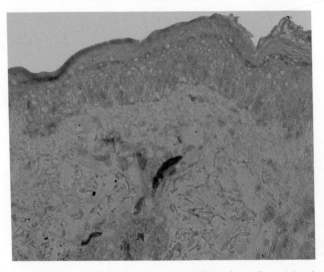

Fig. 19.4. E-selectin expression on upper dermal vessels. Staining is seen also without surrounding infiltrate. UV-induced lesion in a patient with chronic CLE (×250)

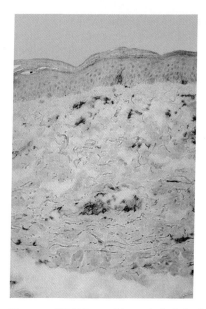

Fig. 19.5. VCAM-1 positive endothelial cells and some infiltrating cells in a patient with chronic CLE 14 days after UVB photoprovocation (×250)

induce the up-regulation of ICAM-1. Most UVB wavelengths do not penetrate the epidermis, and yet UVB induces reactions in the skin of patients with CCLE, perhaps indicating a role for the isomerization of *trans-* to *cis* urocanic acid, and the concomitant release of TNF-α. However, the *cis*-form of urocanic acid was found to be lower in light-protected skin of patients with DLE compared with patients with PLE and controls (Hasan et al. 1999). Our impression of biopsy samples from induced lesions in patients with LE is that the E-selectin-positive vessels are mostly found in upper and mid-dermis (data not shown). Endothelial CAMs were up-regulated also in nonlesional skin of our patients with LE in accordance with earlier studies in which it was suggested that activated endothelial cells are a common denominator for the diverse symptoms in LE (Belmont et al. 1994). VLA-4 (the counterreceptor for VCAM-1) and lymphocyte function–associated antigen 1 (the counterreceptor for ICAM-1) have been reported to be overexpressed on lymphocytes from patients with SLE, VLA-4 only in patients with vasculitis (Tsokos 1996).

Soluble CAMs

Circulating, soluble isoforms of CAMs are biologically active in that they retain their binding function (Seth et al. 1991). It is regarded as most likely that the circulating forms of ICAM-1 and E-selectin are proteolytically cleaved at the cell membrane (Leeuwenberg et al. 1992). Possible physiologic roles for soluble CAMs are inhibition of binding by competition, or that the shedding of surface molecules is a process that serves to down-regulate the adhesion of the relevant ligand (Gearing and Newman 1993, Trefzer and Krutmann 1995).

Elevated levels of soluble (s)E-selectin were found in serum samples from 25 patients with active, widespread CLE lesions and without systemic symptoms. Most patients had a history of PLE (Nyberg 1997, Nyberg and Stephansson 1999, Nyberg et al. 1997). E-selectin is a specific marker for activated endothelial cells, which indicates that endothelial cells play a more central role in CLE than previously assumed. E-selectin is mainly expressed on the luminar surface of cytokine-activated endothelium, only in postcapillary venules but not by arterioles (Walsh et al. 1990). Hence, the conflicting results reported on (s)E-selectin in patients with vasculitis (Mrowka and Sieberth 1994, Spronk et al. 1994) can be due to involvement of vessels with different calibers.

Increased levels of sICAM-1 and sVCAM-1 were found in patients with SLE and SCLE (Nyberg 1997, Nyberg and Stephansson 1999). Increased levels of VCAM-1 in SLE serum have been reported by several authors and have been correlated to disease activity (Mrowka and Sieberth 1994, 1995). In one study, VCAM-1 levels were elevated in patients with SLE and also in patients with DLE, although to a lesser extent than in those with SLE (Koide et al. 1996).

Soluble E-selectin might be useful clinically as an activity marker in CLE. Blocking of (s)E-selectin might be considered as possible therapy. An analogy is treatment with anti-ICAM-1 antibody that has decreased the rejection of skin grafts in experimental animal models (Trefzer and Krutmann 1995) and prevented neurologic symptoms and vasculitic skin lesions in SLE-prone mice (Brey et al. 1997).

Hypothetically, an altered CAM expression, induced by an unbalanced cytokine network brought about by an altered T-cell/B-cell repertoire in genetically susceptible individuals, could be a unifying concept for the related studies. It is possible, that studies of CAMs or certain subsets of T cells are useful in the evaluation of clinically doubtful, sunlight-induced cutaneous reactions.

References

Alaibac M, Morris J, Yu R, Chu A (1992) T lymphocytes bearing the gamma-delta T-cell receptor: a study in normal human skin and pathological skin conditions. Br J Dermatol 127: 458–462.

Andrews B, Schenk A, Barr R, Frious G, Mirick G, Ross P (1986) Immunopathology of cutaneous human lupus erythematosus defined by murine monoclonal antibodies. J Am Acad Dermatol 15:474–481

Baadsgard O, Fox D, Cooper K (1988) Human epidermal cells from ultraviolet light-exposed skin preferentially activate autoreactive CD4+2H4+ suppressor-inducer lymphocytes and CD8+ suppressor/cytotoxic lymphocytes. J Immunol 140:1738–1744

Behrendt A, Simmons D, Tansey J, Newbold C, Marsh K (1989) Intercellular adhesion molecule-1 is an endothelial cell receptor for plasmodium falciparum. Nature 341:57–59

Belmont H, Abramson S (1997) Mechanisms of acute inflammation and vascular injury in systemic lupus erythematosus. In: Pine J (ed) Dubois' lupus erythematosus. Baltimore, pp 263–278

Belmont M, Buyon J, Giorno R, Abramson S (1994) Up-regulation of endothelial cell adhesion molecules characterizes disease activity in systemic lupus erythematosus. The Shwartzman phenomenon revisited. Arthritis Rheum 37:376–383

Bennion S, Norris D (1997) Ultraviolet light modulation of autoantigens, epidermal cytokines and adhesion molecules as contributing factors of the pathogenesis of cutaneous LE. Lupus 6:181–192

Bennion S, Middleton M, David-Bajar K, Brice S, Norris DA (1995) In three types of interface dermatitis, different patterns of expression of intercellular adhesion molecule-1 indicate different triggers of disease. J Invest Dermatol 105:71S–79S

Blakemore A, Tarlow Y, Cork M, Gordon C, Emery P, Duff G (1994) Interleukin-1 receptor antagonist gene polymorphism as a disease severity factor of systemic lupus erythematosus. Arthritis Rheum 37:1380–1385

Bos J, Teunissen M, Cairo I, Krieg S, Kapsenberg M, Das P, Borst J (1990) T-cell receptor gamma-delta bearing cells in normal human skin. J Invest Dermatol 94:37–42

Brey R, Amato A, Kagan-Hallet K, Rhine C, Stallworth C (1997) Anti-intercellular adhesion molecule-1 (ICAM-1) antibody treatment prevents central and peripheral nervous system disease in autoimmune-prone mice. Lupus 6:645–651

Butcher E (1991) Leukocyte-endothelial cell recognition: three (or more) steps to specificity and diversity. Cell 67:1033–1036

Butcher E, Lewinsohn D, Duijvestijn A, Bargatze R, Wu N, Jalkanen S (1986) Interactions between endothelial cells and leukocytes. J Cell Biochem 30:121–131

Callen JP, Klein J (1988) Subacute cutaneous lupus erythematosus. Clinical, serologic, immunogenetic, and therapeutic considerations in seventy-two patients. Arthritis Rheum 31:1007–1013

Casciola-Rosen L, Rosen A (1997) Ultraviolet light-induced keratinocyte apoptosis: a potential mechanism for the induction of skin lesions and autoantibody production in LE. Lupus 6:175–180

Chan O, Paliwal V, McNiff J, Park S, Bendelac A, Shlomchik M (2001) Deficiency in beta(2)-microglobulin, but not CD1, accelerates spontaneous lupus skin disease while inhibiting nephritis in MRL-Fas(lpr) nice: an example of disease regulation at the organ level. J Immunol 167:2985–2990

Chapman P, Haskard DO (1995) Leukocyte adhesion molecules. Br Med Bull 51:296–311

Cornelius L, Taylor J, Degitz K, Li L, Lawley T, Caughman S (1993) A 5′ portion of the ICAM-1 gene confers tissue-specific differential expression levels and cytokine responsiveness. J Invest Dermatol 100:753–758

Cornelius L, Sepp N, Li L, Degitz K, Swerlick R, Lawley T, Caughman S (1994) Selective upregulation of intercellular adhesion molecule (ICAM-1) by ultraviolet B in human dermal microvascular endothelial cells. J Invest Dermatol 103:23–28

Denfeld R, Kind P, Sontheimer R, Schopf E, Simon J (1997) In situ expression of B7 and CD28 receptor families in skin lesions of patients with lupus erythematosus. Arthritis Rheum 40:814–821

Di Nuzzo S, Sylva-Steenland R, De Rie M, Das P, Bos J, Teunissen M (1998) UVB radiation preferentially induces recruitment of memory CD4+ cells in normal human skin: long term effect after a single exposure. J Invest Dermatol 110:978–981

Dustin M, Rothlein R, Bhan A, Dinarello C, Springer T (1986) Induction of IL-1 and interferon-gamma: tissue distribution, biochemistry, and function of a natural adherence molecule (ICAM-1). J Immunol 137:245–254

Farkas L, Beiske K, Lund-Johansen F, Brandtzaeg P, Jahnsen F (2001) Plasmacytoid dendritic cells (natural interferon- alpha/beta-producing cells) accumulate in cutaneous lupus erythematosus lesions. Am J Pathol 159:237–243

Fivensson D, Rheins L, Nordlund J, Pomaranski M, Douglass M, Krull E (1991) Thy-1 and T-cell receptor antigen expression in mycosis fungoides and benign inflammatory dermatoses. J Natl Cancer Inst 83:1088–1092

Flier J, Boorsma D, van Beek P, Nieboer C, Stoof T, Willemze R, Tensen C (2001) Differential expression of CXCR3 targeting chemokines CXCL10, CXCL9 and CXCL11 in different types of skin inflammation. J Pathol 194:398–405

Frenette PS, Wagner D (1996) Adhesion molecules – Parts I and II. N Engl J Med 334:1526–1529, 335:43–45

Furukawa F, Tokura Y, Matsushita K, Iwaskai-Inuzuka K, Onagi-Suzuki K, Yagi H, Wakita H, Takigawa M (1996) Selective expansions of T cells expressing Vβ8 and Vβ13 in skin lesions of patients with chronic cutaneous lupus erythematosus. J Dermatol 23:670–676

Gearing AJ, Newman W (1993) Circulating adhesion molecules in disease. Immunol Today 14:506–512

Grether-Beck S, Olaziola-Horn S, Schmitt H, Grewe M, Jahnke A, Johnson J, Briviba K, Sies H, Krutmann J (1996) Activation of transcription factor AP-2 mediates UVA radiation and singlet oxygen-induced expression of the human intercellular adhesion molecule 1 gene. Proc Natl Acad Sci U S A 93:14586–14591

Greve J, Favis G, Meyer A, Forte C, Yost S, Marlow C, Kamarck M, McClelland A (1989) The major human rhinovirus receptor is ICAM-1. Cell 56:839–847

Hasan T, Nyberg F, Stephansson E, Puska P, Häkkinen M, Sarna S, Ros AM, Ranki A (1997) Photosensitivity in lupus erythematosus, UV photoprovocation results compared with history of photosensitivity and clinical findings. Br J Dermatol 136:699–675

Hasan T, Pasanen P, Jansen C (1999) Epidermal urocanic acid in discoid lupus erythematosus. Acta Derm Venereol 79:411–412

Hasan T, Stephansson E, Ranki A (1999) Distribution of naive and memory T-cells in photoprovoked and spontaneous skin lesions of discoid lupus erythematosus and polymorphous light eruption. Acta Derm Venereol 79:437–442

Heckmann M, Eberlein-Konig B, Wollenberg A, Przybilla B, Plewig G (1994) Ultraviolet-A radiation induces adhesion molecule expression on human dermal microvascular endothelial cells. Br J Dermatol 131:311–318

Janeway C, Travers P (1994) Immunobiology, the immune system in health and disease. Current Biology/Garland Publishing, London/New York

Jerdan MS, Hood AF, Moore GW, Callen JP (1990) Histopathologic comparison of the subsets of lupus erythematosus. Arch Dermatol 126:52–55

Johansson-Stephansson E, Partanen J, Kariniemi A (1989) Subacute cutaneous lupus erythematous: genetic markers and clinical and immunological findings in patients. Arch Dermatol 125:791–796

Jones S, Mathew C, Dixey J, Lovell C, McHugh N (1996) VCAM-1 expression on endothelium in lesions from cutaneous lupus erythematosus is increased compared with systemic and localized scleroderma. Br J Dermatol 135:678–686

June C, Bluestone L, Thompson C (1994) The B7 and CD28 receptor families. Immunol Today 15:321–333

Kalish R, Askenase P (1999) Molecular mechanisms of CD8+ T cell-mediated delayed hypersensitivity: implications for allergies, asthma and autoimmunity. J Allergy Clin Immunol 103:192–199

Kita Y, Kuroda K, Mimori T (1998) T cell receptor clonotypes in skin lesions from patients with systemic lupus erythematosus. J Invest Dermatol 110:41–46

Koide M, Furukawa F, Wakita H, Tokura Y, Muso E, Takigawa M (1996) Soluble form of vascular cell adhesion molecule-1 in systemic lupus erythematosus and discoid lupus erythematosus. J Dermatol Science 12:73–75

Kristensson K, Borrebaeck C, Carlsson R (1992) Human CD4+ T cells expressing CD45RA acquire the lymphokine gene expression of CD45RO+ -helper cells after activation in vitro. Immunology 76:103–109

Krutmann J, Kock A, Schauer E, Parlow F, Moller A, Kapp A, Forster E, Schopf E, Luger T (1990) Tumor necrosis factor beta and ultraviolet radiation are potent regulators of human keratinocyte ICAM-1 expression. J Invest Dermatol 95:127–131

Krutmann J, Parlow F, Schopf E, Elmets C (1991) Posttranscriptional modification of ICAM-1 expression on human antigen presenting cells by ultraviolet B (UVB) radiation. Clin Res 39:1029

Krutmann J, Bohnert E, Jung G (1994) Evidence that DNA damage is a mediate in ultraviolet B radiation induced inhibition of human gene expression: ultraviolet B radiation effects on intercellular adhesion molecule-1 expression. 102:428–432

Kuhn A, Fehsel K, Lehmann P, Krutmann J, Ruzicka T, Kolb-Bachofen V (1998) Aberrant timing in epidermal expression of inducible nitric oxide synthase after UV irradiation in cutaneous lupus erythematosus. J Invest Dermatol 111:149–153

Lai K, Leung J, Lai K, Wong K, Lai C (1996) Upregulation of adhesion molecule expression on endothelial cells by anti-DNA autoantibodies in systemic lupus erythematosus. Clin Immunol Immunopathol 81:229–238

Lee L, Roberts C, Frank B, McCubbin V, Rice D, Reichlin M (1993) Autoantibody markers of cutaneous lupus erythematosus. J Invest Dermatol 100:573

Leeuwenberg JF, Neefjes JJ, Shaffer MA, Cinek T, Jenhomme TM, Hern TJ, Buurman WA (1992) E-selectin and intercellular adhesion molecule-1 are released by activated human endothelial cells in vitro. Immunology 77:543–549

McMurray R (1996) Adhesion molecules in autoimmune disease. Semin Arthritis Rheum 25:215–233

Meunier L, Bata-Csorgo Z, Cooper K (1995) In human dermis, ultraviolet radiation induces expansion of a CD36+ CD11b+ CD1– macrophage subset by infiltration and proliferation, CD1+ Langerhans-like dendritic antigen-presenting cells are concomitantly depleted. J Invest Dermatol 105:782–788

Mommaas A, Mulder A, Vermeer M, Boom B, Tseng C, Taylor J, Streilein J (1993) Ultrastructural studies bearing on the mechanism of UVB-impaired induction of the hypersensitivity to DNCB in man. Clin Exp Immunol 92:487–493

Mori M, Pimpinelli N, Romagnoli P, Bernacchi E, Fabbri P, Gianotti B (1994) Dendritic cells in cutaneous lupus erythematosus: a clue to the pathogenesisof lesions. Histopathology 24:311–321

Morimoto C, Letvin N, Boyd A, Hagan M, Brown H, Kornacki M, Schlossman S (1985a) The isolation and characterization of the human helper inducer T cell subset. J Immunol 134:3762–3769

Morimoto C, Letvin N, Distaso J, Aldrich W, Schlossman S (1985b) The isolation and characterization of the human suppressor inducer T-cell subset. J Immunol 134:1508–1515

Morimoto C, Schlossman S (1993) Human naive and memory T cells revisitetd: new markers (CD31 and CD27) that help define CD4+ subsets. Clin Exp Rheumatol 11:241–247

Morita A, Werfel T, Stege H, Ahrens C, Karmann K, Grewe M, Grether-Beck S, Ruzicka T, Kapp A, Klotz L, Sies H, Krutmann J (1997) Evidence that singlet-oxygen-induced human T-helper cell apoptosis is the basic mechanism of ultraviolet-A radiation phototherapy. J Exp Med 186:1763–1768

Mrowka C, Sieberth HG (1994) Circulating adhesion molecules ICAM-1, VCAM-1 and E-Selectin in systemic vasculitis: marked differences between Wegener's granulomatosis and systemic lupus erythematosus. Clin Investig 72:762–768

Mrowka C, Sieberth HG (1995) Detection of circulating adhesion molecules ICAM-1, VCAM-1 and E-Selectin in Wegener's granulomatosis, systemic lupus erythematosus and chronic renal failure. Clin Nephrol 43:288–296

Muller S, Kammerbauer C, Simons U, Shibagaki N, Li L-J, Caughman S, Degitz K (1995) Transcriptional regulation of intercellular adhesion molecule-1: PMA-Induction is mediated by NFKB. J Invest Dermatol 104:970–975

Norris D (1993) Pathomechanisms of photosensitive lupus erythematosus. J Invest Dermatol 100:58S–68S

Norris D (1995) Photoimmunology of lupus erythematosus. In: Krutmann J, Elmets CA (eds) Photoimmunology. Blackwell Science, Oxford, pp 209–227

Norris D, Bennion S, David-Bajar K (1997) Pathomechanisms of cutaneous lupus erythematosus. In: Wallace D, Hahn H (eds) Dubois' lupus erythematosus. Williams & Wilkins, Baltimore, pp 549–567

Norris P, Barker J, Allen M (1992) Adhesion molecule expression in polymorphic light eruption. J Invest Dermatol 99:504–508

Norris P, Poston RN, Thomas S, Thornhill M, Hawk J, Haskard O (1991) The expression of endothelial leukocyte adhesion molecule-1 (ELAM-1), intercellular adhesion molecule-1 (ICAM-1), and vascular cell adhesion molecule-1 (VCAM-1) in experimental cutaneous inflammation: a comparison of ultraviolet B erythema and delayed hypersensitivity. J Invest Dermatol 96:763–770

Nyberg F, Acevedo F, Stephansson E (1997) Different patterns of soluble adhesion molecules in systemic and cutaneous lupus erythematosus. Exp Dermatol 6:230–235

Nyberg F, Hasan T, Puska P, Stephansson E, Hakkinen M, Ranki A, Ros AM (1997) Occurrence of polymorphous light eruption in lupus erythematosus. Br J Dermatol 136:217–221

Nyberg F, Hasan T, Skoglund C, Stephansson E (1999) Early events in ultraviolet light-induced skin lesions in lupus erythematosus: expression patterns of adhesion molecules ICAM-1, VCAM-1 and E-selectin. Acta Derm Venereol 79:431–436

Nyberg F, Stephansson E (1999) Elevated soluble E-selectin in cutaneous lupus erythematosus. In: Mallia C, Uitto J (eds) Rheumaderm, current issues in rheumatology and dermatology. Kluwer Academic/Plenum Publishers, New York, pp 153–159

Orteu C, Sontheimer R, Dutz J (2001) The pathophysiology of photosensitivity in lupus erythematosus. Photoderm Photoimmunol Photomed 17:95–113

Picker L, Kishimoto T, Smith C, Warnock R, Butcher E (1991) ELAM-1 is an adhesion molecule for skin-homing T Cells. Nature 349:796–799

Prinz J, Meurer M, Reiter C, Rieber E, Plewig G, Riethmuller G (1996) Treatment of severe cutaneous lupus erythematosus with a chimeric CD4 monoclonal antibody, cM-T412. J Am Acad Dermatol 34:244-252

Rhodes L, Joyce M, West D, Strickland I, Friedmann P (1996) Comparison of changes in endothelial adhesion molecule expression following UVB irradiation of skin and a human microvascular cell line (HMEC-1). Photodermatol Photoimmunol Photomed 12:114–121

Robak E, Niewiadomska H, Robak T, Bartkowiak J, Blonski J, Wozniacka A, Pomorski L, Sysa-Jedrzejowska A (2001) Lymphocytes T-gamma-delta in clinically normal skin and peripheral blood of patients with systemic lupus erythematosus and their correlation with disease activity. Mediators Inflamm 10:179–189

Rohde D, Schluter-Wigger W, Mielke V, von den Driesch P, von Gaudecker B, Sterry W (1992) Infiltration of both T cells and neutrophils in the skin is accompanied by the expression of endothelial leukocyte adhesion molecule-1 (ELAM-1): an immunohistochemical and ultrastructural study. J Invest Dermatol 98:794–799

Seth R, Raymond F, Makgoba M (1991) Circulating ICAM-1 isoforms: diagnostic prospects for inflammatory and immune disorders. Lancet 338:83–84

Shimizu Y, Newman W, Tanaka, Shaw S (1992) Lymphocyte interactions with endothelial cells. Immunol Today 13:106–112

Shiohara T, Moriya N, Nagashima M (1992) Induction and control of lichenoid tissue reactions. Springer Semin Immunopathol 13:369–385

Simon MM, Aragane Y, Schwarz A, Luger TA, Schwarz T (1994) UVB light induces nuclear factor kappa B (NF kappa B) activity independently from chromosomal DNA damage in cell-free cytosolic extracts. J Invest Dermatol 102:422–427

Sontheimer RD (1996) Photoimmunology of lupus erythematosus and dermatomyositis: a speculative review. Photochem Photobiol 63:583–594

Sontheimer RD, Bergstresser PR (1982) Epidermal Langerhans cell involvement in cutaneous lupus erythematosus. J Invest Dermatol 79:237–243

Sontheimer RD, Maddison PJ, Reichlin M, Jordon RE, Stastny P, Gilliam JN (1982) Serologic and HLA associations of subacute cutaneous lupus erythematosus, a clinical subset of lupus erythematosus. Ann Intern Med 97:664–671

Springer TA (1990) Adhesion receptors of the immune system. Nature 346:425–434

Spronk P, Ootsma H, Huitema M, Limburg P, Kallenberg M (1994) Levels of soluble VCAM-1, soluble ICAM-1 and soluble E-Selectin during disease exacerbations in patients with systemic lupus erythematosus (SLE): a long time prospective study. Clin Exp Immunol 97:439–444

Staunton D, Merluzzi V, Rothlein R, Barton R, Marlin S, Springer T (1989) A cell adhesion molecule, ICAM-1, is the major surface receptor for rhinoviruses. Cell 56:849–853

Stein L, Saed G, Fivensson D (1997) T-Cell cytokine network in cutaneous lupus erythematosus. J Am Acad Dermatol 37:191–196

Stephansson E, Ros AM (1993) Expression of ICAM-1 and OKM-5 in patients with LE and PMLE. Arch Dermatol Res 285:328–222

Stevens G, Bergstresser P (1998) Photoimmunology. In: Hawk J (ed) Photodermatology. Chapman & Hall, London, pp 53–67

Sugerman P, Bigby M (2000) Preliminary functional analysis of human epidermal T cells. Arch Dermatol Res 292:9–15

Tebbe B, Mazur L, Stadler R, Orfanos C (1994) Immunohistochemical analysis of chronic discoid and subacute cutaneous lupus erythematosus – relation to immunopathological mechanisms. Br J Dermatol 132:25–31

Torimoto Y, Rothstein DM, Dang NH, Schlossman SF, Morimoto C (1992) CD31, a novel cell surface marker for CD4 cells of suppressor lineage, unaltered by state of activation. J Immunol 148:388–396

Trefzer U, Krutmann J (1995) Adhesion molecules as molecular targets in ultraviolet B radiation (290–315 nm)-induced immunomodulation: UVB radiation effects on the expression of intercellular adhesion molecule-1 in human cells. In: Krutmann J, Elmets C (eds) Photoimmunology. Blackwell Science, Berlin, pp 77–89

Treina G, Scaletta C, Fourtainer A, Seité S, Frenk E, Applegate L (1996) Expression of intercellular adhesion molecule-1 in UVA-irradiated human skin cells in vitro and in vivo. Br J Dermatol 135:241–247

Tsokos G (1996) Lymphocytes, cytokines, inflammation and immune trafficking. Curr Opin Rheumatol 8:395–402

Tsokos G, Liossis S (1998) Lymphocytes, cytokines, inflammation, and immune trafficking. Curr Opin Rheumatol 10:417–425

Walsh LJ, Lavker RM, Murphy GF (1990) Determinants of immune cell trafficking in the skin. Lab Investig 63:592–600

Wangel A, Johansson E, Ranki A (1984) Polyclonal B-cell activation and increased lymphocyte helper-suppressor ratios in discoid lupus erythematosus. Br J Dermatol 110:665–669

Velthuis PJ, van Weelden H, van Wichen D, Baart de la Faille H (1990) Immunohistopathology of light-induced skin lesions in lupus erythematosus. Acta Derm Venereol 70:93–98

Viljaranta S, Ranki A, Kariniemi A, Nieminen P, Johansson E (1987) Distribution of natural killer cells and lymphocyte subclasses in Jessner's lymphocytic infiltration of the skin and in cutaneous lesions of discoid and systemic lupus erythematosus. Br J Dermatol 116:831–838

Volc-Platzer B, Anegg B, Milota S, Pickl W, Fischer G (1993) Accumulation of gamma-delta T cells in chronic cutaneous lupus erythematosus. J Invest Dermatol 100:84S–91S

Werth V, Dutz J, Sontheimer R (1997) Pathogenetic mechanisms and treatment of cutaneous lupus erythematosus. Curr Opin Rheumatol 9:400–409

Wilson A, de Vries N, Pociot F, di Giovine F, van der Putte L, Duff G (1993) An allelic polymorphism within the human tumor necrosis factor alpha promoter region is strongly associated with HLA A1, 8 and DR3 alleles. J Exp Med 177:557–560

Wilson A, Duff G (1995) Malaria or systemic lupus erythematosus? BMJ 310:1482–1483

Zimmerman G, Prescott S, McIntyre T (1992) Endothelial cell interactions with granulocytes: tethering and signaling molecules. Immunol Today 13:93–99

CHAPTER 20

The Role of Dendritic Cells in Cutaneous Lupus Erythematosus

ANDREAS WOLLENBERG, STEFANIE WETZEL

Lupus erythematosus (LE) is an autoimmune disorder associated with specific and nonspecific skin lesions, UV sensitivity, anti-DNA antibodies, and increased interferon (IFN)-α/β production. Although the histopathology of LE is well defined, the pathogenesis of skin lesions in LE is still insufficiently understood and does not explain all the clinical aspects of LE. Approximately 55% of patients with systemic LE (SLE) develop clinically distinctive skin lesions, whereas patients with specific LE skin disease, such as subacute cutaneous LE (SCLE) or chronic discoid LE, may never develop systemic manifestations (Dubois and Tuffanelli 1964). LE is considered an autoimmune disease. Because several autoimmune processes have been described in LE, it also has been assumed that the cutaneous lesions are based on an autoimmune etiology.

Dendritic cells (DCs) of the skin are believed to present relevant autoantigens to T cells, thus starting the unwanted immune responses of CLE. Several studies have investigated and found alterations in DCs in the skin lesions of LE. This chapter covers our current knowledge of the different types of DCs in the pathogenesis of CLE.

An Introduction to Cutaneous DCs

DCs, a growing family of morphologically and functionally defined cells, can be found in small percentages in most organs of the human body and may be further divided into a myeloid and a lymphoid type (Banchereau et al. 1998, Steinman 1991). DCs are considered to be the most potent antigen-presenting cells (APCs) of the human body and are capable of initiating both primary and secondary immune responses. The term "dendritic cells" was coined in 1973, when Steinmann et al. (Steinman et al. 1973) described a novel cell population in murine spleen cell suspensions. As a rule, T cells require efficient stimulation by APCs to become effector cells and to become involved in pathophysiologic processes. DCs originate from bone marrow precursors and are found in small amounts in most organs of the human body. Studies have shown that DCs can differentiate in vitro from human blood monocytes (Sallusto and Lanzavecchia 1994).

Two major DC types are found in normal human skin: epidermal Langerhans' cells (LCs) and dermal DCs (DDCs). In contrast, inflammatory skin may harbor considerable numbers of two additional major types of DCs: inflammatory dendritic epidermal cells (IDECs) and plasmocytoid DCs (PDCs) (Wollenberg et al. 1996, 2002) (Fig. 20.1). Although LCs, IDECs, and PDCs are well-defined entities, the pool of DDCs probably comprises a heterogenous mixture of different cell types. In addition, any

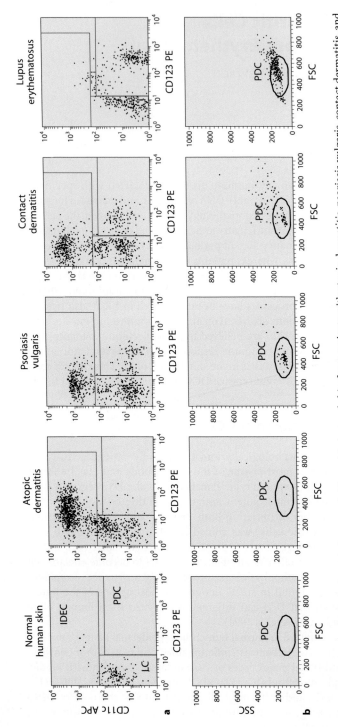

Fig. 20.1a, b. PDCs, LCs, and IDECs in normal skin and in lesional skin from patients with atopic dermatitis, psoriasis vulgaris, contact dermatitis, and lupus erythematosus. Epidermal single cell suspensions were prepared from biopsies of normal skin and of lesional skin from patients with atopic dermatitis, psoriasis vulgaris, contact dermatitis, and lupus erythematosus. **a** Subsets of DCs (PDCs, IDECs, and LCs) were quantified by four-color-staining with HLA-DR (PerCP), lineage markers (FITC), CD11c (APC), and CD123 (PE). **b** The identity of PDCs is confirmed by the FSC and SSC characteristics known from peripheral blood derived PDCs (modified from Wollenberg et al. 2002). APCs, antigen presenting cells; DCs, dendritic cells; FITC, fluoresceinisothiocyanate; FSC, forward light scatter; IDECs, inflammatory dendritic epidermal cells; LCs, Langerhans' cells; PDCs, plasmacytoid dendritic cells; PE, phycoerythrine; SSC, side light scatter

epidermal nonkeratinocyte without cytoplasmic features such as melanosomes, Birbeck granules, or Merkel cell granules may be labeled as "indeterminate cells" (Breathnach 1975). In normal skin, indeterminate cells are rare.

Langerhans' Cells

LCs were discovered by Paul Langerhans in 1868 when he applied a gold chloride stain to cutaneous tissue. Based on the available knowledge, he considered them to be of neural origin because of their dendritic shape (Langerhans 1868). Later, LCs were recognized as professional APCs capable of initiating primary and secondary responses in the skin immune system (Silberberg-Sinakin et al. 1976). Today, LCs are considered the prototype of immature DCs and represent the only major DC type in the normal human epidermis (Wollenberg and Bieber 2002).

Definition

LCs are defined as bone marrow-derived, epidermally located, dendritically shaped, Birbeck granule-containing APCs that express CD1a and major histocompatibility complex (MHC) class II molecules (Wollenberg and Bieber 2002). They are regarded as the prototype of immature skin DCs and are subclassified as myeloid DCs. LCs are located in the basal and suprabasal layers of the normal, uninflamed epidermis and are regarded as the first barrier of the skin toward the environment. All antigens penetrating the human body as well as locally produced self-antigens have to pass this first immunologic wall of defense. A small percentage of Birbeck granule-positive CD1a-expressing DCs can also be found in the dermis and are considered to be migrating LCs (Meunier et al. 1993).

Distribution

The distribution of LCs in normal human skin is homogenous at a density of approximately 450/mm^2 along the entire body; only the palms and soles show lower cell densities of approximately 60/mm^2 (Berman et al. 1983). In normal human skin, LC frequency varies between 0.5% and 2.0% of all epidermal cells (Wollenberg and Bieber 2002).

The number of LCs is decreased in lesional skin of patients with LE compared with their nonlesional or perilesional skin, other inflammatory skin diseases, or normal skin (Bos et al. 1986, Shiohara et al. 1988, Sontheimer and Bergstresser 1982, Wollenberg et al. 2002). In another study, LCs were found to be reduced only in atrophic areas of the lesions (Mori et al. 1994). In perilesional epidermis, the numbers of CD1a$^+$ and HLA-DR$^+$ DCs are similar or identical to those in normal skin of healthy individuals (Mori et al. 1994).

Light sensitivity is an important clinical characteristic of LE, which is mirrored by immunohistochemical abnormalities after light irradiation. In the lesional epidermis of patients with light-induced LE and patients with polymorphous light eruption, the number of CD1a$^+$ cells is diminished compared with that in nonirradiated skin (Velthuis et al. 1990). Although a relatively high number of DCs is found in the dermis of patients with polymorphous light eruption, only a small number of LCs is seen in light-induced LE lesions (Velthuis et al. 1990).

Other skin diseases with reduced LC numbers include chronic graft-vs-host disease, sarcoidosis, and acquired immunodeficiency syndrome (Aractingi et al. 1997, Belsito et al. 1984, Fox et al. 1983). In graft-vs-host disease, the reduced number of LCs may imply an attack by donor T cells (Suitters and Lampert 1983). The increase in CD1a-expressing epidermal DCs in inflammatory skin diseases such as atopic dermatitis and psoriasis, which has frequently been attributed to LC, is due to IDECs, a non-LC DC population (Wollenberg et al. 1999). Immunosuppressive treatment such as glucocorticosteroids or psoralen-UVA therapy may reduce LC numbers in the epidermis (Ashworth et al. 1989, Berman et al. 1983).

Ultrastructure

On electron microscopic analysis, LCs appear as dendritically shaped cells with a clear cytoplasm and a lobulated nucleus. The cytoplasm of LCs contains the specific tennis racket-shaped organelles with the characteristic trilamellar handle known as LC granules or Birbeck granules (Birbeck et al. 1961). Desmosomes and other identifying cytoplasmic features such as melanosomes or Merkel cell granules are absent. Birbeck granules contain the LAG antigen CD207, which is a 40-kDa glycoprotein that can be stained with the monoclonal LAG antibody (Kashihara et al. 1986). The function of the Birbeck granules is still unknown, but they may play a role in the antigen-presenting function of LCs.

Immunophenotype

The immunophenotype of LCs has been studied extensively in normal and inflamed skin by us and others using immunohistochemistry and flow cytometry. It is important to distinguish between normal and inflamed human skin because the immunophenotype of LC is subject to highly complex regulatory mechanisms: (a) freshly isolated LC change their phenotype (and function) during short-term culture toward highly stimulatory mature DCs, (b) the inflammatory microenvironment as such alters the immunophenotype of the LC in situ, and (c) in some skin diseases, for example, atopic dermatitis, a subset of membrane receptors shows evidence for disease-specific regulation (Wollenberg et al. 1999).

A variety of immunoglobulin receptors, MHC class I and class II molecules, and multiple adhesion molecules are the immunophenotypic hallmark of normal LCs. The nonclassic MHC class Ib molecule CD1a is regarded as the most specific LC marker for normal human skin currently available (Fithian et al. 1981). This does not apply to inflammatory skin conditions because another CD1a-expressing population cell (IDEC) is present in the epidermis and may be mistaken for LCs (Wollenberg et al. 1996).

In the lesional epidermis of LE, a reduction in HLA-DR$^+$ DCs compared with CD1a$^+$ cells suggests reduced expression of HLA-DR antigen by CD1a$^+$ DCs (Mori et al. 1994, Sontheimer and Bergstresser 1982). In vivo studies of LCs in LE show altered morphologic characteristics when examined by cell surface ATPase activity, HLA-DR antigens, and OKT-6 antigens (Sontheimer and Bergstresser 1982). The most important of these changes were reduced surface density, loss of dendritic processes, and bizarre shapes (Sontheimer and Bergstresser 1982). The morphologic and density alterations are said not to be associated with a decreased alloantigen-presenting capacity of LCs. Yet, a newer study revealed a diminished T-cell stimulatory capacity in the allogeneic mixed lymphocyte reaction in DC-enriched APCs from patients with SLE compared with healthy individuals (Scheinecker et al. 2001).

Function

After antigen uptake in the epidermis, LCs migrate into the T-cell areas of the lymph nodes, where they present their antigens to the T cells. The considerable changes in the immunophenotype, which occur during this migration in vivo, may be studied in vitro by investigating freshly isolated cells during short-term culture (Romani et al. 1989). Although LCs lose their characteristic BG and CD1a expression, several other surface molecules required for the initiation of immune responses are expressed de novo. This involves the up-regulation of MHC class I and II molecules, of adhesion molecules (e. g., intercellular adhesion molecule-1), and of co-stimulatory molecules such as CD80 and CD86 (Romani et al. 1989, Schuller et al. 2001, Teunissen et al. 1990).

LCs may play a role in the pathogenesis of LE (Bos et al. 1986, Mori et al. 1994, Sontheimer and Bergstresser 1982), atopic dermatitis (Bruynzeel-Koomen et al. 1986), allergic contact eczema (Silberberg et al. 1973), psoriasis vulgaris (Bos et al. 1983), and mycosis fungoides (Pimpinelli et al. 1994) by presentation of (auto)antigens to T cells.

Outlook

At present, it is not clear which factors reduce the number of LCs in the skin lesions of LE and whether this decrease causes any of the clinical and histologic features of CLE. The possible significance of other DC types remains to be demonstrated.

Dermal DCs

Definition

In 1986, Headington (Headington 1986) described the dermal dendrocyte as DCs of the human dermis. These DDCs appear nowadays as an ill-defined, probably heterogenous, dendritically shaped cell type within the dermal compartment exhibiting a considerable degree of immunophenotypic and functional heterogeneity. Some aspects of DDCs have been studied, for example, in psoriasis (Nestle et al. 1994), but no general or unifying concept of DDC biology has been established. The role of DDCs in the pathogenesis of inflammatory skin diseases is currently unclear.

Distribution

DDCs are located in the papillary dermis predominantly around the capillary vessels (Teunissen et al. 1997). In lesional dermis of LE, DDCs can be present in higher numbers than in perilesional dermis or normal skin (Mori et al. 1994).

Ultrastructure

The ultrastructure of DDCs shows a dendritic shape but no Birbeck granules. In other aspects, they mostly resemble IDECs. Whereas DDCs exhibit a dendritic profile in two-dimensional sections, three-dimensional sections reveal the protrusion of thin membrane flaps.

Immunophenotype

Characteristically, DDCs express the blood clotting enzyme factor XIII (Cerio et al. 1990) and several surface markers, such as HLA-DR, but lack the typical LC markers CD1a, Birbeck granules, and ATPase, suggesting a closer relation of DDCs to macrophages than to other DCs (Headington 1986, Teunissen et al. 1997).

Another more detailed study showed that normal skin contains at least three separate populations of DDCs by immunophenotypic analysis using a broad panel of 45 different antibodies based on the expression of blood clotting enzyme factor XIIIa that have distinctive phenotypic markers and immunologic capabilities (Nestle et al. 1993). By triple color staining, the relative distribution of factor XIIIa+ DDCs is as follows: subset 1 (65%–70% of total DDCs) expresses neither CD1a nor CD14; subset 2 (15%–20% of total DDCs) expresses CD1a but not CD14, and subset 3 (10%–15% of total DDCs) expresses CD14 but not CD1a.

Function

A major function of DDCs is their capacity to phagocytose large antigen-antibody complexes. This extensive phagocytic function is also demonstrated by their capacity to take up carbon particles, hemosiderin, or melanin and distinguishes them from LCs (Headington 1986).

The function of DDCs in the pathogenesis of LE is unclear. In psoriasis plaques, many DDCs have been identified that were able to induce T helper (Th) 1–type cytokines on phytohemagglutinin (PHA) addition, suggesting an important autostimulatory capacity (Nestle et al. 1994).

Inflammatory Dendritic Epidermal Cells

IDECs are a non-LC DC population that accumulates in the inflamed epidermis and is best characterized in atopic dermatitis skin. These cells have been observed for many years by different research groups (Baadsgaard et al. 1987, Bani et al. 1988, Taylor et al. 1991), but ultrastructural and immunophenotypic delineation of LCs and IDECs as two different cell types has been achieved only recently in atopic dermatitis (Wollenberg et al. 1996).

Definition

IDECs are defined as epidermally located, dendritically shaped cells with moderate CD1a but high CD11b expression that lack the LC-specific Birbeck granules (Wollenberg et al. 1996). IDECs may be regarded as a well-characterized subset of indeterminate cells. IDECs have been described in many inflammatory skin diseases but do not reach significant numbers in normal human epidermis. The ontogenesis of IDECs is unclear, but there is indirect evidence for a monocyte-derived origin of these cells.

Distribution

Whereas LCs are resident DCs of the epidermis, IDECs are assumed to migrate de novo in the epidermis after chemotactic stimuli (Wollenberg and Bieber 2002). IDECs typically represent 30%–80% of the total epidermal DCs in inflammatory skin diseases such as atopic dermatitis, psoriasis, and contact dermatitis but are almost absent in lesional skin of patients with LE (Wollenberg et al. 1996, 2002). The reduced number of LCs and IDECs in LE may result from an attack of cytotoxic T cells, but the exact cause is unknown.

Ultrastructure

The ultrastructure of IDECs shows a clear cytoplasm and a lobulated nucleus but no Birbeck granules, melanosomes, Merkel cell granules, or desmosomes (Wollenberg et al. 1996). Consequently, the immunohistochemical or flow cytometric analysis of epidermal DCs for the Birbeck granule–specific Langerin (LAG antigen, CD207) represents an alternative technique to the ultrastructural analysis for delineation of IDECs and LCs (Wollenberg et al. 1996). Close to the cell membrane, IDECs show areas with numerous coated pits and coated and uncoated vesicles. These seem to be fusing with endosomes, thus confirming the endocytotic activity (Wollenberg et al. 2002).

Immunophenotype

The immunophenotype of IDEC has been thoroughly investigated and includes Fc receptors, MHC molecules, adhesion molecules, chemokine receptors, co-stimulatory molecules, the thrombospondin receptor CD36, and the mannose receptor CD206. All IDECs express moderate CD1a but high CD11b and CD11 c levels (Bieber et al. 2000, Wollenberg et al. 1996). Based on the results of these experiments, IDECs resemble the immunophenotype of immature myeloid DCs of the interstitial type (Banchereau et al. 1998). Thus, all essential structures for DC function have been identified on IDECs.

Some key features of epidermal DCs in atopic dermatitis lesions, such as in situ IgE binding and expression of the high-affinity IgE receptor FcεRI, are shared by IDECs and LCs (Wollenberg et al. 1999). The demonstration of IgE molecules on the surface of epidermal DCs, which has initially been attributed to the LC population, is in fact mostly due to the IDECs and the fact that IDECs and not LCs are the relevant FcεRI-expressing epidermal DC population in the epidermis (Wollenberg and Bieber 2002). The same holds true for the expression of the co-stimulatory molecules CD80 and CD86 (Schuller et al. 2001).

Phenotypic analysis of IDECs in LE is hampered by the striking scarcity of IDECs in LE, which may be due to either lack of selective chemotactic recruitment or IDEC-specific apoptosis in LE lesions (Wollenberg et al. 1996, 2002).

Function

Functional aspects of IDECs have been investigated in atopic dermatitis by different research groups, but there are no data or evidence for a direct functional role of IDECs in LE at this time.

Plasmacytoid Dendritic Cells

Definition

PDCs are a distinct DC subset best characterized in human peripheral blood. These cells produce large amounts of type 1 IFN (IFN-α and IFN-β) on recognition of viral infection and thus are important players in the antiviral defense strategy of the immune system (Cella et al. 1999, Siegal et al. 1999).

PDCs were originally described as plasmacytoid T cells or plasmacytoid monocytes (Facchetti et al. 1988) and are identical to the "natural type 1 IFN-producing cell" (Cella et al. 1999, Siegal et al. 1999) described many years ago as a rare CD4$^+$/MHC II$^+$ population (Abb et al. 1983, Chehimi et al. 1989, Fitzgerald-Bocarsly et al. 1993). On maturation, this cell type develops characteristic features of DCs (Cella et al. 1999, Siegal et al. 1999).

There are hints that PDCs may be involved in the pathogenesis of LE (Ronnblom et al. 2001), allergy (Jahnsen et al. 2000), viral infections (Feldman et al. 2001), and cancer (Zou et al. 2001).

Distribution

Low percentages of PDCs circulate in the human peripheral blood ($< 0.3\%$) and also constitute a cell subset in organized lymphoid tissue. Under special conditions they may accumulate in the skin: PDCs apparently have the capacity to migrate into the inflammatory skin lesions of patients with LE, where they produce and secrete high amounts of type 1 IFN. PDCs are also present in skin lesions of patients with psoriasis and contact dermatitis, where they were demonstrated as frequently as in peripheral blood (Wollenberg et al. 2002). PDCs were reduced or absent in lesional skin of patients with atopic dermatitis and in normal skin (Wollenberg et al. 2002), whereas the PDC frequency is increased in peripheral blood of patients with atopic dermatitis.

In skin sections of LE, PDCs predominantly accumulate along the dermoepidermal junction, around hair follicles, and perivascularly (Farkas et al. 2001). Whereas the number of PDCs is decreased in peripheral blood of patients with LE, their numbers were increased in lesional skin of patients with LE, indicating their capacity to migrate into LE lesions, where they produce and secrete IFN-α (Farkas et al. 2001, Wollenberg et al. 2002).

There is an apparent dichotomy of PDC and IDEC accumulation in skin, which depends on the diagnosis. The extremes are, on the one hand, atopic dermatitis, with many IDECs and few if any PDCs, and, on the other hand, LE lesions, with a pronounced infiltrate of PDCs but very few IDECs (Wollenberg et al. 2002).

Immunophenotype

The simultaneous expression of cell surface antigens and intracellular IFN-α in herpes simples virus-stimulated PDCs was examined by flow cytometry. PDCs were confirmed to lack leukocyte lineage-specific markers and to express CD4, CD36, and HLA-DR (Svensson et al. 1996). Furthermore, high levels of CD44, CD45RA, and CD45RB and moderate levels of CD40, CD45R0, CD72, and CD83 were detected. Expression of CD13, CD33, and FcεRI was weak, whereas no CD5, CD11b, CD16, CD64, CD80, or CD86 was detected at all (Svensson et al. 1996). Today it is clear that the immunophenotype of PDCs somewhat resembles that of immunoglobulin-secreting plasma cells. Common gating strategies for PDCs from peripheral blood are based on a class II-positive (HLA-DR$^+$), lineage-negative (CD3$^-$, CD14$^-$, CD16$^-$, CD19$^-$, CD20$^-$, CD56$^-$), interleukin (IL)-3 receptor α-chain-positive (CD123$^+$), CD11 c$^-$ cell population (Wollenberg et al. 2002).

In skin sections of patients with discoid LE and SLE, PDCs are easily identified by their high expression of CD123 and HLA-DR and co-expression of CD45RA and CD68 (Farkas et al. 2001). The density of PDCs correlates with the presence of a high number of cells expressing the IFN-α- and IFN-β-inducible protein MxA (Farkas et al. 2001).

Flow cytometric detection of PDCs from different inflammatory skin lesions has recently been described and may be performed by gating strategies for either HLA-DR$^+$, lineage-negative, CD123$^+$, CD11 c-negative cells or for HLA-DR$^+$, lineage- negative, BDCA-2-positive cells (Wollenberg et al. 2002). The BDCA-2 antibody is directed against a recently identified C-type lectin, which is expressed weakly but very specifically on PDCs in peripheral blood and inflamed skin (Dzionek et al. 2001).

Function

PDCs may induce Th1- or Th2-predominated immune responses. In the presence of IL-3 and CD40 ligand, PDCs develop into mature DCs and induce naive T cells to produce Th2 cytokines (Rissoan et al. 1999). On the other hand, virus-triggered PDCs can induce a Th1 response by activating naive CD4$^+$ T cells to produce IFN-γ and IL-10 (Cella et al. 2000, Kadowaki et al. 2000). Thus, PDCs may play an important role in several inflammatory skin diseases.

Patients with LE have high systemic IFN-α levels that are associated with disease activity. PDCs have been proposed to be the main source of IFN-α in LE (Kim et al. 1987). Anti-double-stranded DNA antibodies in combination with immunostimulatory plasmid DNA mimic an endogenous IFN-α inducer in SLE (Vallin et al. 1999). PDCs have been found to produce IFN-α in response to plasmid DNA/anti-DNA-antibody complexes (Dzionek et al. 2001).

Considering the many immunoregulatory actions of IFN-α, prolonged endogenous production of this cytokine may be an important pathogenic factor in LE. Although IFN-γ modulates several immunologic processes, including inhibiting the granulocyte macrophage-colony-stimulating factor-induced expression of CD80 on LCs (Ozawa et al. 1996), it is not yet clear whether high levels of IFN-α may also have a direct effect on LCs. Although IFN-α-induced LE has not yet been described, SLE-like syndrome has been reported in a patient with malignant carcinoid tumor undergoing IFN-α therapy (Ronnblom et al. 1990).

High IL-10 levels, which may be secreted by PDC-stimulated CD4+ T cells, may also prevent the maturation of monocytes into DCs (Allavena et al. 1998).

Outlook on Lupus Erythematosus and DCs

Studies have confirmed the presence of large numbers of T lymphocytes in the dermis of LE (Synkowski et al. 1983). LCs are diminished and IDECs are almost absent in the epidermis of LE lesions. Instead, PDCs seem to accumulate in lesional epidermis and dermis (Farkas et al. 2001, Wollenberg et al. 2002). In the dermal compartment, DDC numbers are increased (Mori et al. 1994).

In terms of LE pathophysiology, PDCs may be regarded as the most interesting DC type because of their accumulation in the skin lesions of LE as well as their capability to produce type 1 IFN. It is unclear whether the decreased number of LCs and IDECs in the inflamed epidermis is causally linked with the epidermal accumulation of PDCs. Further investigations are warranted to clarify the complex and difficult interplay of several immunologic factors and cells in the pathogenesis of LE.

References

Abb J, Zander H, Abb H, Albert E, Deinhardt F (1983) Association of human leucocyte low responsiveness to inducers of interferon alpha with HLA-DR 2. Immunology 49:239–244

Allavena P, Piemonti L, Longoni D, Bernasconi S, Stoppacciaro A, Ruco L, Mantovani A (1998) IL-10 prevents the differentiation of monocytes to dendritic cells but promotes their maturation to macrophages. Eur J Immunol 28:359–369

Aractingi S, Gluckman E, Dauge-Geffroy MC, Le Goue C, Flahaut A, Dubertret L, Carosella E (1997) Langerhans' cells are depleted in chronic graft versus host disease. J Clin Pathol 50:305–309

Ashworth J, Kahan MC, Breathnach SM (1989) PUVA therapy decreases HLA-DR+ CDIa+ Langerhans cells and epidermal cell antigen-presenting capacity in human skin, but flow cytometrically-sorted residual HLA-DR+ CDIa+ Langerhans cells exhibit normal alloantigen-presenting function. Br J Dermatol 120:329–339

Baadsgaard O, Cooper KD, Lisby S, Wulf HC, Wantzin GL (1987) Dose response and time course for induction of T6- DR+ human epidermal antigen-presenting cells by in vivo ultraviolet A, B, and C irradiation. J Am Acad Dermatol 17:792–800

Banchereau J, Steinman RM, Wollenberg A, Kraft S, Hanau D, Bieber T (1998) Dendritic cells and the control of immunity. Nature 392:245–252

Bani D, Moretti S, Pimpinelli N, Gianotti B (1988) Differentiation of monocytes into Langerhans cells in human epidermis. An ultrastructural study. In: Thivolet J, Schmitt D (eds) The Langerhans cell. John Libbey Eurotext, Paris/London, pp 75–83

Belsito DV, Sanchez MR, Baer RL, Valentine F, Thorbecke GJ (1984) Reduced Langerhans' cell Ia antigen and ATPase activity in patients with the acquired immunodeficiency syndrome. N Engl J Med 310:1279–1282

Berman B, Chen VL, France DS, Dotz WI, Petroni G (1983) Anatomical mapping of epidermal Langerhans cell densities in adults. Br J Dermatol 109:553–558

Berman B, France DS, Martinelli GP, Hass A, Ashworth J, Kahan MC, Breathnach SM (1983) Modulation of expression of epidermal Langerhans cell properties following in situ exposure to glucocorticosteroids. J Invest Dermatol 80:168–171

Bieber T, Kraft S, Geiger E, Wollenberg A, Koch S, Novak N (2000) Fc epsilon RI expressing dendritic cells: the missing link in the pathophysiology of atopic dermatitis? J Dermatol 27:698–699

Birbeck M, Breathnach A, Everall J (1961) An electron microscopic study of basal melanocytes and high level clear cells (Langerhans cells) in vitiligo. J Invest Dermatol 37:51

Bos JD, Hulsebosch HJ, Krieg SR, Bakker PM, Cormane RH, Romagnoli P, Giannotti B (1983) Immunocompetent cells in psoriasis. In situ immunophenotyping by monoclonal antibodies. Arch Dermatol Res 275:181–189

Bos JD, van Garderen ID, Krieg SR, Poulter LW (1986) Different in situ distribution patterns of dendritic cells having Langerhans (T6+) and interdigitating (RFD1+) cell immunophenotype in psoriasis, atopic dermatitis, and other inflammatory dermatoses. J Invest Dermatol 87:358–361

Breathnach AS (1975) Aspects of epidermal ultrastructure. J Invest Dermatol 65:2–15

Bruynzeel-Koomen C, van Wichen DF, Toonstra J, Berrens L, Bruynzeel PL (1986) The presence of IgE molecules on epidermal Langerhans cells in patients with atopic dermatitis. Arch Dermatol Res 278:199–205

Cella M, Jarrossay D, Facchetti F, Alebardi O, Nakajima H, Lanzavecchia A, Colonna M (1999) Plasmacytoid monocytes migrate to inflamed lymph nodes and produce large amounts of type I interferon. Nat Med 5:919–923

Cella M, Facchetti F, Lanzavecchia A, Colonna M (2000) Plasmacytoid dendritic cells activated by influenza virus and CD40L drive a potent TH1 polarization. Nat Immunol 1:305–310

Cerio R, Spaull J, Oliver GF, Jones WE (1990) A study of factor XIIIa and MAC 387 immunolabeling in normal and pathological skin. Am J Dermatopathol 12:221–233

Chehimi J, Starr SE, Kawashima H, Miller DS, Trinchieri G, Perussia B, Bandyopadhyay S (1989) Dendritic cells and IFN-alpha-producing cells are two functionally distinct non-B, non-monocytic HLA-DR+ cell subsets in human peripheral blood. Immunology 68:488–490

Dubois E, Tuffanelli D (1964) Clinical manifestations of systemic lupus erythematosus. JAMA 190:104–111

Dzionek A, Sohma Y, Nagafune J, Cella M, Colonna M, Facchetti F, Gunther G, Johnston I, Lanzavecchia A, Nagasaka T, Okada T, Vermi W, Winkels G, Yamamoto T, Zysk M, Yamaguchi Y, Schmitz J (2001) BDCA-2, a novel plasmacytoid dendritic cell-specific type II C-type lectin, mediates antigen capture and is a potent inhibitor of interferon alpha/beta induction. J Exp Med 194:1823–1834

Facchetti F, De Wolf-Peeters C, van den Oord JJ, De vos R, Desmet VJ (1988) Plasmacytoid T cells: a cell population normally present in the reactive lymph node. An immunohistochemical and electronmicroscopic study. Hum Pathol 19:1085–1092

Farkas L, Beiske K, Lund-Johansen F, Brandtzaeg P, Jahnsen FL (2001) Plasmacytoid dendritic cells (natural interferon- alpha/beta-producing cells) accumulate in cutaneous lupus erythematosus lesions. Am J Pathol 159:237–243

Feldman S, Stein D, Amrute S, Denny T, Garcia Z, Kloser P, Sun Y, Megjugorac N, Fitzgerald-Bocarsly P (2001) Decreased interferon-alpha production in HIV-infected patients correlates with numerical and functional deficiencies in circulating type 2 dendritic cell precursors. Clin Immunol 101:201–210

Fithian E, Kung P, Goldstein G, Rubenfeld M, Fenoglio C, Edelson R (1981) Reactivity of Langerhans cells with hybridoma antibody. Proc Natl Acad Sci USA 78:2541–2544

Fitzgerald-Bocarsly P, Perussia B, Bandyopadhyay S (1993) Human natural interferon-alpha producing cells. Pharmacol Ther 60:39–62

Fox JL, Berman B, Teirstein AS, France DS, Reed ML (1983) Quantitation of cutaneous Langerhans cells of sarcoidosis patients. J Invest Dermatol 80:472–475

Headington J (1986) The dermal dendrocyte. In: Callen J, Dahl M, Golitz L, Rassumssen J, Stegmen S (eds) Advances in dermatology. Yearbook Medical, Chicago, IL, pp 159–171

Jahnsen FL, Lund-Johansen F, Dunne JF, Farkas L, Haye R, Brandtzaeg P (2000) Experimentally induced recruitment of plasmacytoid (CD123 high) dendritic cells in human nasal allergy. J Immunol 165:4062–4068

Kadowaki N, Antonenko S, Lau JY, Liu YJ (2000) Natural interferon alpha/beta-producing cells link innate and adaptive immunity. J Exp Med 192:219–226

Kashihara M, Ueda M, Horiguchi Y, Furukawa F, Hanaoka M, Imamura S (1986) A monoclonal antibody specifically reactive to human Langerhans cells. J Invest Dermatol 87:602–607

Kim T, Kanayama Y, Negoro N, Okamura M, Takeda T, Inoue T (1987) Serum levels of interferons in patients with systemic lupus erythematosus. Clin Exp Immunol 70:562–569

Langerhans P (1868) Über die Nerven der menschlichen Haut. Virchows Arch Path Anat 44:325

Meunier L, Gonzalez-Ramos A, Cooper KD (1993) Heterogeneous populations of class II MHC+ cells in human dermal cell suspensions. Identification of a small subset responsible for potent dermal antigen-presenting cell activity with features analogous to Langerhans cells. J Immunol 151:4067–4080

Mori M, Pimpinelli N, Romagnoli P, Bernacchi E, Fabbri P, Giannotti B (1994) Dendritic cells in cutaneous lupus erythematosus: a clue to the pathogenesis of lesions. Histopathology 24:311–321

Nestle FO, Zheng XG, Thompson CB, Turka LA, Nickoloff BJ (1993) Characterization of dermal dendritic cells obtained from normal human skin reveals phenotypic and functionally distinctive subsets. J Immunol 15:6535–6545

Nestle FO, Turka LA, Nickoloff BJ (1994) Characterization of dermal dendritic cells in psoriasis: autostimulation of T lymphocytes and induction of Th1 type cytokines. J Clin Invest 94: 202–209

Ozawa H, Aiba S, Nakagawa, Tagami H (1996) Interferon-gamma and interleukin-10 inhibit antigen presentation by Langerhans cells for T helper type 1 cells by suppressing their CD80 (B7–1) expression. Eur J Immunol 26:648–652

Pimpinelli N, Santucci M, Romagnoli P, Giannotti B (1994) Dendritic cells in T- and B-cell proliferation in the skin. Dermatol Clin 12:255–270

Rissoan MC, Soumelis V, Kadowaki N, Grouard G, Briere F, de Waal Malefyt R, Liu YJ (1999) Reciprocal control of T helper cell and dendritic cell differentiation. Science 283:1183–1186

Romani N, Lenz A, Glassel H, Stossel H, Stanzl U, Majdic O, Fritsch P, Schuler G (1989) Cultured human Langerhans cells resemble lymphoid dendritic cells in phenotype and function. J Invest Dermatol 93:600–609

Ronnblom LE, Alm GV, Oberg KE (1990) Possible induction of systemic lupus erythematosus by interferon-alpha treatment in a patient with a malignant carcinoid tumour. J Intern Med 227:207–210

Ronnblom L, Alm GV, Hemmi H, Takeuchi O, Kawai T, Kaisho T, Sato S, Sanjo H, Matsumoto M, Hoshino K, Wagner H, Takeda K, Akira S (2001) A pivotal role for the natural interferon alpha-producing cells (plasmacytoid dendritic cells) in the pathogenesis of lupus. J Exp Med 194:F59–63

Sallusto F, Lanzavecchia A (1994) Efficient presentation of soluble antigen by cultured human dendritic cells is maintained by granulocyte/macrophage colony stimulating factor plus interleukin 4 and downregulated by tumor necrosis factor alpha. J Exp Med 179:1109–1118

Scheinecker C, Zwolfer B, Koller M, Manner G, Smolen JS (2001) Alterations of dendritic cells in systemic lupus erythematosus: phenotypic and functional deficiencies. Arthritis Rheum 44:856–865

Schuller E, Teichmann B, Haberstok J, Moderer M, Bieber T, Wollenberg A (2001) In situ expression of the costimulatory molecules CD80 and CD86 on Langerhans cells and inflammatory dendritic epidermal cells (IDEC) in atopic dermatitis. Arch Dermatol Res 293:448–454

Shiohara T, Moriya N, Tanaka Y, Arai Y, Hayakawa J, Chiba M, Nagashima M (1988) Immunopathologic study of lichenoid skin diseases: correlation between HLA-DR-positive keratinocytes or Langerhans cells and epidermotropic T cells. J Am Acad Dermatol 18:67–74

Siegal FP, Kadowaki N, Shodell M, Fitzgerald-Bocarsly PA, Shah K, Ho S, Antonenko S, Liu YJ (1999) The nature of the principal type 1 interferon-producing cells in human blood. Science 284:1835–1837

Silberberg I, Pimpinelli N, Santucci M, Romagnoli P, Giannotti B (1973) Apposition of mononuclear cells to Langerhans cells in contact allergic reactions. An ultrastructural study. Acta Derm Venereol 53:1–12

Silberberg-Sinakin I, Thorbecke GJ, Baer RL, Rosenthal SA, Berezowsky V (1976) Antigen-bearing Langerhans cells in skin, dermal lymphatics and in lymph nodes. Cell Immunol 25:137–151

Sontheimer RD, Bergstresser PR (1982) Epidermal Langerhans cell involvement in cutaneous lupus erythematosus. J Invest Dermatol 79:237–243

Steinman RM (1991) The dendritic cell system and its role in immunogenicity. Annu Rev Immunol 9:271–296

Steinman RM, Kaplan G, Witmer MD, Cohn ZA (1973) Identification of a novel cell type in peripheral lymphoid organs of mice. V. Purification of spleen dendritic cells, new surface markers, and maintenance in vitro. J Exp Med 149:1–16

Suitters AJ, Lampert IA (1983) The loss of Ia$^+$ Langerhans' cells during graft-versus-host disease in rats. Transplantation 36:540–546

Svensson H, Johannisson A, Nikkila T, Alm GV, Cederblad B (1996) The cell surface phenotype of human natural interferon-alpha producing cells as determined by flow cytometry. Scand J Immunol 44:164–172

Synkowski DR, Provost TT, Norris DA, Lee LA (1983) Characterization of the inflammatory infiltrate in lupus erythematosus lesions using monoclonal antibodies. J Rheumatol 10:920–924

Taylor RS, Baadsgaard O, Hammerberg C, Cooper KD (1991) Hyperstimulatory CD1a$^+$CD1b$^+$CD36$^+$ Langerhans cells are responsible for increased autologous T lymphocyte reactivity to lesional epidermal cells of patients with atopic dermatitis. J Immunol 147:3794–3802

Teunissen MB, Wormmeester J, Krieg SR, Peters PJ, Vogels IM, Kapsenberg ML, Bos JD (1990) Human epidermal Langerhans cells undergo profound morphologic and phenotypical changes during in vitro culture. J Invest Dermatol 94:166–173

Teunissen M, Kapsenberg M, Bos J (1997) Langerhans cells and related skin dendritic cells. In: Bos J (ed) Skin immune system (SIS). CRC Press LLC, Boca Raton, FL

Vallin H, Perers A, Alm GV, Ronnblom L (1999) Anti-double-stranded DNA antibodies and immunostimulatory plasmid DNA in combination mimic the endogenous IFN-alpha inducer in systemic lupus erythematosus. J Immunol 163:6306–6313

Velthuis PJ, van Weelden H, van Wichen D, Baart de la Faille H (1990) Immunohistopathology of light-induced skin lesions in lupus erythematosus. Acta Derm Venereol 70:93–98

Wollenberg A, Bieber T (2002) Antigen-presenting cells. In: Bieber T, Leung D (eds) Atopic dermatitis. Marcel Dekker, New York, pp 267–283

Wollenberg A, Kraft S, Hanau D, Bieber T (1996) Immunomorphological and ultrastructural characterization of Langerhans cells and a novel, inflammatory dendritic epidermal cell (IDEC) population in lesional skin of atopic eczema. J Invest Dermatol 106:446–453

Wollenberg A, Wen S, Bieber T (1999) Phenotyping of epidermal dendritic cells: clinical applications of a flow cytometric micromethod. Cytometry 37:147–155

Wollenberg A, Mommaas M, Oppel T, Schottdorf EM, Gunther S, Moderer M (2002) Expression and function of the mannose receptor CD206 on epidermal dendritic cells in inflammatory skin diseases. J Invest Dermatol 118:327–334

Wollenberg A, Wagner M, Gunther S, Towarowski A, Tuma E, Moderer M, Rothenfusser S, Wetzel S, Endres S, Hartmann G (2002) Plasmacytoid dendritic cells: a new cutaneous dendritic cell subset with distinct role in inflammatory skin diseases. J Invest Dermatol 119:1096–1102

Zou W, Machelon V, Coulomb-L'Hermin A, Borvak J, Nome F, Isaeva T, Wei S, Krzysiek R, Durand-Gasselin I, Gordon A, Pustilnik T, Curiel DT, Galanaud P, Capron F, Emilie D, Curiel TJ (2001) Stromal-derived factor-1 in human tumors recruits and alters the function of plasmacytoid precursor dendritic cells. Nat Med 7:1339–1346

CHAPTER 21

Histologic Findings in Cutaneous Lupus Erythematosus

CHRISTIAN A. SANDER, AMIR S. YAZDI, MICHAEL J. FLAIG, PETER KIND

Lupus erythematosus (LE) is a chronic inflammatory disease that can be clinically divided into three major categories: chronic cutaneous LE (CCLE), subacute cutaneous LE (SCLE), and systemic LE (SLE). In general, LE represents a spectrum of disease with some overlap of these categories. Classification is based on clinical, histologic, serologic, and immunofluorescent (see Chap. 22) features. Consequently, histologic findings alone may not be sufficient for correct classification. In addition, these categories can be subdivided into numerous variants affecting different levels of the skin and subcutaneous tissue.

Chronic Cutaneous Lupus Erythematosus

Discoid Lupus Erythematosus

Discoid LE (DLE) is the most common form of LE. Clinically, the head and neck region is affected in most cases. On the face, there may be a butterfly distribution. However, in some cases, the trunk and upper extremities can be also involved. Lesions consist of erythematous scaly patches and plaques.

Histologically, in DLE the epidermis and dermis are affected, and the subcutaneous tissue is usually spared. However, patchy infiltrates may be present. Characteristic microscopic features are hyperkeratosis with follicular plugging, thinning, and flattening of the epithelium and hydropic degeneration of the basal layer (liquefaction degeneration) (Fig. 21.1). In addition, there are scattered apoptotic keratinocytes (Civatte bodies) in the basal layer or in the epithelium. Particularly in older lesions, thickening of the basement membrane becomes obvious in the periodic acid-Schiff stain. In the dermis, there is a lichenoid or patchy lymphocytic infiltrate with accentuation of the pilosebaceous follicles. There is interstitial mucin deposition and edema, and usually no eosinophils and neutrophils are present.

Hypertrophic lesions have acanthosis and hyperkeratosis of the epidermis (Weedon 2002). Direct immunofluorescence is an important test that should be performed in this subtype. Usually, there is deposition of IgG and IgM in 50%–90% of cases. The differential diagnosis includes drug reaction, dermatomyositis, graft-vs-host disease, and mycosis fungoides. Jessner's lymphocytic infiltration of the skin usually does not involve the epidermis as hydropic degeneration of the basal layer and scattered apoptotic keratinocytes do not occur. Otherwise, the dermal infiltrate is identical to LE. Consequently, Jessner's lymphocytic infiltration of the skin is regarded as a variant of LE by some authors. In a drug reaction there are frequently eosinophils that are not

Fig. 21.1. Discoid lupus erythematosus. Hydropic degeneration of the basal layer

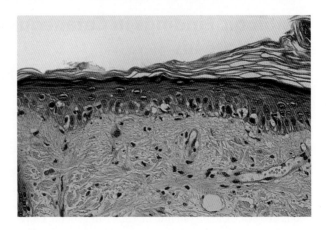

seen in DLE. In graft-vs-host disease, there is usually not a prominent lymphocytic infiltrate involving the dermis. Early-stage dermatomyositis can be histologically difficult to distinguish from DLE because it can exhibit identical changes. Consequently, clinical features should be considered for diagnosis. In mycosis fungoides, lymphocytes frequently exhibit nuclear atypia.

Subacute Cutaneous Lupus Erythematosus

The term "subacute cutaneous lupus erythematosus" was coined in 1977 by Gilliam (Gilliam 1977) and further characterized by Sontheimer et al. (Sontheimer et al. 1979) in 1979. The authors introduced a previously undescribed variant of LE with skin lesions at the neck, shoulders, upper thorax, and arms. Clinically, recurrent annular polycyclic or papulosquamous lesions involve the upper trunk, extensor regions of the arms, and face and neck region.

The histopathologic features of SCLE are almost identical to those of DLE (Fig. 21.2). In individual cases, in particular in early lesions, differentiation by histopathologic features alone may be difficult or impossible. However, usually in SCLE there are more prominent changes at the dermoepidermal interface such as hydropic degeneration of the basal epithelial layer. Forming clefts or vesicles, epidermal atrophy, and dermal edema may be also more prominent as in DLE, and there may be extravasation of erythrocytes and dermal fibrin deposits. Apoptotic keratinocytes (Civatte bodies) in the epidermis may be numerous. In addition, the lymphocytic infiltrate is more confined to the upper dermis and bandlike compared with DLE.

Compared with DLE, SCLE has less hyperkeratosis, atrophy of pilosebaceous units, follicular plugging, and thickening of the basal layer (Bangert et al. 1984, Jerdan et al. 1990). The lupus band test result is positive in approximately 60% of cases.

Fig. 21.2A–C. Subacute cutaneous lupus erythematosus.
B Hydropic degeneration of the basal layer and apoptotic keratinocytes in the epidermis.
C Mucin deposition in the dermis

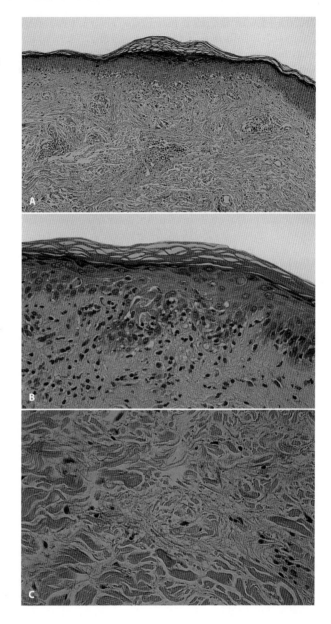

Systemic Lupus Erythematosus

Clinically, in SLE there are erythematous patches. In early lesions, histopathologic changes of SLE can show indifferent changes that may be unspecific, including discrete vacuolar degeneration of the basal layer, edema, and a discrete lymphocytic infiltrate in the upper dermis. Well-established lesions show prominent vacuolar degeneration of the basal membrane, edema, extravasation of erythrocytes, and a lymphocytic infiltrate in the upper dermis. Neutrophils are sometimes present in early lesions at the dermoepidermal junction. Fibrinoid material may be present in the dermis around vessels and between collagen strands. In individual cases, distinction from leukocytoclastic vasculitis is impossible because all of the signs of leukocytoclastic vasculitis may be present, including nuclear dust, fibrinoid necrosis of vessel walls, neutrophilic infiltrate, and extravasation of erythrocytes. Eosinophils may be present in some drug-induced cases. Mucin can be present in larger amounts in the dermis and can be verified by using special stains (Alcian blue). The subcutaneous fat is frequently involved, with changes that are similar to those seen in LE profundus (see the following section).

The differential diagnosis includes polymorphous light eruption that usually does not exhibit larger amounts of mucin. Leukocytoclastic vasculitis does not show prominent mucin deposition or vacuolar degeneration of the basal layer.

Variants of Lupus Erythematosus

Lupus Erythematosus Tumidus

LE tumidus (LET) usually affects sun-exposed areas such as the face, back, and V area of the neck. Clinically, there are erythematous, succulent, edematous, nonscarring plaques (Kuhn et al. 2000). Histologically, LET is characterized by patchy lymphocytic infiltrates in the dermis. Mucin deposits are observed between the collagen fibers. The epidermis and the subcutaneous tissue are usually not involved (Kuhn et al. 2003).

Direct immunofluorescence depends on the duration of the lesion. In long-lasting lesions, usually there is deposition of IgG and IgM along the basement membrane (Kind et al. 1992). The differential diagnosis includes polymorphous light eruption, Jessner's lymphocytic infiltration of the skin, and pseudolymphoma (reactive lymphocytic infiltrate). Furthermore, reticular erythematous mucinosis (Steigleder et al. 1974) is regarded by Ackerman as a variant of LE.

Lupus Erythematosus Profundus

LE profundus is a variant of LE described by Kaposi (Kaposi 1883) in 1883 and in more detail by Irgang in 1940 (Irgang 1940). LE profundus is a panniculitis, also termed "lupus panniculitis". Clinically, LE profundus has a predilection for the face, neck, proximal extremities, trunk, and lower back (Tuffanelli 1985).

Histologically, the epidermis and dermis may be involved, with vacuolar degeneration and dermal lymphocytic infiltration (Fig. 21.3). However, the key feature is the prominent lobular panniculitis. There is a diffuse lymphocytic infiltrate with nuclear dust (Sanchez et al. 1981), and fat necrosis may develop later on in hyalinization of adipose lobules. Areas with fat necrosis have plasma cells, histiocytes, and neutrophils. Eosinophils may be present in approximately 25% of cases (Peters et al. 1991). Vascular involvement includes arteries and veins with endothelial cell hypertrophy, edema, and, in some cases, thrombosis or calcification. Perivascular fibrosis (onion-skin configuration) can be observed in the surroundings of vessels.

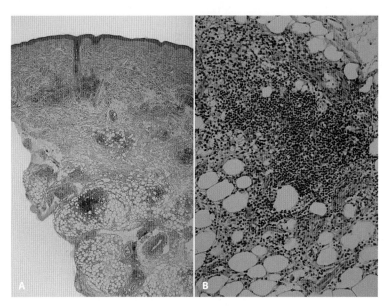

Fig. 21.3A, B. Lupus erythematosus profundus. Patchy lymphocytic infiltrates in the dermis and subcutaneous tissue

Another characteristic feature is the presence of reactive lymphoid follicles. Lymphoid follicles are rare in panniculitis but may be seen in rare cases of erythema nodosum, erythema induratum, and morphea (Harris et al. 1979). These entities are also part of the differential diagnosis of LE profundus. However, erythema induratum is usually on the calves of women, a location that is not common in LE profundus. In morphea, there are thickened collagen bundles, which are not present in LE profundus. Erythema nodosum usually does not display the histologic changes in the epidermis that may be seen in LE profundus. Another important differential diagnosis is subcutaneous panniculitis-like T-cell lymphoma, which is a cytotoxic T-cell malignancy. The neoplastic cells infiltrate the subcutaneous tissue and rim individual fat cells. Angioinvasion and necrosis may be prominent. T-cell receptor gene rearrangement studies are useful in diagnosis, as benign panniculitis does not show a monoclonal population (Sander et al. 2001).

Neonatal Lupus Erythematosus

NLE is a rare disease presenting in the neonatal period that resolves in the first 6 months of life. Associated disorders include transient thrombocytopenia, leukopenia, and a congenital heart block. Affected are children of mothers suffering from SLE. Clinically, children exhibit lesions as seen in SCLE. The causative agents are maternal IgG antinuclear antibodies (usually anti-Ro/SSA, less frequently anti-La/SSB, α-fodrin, and U1-RNP).

Histologic changes are similar to those of SCLE. However, infiltration at the dermoepidermal interface and vacuolar degeneration of the basal layer are more pronounced, sometimes with formation of clefts and edema of the dermis.

Fig. 21.4A, B. Bullous
lupus erythematosus.
Blister formation

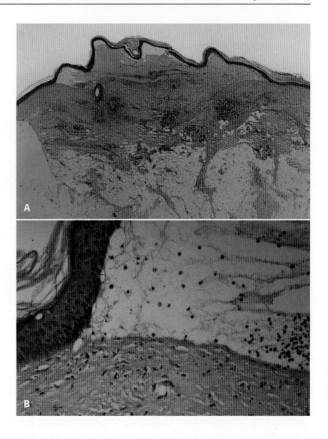

Bullous Lupus Erythematosus

In BLE, patients present with blisters that can resemble dermatitis herpetiformis or
bullous pemphigoid. Histologically, BLE can present with two different variants: in
one variant the infiltrate consists of neutrophils and in the other of mononuclear
cells. There is a pronounced neutrophilic infiltrate in the dermis with the formation
of papillary dermal abscesses, resembling dermatitis herpetiformis or linear IgA bullous disease. In addition, there is blister formation and dermal edema. Nuclear dust
is seen in the papillary dermal abscesses. In the second variant, there is a mononuclear
infiltrate with formation of blisters believed to represent a long-standing lesion of LE
(Fig. 21.4).

References

Bangert JL, Freeman RG, Sontheimer RD, Gilliam JN (1984) Subacute cutaneous lupus erythe-
    matosus and discoid lupus erythematosus. Comparative histopathologic findings. Arch Der-
    matol 120:332–337
Gilliam JN (1977) The cutaneous signs of lupus erythematosus. Cont Educ Fam Phys 6:34–70

Harris RB, Duncan SC, Ecker RI, Winkelmann RK (1979) Lymphoid follicles in subcutaneous inflammatory disease. Arch Dermatol 115:442–443

Irgang S (1940) Lupus profundus. Report of an example with clinical resemblance to Darier-Roussy sarcoid. Arch Dermatol Syphil 42:97–108

Kaposi M (1883) Pathologie und Therapie der Hautkrankheiten, 2nd ed. Urban & Schwarzenberg, Vienna, p 642

Jaworsky C (1997) Connective tissue diseases. In: Elder D (ed) Histopathology of the skin. Churchill Livingston, Philadelphia, pp 253–285

Jerdan JS, Hood AF, Moore GW, Callan JP (1990) Histopathologic comparison of the subsets of lupus erythematosus. Arch Dermatol 126:52–55

Kind P, Schuppe HC, Goerz G (1992) Kutaner Lupus erythematodes. Dtsch Ärztebl 89:1138–1139

Kind P, Lehmann P (1990) Photobiologie des Lupus erythematodes. Hautarzt 41:66–71

Kuhn A, Richter-Hintz D, Oslislo C, Ruzicka T, Megahed M, Lehmann P (2000) Lupus erytematosus tumidus – a neglected subset of cutaneous lupus erytematosus: report of 40 cases. Arch Dermatol 136:1033–1041

Kuhn A, Sonntag M, Ruzicka T, Lehmann P, Megahed M (2003) Histopathologic findings in lupus erythematosus tumidus: review of 80 patients. J Am Acad Dermatol 48:901–908

Peters MS, Su WPD (1991) Eosinophils in lupus panniculitis and morphea profunda. J Cutan Pathol 18:189–192

Sánchez NP, Peters MS, Winkelmann RK (1981) The histopathology of lupus erythematosus panniculitis. J Am Acad Dermatol 5:673–680

Sander CA, Flaig MJ, Jaffe ES (2001) Cutaneous manifestations of lymphoma: a clinical guide based on the WHO Classification. Clin Lymphoma 2:86–100

Sontheimer RD, Thomas JR, Gilliam JN (1979) Subacute cutaneous lupus erythematosus. A cutaneous marker for a distinct lupus erythematosus subset. Arch Dermatol 115:1409–1415

Steigleder GK, Gartmann H, Linker U (1974) REM-syndrome: reticular erythematous mucinosis (round-cell erythematosis), a new entity? Br J Dermatol 91:191–199

Tomaszewski MM, May DL (1995) Skin manifestations of systemic lupus erythematosus. In: Antonovych TT (ed) Pathology of systemic lupus erythematosus. Armed Forces Institute of Pathology, pp 45–58

Tuffanelli DL (1985) Lupus panniculitis. Semin Dermatol 4:79–81

Weedon D (2002) Skin pathology. Churchill Livingston, London, pp 47–52

CHAPTER 22

Immunopathology
of Cutaneous Lupus Erythematosus

Michael Meurer

Immunodermatologic research started in 1963 with the description of the lupus band test (LBT) in lesional skin of patients with systemic lupus erythematosus (SLE) or discoid LE (DLE) independently by Burnham et al. (Burnham et al. 1963) and Cormane (Cormane 1964). Two years later, in 1965, Braun-Falco and Vogell (Braun-Falco and Vogell 1965), studying the skin of patients with LE with histochemical techniques, had observed periodic acid-Schiff (PAS)-positive precipitates along the dermoepidermal junction (DEJ) and had suggested using the then innovative direct immunofluorescence microscopy technique to further analyze these precipitates. Since then, much has been published about the clinical and diagnostic relevance of the LBT (Mutasim and Adams 2001), but the pathomechanism of the immunoglobulin deposition beneath the epidermis in lesional or uninvolved skin of patients with LE and the antigens involved are still largely unknown (Sticherling 2001). Immunofluorescence studies in LE have mostly been performed in the skin of patients with typical DLE or subacute cutaneous LE (SCLE) or in acute lupus lesions of patients with SLE; atypical or uncommon manifestations of CLE such as LE tumidus, chilblain lupus, and LE profundus have been only infrequently investigated or have proved negative in immunohistopathologic studies. Equally, the immunopathomechanisms underlying the often widespread cutaneous and mucosal vasculitic lesions observed in more severe cases of SLE or overlap syndromes are still poorly understood (Werth et al. 1997), although they are probably closer related to the pathogenesis of organ, e. g., kidney or central nervous system, lesions in SLE. This chapter, therefore, concentrates on the immunopathology of classic CLE lesions seen in sun-exposed or protected skin.

Immunofluorescence Techniques
in Cutaneous Lupus Erythematosus

Direct immunofluorescence (DIF) is routinely performed according to methods first outlined in detail by Beutner et al. (Beutner et al. 1965). The technique detects deposits of the immunoglobulins IgG, IgA, and IgM as well as of the complement components C1q, C4, and C3 at the DEJ of biopsy specimens taken from lesional or unaffected skin of patients with LE. Results are most reliable in snap-frozen skin biopsy samples. The sensitivity of the method may slightly decrease when fresh tissue, immersed in a suitable transport medium such as Michel's solution, is first mailed to a reference laboratory before being processed for DIF. Since the relative intensity of fluorescence may vary in different biopsy sites and to a great extent depends on the duration and past treatment of a lesion, a standardized protocol is needed to ensure an optimal outcome and comparability of results for diagnostic and research purposes. If possible, facial lesions should not be biopsied since chronically sun-exposed facial skin often shows false-positive DIF results. It is known that the frequency and intensity of a positive LBT result increases with the age of a lesion; therefore, LE lesions should be older than 4 weeks before biopsy – a prerequisite often impossible to meet in SCLE or SLE – and should be left either untreated or spared from previous treatment (e. g., with topical corticosteroids) for longer than 3–4 weeks before biopsy (Dahl 1983).

DIF Findings in Cutaneous Lupus Erythematosus (Table 22.1)

All classes of immunoglobulins, occasionally including IgE and IgD, as well as the complement components C3, C4, C1q, MAC, properdin, and deposits of fibrin can be detected in a positive LBT result (Sontheimer and Provost 1991). The immune deposits most frequently present are IgM, IgG, and C3, and sometimes IgA (Wojna-rowska et al. 1986).

Discoid Lupus Erythematosus

The frequency of immune deposits in DLE depends on the biopsy site, past treatment, and the duration of a lesion. In lesional skin, immune deposits are present in about 60%–95% of DLE biopsy sample. IgG and C3 are most frequently detected. The pattern of the immune deposits can be linear in a continuous thick or thin band (Fig. 22.1) or discontinuous with coarse or fine granular deposits (Fig. 22.2). In addition to the deposits along the DEJ, cytoid bodies can be present in the papillary dermis, with positive staining mostly for IgM and IgA. In nonlesional skin, the LBT result is usually negative in sun-protected areas, eg, in biopsy samples taken from the buttock area of patients with DLE; a recent study, however, described deposits of C3 and IgM in uninvolved skin of some patients with DLE (Cardinali et al. 1999).

Subacute Cutaneous Lupus Erythematosus

The composition and pattern of immune deposits in lesional SCLE skin are similar to those seen in DLE (Meurer and Bieber 1987). The LBT in lesional skin is positive in 60%–100% of biopsy samples from SCLE lesions; the frequency may vary with the

Table 22.1. Direct immunofluorescence findings (IgG) in lupus erythematosus (LE)

Disease	Lesional LBT (%)	Nonlesional, sun-protected LBT (%)
Chronic discoid LE	60–90	0
Subacute cutaneous LE	60–100	0
Systemic LE	90–100	50–90

LBT, lupus band test.

Fig. 22.1. Linear, band-like deposits of IgM along the dermoepidermal junction of a chronic discoid lupus erythematosus lesion

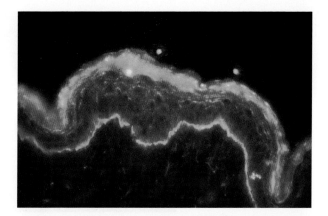

Fig. 22.2. Granular deposits of C3 along the dermoepidermal junction of a chronic discoid lupus erythematosus lesion (a similar pattern is often seen in a false-positive lupus band test result in non-lupus erythematosus inflammatory diseases) (Table 22.2)

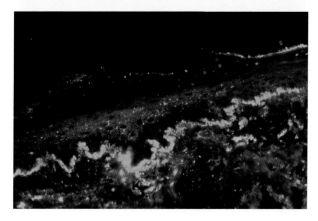

duration of the subacute inflammatory skin lesions and with the anatomic location (Kay and Tuffanelli 1969). Unique to SCLE is a granular fluorescence seen in some patients with SCLE in the cytoplasm and in the nuclei of basal keratinocytes. This fluorescence pattern is thought to be caused by the binding of anti-Ro/SSA or anti-La/SSB antibodies to their respective cytoplasmic or nuclear antigens (Baleski et al. 1992). The LBT result in nonlesional sun-protected skin of patients with SCLE is negative in most cases; positive results, particularly when IgG deposits are found, point to an overlap with SLE (Sontheimer and Provost 1997).

DIF Findings in Systemic Lupus Erythematosus (Table 22.1)

The DIF findings in biopsy samples obtained from typical SLE lesions are similar to those seen in DLE or SCLE: IgG, IgM, IgA, and C3 are most frequently detected, but other complement components and fibrin may be also present. The intensity of the LBT result in lesional skin was shown to correlate with serum titers of anti-DNA antibodies and with disease activity (Sontheimer and Gilliam 1979). As in other forms of

Fig. 22.3. Perivascular
deposits of IgG around
a dermal vessel in
lesional skin (systemic
lupus erythematosus)

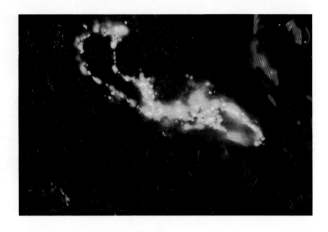

LE, the pattern of immune deposits along the DEJ may be bandlike, linear, or granular. In lesional skin of patients with SLE and active disease before systemic immunosuppressive treatment, the LBT result is positive in 90%–100% of biopsy specimens. A negative DIF finding in lesional skin makes a diagnosis of SLE very unlikely. In affected skin from patients with SLE, immune deposits may also be detected in other areas besides the DEJ: cytoid bodies mostly containing IgM or IgA can be present in the papillary dermis; around superficial dermal blood vessels, precipitates of immunoglobulins and complement may be located as in immune complex vasculitis (Fig. 22.3). These vasculitic changes are specific to SLE and are not seen in DLE or SCLE; they are associated with other systemic immune complex-mediated disease processes, with hypocomplementemia and a serious outcome prognosis (Sontheimer and Provost 1997). In nonlesional sun-protected skin of patients with SLE, the probability of a positive LBT result is much higher than in other LE subtypes and has been reported with a frequency between 50% and 90% (Halberg et al. 1982). The predictive value of a positive LBT result for the diagnosis of SLE is most reliable when deposits of IgG are present along the DEJ in biopsy specimens from uninvolved skin (Dahl 1983).

Immunopathology of the Lupus Band

The exact mechanisms leading to immune deposits along the DEJ in LE are still unknown. Despite numerous experimental attempts, the characterization of putative antigen(s) or specific antibodies within the lupus band have remained largely unsuccessful (Schreiner and Wolff 1970). It is likely that immunoglobulins and complement factors reacting with slowly released nuclear and cytoplasmic cell components from apoptotic keratinocytes are involved in the formation of such deposits (Casciola-Rosen and Rosen 1997). The polyanionic nature of some nuclear antigens such as native DNA may further induce or support a nonspecific binding to immunoglobulin aggregates and complement proteins such as C3 (Meurer and Gigli 1978). It is of interest that in SCLE or mixed connective tissue disease associated with high-titered serum autoantibodies to the nuclear U1RNP and La/SSB antigens or to the cytoplas-

Table 22.2. Diseases with immune deposits along the dermoepidermal junction (false-positive lupus band test result)

Dermatomyositis
Systemic scleroderma
Rheumatoid arthritis
Porphyria cutanea tarda
Lichen ruber planus
Rosacea

mic Ro/SSA antigen, DIF reveals nuclear or intracytoplasmatic fluorescence rather than the typical bandlike immune deposits seen in DLE where no antinuclear antibodies can be detected in the serum.

Diagnostic Relevance of the Lupus Band Test

Before interpreting a positive DIF finding in a presumed case of LE, several reasons for false-positive or false-negative results must be taken into account and excluded. Linear deposits or dust-like particles mostly containing IgM and/or C3 can be seen along the DEJ in a great variety of other inflammatory skin diseases – often in facial or chronically sun-exposed skin (Table 22.2). Continuous deposits of IgG, however, are usually not found in such cases and are conspicuous of true LE. In sun-protected nonlesional skin, DIF findings are always negative in biopsy specimens from patients with the diseases listed in Table 22.2. False-negative results can be obtained when fresh lesions or lesions from patients treated topically or systematically with corticosteroids or immunosuppressants are biopsied (Dahl 1983).

There is common understanding that a positive predictive or confirmatory value of the LBT in lesional skin for the diagnosis of LE is lower than the negative predictive value since a negative DIF finding in lesional skin is rather uncommon, whereas a (false-)positive DIF finding can be found in many other inflammatory skin diseases (Table 22.2). In nonlesional skin, however, a positive LBT result has a far higher positive predictive value than a negative one and clearly points to a diagnosis of LE, especially when deposits of IgG are present. Otherwise, the LBT, in lesional and uninvolved skin, has only little value for the distinction between DLE, SCLE, and SLE. For this purpose, serologic tests with demonstration of subtype-specific antinuclear antibodies are much more sensitive and specific (Conrad et al. 2000).

References

Baleski JE, Kumar V, Forman AB, Beutner EH, Chorzelski TP (1992) A characteristic cutaneous direct immunofluorescent pattern associated with Ro (SS-A) antibodies in subacute cutaneous lupus erythematosus. J Am Acad Dermatol 27:194–198

Beutner EH, Holborow EJ, Johnson GD (1965) A new fluorescent antibody method: Mixed antiglobulin immunofluorescence or labelled antigen indirect immunofluorescence staining. Nature 23:353–355

Braun-Falco O, Vogell W (1965) Elektronenmikroskopische Untersuchungen zur Dynamik der Akantholyse bei Pemphigus vulgaris. 1. Mitteilung: Die klinisch normal aussehende Haut in der Umgebung von Blasen mit positivem Nikolski-Phänomen. Arch Clin Exp Dermol 223:328–346

Burnham TK, Neblett TR, Fine G (1963) The application of the fluorescent antibody technique to the investigation of lupus erythematosus and various dermatoses. J Invest Dermatol 41: 451–456

Cardinali C, Caproni M, Fabbri P (1999) The composition of the lupus band test (LBT) on the sun-protected non-lesional (SPNL) skin in patients with cutaneous lupus erythematosus (CLE). Lupus 8:755–760

Casciola-Rosen L, Rosen L (1997) Ultraviolet light-induced apoptosis: a potential mechanism for the induction of skin lesions and autoantibody production in LE. Lupus 6:175–180

Conrad K, Humbel RL, Meurer M, Shoenfeld Y, Tan EM (2000) Autoantigens and autoantibodies: diagnostic tools and clues to understanding autoimmunity. Pabst Science, Lengrich, Berlin

Cormane RH (1964) "Bound" globulin in the skin of patients with chronic discoid lupus erythematosus and systemic lupus erythematosus. Lancet 1:534–535

Dahl MV (1983) Usefulness of direct immunofluorescence in patients with lupus erythematosus. Arch Dermatol 119:1010–1017

Halberg P, Ullman S, Jorgensen F (1982) The lupus band test as a measure of disease activity in systemic lupus erythematosus. Arch Dermatol 118:572–576

Kay DM, Tuffanelli DL (1969) Immunofluorescent techniques in clinical diagnosis of cutaneous disease. Ann Intern Med 71:753–762

Meurer M, Gigli J (1978) Interaction of DNA with the early components of complement. J Invest Dermatol 70:223

Meurer M, Bieber T (1987) Immunhistologische und serologische Diagnostik von Autoimmunerkrankungen der Haut. Hautarzt 38:59–68

Mutasim DF, Adams BB (2001) Immunofluorescence in dermatology. J Am Acad Dermatol 45:803–822

Schreiner E, Wolff K (1970) Systemic lupus erythematosus: electron microscopic localization of in vivo bound globulins at the dermal-epidermal junction. J Invest Dermatol 55:325–328

Sontheimer RD, Gilliam JN (1979) A reappraisal of the relationship between subepidermal immunoglobulin deposits and DNA antibodies in systemic lupus erythematosus: a study using the crithidia lucillae immunofluorescence anti-DNA assay. J Invest Dermatol 72:29–32

Sontheimer RD, Provost TT (1991) Lupus erythematosus. In: Jordon RE (ed) Immunologic diseases of the skin. Appleton & Lange, Norwalk, pp 355–378

Sontheimer RD, Provost TT (1997) Cutaneous manifestations of lupus erythematosus. In: Wallace DJ, Hahn BH (eds) Dubois' lupus erythematosus, 5th ed. Williams & Wilkins, Baltimore, pp 569–623

Sticherling M (2000) Chronic cutaneous lupus erythematosus. In: Hertl M (ed) Autoimmune diseases of the skin. Springer, Berlin, Heidelberg, New York, pp 169–187

Werth VP, Dutz JP, Sontheimer RD (1997) Pathogenetic mechanisms and treatment of cutaneous lupus erythematosus. Curr Opin Rheumatol 9:400–409

Wojnarowska F, Bhogal B, Black MM (1986) The significance of an IgM band at the dermo-epidermal junction. J Cutan Pathol 13:359–362

CHAPTER 23

Laboratory Features of Cutaneous Lupus Erythematosus

23

Shuntaro Shinada, Daniel J. Wallace

Assuming that patients with cutaneous lupus erythematosus (CLE) do not fulfill the American College of Rheumatology criteria for systemic LE (SLE) (Tan et al. 1982), what laboratory features should the clinician look for? Interestingly, there are several. This chapter attempts to elucidate the laboratory abnormalities associated with CLE, the most common being hematologic (anemia and leukopenia), erythrocyte sedimentation rate (ESR), antinuclear antibodies (ANAs), and antiphospholipid antibodies. These features are compared with those observed in SLE and certain cutaneous clinical subsets that have been studied.

General Approach to Laboratory Testing

When a dermatologist, family practitioner, internist, or rheumatologist first sees a patient with CLE, their principal concern should be to rule out evidence of systemic disease. After all, 15% of patients with CLE progress to SLE in 10–15 years of observation (Rowell 1984). In addition to a complete medical history and physical examination, clinical laboratory findings can be very helpful in this regard. Specifically, a blood chemistry panel allows screening for renal or hepatic involvement. Creatine phosphokinase testing assists in ruling out muscle inflammation. Evidence for autoimmune hemolytic anemia or thrombocytopenia is looked for in the complete blood cell count as well as in the lactic dehydrogenase, reticulocyte count, Coombs' direct antibody testing, serum haptoglobin, and antiplatelet antibodies. A routine urinalysis free of cellular casts or protein makes it highly unlikely that the kidney is involved. Specific autoantibodies, almost never observed in CLE, if found, can suggest central nervous system disease (antiribosomal P, antineuronal), mixed connective tissue disease (anti-RNP), or other disease subsets. In our practice, all patients have annual chest radiographs and electrocardiograms, since there are no blood tests to screen for cardiac or pulmonary involvement. Finally, additional imaging or electrical tests (electromyography, nerve conduction studies, 2-D echocardiography with Doppler) are occasionally ordered, and the results should be normal in CLE. If not, muscle, nerve, cardiac, or pulmonary disease representing visceral involvement should be ruled out.

This chapter assumes that the presence of systemic disease is not under consideration. The question remains, are there any laboratory tests worth ordering to monitor or better characterize CLE?

Medications Used to Manage Cutaneous Lupus Erythematosus Warrant Periodic Laboratory Monitoring

Although the different therapeutic options for CLE are discussed in later chapters, it is valuable to note the laboratory abnormalities associated with the medications used to treat CLE (Table 23.1).

Table 23.1. Laboratory abnormalities associated with use of drugs for cutaneous lupus erythematosus

Medication	Laboratory side effects	Laboratory monitoring
Antimalarials		Monitor CBC, serum creatinine, and LFT every 2 months
Chloroquine	Hemolysis secondary to G-6-PD deficiency, decreased creatinine clearance	
Hydroxychloroquine	Decreased creatinine clearance, decreased cholesterol profile, agranulocytosis (rare)	
Quinacrine	Aplastic anemia	
Antileprosy drugs		
Dapsone	Sulfhemoglobinemia, methemoglobinemia, hemolysis secondary to G-6-PD deficiency, hepatotoxicity	Monitor baseline G-6-PD levels. Monitor CBC every 2 weeks for the first 3 months, then every 2 months thereafter. Monitor baseline LFTs then every 2 months thereafter
Thalidomide	Highly teratogenic, neutropenia	Baseline pregnancy test, then weekly for the first month, then monthly thereafter. Monitor CBC every 2 months
Methotrexate	Blood dyscrasias, hepatotoxicity	Monitor baseline LFTs, CBC, serum creatinine, then weekly until dose stabilized, then every 1–2 months thereafter
Cyclosporine	Increased serum creatinine level	Monitor 2 baseline creatinines, then every 2 weeks for the first 3 months, then every month thereafter
Azathioprine	Thrombocytopenia, neutropenia, hepatotoxicity	Monitor baseline CBC, LFTs, then every 2 weeks for the first month, then every 1–3 months thereafter
Glucocorticosteroids	Increased serum glucose level; increased VLDL-C, HDL-C, and TG levels	Monitor baseline lipid panel, CBC, serum glucose and potassium, then monitor serum/urine glucose every 3–6 months

CBC, complete blood cell count; G-6-PD, glucose-6-phosphate dehydrogenase; HDL-C, high-density lipoprotein cholesterol; LFTs, liver function tests; TG, triglyceride; VLDL-C, very-low-density lipoprotein cholesterol.

Antimalarials

The three antimalarials available at this time for the treatment of CLE are chloroquine, hydroxychloroquine, and quinacrine. Overall, these drugs are relatively safe, but there are some laboratory abnormalities to consider. Chloroquine slightly decreases creatinine levels in half of its users, most likely by raising plasma aldosterone levels (Musabayane 1994). Forty-five percent of hydroxychloroquine is excreted in the kidneys, and the drug is associated with up to a 10% decrease in creatinine clearance (Landewe et al. 1995). Therefore, the dosage should be adjusted for patients with renal impariment. Antimalarials also have a beneficial antihyperlipidemic effect. Hydroxychloroquine induces a 15%–20% decrease in total cholesterol, triglyceride, and LDL levels (Wallace et al. 1990). It is associated with only one case of agranulocytosis, in a patient who was given 1,200 mg daily, which is up to six times the current recommended dosage (Polano et al. 1965), and a handful of case reports of various blood dyscrasias, such as aplastic anemia, leukopenia, thrombocytopenia, and hemolysis in individuals with glucose-6-phosphate dehydrogenase (G-6-PD) deficiency.

Chloroquine has been implicated in rare reports of G-6-PD deficiency hemolysis (Choudhry et al. 1978) and with agranulocytosis (Kersly and Palin 1959). Since chloroquine is known to concentrate in the liver, it should be used with caution in patients with hepatic disease or alcoholism or in conjunction with known hepatotoxic drugs.

The prevalence of aplastic anemia among US soldiers in the Pacific during World War II rose from 0.66 to 2.84 per 100,000 after quinacrine's introduction (Custer 1946). This represented 58 patients, 48 of whom received quinacrine. Of these, 16 were associated with overdoses, and two received marrow-suppressant drugs concurrently (Wallace 1989). It is therefore recommended that patients receiving antimalarial treatment have a complete blood cell count and a serum creatinine test every few months during therapy. Patients taking chloroquine or hydroxychloroquine should undergo ophthalmologic examination at 6- or 12-month intervals, respectively.

Antileprosy Drugs

Dapsone
Dapsone's use is limited by its toxic effects, which include sulfhemoglobinemia and methemoglobinemia, a dose-related hemolytic anemia, a "dapsone hypersensitivity syndrome," and aplastic anemia (Meyerson and Cohen 1994, Mok et al. 1998). All patients treated with dapsone should have their baseline G-6-PD level checked. The drug should not be given to patients with low levels. Complete blood cell counts should be checked every 2 weeks for the first 3 months, then every 2 months thereafter. Toxic hepatitis and cholestatic jaundice have been reported early in therapy. Hyperbilirubinemia may occur more often in G-6-PD-deficient patients. Baseline and subsequent monitoring of liver function is recommended.

Thalidomide
Thalidomide is a highly teratogenic drug with antileprosy and antilupus effects via various mechanisms. Side effects include teratogenicity, fatigue, dizziness, weight gain, constipation, amenorrhea, dry mouth, and a non-dose-related polyneuropathy that is associated with chronic administration (Ludolph and Matz 1982). Because thalido-

mide is so highly teratogenic, women of childbearing potential should have pregnancy testing. The test should be performed within 24 h of beginning thalidomide therapy and at regular intervals when appropriate. Pregnancy testing should also be performed if a patient misses her period or if there is any abnormality in menstrual bleeding.

Decreased white blood cell counts, including neutropenia, have been infrequently reported in association with the clinical use of thalidomide. White blood cell count and differential should be monitored on an ongoing basis, especially in patients who may be more prone to neutropenia. Higher doses of thalidomide may predispose patients to coagulopathies.

Methotrexate

Although serious and sometimes fatal blood dyscrasias are a well-known consequence of high-dose methotrexate therapy, the Committee on Safety of Medicines in the United Kingdom (Dodd et al. 1985) stated in September 1997 that it was also aware of 83 reports of blood dyscrasias associated with low-dose methotrexate used to treat psoriasis or rheumatoid arthritis; there were 36 fatalities. Megaloblastic anaemia, usually with marked macrocytosis, has been reported in mainly elderly patients receiving long-term weekly methotrexate therapy (Dahl 1984).

Methotrexate has been associated with periportal fibrosis and cirrhosis (Neuberger 1995), and its potential for hepatotoxicity has been a source of some concern given its use in nonmalignant disorders such as psoriasis and rheumatoid arthritis. It is recommended that liver function tests (LFTs) (as well as blood cell counts and renal function tests) be checked before beginning therapy then repeated weekly until therapy is stabilized, and thereafter every 2–3 months (Committee on Safety of Medicines/Medicines Control Agency 1994). The American College of Rheumatology recommends checking baseline LFTs, along with complete blood cells counts, creatinine levels, and hepatitis B and C serologies, before initiating treatment; then, at intervals of 4–8 weeks, LFTs should be monitored (Kremer et al. 1994). Methotrexate should be used with great care in patients with bone marrow, hepatic, or renal impairment. Methotrexate is a potent teratogen, and its use should be avoided in pregnancy.

Cyclosporine

Before initiating treatment, a careful physical examination, including blood pressure measurements (on at least two occasions) and two creatinine levels to estimate baseline status should be performed. Blood pressure and serum creatinine levels should be evaluated every 2 weeks during the initial 3 months and then monthly if the patient is stable. It is advisable to monitor serum creatinine levels and blood pressure always after an increase of the dose of nonsteroidal anti-inflammatory drugs and after initiation of new nonsteroidal anti-inflammatory drug therapy in those receiving cyclosporine treatment.

Azathioprine

Thrombocytopenia and leukopenia are dose dependent and may be reversed by reducing the dose or temporarily discontinuing use of azathioprine. Other reported hematologic adverse effects include eosinophilia, leukocytosis, neutropenia, anemia, aplastic anemia, and fatal myelogenous leukemia.

Results of one small study suggest that analysis of thiopurine methyltransferase genotype may allow identification of patients who are at risk for azathioprine hematologic toxic effects. The authors consider testing to be cost-effective compared with the cost of blood monitoring and supportive care for the 2%–12% of patients with this toxic effect (Black et al. 1998).

Data from the National Cooperative Crohn's Disease Study identified six patients (5.3%) with pancreatitis who were treated with azathioprine alone (Sturdevant et al. 1979). Associated symptoms include abdominal pain, elevated amylase and lipase levels, and vomiting.

Azathioprine can be hepatotoxic, and associated symptoms may include anorexia, nausea, fatigue, weight loss, jaundice, pruritis, dark urine, and elevated LFTs. Ideally, LFTs should be monitored every 2 weeks for the first 4 weeks and every 1–3 months thereafter (Gaffney and Scott 1998).

Glucocorticosteroids

Glucocorticoids (GCs) induce insulin synthesis but oppose its effects on glucose metabolism, thus predisposing to or exacerbating, if present, diabetes mellitus. These effects take place because of decreased peripheral utilization of glucose and increased gluconeogenesis induction in the liver. GC enhances effects on lipolysis and protein catabolism, thus increasing the substrates for gluconeogenesis (Schimmer and Parker 1996). GCs have an impact on lipid metabolism by enhancing the lipolytic effect of catecholamines and growth hormone, and they induce a centripetal body fat redistribution (Orth and Kovacs 1998). One study showed that the administration of prednisone for 14 days in healthy men increased the levels of very-low-density lipoprotein cholesterol, high-density lipoprotein cholesterol, and triglycerides (Ettinger and Hazzard 1988). Another study showed that increasing the prednisone dose by 10 mg daily was associated with a 7.5-mg/dL increase in cholesterol levels (Petri et al. 1994). GCs induce peripheral neutrophilia and elevate white blood cell counts by reducing neutrophil migration to tissues (Boumpas et al. 1993). Because of these effects of GCs, before starting therapy, it is recommended to check the baseline lipid panel (total cholesterol, low-density lipoprotein cholesterol, very-low-density lipoprotein cholesterol, and triglyceride levels), complete blood cell count, and serum glucose and potassium levels. Thereafter, serum or urine glucose levels should be checked every 3–6 months. Since corticosteroids promote the excretion of water, some of its mineralocorticoid effects include hypokalemia, which should also be monitored.

Specific Laboratory Tests that Can Be Abnormal in Cutaneous Lupus Erythematosus

Please refer to Tables 23.2 and 23.3.

Hematologic Abnormalities

Hematologic abnormalities are common in SLE and may often be its presenting manifestation. Although hematologic abnormalities are seen in CLE, they are not as

Table 23.2. Laboratory Differences Between the various subtypes of cutaneous lupus erythematosus (CLE). Modified from Sontheimer and Provost 1997

Disease features	ACLE	SCLE	DLE
Antinuclear antibodies	+++	++	+
Ro/SSA antibodies			
By immunodiffusion →	+	+++	0
By ELISA →	++	+++	+
Antinative DNA antibodies	+++	+	0
Hypocomplementemia	+++	+	+
Risk for developing SLE	+++	++	+

ACLE, acute CLE; DLE, discoid LE; ELISA, enzyme-linked immunosorbent assay; SCLE, subacute CLE; SLE, systemic LE.
+++, strongly associated; ++, moderately associated; +, weakly associated; 0, negative, no association.

common as in SLE. Patients with CLE had anemia ranging from 2% to 27% of the time, whereas patients with SLE had anemia 30% of the time. Eight percent of patients with SLE have hemolytic anemia, whereas it does not occur in patients with CLE (Pistiner et al. 1991). Between 0% and 30% of patients with CLE have leukopenia vs 51% of patients with SLE. Thrombocytopenia occurs in 2%–4% of patients with CLE as opposed to in 16% of those with SLE.

Erythrocyte Sedimentation Rate

The ESR is a nonspecific marker for increased immunologic activity and is often time elevated in various types of inflammatory processes. The ESR is elevated in 20%–56% of patients with CLE, whereas it is elevated in most patients with SLE.

Antinuclear Antibodies

The ANA test is a helpful serologic marker in the diagnosis of LE and other rheumatologic conditions. Approximately 96% of patients with SLE are positive for ANA, whereas 4%–63% of patients with CLE are positive for ANA. When reference laboratories switched from using animal substrates to the HEp-2 cell line in the mid-1980s to detect ANA, many ANA-negative patients became positive. This may help explain why in studies done earlier than the mid-1980s, patients with CLE had lower ANA positivity rates than in those done after the mid-1980s.

Anticardiolipin Antibodies

The anticardiolipin antibody is one of the serologic markers used to diagnose the antiphospholipid syndrome. The anticardiolipin antibody was positive in 31% of patients with CLE, whereas in patients with SLE its prevalence is slightly higher. Although anticardiolipin antibody is seen in 30%–40% of patients with SLE and CLE, it has not been associated with any complications (e.g., spontaneous abortions or arterial and/or venous occlusive disease) in CLE (Mayou et al. 1988).

Table 23.3. Laboratory data comparing cutaneous lupus erythematosus (CLE) and systemic LE (SLE)

Parameter	Prystowski et al. 1975	O'Loughlin et al. 1978	Millard and Rowell 1979	Callen 1982	Wallace et al. 1992	Pistiner et al. 1991	CLE vs SLE P Value, Wallace et al. 1992	Tebbe et al. 1997
Cases (n)	80 CLE	69 CLE	92 CLE	56 CLE	67 CLE	464 SLE	–	245 CLE
Year	1975	1978	1979	1982	1990	1991	1991	1997
Anemia (%)	2	10	27	0	7	30	0.0001	–
Hemolytic anemia (%)	–	–	–	0	0	8	0.009	–
Leukopenia (%)	0	14	12	10	30	51	0.002	–
Thrombocytopenia (%)	–	–	4	–	2	16	0.0001	–
Positive ANAs (%)	4	49	25	22	63	96	0.0001	29
Low C3 (%)	8	0	–	0	10	39	0.0001	–
High anti-ds-DNA (%)	0	0	–	4	8	40	0.0001	35
Positive anti-RNP (%)	–	–	–	5	2	14	0.081	–
Positive RF (latex fixation) (%)	1	6	13	21	9	23	0.02	–
Positive anti-RoSSA (%)	–	–	–	–	4	18	0.003	–
Positive anticardiolipin antibody (%)	–	–	–	–	31	38	0.53	–
High sedimentation rate (%)	56	45	20	43	31	54	0.001	56

ANAs, antinuclear antibodies; ds, double-stranded; RF, rheumatoid factor.

Anti-Ro/SSA Antibody

Anti-Ro/SSA antibodies are present in the serum of patients with SLE and Sjögren's syndrome and in 1 in 1,000 healthy people. The anti-Ro/SSA antibody is directed against ribonucleoproteins consisting of a 60-kDa peptide and an antigenically distinct 52-kDa polypeptide. Positive anti-Ro/SSA antibody has been seen in 4% of patients with CLE, whereas in patients with SLE the prevalence is 18%–30%, depending on whether immunoblotting or double diffusion methods are used. In a 1998 report by Chelbus et al. (Chelbus et al. 1998), there was similar frequency of both anti-Ro/SSA and anti-La/SSB in subacute cutaneous LE (SCLE) and SLE (approximately 70%). In another study, approximately 75% of patients with SCLE had anti-Ro/SSA precipitins (Sontheimer et al. 1982). Patients with SCLE have higher prevalence and titers of antibodies to both native 60-kDa Ro/SSA and 52-kDa Ro/SSA than those with chronic CLE (Lee et al. 1994).

Anti-double-stranded DNA Antibodies

Autoantibodies to DNA are classically associated with SLE. Wallace et al. (Wallace et al. 1992) reported that 4%–8% of patients with CLE had high anti-double-stranded (ds) DNA antibodies (Farr assay) as opposed to 40% with SLE. Chelbus et al. (Chelbus et al. 1988) noted that 1.2% of patients with SCLE had high anti-ds-DNA antibodies compared with 34% of patients with SLE.

Abnormal Testing Associated with Cutaneous Lupus Erythematosus Subsets

Acute Cutaneous Lupus Erythematosus

ACLE refers to the acute inflammatory rashes in patients with SLE and as such, has not been studied as a separate entity. Wysenbeek et al. (Wysenbeek et al. 1992) noted that the nonspecific "rash" of SLE was associated with the presence of anti-ds-DNA antibodies and low serum complement.

Chronic Cutaneous Lupus Erythematosus

Only a few patients with chronic CCLE without evidence of systemic involvement will have autoantibodies (Prystowsky et al. 1975). Of patients with CCLE, 30%–40% may exhibit low titers of ANA. However, fewer than 5% of patients with CCLE will have the higher levels of ANA that are seen in patients with severe SLE. Antibodies to single-stranded DNA are fairly common in CCLE, whereas antibodies to ds-DNA are uncommon (Callen et al. 1985). Patients whose disease course is dominated by discoid LE (DLE) lesions and who have evidence of mild SLE and overlapping connective tissue disease occasionally have precipitating antibodies to U1RNP (Callen 1982). Sometimes precipitating antibodies to Ro/SSA are seen in CCLE (Lee et al. 1994), and less frequently precipitating La/SSB and Sm antibodies (Provost and Ratrie 1990). Less than 10% of patients with CCLE have IgG isotype cardiolipin antibodies (Mayou et al. 1988).

A small percentage of patients with CCLE will have a false-positive serologic test for syphilis (VDRL), positive rheumatoid factor, slight depression of serum complement levels, modest elevations in gamma globulin levels, or modest leukopenia.

Subacute Cutaneous Lupus Erythematosus

SCLE occurs in 7%–27% of patients with LE (Cohen and Crosby 1994). Studies have shown that SCLE occurs mostly in white female patients in all age groups. Of patients with SCLE, 60%–81% have positive ANAs when human tissue substrate is used (Callen and Klein 1988). With immunodiffusion techniques, anti-Ro/SSA antibodies have been detected in 40%–100% of patients with SCLE (Lee et al. 1994). Anti-La/SSB antibodies by gel double diffusion have been observed in 12%–42% of patients with SCLE (Johansson-Stephansson et al. 1989). However, higher percentages of anti-La/SSB antibody levels have been seen in several studies outside the United States (Shou-yi et al. 1987). It has been reported that patients with SCLE have anti-ds-DNA at a prevalence of 1.2% (Chelbus et al. 1998).

A false-positive syphilis serologic test result is detected in 17%–33% of patients with SCLE (Sontheimer 1989), and ca. 10%–16% of patients with SCLE have anticardiolipin antibodies (Fonesca et al. 1992). Rheumatoid factor is present in approximately one third of patients (Sontheimer 1989). Only 10% of patients with SCLE have anti-ds-DNA, anti-SmRNP, or anti-U1RNP antibodies (Sontheimer 1989). Approximately one third of patients with SCLE have antilymphocyte antibodies, and 18%–44% of patients with SCLE are reported to possess antithyroid antibodies (Callen et al. 1986, Konstadoulakis et al. 1993).

Other Cutaneous Lupus Erythematosus Subsets

Lupus Erythematosus Profundus/Lupus Erythematosus Panniculitis
LE profundus/LE panniculitis is another rare form of CCLE characterized by inflammatory lesions in the lower dermis and the subcutaneous tissue. Of these patients, 70%–75% have positive ANA, but anti-ds-DNA antibodies are uncommon (Sanchez et al. 1982).

Chilbain Lupus Erythematosus/Lupus Pernio
Chilbain LE/lupus pernio is another variant of CLE consisting of red-purple patches and plaques on patients' faces, fingers, and toes that are precipitated by cold, damp climates. One study in 1998 found that eight of nine patients with chilbains lupus had anti-Ro/SSA antibodies (Franceschini et al. 1998). Most of these patients also complained of photosensitivity and Raynaud's phenomenon.

Lupus Erythematosus Tumidus (LET), Hypertrophic Lupus Erythematosus, Mucosal Lupus Erythematosus
LE tumidus (LET) is a subset of CLE seen when there is excessive accumulation of dermal mucin early in the course of a CLE lesion. The result is edematous, urticarial-appearing plaques of LE tumidus. Hypertrophic HLE (i.e., hyperkeratotic HLE, verrucous HLE) is a rare variant of CLE in which the hypekeratosis that is usually present in classic DLE is greatly exaggerated. Mucosal DLE is a variant of chronic

cutaneous DLE involving most frequently the oral mucosa, as well as the nasal, conjunctival, and genital mucosal surfaces. The laboratory features of these three subsets of CLE are not well delineated.

Laboratory Testing and Progress to Dissemination of Systemic Lupus Erythematosus

Approximately 15% of patients with CLE eventually progress to SLE (Rowell 1984). Several studies have been undertaken to determine the clinical and laboratory features that may predict such a pattern of disease progression. Clinically, patients with generalized DLE are at higher risk of developing SLE, oftentimes with more severe manifestations (Callen 1982). Laboratory tests associated with the development of SLE in patients with DLE include severe leukopenia, unexplained anemia, false-positive serologic tests for syphilis, persistently positive, high-titer ANA, anti-single-stranded DNA antibody, hypergammaglobulinemia, an elevated ESR greater than 50 mm/h, and a positive lupus band test (Callen 1982). A study in 1997 showed that in SCLE and/or DLE, patients with evidence of nephropathy, arthralgias, or ANA titer of 1:320 were at significantly higher risk of having systemic disease (Tebbe et al. 1997). This study did not find ESR and anti-ds-DNA antibodies to be useful in distinguishing patients with or without systemic disease. Another recent study suggests that elevated soluble interleukin 2 receptor levels might correlate with patients with SLE and discoid lupus lesions (Blum et al. 1993).

Summary and Recommendations

Although there are laboratory features that are more prevalent in CLE vs SLE, there are no specific serologic tests that differentiate the two diseases. Clinical correlation is indispensable in distinguishing them. There are also important laboratory values that need to be monitored at the onset and during treatment of CLE with medications.

References

Black AJ, McLeod HL, Capell HA, Powrie RH, Matowe LK, Pritchard SC, Collie-Duguid ES, Reid DM (1998) Thiopurine methyltransferase genotype predicts therapy-limiting severe toxicity from azathioprine. Ann Intern Med 129:716–718

Blum C, Zillikens D, Tony HP, Hartmann AA, Burg A (1993) Soluble interleukin-2 receptor as activity parameter in serum of systemic and discoid lupus erythematosus. Hautarzt 44:290–295

Boumpas DT, Chrousos GP, Wilder RL, Cupps TR, Balow JE (1993) Glucocorticoid therapy for immune-mediated diseases: basic and clinical correlates. Ann Intern Med 119:1198–1208

Callen JP (1982) Chronic cutaneous lupus erythematosus: clinical, laboratory, therapeutic, and prognostic examination of 62 patients. Arch Dermatol 118:412–416

Callen JP, Klein J (1988) Subacute cutaneous lupus erythematosus. Clinical, serologic, immunogenetic, and therapeutic considerations in 72 patients. Arthritis Rheum 31:1007–1013

Callen JP, Fowler JF, Kulick KB (1985) Serologic and clinical features of patients with discoid lupus erythematosus: relationship of antibodies to single-stranded deoxyribonucleic acid and of other antinuclear antibody subsets to clinical manifestations. J Am Acad Dermatol 13:748–755

Callen JP, Kulick KB, Stelzer G, Fowler JF (1986) Subacute cutaneous lupus erythematosus. Clinical, serologic, and immunogenetic studies of 49 patients seen in a non-referral setting. J Am Acad Dermatol 15:1227–1237

Chelbus E, Wolska H, Blaszyk M, Jablonska S (1998) Subacute cutaneous lupus erythematosus versus systemic lupus erythematosus: diagnostic criteria and therapeutic implications. J Am Acad Dermatol 38:405–412

Choudhry V, Madan N, Sood SK, Ghai OP (1978) Chloroquine-induced haemolysis and acute renal failure in subjects with G-6-PD deficiency. Trop Geogr Med 30:331–335

Cohen MR, Crosby D (1994) Systemic disease in subacute cutaneous lupus erythematosus: a controlled comparison with systemic lupus erythematosus. J Rheumatol 21:1665–1669

Committee on Safety of Medicines/Medicines Control Agency (1997) Blood dyscrasias and other ADRs with low-dose methotrexate. Current Problems 23:12–18

Custer RP (1946) Aplastic anemia in soldiers treated with Atabrine (quinacrine). Am J Med Sci 212:211–224

Dahl MGC (1984) Folate depletion in psoriatics on methotrexate. Br J Dermatol 111(Suppl 26):18

Dodd HJ, Kirby JD, Munro DD (1985) Megaloblastic anaemia in psoriatic patients treated with methotrexate. Br J Dermatol 112:630–631

Ettinger WH, Hazzard WR (1988) Prednisone increases very low density lipoprotein and high density lipoprotein in healthy men. Metabolism 37:1055–1058

Fonseca E, Alvarez R, Gonzalez MR, Pascual D (1992) Prevalence of anticardiolipin antibodies in subacute cutaneous lupus erythematosus. Lupus 1:265–268

Franceschini F, Calzavara-Pinton P, Quinzanini M, Cavazzana I, Bettoni L, Zane C, Facchetti F, Airo P, McCauliffe DP, Cattaneo R (1998) Chilbains lupus erythematosus is associated with antibodies to SSA/Ro. Lupus 8:215–219

Gaffney K, Scott DG (1998) Azathioprine and cyclophasphamide in the treatment of rheumatoid arthritis. Br J Rheum 37:824–836

Johansson-Stephansson E, Koskimes S, Partanen J, Kariniemi AL (1989) Subacute cutaneous lupus erythematosus: genetic markers and clinical and immunological findings in patients. Arch Dermatol 125:791–796

Kersley GD, Palin AG (1959) Amodiaquine and hydroxychloroquine in rheumatoid arthritis. Lancet ii:886–888

Konstadoulakis MM, Kroubouzos G, Tosca A, Piperingos G, Marafelia P, Konstadoulakis M, Varelzidis A, Koutras DA (1993) Thyroid autoantibodies in the subsets of lupus erythematosus: correlation with other autoantibodies and thyroid function. Thyroidol Clin Exp 5:1–7

Kremer JM, Alarcon GS, Lightfoot RW Jr, Willkens RF, Furst DE, Williams HJ, Dent PB, Weinblatt ME (1994) Methotrexate for rheumatoid arthritis. Suggested guidelines for monitoring liver toxicity. American College of Rheumatology. Arthritis Rheum 37:1829–1830

Landewe RB, Vergouwen MS, Goeei The SG, Van Rijthoven AW, Breedveld FC, Dijkmans BA (1995) Antimalarial drug induced decrease in creatinine clearance. J Rheumatol 22:34–37

Lee LA, Roberts CM, Frank MB, McCubbin VR, Reichlin M (1994) The autoantibody response to Ro/SSA in cutaneous lupus erythematosus. Arch Dermatol 130:1262–1268

Ludolph A, Matz DR (1982) Electrophysiologic changes in thalidomide neuropathy under treatment for discoid LE. EEG EMG 13:167–170

Mayou SC, Wojnorowska F, Lovell CR, Asherson RA, Leigh IM (1988) Anticardiolipin and anti-nuclear antibodies in discoid lupus erythematosus – their clinical significance. Clin Exp Dermatol 13:389–392

Meyerson MA, Cohen PR (1994) Dapsone-induced aplastic anemia in a woman with bullous systemic lupus erythematosus. Mayo Clin Proc 69:1159–1162

Millard LG, Rowell NR (1979) Abnormal laboratory test results and their relationship to prognosis in discoid lupus erythematosus. A long-term follow-up study of 92 patients. Arch Dermatol 115:1055–1058

Mok CC, Lau CS, Woon Sing Wong R (1998) Toxicities of dapsone in the treatment of cutaneous manifestations of rheumatic diseases. J Rheumatol 25:1246–1247

Musabayane CT, Ndhlovu CE, Balment RJ (1994) The effects of oral chloroquine administration on kidney function. Renal Fail 16:221–228

Neuberger J (1995) Methotrexate and liver disorders. Prescribers' J 35:158–63

O'Loughlin S, Schroeter AL, Jordan RE (1978) A study of lupus erythematosus with particular reference to generalized discoid lupus. Br J Dermatol 99:1–11

Orth DN, Kovacs WJ (1998) The adrenal cortex. In: Wilson JD, Foster DW, Kronenberg HM, Larsen PR (eds) Williams textbook of endocrinology, 9th ed. WB Saunders, Philadelphia, pp 517–664

Petri M, Lakatta C, Magder L, Goldman D (1994) Effects of prednisone and hydroxychloroquine on coronary artery disease rise factors in systemic lupus erythematosus: a longitudinal data analysis. Am J Med 96:254–259

Pistiner M, Wallace DJ, Nessim S, Metzger AL, Klinenberg JR (1991) Lupus erythematosus in the 1980s: a survey of 570 patients. Semin Arthritis Rheum 21:55–64

Polano MK, Cats A, van Olden GAJ (1965) Agranulocytosis following treatment with hydroxy-chloroqine sulfate. Lancet 1:1275

Provost TT, Ratrie H (1990) Autoantibodies and autoantigens in lupus erythematosus and Sjogren's syndrome. Curr Probl Dermatol 2:150–208

Prystowsky SD, Kerndon JH, Gilliam JN (1975) Chronic cutaneous lupus erythematosus (DLE): a clinical and laboratory investigation of 80 patients. Medicine 55:183–191

Rowell NR (1984) The natural history of lupus erythematosus. Clin Exp Dermatol 9:217–231

Sanchez NP, Peters MS, Winkelmann RK (1981) The histopathology of lupus erythematosus panniculitis. J Am Acad Dermatol 5:673–680

Schimmer BP, Parker KL (1996) Adrenocorticotropic hormone; adrenocortical steroids and their synthetic analogs; inhibitors of the synthesis and actions of adrenocortical hormones. In: Hardman JE, Limbird LE, Molinoff PB, Ruddon RW, Gilman AG (eds) The pharmacological basis of therapeutics, 9th ed. McGraw-Hill, New York, pp 1459–1485

Shi SY, Feng SF, Liao KH, Fang L, Kang KF (1987) Clinical study of 30 cases of subacute cutaneous lupus erythematosus. Chin Med J 100:45–48

Sontheimer RD (1989) Subacute cutaneous lupus erythematosus: a decade's perspective. Med Clin North Am 73:1073–1090

Sontheimer RD, Provost TT (1997) Cutaneous manifestations of lupus erythematosus. In: Wallace DJ, Hahn BH (eds) Dubois' lupus erythematosus, 5th ed. Williams & Wilkins, Philadelphia, pp 569–623

Sontheimer RD, Maddison PJ, Richlin M, Jordon RE, Stasny P, Gilliam JN (1982) Serologic and HLA associations in subacute cutaneous lupus erythematosus: a clinical subset of lupus erythematosus. Ann Intern Med 97:664–671

Sturdevant RA, Singleton JW, Derern JL, Law DH, McCleery JL (1979) Azathioprine-related pancreatitis in patients with Crohn's disease. Gastroenterology 77:883–886

Tan EM, Cohen AS, Fries JF, Masi AT, McShane DJ, Rothfield NF, Schaller JG, Talal N, Winchester RJ (1982) Special article: the 1982 revised criteria for the classification of systemic lupus erythmatosus. Arthritis Rheum 25:1271–1277

Tebbe B, Mansmann U, Wollina U, Auer-Grumbach P, Licht-Mbalyohere A, Arensmeier M, Orfanos CE (1997) Markers in cutaneous lupus erythematosus indicating systemic involvement – a multicenter study on 296 patients. Acta Derm Venereol 77:305–308

Wallace DJ (1989) The use of quinacrine (Atabrine) in rheumatic diseases: a reexamination. Semin Arthritis Rheum 18:282–296

Wallace DJ, Metzger AL, Stecher VJ, Turnbull BA, Kern PA (1990) Cholesterol-lowering effects of hydroxychloroquine in patients with rheumatic disease: reversal of deleterious effects of steroids on lipids. Am J Med 89:322–326

Wallace DJ, Pistiner M, Nessim S, Metzger AL, Klinenberg JR (1992) Cutaneous lupus erythematosus without systemic lupus erythematosus: clinical and laboratory features. Semin Arthritis Rheum 21:221–226

Winkelmann RK, Peters MS (1982) Lupus panniculitis. Dermatol Update 135

Wysenbeek AJ, Guedj D, Amit M, Weinberger A (1992) Rash in systemic lupus erythematosus: prevalence and relation to cutaneous and non-cutaneous disease manifestations. Ann Rheum Dis 51:717–719

Antinuclear Autoantibodies in Cutaneous Lupus Erythematosus: Biochemical and Cell Biological Characterization of Ro/SSA

24

Anna von Mikecz

Humoral Autoimmune Responses Against Nuclear Proteins

Patients with systemic rheumatic diseases such as systemic lupus erythematosus (SLE), scleroderma, and Sjögren's syndrome characteristically produce antinuclear antibodies (ANAs) that recognize intracellular nucleoprotein complexes. Systemic rheumatic diseases constitute chronic, life-threatening, multiorgan autoimmune disorders (Reichlin 1998). Their etiology is unknown, but genetic, hormonal, and environmental factors are involved. SLE is best characterized as a systemic immune complex vasculitis due to continued production of autoantibodies directed against nucleoplasmic antigens (e. g., DNA, histones, spliceosomal components, ribonucleoproteins), whereas scleroderma-associated autoantibodies primarily detect nucleolus-associated proteins such as DNA topoisomerase I (Scl-70) and centromeres. Autoantibodies target evolutionary, conserved epitopes of nucleoprotein complexes, which often constitute the functional regions (Tan 1989). Thus, the immunofluorescence staining patterns observed with autoantibody-containing serum samples can be regarded as an autoantigenic map that provides information on the subcellular distribution and function of the target antigens (Hemmerich and von Mikecz 2000, Tan 1991). Humoral autoimmune responses seem to be antigen driven and T-cell dependent (Lanzavecchia 1995). However, the molecular mechanisms responsible for stimulating autoreactive B and T cells, as well as for the generation of a systemic autoimmune response against the cell nucleus, remain unclear and represent an intensively investigated topic of current immunology.

ANAs in Cutaneous Lupus Erythematosus

SLE is a multisystem disorder with symptoms spanning from relatively benign cutaneous eruption to a severe, in some cases fatal, systemic disease. Although SLE can affect virtually every organ, abnormalities of the skin or mucous membranes are very frequent, being the second most common manifestation of SLE. Cutaneous lesions occur in approximately 85% of patients with SLE and are associated with photosensitivity, which may be linked to the pathogenesis of the underlying autoimmune response. The idea is that ultraviolet (UV) irradiation of the skin may expose previously cryptic antigens on the cell surface of epidermal cells, which, in turn, may be recognized by autoantibodies and T cells as foreign components, leading to (a) a systemic autoimmune response and (b) production of lupus skin lesions.

Four subsets of cutaneous LE (CLE) have been defined: acute CLE (ACLE), subacute CLE (SCLE), chronic CLE (CCLE), and neonatal LE (NLE). In SCLE and NLE, the
occurrence of specific autoantibodies against components of the cell nucleus has
been observed. SCLE is defined by a nonscarring skin eruption in association with
autoantibodies against Ro/SSA (Fig. 24.1) (Gilliam 1977, Sontheimer et al. 1979). Fifty
percent of these patients fulfill the criteria of the American Rheumatism Association
for SLE established in 1982 (Tan et al. 1982). Depending on the detection method, 60%
to 95% of patients with SCLE have anti-Ro/SSA antibodies in their serum.

NLE is a rare disease with skin manifestations resembling those seen in SCLE (Lee
1993). Approximately one half of the NLE cases exhibit skin disease, the other half

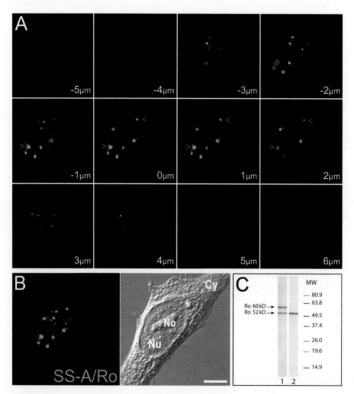

Fig. 24.1. Subcellular distribution of Ro/SSA. **A** Indirect immunofluorescence and confocal
microscopy of HEp-2 cells with subacute cutaneous lupus erythematosus (SCLE) autoantibodies against Ro/SSA revealed bright speckles embedded in a weaker homogeneous staining
pattern (*green*) within the nucleoplasm. Confocal sectioning was conducted by recording focal
planes from the bottom to the top of one cell (intervals, 1 μm). Note that single Ro speckles occur
in three to four focal planes (*red arrows*). **B** Focal sections displayed in **A** were fused to one
stack (left micrograph, *green*). The morphology of the cell was recorded simultaneously by
differential interference contrast (right micrograph, *gray*). Nu, nucleoplasm; No, nucleolus;
Cy, cytoplasm. Bar, 5 μm. **C** Immunoblotting of patient sera against Ro60 and Ro52. Patient
serum 1 recognizes both, Ro60 and Ro52, whereas serum 2 is exclusively directed against
Ro52. Confocal microscopy was conducted with serum 2. Molecular weight (*MW*) is given in
kilodaltons

have congenital heart block (Michaelsson and Engle 1972), and approximately 10% have both skin disease and congenital heart block. The hallmark of NLE is that in approximately 95% of the cases, the serum of both the baby and the mother contains autoantibodies directed against Ro/SSA (Franco et al 1980, Lee and Weston 1988). In contrast, other ANA specificities are rarely found (Provost et al. 1987). Anti-Ro/SSA autoantibodies are so characteristically prevalent in SCLE and NLE that clinicians usually use these ANA specificities as a confirmatory diagnostic test in patients who present with symptoms of the disorders.

However, the presence of these antibodies is not simply a matter of diagnostic or academic interest. Anti-Ro/SSA antibodies have been eluted from kidneys of patients with SLE (Maddison and Reichlin 1979) and are commonly associated with photo-sensitive rashes. Antibodies to Ro/SSA can cross the placenta and induce in approximately 1 of 20 cases NLE. Therefore, many investigators have explored the structure, origins, and precise targets of anti-Ro/SSA autoantibodies.

Discovery of Ro/SSA Antigens

In 1961, two precipitating autoantibody specificities known as SjD and SjT were described in patients with Sjögren's syndrome (Anderson et al. 1961). SjD antigen was reported to be insensitive to trypsin or heat treatment, whereas SjT antigen could be destroyed by the same treatment. In 1969, Clark et al. (Clark et al. 1969) reported a novel antibody specificity known as Ro in 40% of patients with SLE. The Ro antigen was described as a protease-, RNase-, and DNase-resistant cytoplasmic antigen observed in various tissue extracts. Six years later, in 1975, Alspaugh and Tan (Alspaugh and Tan 1975) described precipitin lines for two distinct autoantibody specificities termed "SSA" and "SSB" occurring predominantly in serum from patients with Sjögren's syndrome. It was not until 1979 that SSA and Ro were shown to be identical (Alspaugh and Maddison 1979); since then, this antigen system has been referred to as Ro/SSA. However, in the research areas of molecular biology and cell biology, this system is exclusively referred to as Ro ribonucleoprotein (RoRNP), since Ro antigens were shown to be associated with small RNAs (Lerner et al. 1981). Within the RoRNP complex, human serum containing anti-Ro/SSA antibodies recognizes two proteins with the molecular weight of 52 and 60 kDa (Fig. 24.1C). The 60-kDa Ro/SSA protein binds to a subpopulation of small RNAs, termed "hY RNAs" (Wolin and Steitz 1984). Antibodies to the Ro-associated RNA molecule hY5 RNA have also been detected (Granger et al. 1996), supporting the importance of the whole RoRNP particle in the autoimmune response.

Biochemical/Cell Biological Properties of Ro/SSA

The RoRNP complex in mammalian cells was first described as being composed of one of at least four hY RNAs associated with two proteins of 52 kDa (Ro/SSA52) and 60 kDa (Ro/SSA60) (Ben-Chetrit et al 1988, Rader et al. 1989). hY RNAs are small RNAs known as hY1, hY2, hY3, hY4, and hY5 RNA ranging from 84 to 112 nucleotides and are present in about 1 to 5×10^5 copies per cell (Wolin and Steitz 1984). All Y RNAs can be folded into a structure containing a large internal loop and a long stem formed by base pairing the 5' and 3' ends (Van Horn et al. 1995). Within the stem is a highly conserved bulged helix that is the binding site for the Ro/SSA protein (Green et al. 1998). In human cells, RoRNPs consist of one of the four hY RNAs and two core proteins: Ro/SSA60 and La/SSB. Physicochemical studies on native RoRNPs indicate that the particles segregate into three discrete subpopulations, one containing hY5, another containing hY4, and a third containing hY1, hY3, and hY4 (Boire and Craft 1989). Initially, it seemed that the 60-kDa Ro/SSA polypeptide was the exclusive protein component in the complex, but Boire and Craft (Boire and Craft 1990) were able to biochemically isolate RoRNPs in which the autoantigen La/SSB was a stable component.

Taken together, biochemical characterization of the RoRNP complex lead to the following model: the hY RNA is noncovalently bound to the 60-kDa Ro/SSA via the lower stem of the RNA formed by base pairing their 5' and 3' ends (Wolin and Steitz 1984), whereas La/SSB binds to the 3' oligo uridylate residues of hY RNAs (Fig. 24.2) (van Venrooij et al. 1993). In addition to the two core proteins, conditional association of other proteins such as calreticulin (Rokeach et al. 1991), Ro/SSA52 (Slobbe et al. 1992), RoBPI, and the RNA-binding protein nucleolin (Fournaux et al. 2002) to the RoRNP complex has been reported. However, these associations seem to be dependent on the structure of the hY RNA.

Although the evolutionarily conserved RoRNPs have been the subject of investigation in a number of laboratories for many years, their precise molecular definition, function, and subcellular localization remained unclear. The cellular distribution of Ro/SSA has been a matter of controversy since the early description of the autoantigen, because the Ro/SSA antigen seems to be present in both the cytoplasm and the nucleus. Although reports on association of Ro with cytoplasmic hY RNAs suggested

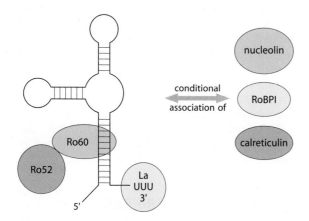

Fig. 24.2. The structure of the Ro ribonucleoprotein (RoRNP) particle (schematic diagram). In most higher eukaryotic cells, the Ro60 kDa protein is complexed with one of several small cytoplasmic RNAs known as Y RNAs. The Y RNA is folded into a structure containing internal loops and a long stem formed by base pairing the 5' and 3' ends. The 3' end of Y RNA is stably associated with the La protein, whereas the association of Ro52, nucleolin, RoBPI, and calreticulin is conditional

that RoRNPs are cytoplasmic RNP particles (Lerner et al. 1981, Peek et al. 1993), the study of Harmon et al. (Harmon et al. 1984) (see also Fig. 24.1) clearly showed that specific Ro/SSA antibodies predominantly detect nucleoplasmic speckles. Corroborating the idea of nuclear Ro/SSA location, rabbit anti-Ro/SSA60 antibodies displayed a speckled nucleoplasmic immunofluorescence staining pattern, which could be completely abolished by addition of purified Ro/SSA60 protein in serologic competition experiments (Mamula et al. 1989). Moreover, Ro/SSA52 contains transcription factor-like motifs, for example, leucine zippers, which have been shown to promote protein dimer formation and to contribute to inhibition of transcriptional activity in vitro (Wang et al. 2001).

Cloning of complementary DNAs (cDNAs) for Ro/SSA allowed further characterization of the proteins. The complete cDNA and protein sequence of Ro/SSA52 (GenBank/EBML accession numbers M35041) revealed that the open reading frame consists of 475 amino acid residues with a predicted molecular mass of 54 Kda and pI of 6.35. Based on the amino acid sequence, Ro/SSA52 is expected to contain three domains: (a) an N-terminal zinc finger domain, (b) a central coiled-coil (leucine zipper) domain, and (c) a C-terminal rfp-like domain. The N-terminal zinc finger domain is a member of the previously described 'Ring' finger proteins (Reddy et al. 1992), and the C-terminal rfp-like domain belongs to a second protein domain superfamily named after the rfp protein (Takahashi et al. 1988). It is important to note that all sequence motifs of Ro/SSA52 represent DNA and/or RNA-binding motifs. The full-length cDNA sequences of the 60-kDa Ro/SSA protein has been published by Deutscher et al. (Deutscher et al. 1988) and Ben-Chetrit et al. (Ben-Chetrit et al. 1989) and showed identical sequences except the C-terminal nucleotides. Ro/SSA60, like Ro/SSA52, contains nucleic acid binding motifs. The N-terminal RNA binding domain is highly conserved between Xenopus and human Ro/SSA60 sequences (O'Brian et al. 1993) and may account for the binding of the 60-kDa protein to hY RNAs. In contrast, the function of the Ro/SSA60 zinc finger domain has not yet been characterized.

The genes for Ro/SSA52 and Ro/SSA60 have not been published yet. However, using cDNA probes it was demonstrated that the human Ro/SSA52 gene is located on chromosome 11 (Frank et al. 1993), and the human Ro/SSA60 gene has been localized to gene locus 1q31 by fluorescence in situ hybridization (Chan et al. 1994).

Detection of Anti-Ro/SSA Antibodies

A hallmark of eukaryotic cells is their separation into subcellular compartments. The nucleus contains many internal nuclear domains, including the nuclear envelope, the nucleolus (Carmo-Fonseca et al. 2000), splicing speckles (Spector 1993), and a variety of nuclear bodies (Gall 2000, Zhong et al. 2000). This spatial organization reflects the requirement for spatial and temporal coordination of nuclear processes: Nuclear proteins with related functions, such as DNA replication, transcription of RNA, or subsequent RNA splicing, are assembled in multiprotein/nucleic acid complexes and thus colocalize at the cytological level.

During the past 25 years, characterization of ANAs has helped to identify many nuclear proteins by their subcellular localization. The commonly used technique for detection of ANA, immunofluorescence microscopy, represents a valuable tool for both the clinician to identify certain autoantibody specificities to diagnose subsets of systemic autoimmune diseases and the biomedical researcher to analyze the architecture and function of the cell nucleus. Immunofluorescence enables the visualization of antigens and the identification of structures in cells and tissues. The emitted signal of excited fluorochromes is viewed against a black background, thus providing high contrast. In addition, fluorescence imaging delivers superb specificity. These advantages of immunofluorescence techniques can be further enhanced by confocal laser scanning microscopy. Confocal microscopes differ from conventional (widefield) microscopes because they fade out out-of-focus signals. In a confocal microscope, most of the out-of-focus light is excluded from the final image, which greatly increases the contrast and the visibility of fine details in the specimen. Thus, confocal microscopy may lead to refined analyses of nuclear autoantigens as well as new opportunities for differential diagnosis of systemic rheumatic diseases and identification of (new) autoantigens, which might have been missed by conventional epifluorescence microscopy (Hemmerich and von Mikecz 2000).

Figure 24.1 shows confocal imaging of an autoantibody that is specifically directed against Ro52 (Fig. 24.1C, lane 2). Confocal sectioning of a human epidermal cell line (HEp-2) reveals a unique staining pattern of bright speckles embedded in a weak homogeneous staining of the nucleoplasm (Fig. 24.1A, B, green color), whereas nucleoli as well as the cytoplasm are not labeled. The typical feature of a confocal Ro/SSA image is the visibility of one speckle in three to four focal planes (Fig. 24.1A, arrows), suggesting that nucleoplasmic Ro/SSA speckles have a size of approximately 2 μm. Thus, Ro/SSA speckles can be easily and unmistakably distinguished from splicing speckles, which occupy a larger subnuclear area, and from other nuclear structures, such as nucleoli, centromeres, and nuclear bodies; the latter display a staining pattern of smaller dots.

Many clinical laboratories still use immunodiffusion or counterimmunoelectrophoresis for the detection of anti-Ro/SSA antibodies, whereas biomedical research laboratories apply immunofluorescence, immunoblotting, immunoprecipitation, and enzyme-linked immunosorbent assay (ELISA) techniques. The early work leading to the discovery of anti-Ro/SSA antibodies was based on immunodiffusion using extracts from human thyroid, spleen, and calf thymus (Clark et al. 1969, Alspaugh and Tan 1975). The method is easy and quick; however, the substrates are rather unspecific and thus may lead to misleading results, especially when appropriate control sera are not available. In terms of specificity, immunoblotting and immunprecipitation are the methods of choice. Extracts of MOLT-4 and HeLa cell lines have been used successfully for the detection of Ro/SSA antigens by immunoblotting (Ben-Chetrit et al. 1988, Rader et al. 1989). Immunoblotting enables the exact identification of the target antigens by determination of their molecular weight. With the cloning of Ro/SSA52 and Ro/SSA60 proteins, purified recombinant proteins have become the preferred substrates in ELISAs (Chan et al. 1991). However, ELISAs are expensive and prone to false-positive results, since the technique does not allow definition of molecular and cell biological properties of the substrate.

In contrast, a combination of immunofluorescence and immunoblotting provides information on the subcellular distribution and molecular weight (= integrity) of target antigens, and thus allows exact identification of ANA specificities. Moreover, the use of confocal microscopes delivers subnuclear immunofluorescent staining patterns in such detail that nuclear autoantigens can be distinguished by exclusive employment of this imaging technique (see previously). Since the new instruments are easy to use and become less and less expensive, it is safe to assume that confocal laser scanning microscopy will find its way from the research laboratories to the clinical routine laboratories.

B-Cell Epitopes of Ro/SSA

A major goal of immunochemistry is to define the molecular basis of receptor recognition, which requires the analysis of structure and function of (1) the receptor, (2) the ligand, and (3) the interface between the two. The portion of the antigen that is recognized by an antibody during the binding reaction is called "antigenic determinant" or "epitope". Structurally defined antibody-protein complexes share common features: 15–22 amino acid residues contact each other on both antibody and antigen molecules (Laver et al. 1990, Smith-Gill 1994). Epitopes are usually classified as either continuous or discontinuous, consisting of linear peptides or amino acid residues brought together by folding of the polypeptide chain, respectively.

Patients with autoimmune connective tissue diseases such as SLE characteristically produce autoantibodies that recognize continuous or discontinuous B-cell epitopes. A considerable heterogeneity of epitopes has been targeted by patient sera (Chou et al. 1992, van Venrooij et al. 1994). Properties of autoantigenic epitopes seem to be similar to those of foreign protein antigens in that they reside in hydrophilic and highly conserved domains (Elkon et al. 1988). However, ANAs are often directed against functional regions of the conserved antigenic molecules (Chan and Tan 1989), and autoantigens of systemic rheumatic diseases are generally either basic or contain extended, multivalent, charge-rich sequence motifs such as coiled-coils (Dohlman et al. 1993).

Numerous studies described the definition of important epitopes on the RoRNP complex. Autoepitopes of Ro/SSA60 have been reported by several authors using different biochemical methods. The most commonly used methods are to test autoimmune sera (a) with successively truncated recombinant fragments of the autoantigen by immunoblot or immunoprecipitation or (b) with overlapping synthetic peptides in ELISA. Although detection techniques differed between the studies, positions of major epitopes within Ro/SSA60 and Ro/SSA52 were found to be consistent. The major antigenic region of Ro/SSA60 resides in the middle of the protein, between amino acid residues 150 and 320 (Saitta et al. 1994, Scofield and Harley 1991, Wahren et al. 1996). Accordingly, sera from most patients with NLE, SCLE, and Sjögren's syndrome recognized an epitope within residues 139 and 326 (McCauliffe et al. 1994). The major epitope of Ro/SSA52 has been mapped to the center of the protein within residues 136–292 (Buyon et al. 1994, Frank et al. 1994, Kato et al. 1995, Dorner et al. 1996). It turned out that the major antigenic determinant of the Ro/SSA60 antigen is the most hydrophilic and presumably the most exposed part of the protein. The most frequently identified antigenic domains of Ro/SSA52 contain a putative coiled-coil domain (Kastner et al. 1992) and a leucine zipper motif (Chan et al. 1991, Itoh et al. 1991). Taken together, the data suggest that the similarities in the autoimmune response against Ro/SSA as observed with different (a) patient sera and (b) detection methods results from an immune response that is stimulated by endogenous autoantigens. Such immune responses are also referred to as antigen driven.

The idea that Ro/SSA autoantibodies generate during antigen-driven immune responses is corroborated by results from animal experiments. In contrast to the epitope mapping with patient sera, monoclonal antibodies raised in mice recognized various antigenic regions on Ro/SSA60 and Ro/SSA52 that were not confined to the middle part but that are distributed all over the proteins (Schmitz et al. 1997, Veldhoven et al. 1995). Immunization of mice (Topfer et al. 1995) and rabbits (Scofield et al. 1996) with recombinant Ro/SSA antigens or synthetic Ro/SSA peptides leads to intramolecular and intermolecular spreading of the immune reactivity, referred to as epitope spreading. It is thought that once an autoimmune response to one antigenic determinant has developed it might spread to associated proteins. However, to date, it is far from clear whether such an epitope spreading (a) occurs in patients during the onset of systemic autoimmune responses or (b) merely represents an artifact resulting from immunization of animals with exogenous proteins.

To address the issue of discontinuous epitopes on the RoRNP particle, Saitta et al. (Saitta et al. 1994) generated 10 overlapping recombinant polypeptides of the human 60-kDa Ro/SSA protein and compared their reactivities to immunoprecipitation of in vitro translated, native Ro60. Patient sera that immunoprecipitated full-length Ro/SSA60 had low or undetectable anti-Ro/SSA60 titers by ELISA and immunoblotting using recombinant antigens. These results suggest that discontinuous epitopes are the predominant targets of anti-Ro/SSA60 autoantibodies. It is important to note that during immunoprecipitation and immunofluorescence, the autoantigens retain their native structure, whereas in ELISA and immunoblotting, the substrate proteins are more or less denatured, which favors the exclusive detection of linear epitopes. Since ANAs in general represent very useful tools for immunoprecipitation, it was concluded that they preferentially recognize discontinuous epitopes on RNP complexes. Using ribonuclease protection assays, Wolin and Steitz (Wolin and Steitz 1984) discovered the major epitope of anti-Ro/SSA antibodies on the RoRNP particle. For each of the three human Ro RNAs whose sequence was known at that time, the most highly protected portion was found in immunoprecipitates corresponding to the lower section of the stem formed by base pairing the 5' and 3' ends of the RNA (see Fig. 24.2). These results confirmed that the complex of Ro/SSA60 and the lower stem of Ro RNA forms a major, discontinuous epitope for anti-Ro/SSA autoantibodies.

Outlook/Perspectives

Although the structure of Ro/SSA autoantigens and the antigenic targets (epitopes) for anti-Ro/SSA autoantibodies have been characterized in detail, two important challenges should be addressed in future research: (a) the function of the RoRNP particle is still unknown and (b) the molecular causes and mechanisms leading to systemic autoimmune responses against RoRNPs remain to be identified.

Since autoantibodies cannot penetrate into the cells, the central question is: How is an immune response against intracellular, nuclear proteins generated? Processing and presentation of antigens represents the prerequisite for every antigen-driven (auto)immune response. To date, little information exists on how nuclear autoantigens are processed and where this processing takes place in the cell, in situ. Recent evidence suggests that nuclear autoantigens are subjected to proteasomal proteolysis (Desai et al. 1997, Everett et al. 1999) within the nucleus (Chen et al. 2002, Rockel and von Mikecz 2002). Since proteasomes constitute a major proteolytic system that delivers peptides to antigen presentation, these new findings are the basis for the following hypothesis on the generation of systemic autoimmune responses: alteration of nuclear structure and function may result in recruitment of autoantigens to antigen-processing proteases, for example, the proteasome system. Previously cryptic nuclear proteins may be efficiently processed into peptides and subjected to antigen presentation. Thus, new antigenic peptides might appear on the surface of antigen-presenting cells, which are mistakenly interpreted as "non self" or foreign by T lymphocytes, and an autoimmune response is initiated against components of the body's own cells.

Sensitivity to sun is a cardinal feature of SLE, and UV light may be involved in its pathogenesis (Chen et al. 2000). In this respect, it is intriguing that the presence of anti-Ro/SSA antibodies in patients suffering from rheumatic disease is highly correlated with photosensitive dermatitis (von Muhlen and Tan 1995). According to the above-mentioned hypothesis, UV irradiation might induce recruitment of Ro/SSA to proteasomal proteolysis. Thus, future investigations on processing and presentation of RoRNPs and their intracellular trafficking may permit more insight into the molecular mechanisms that cause the generation of autoimmune responses and the production of anti-Ro/SSA antibodies.

References

Alspaugh MA, Tan EM (1975) Antibodies to cellular antigens in Sjogren's syndrome. J Clin Invest 55:1067–1073

Ben-Chetrit E, Chan EKL, Sullivan KF, Tan EM (1988) A 52-kD protein is a novel component of the SS-A/Ro antigenic particle. J Exp Med 167:1560–1571

Ben-Chetrit E, Gandy BJ, Tan EM, Sullivan KF (1989) Isolation and characterization of a cDNA clone encoding the 60-kD component of the human SS-A/Ro ribonucleoprotein autoantigen. J Clin Invest 83:1284–1292

Boire G, Craft J (1989) Biochemical and immunological heterogeneity of the Ro ribonucleoprotein particles. J Clin Invest 84:270–279

Boire G, Craft J (1990) Human Ro ribonucleoprotein particles: characterization of native structure and stable association with the La polypeptide. J Clin Invest 85:1182–1190

Buyon JP, Slade SG, Reveille JD, Hamel JC, Chan EKL (1994) Autoantibody responses to the "native" 52-kDa SS-A/Ro protein in neonatal lupus syndromes, systemic lupus erythematosus, and Sjögren's syndrome. J Immunol 152:3675–3684

Carmo-Fonseca M, Mendes-Soares L, Campos I (2000) To be or not to be in the nucleolus. Nature Cell Biology 2:E107–E111

Chan EKL, Hamel JC, Buyon JP, Tan EM (1991) Molecular definition and sequence motifs of the 52-kD component of human SS-A/Ro autoantigen. J Clin Invest 87:68–76

Chan EKL, Tan EM (1989) Epitopic targets for autoantibodies in systemic lupus erythematosus and Sjögren's syndrome. Curr Opin Rheumatol 1:376–381

Chan EKL, Tan EM, Ward DC, Matera AG (1994) Human 60-kDa SS-A/Ro ribonucleoprotein autoantigen gene (SSA2) localized to 1q31 by fluorescence in situ hybridization. Genomics 23:298–300

Chen M, Rockel T, Steinweger G, Hemmerich P, Risch J, von Mikecz A (2002) Subcellular recruitment of fibrillarin to nucleoplasmic proteasomes: implications for processing of a nucleolar autoantigen. Mol Biol Cell 13:3576–3587

Chen X, Quinn AM, Wolin SL (2000) Ro ribonucleoproteins contribute to the resistance of Deinococcus radiodurans to ultraviolet irradiation. Genes Dev 14:777–782

Chou CH, Satoh M, Wang J, Reeves WH (1992) B-cell epitopes of autoantigenic DNA-binding proteins. Mol Biol Rep 16:191–198

Clark G, Reichlin M, Tomasi TB (1969) Characterization of a soluble cytoplasmic antigen reactive with sera from patients with systemic lupus erythmatosus. J Immunol 102:117–122

Desai SD, Liu LF, Vazquez-Abad D, D'Arpa P (1997) Ubiquitin-dependent destruction of topoisomerase I is stimulated by the antitumor drug camptothecin. J Biol Chem 272:24159–24164

Deutscher SL, Harley JB, Keene JD (1988) Molecular analysis of the 60-kDa human Ro ribonucleoprotein. Proc Natl Acad Sci USA 85:9479–9483

Dohlman JG, Lupas A, Carson M (1993) Long, charge-rich alpha-helices in systemic autoantigens. Biochem Biophys Res Commun 195:686–696

Dorner T, Feist E, Wagenmann A, Kato T, Yamamoto K, Nishioka K, Burmester GR, Hiepe F (1996) Anti-52 kDa Ro(SSA) autoantibodies in different autoimmune diseases preferentially recognize epitopes on the central region of the antigen. J Rheumatol 23:462–468

Elkon, K, Bonfa E, Llovet R, Danho W, Weissbach C, Brot N (1988) Properties of the ribosomal P2 autoantigen are similar to those of foreign protein antigens. Proc Natl Acad Sci USA 85:5186–5189

Everett RD, Earnshaw WC, Finlay J, Lomonte P (1999) Specific destruction of kinetochore protein CENP-C and disruption of cell division by herpes simplex virus immediate-early protein Vmw110. EMBO J 18:1526–1538

Fouraux MA, Bouvet P, Verkaart S, van Venrooij, Pruijn GJ (2002) Nucleolin associates with a subset of the human Ro ribonucleoprotein complexes. J Mol Biol 320:475–488

Franco HL, Weston WL, Tan EM, Peebles C, Forstot SL, Kohler PF (1980) Association of antibodies to sicca syndrome antigens in newborn with lupus erythematosus and their mothers. Clin Res 28:134A

Frank MB, Itoh K, Fujisaku A, Pontarotti P, Mattei MG, Neas BR (1993) The mapping of the human 52-kD Ro/SSA autoantigen gene to human chromosome 11, and its polymorphisms. Am J Hum Genet 52:183–191

Frank MB, Itoh K, McCubbin V (1994) Epitope mapping of the 52-kD Ro/SSA autoantigen. Clin Exp Immunol 95:390–396

Gall J (2000) Cajal bodies: the first 100 years. Annu Rev Cell Dev Biol 16:273–300

Gilliam JN (1977) The cutaneous signs of lupus erythematosus. Continuing education. Fam Physician 6:34–70

Granger D, Tremblay A, Boulanger C, Chabot B, Menard HA, Boire G (1996) Autoantigenic epitopes on hY5 Ro RNA are distinct from regions bound by the 60-kDa Ro and La proteins. J Immunol 157:2193–2200

Green CD, Long KS, Shi H, Wolin SL (1998) Binding of the 60-kDa Ro autoantigen to Y RNAs: Evidence for recognition in the major groove of a conserved helix. RNA 4:750–765

Harmon CE, Deng JS, Peebles CL, Tan EM (1984) The importance of tissue substrate in the SS-A/Ro antigen-antibody system. Arthritis Rheum 27:166–173

Hemmerich P, von Mikecz A (2000) Antinuclear autoantibodies: fluorescent highlights on structure and function in the nucleus. Int Arch Allergy Immunol 123:16–27

Itoh K, Itoh Y, Frank MB (1991) Protein heterogeneity in the human Ro/SSA ribonucleoproteins. The 52- and 60-kD Ro/SSA autoantigens are encoded by separate genes. J Clin Invest 87:177–186

Kastner K, Perez A, Lutz Y, Rochette-Egly C, Gaub MP, Durand B, Lanotte M, Berger R, Chambon P (1992) Structure, localization and transcriptional properties of two classes of retinoic acid receptor alpha fusion proteins in acute promyelocytic leukemia (APL): structural similarities with a new family of oncoproteins. EMBO J 11:629–642

Kato T, Sasakawa H, Suzuki S, Shirako M, Tashiro F, Nishioka K, Yamamoto K (1995) Autoepitopes of the 52-kd SS-A/Ro molecule. Arthritis Rheum 38:990–998

Lanzavecchia A (1995) How can cryptic epitopes trigger autoimmunity? J Exp Med 181:1945–1948

Laver WG, Air GM, Webster RG, Smith-Gill SJ (1990) Epitopes on protein antigens: misconceptions and realities. Cell 61:553–556

Lee LA (1993). Neonatal lupus erythematosus. J Invest Dermatol 100 (Suppl):9S–13S

Lee LA, Weston WL (1988) Neonatal lupus erythematosus. Semin Dermatol 7:66–72

Lerner MR, Boyle JA, Hardin JA, Steitz JA (1981) Two novel classes of small ribonucleoproteins detected by antibodies associated with lupus erythematosus. Science 211:400–402

Maddison PJ, Reichlin M (1979) Deposition of antibodies to a soluble cytoplasmic antigen in the kidneys of patients with systemic lupus erythematosus. Arthritis Rheum 22:858–863

Mamula MJ, Silverman ED, Laxer RM, Bentur L, Isacovics B, Hardin JA (1989) Human monoclonal anti-La antibodies. The La protein resides on a subset of Ro particles. J Immunol 143:2923–2928

McCauliffe DP, Yin H, Wang L-X, Lucas L (1994) Autoimmune sera react with multiple epitopes on recombinant 52 and 60 kDa Ro(SSA) proteins. J Rheumatol 21:1073–1078

Michaelsson M, Engle MA (1972) Congenital complete heart block: An international study of natural history. In: Brest AN (ed) Pediatric cardiology. Davis, Philadelphia, pp 85–101

O'Brian CA, Margelot K, Wolin SL (1993) Xenopus Ro ribonucleoproteins: members of an evolutionarily conserved class of cytoplasmic ribonucleoproteins. Proc Natl Acad Sci USA 90:7250–7254

Peek R, Pruijn GJM, van der Kemp AJW, van Venrooij WJ (1993) Subcellular distribution of Ro ribonucleoprotein complexes and their constituents. J Cell Sci 106:929–935

Provost TT, Watson R, Gammon WR, Radowsky M, Harley JB, Reichlin M (1987) Neonatal lupus syndrome associated with U1 RNP (nRNP) antibodies. N Engl J Med 316:1135–1138

Rader MD, O'Brian C, Liu YS, Harley JB, Reichlin M (1989) Heterogeneity of the Ro/SSA antigen. Different molecular forms in lymphocytes and red blood cells. J Clin Invest 83:1293–1298

Reddy BA, Etkin LD, Freemont PS (1992) A novel zinc finger coiled-coil domain in a family of nuclear proteins. Trends Biochem Sci 17:344–345

Reichlin M (1998) Systemic lupus erythematosus. In: Rose NR, Mackay IR (eds) The autoimmune diseases. Academic Press, San Diego, pp 283–298

Rockel TD, von Mikecz A (2002) Proteasome-dependent processing of nuclear proteins is correlated with their subnuclear localization. J Struct Biol 140:189–199

Rokeach LA, Haselby JA, Meilof JF, Smeenk RJT, Unnasch TR, Greene BM, Hoch SO (1991) Characterization of the autoantigen calreticulin. J Immunol 147:3031–3039

Saitta MR, Arnett FC, Keene JD (1994) 60-kDa Ro protein autoepitopes identified using recombinant polypeptides. J Immunol 152:4192–4202

Schmitz M, Bachmann M, Laubinger J, Thijssen JP, Pruijn GJ (1997) Characterization of murine monoclonal antibodies against the Ro52 autoantigen. Clin Exp Immunol 110:53–62

Scofield RH, Harley JB (1991) Autoantigenicity of Ro/SSA antigen is related to a nucleocapsid protein of vesicular stomatitis virus. Proc Natl Acad Sci USA 88:3343–3347

Scofield RH, Henry WE, Kurien BT, James JA, Harley JB (1996) Immunization with short peptides from the sequence of the systemic lupus erythematosus-associated 60-kDa Ro autoantigen results in anti-Ro ribonucleoprotein autoimmunity. J Immunol 156:4059–4066

Slobbe RL, Pluk W, van Venrooij W, Pruijn GJM (1992) Ro ribonucleoprotein assembly in vitro. Identification of RNA-protein and protein-protein interactions. J Mol Biol 227:361–366

Smith-Gill SJ (1994) Protein epitopes: functional vs. structural definitions. Res Immunol 145:67–70

Sontheimer MD, Thomas JR, Gilliam JN (1979) Subacute cutaneous lupus erythematosus: a cutaneous marker for a distant lupus erythematosus subset. Arch Dermatol 115:1409–1415

Spector DL (1993) Macromolecular domains within the cell nucleus. Annu Rev Cell Biol 9:265–315

Tan EM, Cohen AS, Fries JF, Masi AT, McShane DJ, Rothfield NF, Schaller JG, Talal N, Wischester RJ (1982) The revised criteria for the classification of systemic lupus erythematosus. Arthritis Rheum 25:1271–1277

Takahashi M, Inaguma Y, Hiai H, Hirose F (1988) Developmentally regulated expression of a human "finger"-containing gene encoded by the 5' half of the ret transforming gene. Mol Cell Biol 8:1853–1856

Tan EM (1989) Antinuclear antibodies: diagnostic markers for autoimmune disease and probes for cell biology. Adv Immunol 44:93–151

Tan EM (1991) Autoantibodies in pathology and cell biology. Cell 67:841–842

Topfer F, Gordon T, McCluskey J (1995) Intra- and intermolecular spreading of autoimmunity involving the nuclear self-antigens La (SS-B) and Ro (SS-A). Proc Natl Acad Sci USA 92:875–879

van Horn DJ, Eisenberg D, O'Brien CA, Wolin SL (1995) Caenorhabditis elegans embryos contain only one major species of Ro RNP. RNA 1:293–303

van Venrooij WJ, Slobbe RL, Pruijn GJ (1993) Structure and function of La and RoRNPs. Mol Biol Rep 18:113–119

van Venrooij WJ, van Gelder CWG (1994) B cell epitopes on nuclear autoantigens: what can they tell us? Arthritis Rheum 37:608–616

Veldhoven CHA, Pruijn GJM, Meilof JF, Thijssen JP, Van der Kemp AW, Van Venrooij WJ, Smeenk RJ (1995) Characterization of murine monoclonal antibodies against 60-kD Ro/SSA and La/SS-B autoantigens. Clin Exp Immunol 101:45–54

von Muhlen CA, Tan EM (1995) Autoantibodies in the diagnosis of systemic rheumatic diseases. Semin Arthritis Rheum 24:323–358

Wahren M, Ruden U, Andersson B, Ringertz NR, Petterson I (1992) Identification of antigenic regions of the human Ro 60 kDa protein using recombinant antigen and synthetic peptides. J Autoimmun 5:319–332

Wang D, Buyon JP, Yang Z, Di Donato F, Miranda-Carus ME, Chan EKL (2001) Leucine zipper domain of 52 kDa SS-A/Ro promotes protein dimer formation and inhibits in vitro transcription activity. Biochim Biophys Acta 1568:155–161

Wolin SL, Steitz JA (1984) The Ro small cytoplasmic ribonucleoproteins: identification of the antigenic protein and its binding site on the Ro RNAs. Proc Natl Acad Sci USA 81:1996–2000

Zhong S, Salomoni P, Pandolfi PP (2000) The transcriptional role of PML and the nuclear body. Nat Cell Biol 2:E85–E90

Part IV
Treatment and Management of Cutaneous Lupus Erythematosus

CHAPTER 25

Topical Treatment of Cutaneous Lupus Erythematosus

Percy Lehmann

Topical treatment of cutaneous lupus erythematosus (CLE) has undergone far less scientific evaluation than systemic therapeutic modalities. Nevertheless, in many cases in which LE is confined to the skin and disease extension is limited to a few areas, local therapy and avoidance of triggering factors may be sufficient to efficaciously control the cutaneous manifestations. In extensive cases and systemic disease with skin involvement, topical therapy is an important addition to systemic therapy in the strategy to keep the complex disease under control. Therefore, management of CLE depends on the subset and on the severity and the extension of the disease in the individual patient, and it usually has to include a combination of local measures and systemic pharmaceuticals (Lo et al. 1989, Ting and Sontheimer 2001, Werth et al. 1997).

The local measures encompass topical medications as well as avoidance of disease-triggering factors, of which ultraviolet (UV) irradiation is the most important and the best studied. Other environmental triggers include cold, heat, and mechanical stress, which also may provoke skin lesions in LE and are far less studied than ultraviolet (UV) irradiation (Baer and Harber 1965, Ueki 1994).

Topical Corticosteroids

Application of topical corticosteroids (CSs) is part of the standard external therapy in CLE. Alone or in combination with systemic anti-inflammatory agents, CSs are very effective in reducing the main symptoms of the skin lesions of LE, namely, redness and squamae. To be effective in LE, intermediate (e. g., triamcinolone acetonide) to potent or superpotent CS preparations (betamethasone dipropionate, halobetasol propionate, fluocinonide, and clobetasol propionate) have to be used to achieve significant amelioration of the skin lesions. Usually, potent CS preparations should not be used on the face since the well-known side effects (atrophy, telangiectasias, steroid dermatitis, and folliculitis) tend to be especially severe in facial skin. However, in view of the risk-benefit ratio, CLE represents an exception to that rule, since the facial skin lesions of LE are often exceedingly disfiguring so that the CS side effects are less troublesome. Twice-daily application for a few weeks followed by a rest period of a few weeks may help minimize the risk of local side effects.

The choice of the vehicle for the CS treatment is important, for example, ointment-based products have a greater effectiveness since they induce stronger hydration of the skin with greater delivery of the CS through the horny layer into the skin. At the same time, these preparations are especially suitable for hypertrophic lesions, as they effectively ameliorate the stubborn hyperkeratosis of LE.

Creams may be cosmetically more acceptable for some patients, but they also may be more irritating owing to the emulsifiers, preservatives, and fragrances that most of them contain. For scalp lesions, CS solutions and gels are best applied since they can also be easily washed off with standard shampoos. For scalp lesions, the CS side effects are less harmful since the skin in this area seems to be less sensitive, especially regarding atrophy and telangiectasias. Potent CS preparations, therefore, may be applied here deliberately.

To enhance the efficacy of CSs, occlusive therapy may be chosen, especially for scalp lesions (e. g., shower cap). Different occlusive techniques exist for the various skin areas, which all can be applied overnight for maximum efficacy. Plastic food wrap (saran wrap) or adhesive gas-permeable surgical dressings (TegaDerm) can be used for larger areas on the trunk and extremities. For the hands, vinyl-over-cotton gloves (two-layered glove technique) can be recommended. If only the fingers are affected, rubber finger cots are available for occlusion.

To further increase CS efficacy and to achieve maximal drug concentrations in the active lesion, intralesional therapy may be chosen. Especially in hyperkeratotic discoid LE (DLE) and other refractory lesions, intralesional CS application may lead to better treatment responses. The concentration of the CS has to be adjusted to the site of injection, that is, 2.5–5 mg/mL triamcinolone acetonide suspension for the face and up to 10 mg/mL for other sites like the scalp or extremities. Intralesional CS application has long-lasting effects and may not be repeated until 4–6 weeks after the previous injections. To avoid subcutaneous atrophy, the injections should be placed in the dermis and not in the subcutaneous fat.

Dermatosurgical and Laser Therapy in Cutaneous Lupus Erythematosus

In patients with treatment-resistant lesions, different surgical techniques may offer additional alternatives. For many years, cryotherapy has been used to treat LE lesions; however, systematic studies are lacking, and the reported numbers in treatment series are low (Ting and Sontheimer 2001). Further surgical techniques that have been reported in individual cases include dermabrasion, laser resurfacing, hair transplantation, and surgical excision of disfiguring lesions. Owing to the disease-specific nature of LE, a test area should probably be treated first so that avoidance of the Koebner phenomenon and adequate healing may be ensured.

Vascular lesions with telangiectasias on visible areas, such as the face, are common in DLE; however, efficient management of these skin lesions can sometimes be difficult. Since argon laser light can specifically coagulate vascular structures, it has been used in the treatment of various vascular skin malformations. Effective use of argon laser has been reported by two groups (Kuhn et al. 2000, Zachariae et al. 1988) (Table 25.1).

Single observations in the literature revealed successful treatment of cutaneous vascular lesions of LE with the carbon dioxide and the pulsed dye laser. In 1986, Henderson and Odom (Henderson and Odom 1986) treated characteristic plaques of

Table 25.1. Treatment of lupus erythematosus (LE) with laser: review of the literature. (Modified after Kuhn et al. 2000)

Year	Authors	Indication (number of patients)	Type of laser	Response	Side effects
1986	Henderson and Odom	DLE (1)	Carbon dioxide laser	Dramatic clinical and cosmetic improvement	Splotchy hypopigmentation
1988	Zachariae et al.	DLE (5)	Argon laser	Cosmetically satisfactory result	60%–70% permanent bleaching
1995	Nunez et al.	LE teleangiectoides (1)	FPDL	Excellent improvement	None
1996	Nunez et al.	SLE (4)	FPDL	Clearance in >75%	Slightly transient hyperpigmentation
1996	Nurnberg et al.	DLE (1)	Argon laser	Clinical and histologic improvement	Hypopigmentation
1999	Raulin et al.	DLE (8) CLE (1) SCLE (1) SLE (2)	FPDL	Clearance rate of 70%	Transient hyperpigmentation
2000	Kuhn et al.	DLE (1)	Argon laser	Complete resolution of lesions	None

CLE, cutaneous LE; DLE, discoid LE; FPDL, flashlamp pulsed dye laser; SCLE, subacute CLE; SLE, systemic LE.

a patient with DLE by using the carbon dioxide laser and observed a dramatic clinical and cosmetic improvement in the cutaneous lesions. Hypopigmentation in the tested areas and reactivation of DLE in the periphery were described as side effects. Nunez et al. (Nunez et al. 1995, 1996) described telangiectatic chronic erythema of cutaneous lesions in four patients with systemic LE (SLE) who had been successfully treated with the flashlamp pulsed dye laser operating at 585 nm. Recently, Raulin et al. (Raulin et al. 1999) described a group of 12 patients with different forms of LE who were treated with the pulsed dye laser. A clearance rate was attained in 70% of the patients, and even in the two patients with SLE, a significant improvement was achieved. None of these patients showed any prolonged laser-induced scarring.

In 1988, Zachariae et al. (Zachariae et al. 1988) reported for the first time the treatment of cutaneous vascular lesions in connective tissue diseases with the argon laser. They noticed significant blanching of the patches, although scarring and hyperpigmentation remained. Since then, only one further report in the German literature (Nurnberg et al. 1996) documented successful treatment with the argon laser of skin lesions on the extensor aspect of the arms in one patient with chronic DLE. In contrast, Wolfe et al. (Wolfe et al. 1997) suggested that overtreatment with an argon laser has the potential to induce DLE since thermal injury seems to have caused the Koebner phenomenon in a patient without any previous history of autoimmune disease. The induction of such isomorphic skin changes after cutaneous injury in previously uninvolved skin has been associated with DLE (Ueki 1994, Wolfe et al. 1997).

The argon laser seems to be a promising alternative for the treatment of vascular DLE skin lesions, with an excellent cosmetic result. However, the indication must be carefully evaluated and the risks and benefits should be precisely documented, as skin texture changes and scarring might occur

Experimental New Topical Therapeutic Agents

Since retinoids have been shown to possess anti-inflammatory and antiproliferative as well as regulatory capacity on keratinocyte differentiation, they are good candidates to be beneficial in LE. In fact, various topical and systemic retinoids have been reported to be effective in patients with subacute CLE (SCLE) and chronic CLE (Werth et al. 1997). However, systematic controlled studies are lacking here too.

Tazarotene, the receptor-selective topical representative of the novel acetylenic retinoids, has been very effective in the treatment of an otherwise untreatable patient with DLE (Edwards et al. 1999). Further studies are needed to evaluate the role of topical retinoids in LE.

Another very promising development in topical dermatotherapy are the calcineurin inhibitors. Tacrolimus and pimecrolimus are prototypes of a class of immunosuppressive agents with a great potential in the treatment of inflammatory skin diseases, atopic dermatitis above all, but also in cutaneous autoimmune diseases. These pharmaceuticals have been shown to act at a point in activation of T lymphocytes that lies between T-cell receptor ligation and the transcription of early genes. Therefore, besides atopic dermatitis, all T-cell-mediated skin diseases, such as lichen planus, represent a potential area of use. Animal studies have demonstrated a beneficial effect of systemic tacrolimus in murine SLE (Furukawa et al. 1995). Similarly, systemic application of tacrolimus was used successfully in patients with SLE whose active disease had been poorly controlled by conventional treatments (Ruzicka et al. 1999). Consequently, topical calcineurin inhibitors were applied to treat the malar rash of SLE, with good results in three patients (Kanekura 2003). Anecdotal reports also demonstrated good efficacy of tacrolimus and pimecrolimus in patients with severe recalcitrant chronic DLE (Furukawa et al. 2002, Walker et al. 2002, Yoshimasu et al. 2002, Zabawski 2002), SCLE (Bohm et al. 2003, Druke et al. 2004), and LE tumidus (Bacman et al. 2003). Taken together, preliminary reports show very promising effects of this highly interesting new generation of topical treatment modality in dermatotherapy for cutaneous autoimmune disease, which urgently needs systematic evidence-based study evaluation.

Sunscreen and Photoprotection: Current Status and Perspectives

Since clinical data, phototesting procedures, and experimental evidence demonstrate unequivocally the detrimental effects of sun irradiation on patients with LE, sunscreens and photoprotection are major issues in the management of patients with LE (Furukawa et al. 1990, Lehmann et al. 1990, Norris 1993, Sontheimer 1996). Photoprotection can be achieved by topical and systemic agents as well as by behavioral measures, which have to be taught to the patient (Gil and Kim 2000, Lehmann 1996, Lehmann and Ruzicka 2001).

Sunscreens

Sunscreens have been developed to prevent the short- and long-term damaging effects of UV irradiation. However, the sun protective factor (SPF), which is defined as the ratio of the minimal erythema dose (MED) of sun-protected skin divided by the MED erythema of non-sun-protected skin, gives only a quantitative level of protection against sunburn and edema. Therefore, there is an ongoing debate on the potency of sunscreens to protect against many other deleterious biological UV effects such as photoimmunosuppression, skin aging, or skin cancer. Recent efforts have been directed toward determining the end points of sunscreen efficacy, such as immune protection factor (IPF), mutation protection factor (MPF), and protection against photocarcinogenesis (Gil and Kim 2000). Although standardized phototest procedures are available and can be used as tools to evaluate the protective effects of sunscreens toward UV induction of LE lesions, studies addressing this important topic are lacking. Sunscreens may be subdivided into products using UV filters on a physical or a chemical base. Physical agents used in sunscreens are titanium dioxide, zinc oxide, talcum, kaolin, bentonide, silica, and mica, which protect against UVB and UVA irradiation. Physical sunscreens show, contrary to chemical filters, no potential for phototoxicity or allergenicity, and they are photostable, cost effective, and applicable to children as well as adults. Most physical sunscreens contain ZnO or TiO_2 and are referred to as physical blockers because they provide at specified concentrations high SPF protection through absorption, scattering, and reflection of UV radiation in a wide spectral range. Especially since the development of micronized formulations of ZnO and TiO_2, the cosmetic acceptability of physical sunscreens has increased, and physical sunscreens have gained growing interest. Chemical agents most often used include aminobenzoates (para-aminobenzoic acid), cinnamates (diethanolamine p-methoxycinnamate [Parsol]), salicylates (2-ethylhexyl salicylate), and benzophenones (dioxybenzone, sulisobenzone, and oxybenzone). Most chemical blockers contain a combination of different filters to block a higher percentage and a broader range of UV rays. Owing to different absorption peaks, chemical filters may protect against UVB alone, UVA alone, or combined UVB and UVA (Table 25.2). There are several hundred sunscreen formulations containing different UV-protective chemicals on the market. However, it is important to have the photoreactivity of a broadband absorbing sunscreen, which protects against UVB as well as UVA and exerts a high SPF (>15). This type of sunscreen has combinations of UVA and UVB filters and sometimes ZnO and TiO_2.

Additional UV-Protective Chemicals

Further compounds are included in sunscreens to exert their effects in different ways than mere absorption and scattering of UV radiation. Since knowledge of the mole-

Table 25.2. Sunscreen Filters

UVB chemical sunscreens
Aminobenzoates
 p-Aminobenzoic acid (PABA)
 Amyl dimethyl PABA
 Glyceryl PABA
 2-ethylhexyl PABA
Cinnamates
 2-ethoxyethyl p-methoxycinnamate (Parsol)
 Diethanolamine p-methoxycinnamate
Salicylates
 Octyl salicylate
 Trolamine salicylate
 2-ethylhexyl salicylate
 Homomenthyl salicylate
 Triethanolamine salicylate
Miscellaneous
 Digalloyl trioleate
 Lawsone with dihydroxyacetone
 Glyceryl aminobenzoate

UVA chemical suncreens
Benzophenones
 Oxybenzone
 Sulisobenzone
 Dioxybenzone
Miscellaneous
 Menthyl anthralinate
 Eusolex 2020
 Dibenzoyl methane (Parsol 1789, Avobenzone)

UVB and UVA physical sunblocks
Kaolin
Magnesium silicate
Magnesium oxide
Red veterinary petrolatum
Titanium dioxide
Iron oxide
Zinc oxide

---

cular events of UV damage is increasing rapidly, a variety of different compounds that may interfere with these events are likely to be used increasingly in sunscreens.

Antioxidants

Since UV-induced generation of oxygen radicals seems to be an important mechanism for a variety of detrimental UV effects, inclusion of antioxidants and scavengers in sunscreens should provide additional UV protection. Vitamin C (ascorbic acid) and vitamin E (α-tocopherol) are the most prominent antioxidants used in sunscreens. Asorbic acid has been reported to prevent UVB-induced radical damage, secretion of proinflammatory cytokines by UVA, UV-induced suppression of systemic contact hypersensitivity, and UV-induced activation of ERK1/2 and p38 activation (Steenvoerden and Beijersbergen van Henegouwen 1999, Tebbe et al. 1997). Tocopherol inhibits UVB-induced erythema, photocarcinogenic DNA damage, and suppression of local contact hypersensitivity, as well as depletion of Langerhans cells (McVean and Liebler 1997, Trevithick et al 1992, Yuen and Halliday 1997).

Tocopherol and ascorbic acid in sunscreens showed a significant effect on the reduction of UV-induced sunburn cells (apoptotic keratinocytes) (Darr et al. 1996). Prophylactic use of the antioxidants of α-glycosylrutin, ferulic acid, and tocopheryl acetate in different concentrations showed a significant reduction in polymorphic light eruption lesions and pruritus, proven by photoprovocation tests (Hadshiew et al. 1997). Although a similar effect in LE seems conceivable, no such study has been published.

Future Developments

Epidermal DNA is probably the molecule that converts the physical energy of UV into a biological signal, thus leading to immunodysregulation. Liposome-encapsuled T4 endonuclease V, which increases the rate of pyrimidine dimer repair, can prevent UV-induced suppression of delayed-type hypersensitivity (Yarosh et al. 1999). Thus, repair of UV radiation-induced DNA damage through topical application of DNA repair enzymes seems to be a promising approach to reverse damaging UV effects. Stege et al. (Stege et al. 2000) demonstrated that application of the DNA repair enzyme photolyase in liposomes after UV irradiation induced dimer reversal and restored normal immune status. Whereas the potential of DNA repair enzymes as adjuvants in sunscreens or after sun lotions to prevent photocarcinogenesis is obvious, the ability of these chemicals to prevent photoinduction of LE remains unclear. Since DNA damage is believed to be crucial for the initiation of UV-induced autoimmunity, this approach is worth testing in UV-induced LE. Therefore, future development of sunscreen products should take the current knowledge of the pathophysiology of UV-induced LE into consideration to achieve more specifically tailored photoprotective agents.

General Photoprotection Measurements

The use of sun-protective clothing is especially recommended for individuals with extreme photosensitivity. The availability of fabrics with a wide choice of colors, weaves, and textures has led to increased popularity of this protective measure. The proven and documented high SPF values of modern sun-protective clothing ensure adequate protection as an adjunctive measure. Tightly knit fabric made of cotton blend is preferable to clothing of synthetic fibers because they lead to high temperature and humidity, which also may adversely affect patients with LE.

Conclusion

As mentioned earlier, many patients with LE are unaware of the detrimental effects of the sun on their disease and are ignorant about simple ways to avoid them. Therefore, education on sun protection, in addition to specific measures like sunscreens and photoprotective clothing, is of special value for patients with LE. Consequent protection against UV and other physical and mechanical injuries may prevent induction and exacerbation of the disease. Although no formal studies exist to demonstrate the beneficial effects of such measures, clinical experience strongly supports this strategy. In view of the available data indicating deleterious effects of UV irradiation on LE, objective evaluation of treatment and prophylactic strategies, e. g., appropriate sunscreens, is urgently needed for better care of the patients. With the development of standardized phototest protocols, excellent tools are available for the performance of such studies. However, photoprotection and skin care in patients with LE go beyond the use of sunscreens taking into consideration that LE-specific lesions can be precipitated in nonlesional skin by a variety of nonspecific injuries (Koebner phenomenon), including mechanical traumas, heat, cold, etc., a poorly studied fact (Walker et al. 2002).

References

Baer RL, Harber LC (1965) Photobiology of lupus erythematosus. Arch Dermatol 92:124–128

Bacman D, Tanbajewa A, Megahed M, Ruzicka T, Kuhn A (2003) Topical treatment with tacrolimus in lupus erythematosus tumidus. Hautarzt 54:977–979

Bohm M, Gaubitz M, Luger TA, Metze D, Bonsmann G (2003) Topical tacrolimus as a therapeutic adjunct in patients with cutaneous lupus erythematosus. A report of three cases. Dermatology 207:381–385

Darr D, Dunston S, Faust H, Pinnell S (1996) Effectiveness of antioxidant (vitamin C and E) with and without sunscreens as topical photoprotectants. Acta Dermatol Venereol (Stockh) 76:264–268

Druke A, Gambichler T, Altmeyer P, Freitag M, Kreuter A (2004) 0.1% Tacrolimus ointment in a patient with subacute cutaneous lupus erythematosus. Dermatolog Treat 15:63–64

Edwards KR, Burke WA (1999) Treatment of localized discoid lupus erythematosus with tazarotene. J Am Acad Dermatol 41:1049–1050

Furukawa F, Kashihara-Sawami M, Lyons MB, Norris DA (1990) Binding of antigens SS-A/Ro and SS-B/La is induced on the surface of human keratinocytes by ultraviolet light (UVL): implications for the pathogenesis of photosensitive cutaneous lupus. J Invest Dermatol 94:77–85

Furukawa F, Imamura S, Takigawa M (1995) FK 506: therapeutic effects on lupus dermatoses in autoimmune-prone MRL/MP-lpr mice. Arch Dermatol Res 287:558–563

Furukawa F, Yoshimasu T, Ohtani T, Ikeda K, Nishide T, Uede K (2002) Topical tacrolimus therapy for lesions of cutaneous lupus erythematosus – reply to the comments of Drs. Walker, Kirby and Chalmers. Eur J Dermatol 12:389

Gil EM, Kim TN (2000) UV-induced immune suppression and sunscreen. Photodermatol Photimmunol Photomed 16:101–110

Hadshiew I, Stab F, Untiedt S, Bohnsack K, Rippke F, Hozle E (1997) Effects of topically applied antioxidants in experimentally provoked polymorphous light eruption. Dermatology 195:362–368

Henderson DL, Odom JC (1986) Laser treatment of discoid lupus. Lasers Surg Med 6:12–15

Kanekura T, Yoshii N, Terasaki K, Miyoshi H, Kanzaki T (2003) Efficacy of topical tacrolimus for treating the malar rash of systemic lupus erythematosus. Br J Dermatol 148:353–356

Kuhn A, Becker-Wegerich PM, Ruzicka T, Lehmann P (2000) Successful treatment of discoid lupus erythematosus with argon Laser. Dermatology 201:175–177

Lehmann P, Holzle E, Kind P, Goerz G, Plewig G (1990) Experimental reproduction of skin lesions in lupus erythematosus by UVA and UVB radiation. J Am Acad Dermatol 22:181–187

Lehmann P (1996) Photosensitivität des Lupus erythematodes. Akt Dermatol 22:52–56

Lehmann P, Ruzicka T (2001) Sunscreens and photoprotection in lupus erythematosus. Dermatol Ther 14:167–173

Lo JS, Berg RE, Tomecki KJ (1989) Treatment of discoid lupus erythematosus. Int J Dermatol 28:497–507

McVean M, Liebler DC (1997) Inhibition of UVB-induced DNA damage in mouse epidermis by topically applied α-tocopherol. Carcinogenesis 18:1617–1622

Norris DA (1993) Pathomechanisms of photosensitive lupus erythematosus. J Invest Dermatol 100:S58–S68

Nurnberg W, Algermissen B, Hermes B, Henz BM, Kolde G (1996) Erfolgreiche Behandlung des chronisch diskoiden Lupus erythematodes mittels Argon-Laser. Hautarzt 47:767–770

Nunez M, Boixeda P, Miralles ES, de Misa RF, Ledo A (1995) Pulsed dye laser treatment in lupus erythematosus telangiectoides. Br J Dermatol 133:1010–1011

Nunez M, Boixeda P, Miralles ES, de Misa RF, Ledo A (1996) Pulsed dye laser treatment of telangiectatic chronic erythema of cutaneous lupus erythematosus. Arch Dermatol 132:354–355

Raulin C, Schmidt C, Hellwig S (1999) Cutaneous lupus erythematosus – treatment with pulsed dye laser. Br J Dermatol 141:1046–1050

Ruzicka T, Assmann T, Homey B (1999) Tacrolimus, the drug for the turn of the millennium? Arch Dermatol 135:574–580

Sontheimer RD (1996) Photoimmunology of lupus erythematosus and dermatomyositis: a speculative review. Photochem Photobiol 63:583–594

Steenvoorden DP, Beijersbergen van Henegouwen G (1999) Protection against UV-induced systemic immunosuppression in mice by a single topical application of the antioxidant vitamins C and E. Int J Radiat Biol 75:747–755

Stege H, Roza L, Vink AA, Grewe M, Ruzicka T, Grether-Beck S, Krutmann J (2000) Enzyme plus light therapy to repair DNA damage in ultraviolet-B-irradiated human skin. Proc Natl Acad Sci USA 97:1790–1795

Tebbe B, Wu S, Geilen CC, Eberle J, Kodelja V, Orfanos CE (1997) L-ascorbic acid inhibits UVA-induced lipid peroxidation and secretion of IL-1 alpha and IL-6 in cultured human keratinocytes in vitro. J Invest Dermatol 108:302–306

Ting WW, Sontheimer RD (2001) Local therapy for cutaneous and systemic lupus erythematosus: Practical and theoretical considerations. Lupus 10:171–184

Trevithick JR, Xiong H, Lee S, Shum DT, Sanford SE, Karlik SJ, Norley C, Dilworth GR (1992) Topical tocopherol acetate reduces post-UVB, sunburn-associated erythema, edema, and skin sensitivity in hairless mice. Arch Biochem Biophys 296:575–582

Ueki H (1994) Koebner-Phänomen bei Lupus erythematodes. Hautarzt 45:154–160

Walker SL, Kirby B, Chalmers RJ (2002) The effect of topical tacrolimus on severe recalcitrant chronic discoid lupus erythematosus. Br J Dermatol 147:405–406

Werth VR, Dutz JP, Sontheimer RD (1997) Pathogenetic mechanisms and treatment of cutaneous lupus erythematosus. Rheumatology 9:400–409

Wolfe JT, Weinberg JM, Elenitsas R, Uberti-Benz M (1997) Cutaneous lupus erythematosus following laser-induced thermal injury. Arch Deramtol 133:392–393

Yarosh DB, O Connor A, Alas L, Potten C, Wolf P (1999) Photoprotection by topical DNA repair enzymes: molecular correlates of clinical studies. Photochem Photobiol 69:136–140

Yoshimasu T, Ohtani T, Sakamoto T, Oshima A, Furukawa F (2002) Topical FK 506 [tacrolimus] therapy for facial erythematous lesions of cutaneous lupus erythematosus and dermatomyositis. Eur J Dermatol 12:50–52

Yuen KS, Halliday GM (1997) α-Tocopherol, and inhibitor of epidermal lipid peroxidation, prevents ultraviolet radiation form suppressing the skin immune system. Photochem Photobiol 65:587–592

Zabawski E (2002) Treatment of cutaneous lupus with Elidel. Dermatol Online J 8:25

Zachariae H, Bjerring P, Cramers M (1988) Argon laser treatment of cutaneous vascular lesions in connective tissue diseases. Acta Derm Venereol 68:179–182

CHAPTER 26

Antimalarials 26

Falk R. Ochsendorf

In 1934, Andersag synthesized chloroquine as a succession to chinine for the prophylaxis and treatment of malaria. Hydroxychloroquine is β-hydroxylated chloroquine. Since 1960, these substances as well as quinacrine, an acridine derivative widely used during World War II as an antimalarial (3 million soldiers for up to 4 years), were also successfully used for the therapy of noninfectious diseases, such as lupus erythematosus (LE) or rheumatoid arthritis. Their side effects, especially the fear of an irreversible retinopathy, limited their use. These unwanted effects, however, are primarily related to an excessive daily dosage and can be prevented by observing the maximal daily dosage of 3.5 (to 4) mg for chloroquine and 6 (to 6.5) mg for hydroxychloroquine per kilogram of *ideal* body weight. If these limits and the following information are taken into consideration, the therapy is rather safe.

These "antimalarials" are losing their primary indication, malaria, owing to the increasing resistance of plasmodia and newer compounds. On the other hand, even today there are new indications for chloroquine and hydroxychloroquine, for example, the treatment of human immunodeficiency virus infections (Boelaert et al. 2001, Savarino et al. 2001) (see also Table 26.1).

Chemistry

Chloroquine (7-chloride-4-[4'-diethyleamino-1'-methyle-butylamino]-chinoline; molecular weight 319.89; chloroquine diphosphate molecular weight 515.9) is a white, crystalline, bitter-tasting powder. It is easily soluble in water and nearly unsoluble in ethanol and chloroform. Hydroxychloroquine is a derivative of chloroquine. As the latter does not significantly differ from chloroquine with respect to mode of action, pharmacokinetics, toxicology, side effects, and indications, both medicaments are discussed together.

One hundred fifty milligrams of the pure chloroquine base corresponds to approximately 250 mg of the commercially available chloroquine diphosphate, and 155 mg of hydroxychloroquine base corresponds to 200 mg of hydroxychloroquine sulfate. The conversion factor from chloroquine diphosphate to the base is approximately 0.6, and from the base to the salt is approximately 1.6. The factors for hydroxychloroquine are 0.77 and 1.29, respectively. The dosages in the text relate to the clinically relevant dosages of the salts.

Quinacrine (Atabrine, mepacrine, atebrin) (6-chloro-9-[1-methyl-4-diethylamine]butylamino-2-methoxyacridine) is available as the dihydrochloride. It is a

Table 26.1. Indications for chloroquine and hydroxychloroquine for the treatment of noninfectious diseases (according to Arneal et al. 2002, Barthel et al. 1996, Dereure and Guilhou 2002, Erhan et al. 2002, Khoury et al. 2003, Nguyen et al. 2002, Reeves et al. 2004, Wallace 1996, Ziering et al. 1993)

	Disease	Proven by
Proven effectivity	Lupus erythematodes	Prospective controlled double-blind studies
	Chronic polyarthritis	Prospective controlled double-blind studies
	Porphyria cutanea tarda	Clinical studies
Strong indications for effectivity	Sarcoidosis (of the skin)	Controlled clinical studies, partially double blind
	Hyperlipidemia (mainly during corticosteroid therapy)	Controlled clinical studies
	Thromboembolic prophylaxis in case of antiphospholipid antibodies or intraoperatively	Controlled clinical studies
	Skin manifestations of dermatomyositis	Large series of patients
	Pseudogout	Controlled double-blind study
Indication for effectivity in individual cases	Primary Sjögren's syndrome	Controlled double-blind study (only laboratory improvement)
	Polymorphous light eruption	Prospective double-blind study
	REM syndrome	Large series of patients
	Lymphocytic infiltration	Large series of patients
	Interstitial or alveolear lung diseases in children	Large series of patients
	Hypercalcemia	Large series of patients
	Autoimmune thrombocytopenia (with steroids)	Patient series
Effectivity may evolve	Chronic fatigue syndrome	Case reports
	Asthma	Open clinical studies
	Giant cell arteriitis	Large series of patients
	Lichen planus mucosae	Open study
	Atopic dermatitis	Open study
	Diabetes	Controlled clinical studies
	Nonrheumatoid forms of inflammatory arthritis	Large series of patients
	Prevention of acute GvHD	Open clinical study
Case records with positive effects	Sideroblastic anemia, chronic ulcerative stomatitis, epidermolysis bullosa, erythema anlare centrifugum, granuloma anulare, granulomatosis disciformis, light urticaria, Lyme disease, morphea, cutaneous mucinoses, panniculitis (Pfeiffer-Weber-Christian), pemphigus, polymyalgia rheumatica, pseudolymphoma, pseudopelade Broq, chronic sinusitis, urticarial vasculitis, Well's syndrome, autoimmune urticaria, necrobiosis lipoidica	

GvHD, graft versus host disease; REM, reticular erythematous mucinosis.

bright yellow, odorless, bitter crystalline, water-soluble powder that contains an approximately 80% quinacrine base. Tablets contain 100 mg of the dihydrochloride.

Mode of Action

The complex mode of action of chloroquine can only be briefly described. For detailed discussions, consult the extensive literature (see Barthel et al. 1996, Zeidler 1995). Chloroquine is an amphiphilic molecule (lipophilic ring structure and hydrophilic side chain). This enables the incorporation in interphases such as phospholipid membranes. The weak basic antimalarials pass the membranes and are protonated in the acidic environment of the lysosomes. As a result, they are unable to penetrate the membranes, and chloroquine accumulates. The following effects can be explained by this mechanism:

- In plasmodia, intralysosomal proteases are inhibited, and heme, toxic for plasmodia, accumulates.
- In lysosomes of human leukocytes, the binding of antigens (low-affine peptides) to the "major histocompatibility complex" is inhibited and, as a result, the stimulation of specific T cells is prevented.
- This inhibition of antigen processing also impairs the production of antibodies, the activity of natural killer cells, and the release of interleukin-1, -2 and tumor necrosis factor-α (Jeong et al. 2002).

Furthermore, chloroquine reduces the generation of reactive oxygen species by neutrophils (Jancinova et al. 2001) and inhibits lymphocyte apoptosis (Liu et al. 2001).

In porphyria cutanea tarda, chloroquine forms complexes with the porphyrines, thus increasing their elimination with urine. In sarcoidosis, chloroquine inhibits the hydroxylation of 1,25,dihydroxy-vitamine D3, thus lowering the high plasma levels of vitamin D. In LE, a sunscreen effect and the inhibition of UV-induced activation of transcription factors are discussed.

Besides these immunologic effects, chloroquine and hydroxychloroquine inhibit the aggregation of thrombocytes without prolongation of the bleeding time (Espinola et al. 2002). Chloroquine increases the binding of insulin to its receptor, changes the metabolism of insulin in the liver, and thus amplifies the insulin action. Antimalarials increase the number of low-density lipoprotein receptors and inhibit the hepatic synthesis of cholesterol, thus lowering total cholesterol, low-density lipoprotein cholesterol, and triglyceride concentrations. Chloroquine also increases the pain threshold, even in healthy persons. This could explain the subjective improvement in joint pain.

The mechanisms of action of quinacrine are multifaceted. They include some of the mentioned effects (inhibition of T-cell response, antioxidant, inhibition of platelet aggregation) as well as antiprostaglandin actions (phospholipase A2 inhibition), lysosome stabilization, blocking of photodynamic actions and increase in light tolerance, sclerosing actions [nonsurgical sterilization by quinacrine pellet instillation into the uterus (Benagiano 2001)], and antimicrobial properties (see references in: Wallace 1989). Quinacrine had a more powerful in vitro anti-inflammatory activity compared with chloroquine and hydroxychloroquine (Ferrante et al. 1986).

Pharmacology

Methods of Analysis

Gas chromatography allows the measurement of chloroquine and its metabolite monodesethylchloroquine in concentrations of 30–60 µg/l (0.1–0.2 µmol/l). High performance liquid chromatography detects plasma concentrations of 3 ng/l (10 nmol/l) with a UV detector and of 0.15 ng/ml (0.5 nmol/l) with a fluorescence detector (Minzi et al. 2003, Walker and Ademowo 1996). The determination of chloroquine concentrations in saliva are not suited for the monitoring of therapy. Such monitoring is possible using hair and gas chromatography/mass spectrometry (Runne et al. 1992).

Because of the strong binding of chloroquine and its main metabolite to thrombocytes and granulocytes as well as the accumulation in erythrocytes (factors 2–5), the concentration in whole blood is 3–10 times higher than that in plasma. Compared with plasma, the chloroquine serum concentrations are higher and more variable because of the release of chloroquine out of thrombocytes during coagulation. To prevent these errors, adequate centrifugation (2000 g, 10–15 min) is required. The binding of chloroquine to glass may lower chloroquine concentrations in standard solutions and analytical jars. The addition of serum prevents this.

Pharmacokinetics

The information in the literature concerning the pharmacokinetics of chloroquine differ considerably with respect to patients, dosage intervals, indications, and mode of application (Carmichael et al. 2003, Ducharme and Farinotti 1996, Krishna and White 1996, Tett et al. 1994).

Resorption
Chloroquine is rapidly and almost completely absorbed after oral administration. Its bioavailability is ca. 0.77 to 0.16 in tablets and 0.88 to 0.16 in solution. In combination with a meal rich in fat and proteins, the resorption is enhanced in contrast to an empty stomach or meals deficient in fat or proteins. The maximum plasma concentrations are reached within 1–2 h. Quinacrine is also very readily absorbed from the intestinal tract. It reaches a peak in 8–12 h.

Distribution
The chloroquine concentrations in plasma depend on the dose taken and on the kidney and liver functions. Even with constant doses of 250 mg, a strong interindividual (0.2–0.8 µmol/ml) as well as intraindividual variation of approximately 30% can be found. Fifty percent to 70% of chloroquine is bound to plasma proteins. In many organs, the concentrations of chloroquine are much higher than in blood, sometimes up to 1,000 times higher. Owing to the strong affinity of chloroquine to melanin, it accumulates in the iris, chorioidea, and inner ear (concentrations are 80 times higher than in the liver). The concentrations decrease from the liver (highest) over spleen, kidney, lung, heart to muscle and brain. In fatty tissues, however, chloroquine is barely accumulated. This characteristic is important for the dosage. Chloroquine concentrations in the skin are approximately 100–200 times higher than in plasma,

whereas the concentration in the epidermis is approximately 3–7 times higher than in the dermis. Chloroquine can be found in the keratinocytes. The concentrations in living epidermis and stratum corneum are the same.

The fictive volume of distribution is high because of this accumulation in deep compartments In blood it reaches a mean±SD value of 115–167±64 l/kg, and in plasma about 800 l/kg. Chloroquine reaches equilibrium between plasma and tissue not before 4 weeks, and hydroxychloroquine not before 6 months.

Quinacrine is widely distributed in the tissues and very slowly liberated. Plasma concentrations increase rapidly during the first week, and 94% equilibrium is attained by the fourth week. Eighty percent to 90% of quinacrine is bound to plasma proteins. The drug accumulates in the same organs as chloroquine (liver: 20 000 times the plasma level; leukocytes, factor 200; erythrocytes, factor 2) and accumulates progressively if chronically administered (Wallace 1989).

Excretion

Chloroquine is eliminated very slowly. The pharmacokinetics of chloroquine excretion can be described with a multicompartmental model. The plasma concentrations fall poly-exponentially, that is, fast in the beginning and then slowly in the terminal phase. This elimination is prolonged with higher dosages. Therefore, the reported half-lives differ between 74.7 and 30.1 h, 146 to 325 h, and 32 days depending on dosage and the reference to the poly-exponential decrease (e. g., early or late terminal half-life time).

Forty percent to 70% of chloroquine is excreted unchanged with urine. The percentage is higher in acidic than in alkaline urine. The mean value of the total clearance of chloroquine reaches 0.35 l/kg per hour. An impaired kidney function prolongs the half-life time significantly. Chloroquine itself and, to a lesser extent, hydroxychloroquine, can impair creatinine clearance by 10%, which can reduce chloroquine excretion, especially in older patients. In these instances, an increased rate of side effects has to be expected owing to the accumulation of chloroquine, and the dosage has to be reduced.

Twenty-five percent to 40% of chloroquine is metabolized in the liver via cytochrome P450 enzymes to the pharmacologically active metabolites desethyl chloroquine and bisdesethyl chloroquine. Their plasma concentrations reach ca. 33%–40% and 10% of the chloroquine concentrations, respectively. Findings from animal experiments hinted at a stereoselectivity with respect to the binding to proteins (S[+]chloroquine 67%, R[-]chloroquine 35%) as well as to the clearance (faster metabolism and excretion of S[+]enantiomers). Corresponding differences in the clinical effects in men, however, were not reported up to now.

Five percent to 10% of chloroquine is excreted unchanged with the feces. The elimination of chloroquine is limited by the back diffusion of the substance from deep compartments into plasma. After a single dose, small amounts of chloroquine can be found in plasma and erythrocytes even after 56 days. After prolonged therapy, chloroquine could be detected in the plasma, erythrocytes, and urine of patients even 5 years after the last intake.

Quinacrine is slowly eliminated from the body. Less than 11% is eliminated in the urine daily. Significant amounts of quinacrine can still be detected in the urine for at least 2 months after therapy is discontinued.

Pharmacodynamics

For chloroquine, the relations of dose and effect are not well defined. For the pro-phylaxis of malaria, the plasma concentrations of chloroquine are regarded as effective if they are greater than 30 nmol/l (>9.6 µg/l) (better 40–100 nmol/l (12.8–32 µg/l). For the treatment of malaria, 300–600 nmol/l (96–192 µg/l) should be reached. To treat inflammatory rheumatic disorders, the recommended plasma concentration is 200 nmol/l (65 µg/l). With respect to the therapeutic effect, no differences in the plasma concentrations between responders and nonresponders were found (Miller et al. 1987, Wollheim et al. 1978). The rate of side effects, however, could be related to the plasma concentrations (not the cumulative total dose). Concentrations greater than 600 nmol/l are associated with an increased incidence of side effects. Furthermore, the acute intoxication symptoms after an overdose can be related to the plasma concentrations. Consequently, chloroquine should not be given intravenously or intra-muscularly to avoid cardiotoxic effects.

Indications

Chloroquine is used for a variety of diseases. For some indications the effectiveness is well established, such as LE, rheumatoid arthritis (O'Dell et al. 1996, [No authors listed] 1995), and prophylaxis and therapy of malaria. In other diseases, studies, small series, or case reports indicate a potential benefit of antimalarials (Table 26.1). Quinacrine is, according to controlled studies, effective in LE and several microbial diseases (giardiasis, tapeworms) (Wallace 1989).

Contraindications

As outlined previously, the severity of the treated disease has to be weighed against the risk of its therapy. Chloroquine and hydroxychloroquine are contraindicated in the case of hyperreactivity to 4-aminoquinolones (exanthema or exfoliative dermati-tis), retinopathy or impaired visual fields (danger of blindness), disorders of the hematopoietic system (risk of anemia, leukopenia, or agranulocytosis), glucose-6-phosphate dehydrogenase deficiency (danger of hemolysis; see previously), myasthe-nia gravis (neuromyopathy), and pregnancy (risk of malformations [exception: malaria and nursing; see previously]).

In the case of a history of porphyria, seizures (in individual cases, exacerbation of seizures), and severe liver or kidney insufficiency (risk of additional kidney damage and impaired chloroquine excretion), limiting chloroquine use is recommended. This also holds true for psoriasis, although in larger patient series no general deterioration of this skin disease was described (see Ochsendorf and Runne 1991).

Table 26.2. Drug interactions of chloroquine and hydroxychloroquine

Combination of chloroquine and hydroxychloroquine with ...			
Has no effect	Decreases bioavailability of	Bioavailability of chloroquine is decreased by	Increases rate of
Acetylsalicylic acid Ranitidine Imipramine	Ampicillin Bacampicillin	Cholestyramine Caolin/pectin Ammonium chloride	*Cutaneous reactions* Phenylbutanoze Pyrimethamin/sulfa-doxin *Sensibilization:* Probenecid *Muscle weakness:* Glucocorticoids Aminoglycosides
Increases side effects of	Increases plasma levels of	Bioavailability of chloroquine is increased by	Decreases effects of
Aurothioglucose Penicillamine Cyclosporine	Digoxin Methotrexate	Cimetidine Ritonavir Quinacrine	Physostigmine Neostigmine Rabies vaccination Typhus vaccination

Drug Interactions

Some possibly relevant drug interactions are summarized in Table 26.2 (Micromedex edition 1994, Rote Liste 2001). There are no data on incidence and actual clinical relevance.

Dosage

Application

Chloroquine can be given orally, intravenously, subcutaneously, and intramuscularly. Parenteral application leads to very high plasma concentrations (mean±SD plasma concentration after 3 mg/kg intramuscularly, 265±149 µg/l; orally, 54±122 µg/l). They are accompanied by unwanted and sometimes dangerous side effects.

A chloroquine daily oral dose of 250 mg leads to therapeutic plasma concentrations not before 3 weeks owing to the long plasma half-life. It was recommended to give a single dose of 1 g initially in adults, that is, four tablets of chloroquine. In our experience, this approach can lead to misunderstanding and an involuntary overdose (Ochsendorf and Runne 1991). Higher doses initially, such 2×250 mg/day for 4 weeks, often lead to unspecific side effects, such as nausea or stomach problems. Therefore, the patient may not accept this effective therapeutic concept any longer. It is recommended that higher doses be used only for a short period if at all. Short-term higher doses, as in malaria prophylaxis, seem to be safe with respect to retinopathy.

Quinacrine is given orally. Doses of 100 mg/day (one tablet) should not be exceeded. If optimal effects are achieved (3 to 6 months), the dose should be tapered 1 day a week every 2 months until maintenance doses of one to three tablets a week are reached. If diarrhea or other adverse reactions occur, the daily dose can be reduced to 25–50 mg. The time until a clinically apparent benefit occurs is approximately 2–3 months with this low dose (Wallace 1989).

Avoidance of Unwanted Effects by Regarding the Maximal Daily Dose

To prevent unwanted effects, especially retinopathy, it was recommended that the cumulative total dose of chloroquine be limited to a maximum of 100–300 g, that the duration of therapy be limited to 1 year, or that patients be treated only intermittently. These recommendations severely restricted the use of chloroquine. Chloroquine is undoubtedly able to induce retinal changes. The incidence, however, depends on neither the duration nor the cumulative dose. It is only related to the maximal daily dose of 3.5 (to 4) mg/kg ideal body weight for chloroquine and 6 (to 6.5) mg/kg ideal body weight for hydroxychloroquine.

Chloroquine has to be given according to the *ideal* body weight (calculation for daily routine: males, [body length (in centimeters) –100] –10%; females, [body length (in centimeters) –15%]), as the substance is not stored in fatty tissues.

Several publications demonstrate that even continuous prolonged therapy for years does not induce retinopathy if these daily doses are not exceeded (Mackenzie 1983, Maksymowych and Russell 1987, Scherbel et al. 1965, Levy et al. 1997). This also holds true for children (Laaksonen et al. 1974). Mackenzie did not observe retinal damage in 900 patients who received chloroquine for a mean of 7 years (cumulative dose, ~608 g). A retinopathy developed only if daily doses 4 mg/kg for chloroquine or 6.5 mg/kg for hydroxychloroquine were given (Mackenzie 1983). Levy et al. did not find evidence of maculopathy in 1207 patients treated with hydroxychloroquine at doses less than 6.5 mg/kg ideal body weight. The authors found one case of retinopathy in a patient treated with high doses (average, 6.98 mg/kg daily) for more than 7 years (Levy et al. 1997). These maximal daily doses should not be exceeded over prolonged periods.

The routine daily dose of one tablet of chloroquine (250 mg) or two tablets of hydroxychloroquine (400 mg) leads to an overdose if the ideal or actual body weight is ≤ 63 kg (Mackenzie 1983; see Table 26.3 and Fig. 26.1). Patients with ideal body weights between 63 and 72 kg receive 3.5–4 mg/kg chloroquine. Only body weights greater than 72 kg pose no problems with a daily dose of one tablet (Tables 26.3, 26.4). Care has to be taken when patients with an actual or ideal body weight less than 63 kg are treated. This concerns small and light persons, mainly women and corpulent short people (Fig. 26.1). If kidney or liver functions are impaired, the doses given in Table 26.3 have to be lowered further.

The maximal daily dose of quinacrine is 100 mg. The higher doses given formerly significantly increased the rate of side effects.

Table 26.3. Recommended daily dose according to ideal body weight (I-bw) for chloroquine and hydroxychloroquine[a]

	Chloroquine		Hydroxychloroquine			Chloroquine		Hydroxychloroquine	
I-bw (kg)	3.5 mg/kg I-bw	4 mg/kg I-bw	6 mg/kg I-bw	6.5 mg/kg I-bw	I-bw (kg)	3.5 kg/kg I-bw	4 mg/kg I-bw	6 mg/kg I-bw	6.5 mg/kg I-bw
30	105	120	180	195	60	210	240	360	390
31	108.5	124	186	201.5	61	213.5	244	366	396.5
32	112	128	192	208	62	217	248	372	403
33	115.5	132	198	214.5	63	220.5	252	378	409.5
34	119	136	204	221	64	224	256	384	416
35	122.5	140	210	227.5	65	227.5	260	390	422.5
36	126	144	216	234	66	231	264	396	429
37	129.5	148	222	240.5	67	234.5	268	402	435.5
38	133	152	228	247	68	238	272	408	442
39	136.5	156	234	253.5	69	241.5	276	414	448.5
40	140	160	240	260	70	245	280	420	455
41	143.5	164	246	266.5	71	248.5	284	426	461.5
42	147	168	252	273	72	252	288	432	468
43	150.5	172	258	279.5	73	255.5	292	438	474.5
44	154	176	264	286	74	259	296	444	481
45	157.5	180	270	292.5	75	262.5	300	450	487.5
46	161	184	276	299	76	266	304	456	494
47	164.5	188	282	305.5	77	269.5	308	462	500.5
48	168	192	288	312	78	273	312	468	507
49	171.5	196	294	318.5	79	276.5	316	474	513.5
50	175	200	300	325	80	280	320	480	520
51	178.5	204	306	331.5	81	283.5	324	486	526.5
52	182	208	312	338	82	287	328	492	533
53	185.5	212	318	344.5	83	290.5	332	498	539.5
54	189	216	324	351	84	294	336	504	546
55	192.5	220	330	357.5	85	297.5	340	510	552.5
56	196	224	336	364	86	301	344	516	559
57	199.5	228	342	370.5	87	304.5	348	522	565.5
58	203	232	348	377	88	308	352	528	572
59	206.5	236	354	383.5	89	311.5	356	534	578.5

[a] Data are given in milligrams. In the case of liver or kidney insufficiency, the doses have to be lowered.

Table 26.4. Recommendations for the practical management of the maximal daily dose of chloroquine (3.5–4 mg/kg ideal body weight)[a]

Ideal body weight (kg)	Chloroquine as a tablet 250 mg	+	81 mg (Junior)	Chloroquine as a syrup (ml)	Measuring spoon[b]	Chloroquine dose (mg)
32–35	1/2		–	5.4	1	125
36–41	1/4	+	1	6.2	1	144
42–46	–		2	7.0	2	162
47–53	3/4		–	8.1	2	188
54–59	1/2	+	1	8.9	2	206
60–65	3/4	+	1/2	9.8	2	228
66–70	–		3	10.5	3	243
>71	1		–	10.8	3 1/10	250

[a] Within the weight classes, the chloroquine dose approximates 4 mg/kg with lighter weights and 3.5 mg/kg with heavier weights. The lowest possible dose should be used. With syrup, an individual dose is possible. Caution is necessary in patients with hepatic or renal disease, in whom a dose reduction may be necessary.
[b] One measuring spoon (3.5 ml)=81 mg chloroquine; the maximal daily dose = 4 mg/kg ideal body weight corresponds to 0.17 ml/kg.

Prescription

For oral therapy, chloroquine tablets (250 mg), junior tablets (81 mg) and, at least in some countries, syrup can be prescribed (Table 26.4). Hydroxychloroquine is only available as tablets (200 mg). For individual doses, the dosing given in Table 26.5 can be used (Canadian rheumatology association 2000). Alternatively, tablets have to be pulverized, weighed, and put into portions. The single dose can be given as a powder, where the bitter taste can be masked by adding marmalade, honey, or apple juice. Alternatively, they can be packed into gelatin capsules. Quinacrine tablets contain 100 mg. For lower doses, they have to be cut.

Toxicology and Side Effects

Acute Overdose

Acute overdosing happens accidentally, mainly in children, or during an attempted suicide. Even a single dose of 750 mg of chloroquine (only three pills) can be lethal in small children (1–4 years old). Doses between 1 g (children) and 4 g (adults) may lead to cardiac arrhythmias, cardiac arrest, and death. Therefore, patients have to be explicitly informed about the absolute necessity of safe storage of these drugs to protect their children. In case of misuse, vomiting should be triggered immediately.

Owing to the accumulation in deep compartments and the inability to remove chloroquine, the treatment of acute chloroquine poisoning is very difficult. A better prognosis was reported with the following regimen: gastric lavage followed by active coal char for prevention of further absorption, early assisted ventilation, diazepam

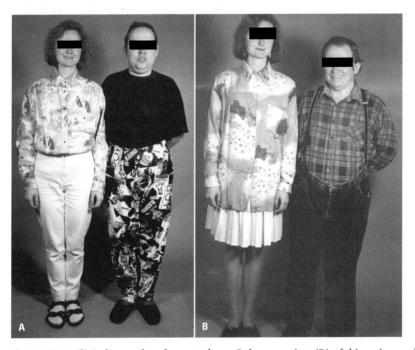

Fig. 26.1A–D. Clinical examples of correct doses. Only one patient (**D**) of this series would not be overdosed with a standard application of 250 mg of chloroquine. **A** The dose of the (index) person on the left has to be calculated according to her actual weight, which is lower than her ideal weight. Although the person on the right is taller and heavier, he still needs less than 250 mg chloroquine per day

	Left	Right
Height (cm)	160	165
Weight (kg)	48	71
Ideal body weight (kg)	51	59
Daily chloroquine dose (mg)	168 (max. 192)	206 (max. 236)
Daily hydroxychloroquine dose (mg)	288 (max. 312)	354 (max. 382)

B The male is smaller than the index person and weighs much more but nevertheless needs about the same daily dose.

	Left	Right
Height (cm)	160	155
Weight (kg)	48	80
Ideal body weight (kg)	51	50
Daily chloroquine dose (mg)	168	175
Daily hydroxychloroquine dose (mg)	288 (max. 312)	300 (max. 325)

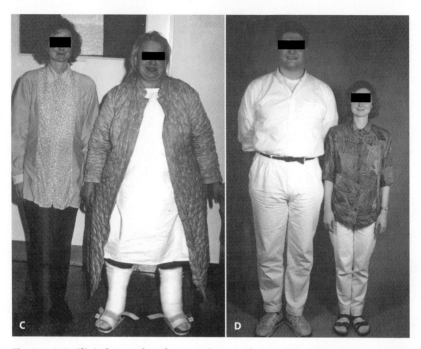

Fig. 26.1A–D. Clinical examples of correct doses. Only one patient (**D**) of this series would not be overdosed with a standard application of 250 mg of chloroquine (continued). **C** Although the lady on the right weighs three times more than the index person, the daily dose is about the same.

	Left	Right
Height (cm)	160	159
Weight (kg)	48	150
Ideal body weight (kg)	51	50
Daily chloroquine dose (mg)	168	175
Daily hydroxychloroquine dose (mg)	288 (max. 312)	300 (max. 325)

D The daily dose of one tablet (250 mg/day of chloroquine) for the man would be no problem and could eventually be increased.

	Left	Right
Height (cm)	196	160
Weight (kg)	125	48
Ideal body weight (kg)	86	51
Daily chloroquine dose (mg)	250 (up to 344)	168
Daily hydroxychloroquine dose (mg)	400 (up to 516, max. 559)	288 (max. 312)

Table 26.5. Recommendations for the practical management of the maximal daily dose of hydroxychloroquine (6–6.5 mg/kg *ideal* body weight). Using 200-mg tablets[a]

Body weight (kg)	Recommendation
31–35	200 mg daily
36–39	400 mg 1 day per week and 200 mg daily for the other 6 days of the week
40–43	400 mg 2 days per week and 200 mg daily for the other 5 days of the week
44–48	400 mg 3 days per week and 200 mg daily for the other 4 days of the week
49–52	200 mg 3 days per week and 400 mg daily for the other 4 days of the week
53–56	200 mg 2 days per week and 400 mg daily for the other 5 days of the week
57–61	200 mg 1 day per week and 400 mg daily for the other 6 days of the week

[a] Caution is necessary in patients with hepatic or renal disease, in whom a dose reduction may be necessary (modified after Canadian rheumatology association 2000).

administration, monitoring of potassium levels and replacement, and, in case of shock, epinephrine administration (Clemessy et al. 1996). The symptoms, clinical course, and treatment of hydroxychloroquine intoxication are the same as those of chloroquine intoxication (Jordan et al. 1999, Marquardt and Albertson 2001).

Side Effects with Therapeutic Doses

Chloroquine/Hydroxychloroquine

The daily dose determines the rate of side effects. If the individual daily doses according to the ideal body weight are not exceeded (Tables 26.3, 26.4), both chloroquine and hydroxychloroquine are tolerated well. Nevertheless, side effects may occur, especially with excessive daily doses or because of an individual hypersensitivity (Ochsendorf and Runne 1991). With the "standard doses" of 250 mg of chloroquine or 400 mg of hydroxychloroquine, approximately 10% of patients may experience one or several of the following side effects. However, as outlined, even these standard doses are too high for many patients. In a retrospective analysis, 20 of 156 patients discontinued therapy because of side effects {gastrointestinal, $n=11$; headache and dizziness, $n=2$; nonretinal eye problem, $n=2$; hearing loss, rash, $n=1$; myopathy, $n=2$ [1.9 cases in 1,000 patient-years]; and retinopathy, $n=1$ [6.5 mg/kg hydroxychloroquine for 6 years (0.95 cases per 1,000 patient-years)]} (Wang et al. 1999).

Unspecific complaints are nausea, abdominal cramps, flatulence, diarrhea, pyrosis, difficulties concentrating, and insomnia. After a pause and a dose reduction, a new and often successful attempt to treat can be made. If a more specific side effects occur, such as eye toxicity, exanthema, neuromyopathy, or hyperexcitability, the therapy has to be stopped.

Several authors believe that hydroxychloroquine is safer than chloroquine with respect to the incidence of side effects but less effective (Avina-Zubieta et al. 1998). It is possible, however, that daily doses were compared that were not equivalent: a comparison of daily doses of 400 mg of hydroxychloroquine with 500 mg of chloroquine revealed a higher incidence of retinopathy with the latter drug. The equivalent dose for therapeutic and unwanted effects, however, is not 500 mg but 250 mg of chloroquine daily (Ochsendorf and Runne 1997). Furthermore, Dubois stated that chloroquine "in much smaller doses than these equivalents produced greater cutaneous improvement and better sense of well-being in the patients with systemic manifestations" (Dubois 1976).

Eye

Chloroquine side effects affecting the eye are the most known and feared: retinopathy, cornea deposits, and difficulties in accommodation.

A *retinopathy* was reported in 0.5%–6% of treated patients; in some older studies, an incidence up to 40% was reported. Retinal changes, such as edema of the macula, narrowing of arterioles, clumping of retinal pigments (the so-called premaculopathy), and the bull's eye macula formerly were reported to be characteristic of chloroquine-induced changes (Maksymowych and Russell 1987). However, up to now, common, generally accepted criteria for the specific diagnosis of chloroquine-induced retinopathy are lacking. There seems to be no single and reliable screening test for retinal toxicity, and so the assessment is subjective (Jones 1999). A critical appraisal of the literature shows that formerly every visible retinal change obviously was regarded as being induced by chloroquine, although baseline investigations, control groups, and functional tests were lacking in many cases. In a controlled study (741 patients mainly with rheumatoid arthritis), Scherbel et al. found the same retinal changes in patients who never received chloroquine (n=333) as in those with long-term chloroquine use (n=408; 250 mg/day for 1–9 years). No functional disturbance was observed (Scherbel et al. 1965). Pinckers and Broekhuyse (Pinkers and Broekhuyse 1983) reported that results of the electro-oculogram, considered a sensitive test of retinal function and suggested as one of the screening tests for ocular damage in antimalarial therapy, were abnormal in 20% of patients with rheumatoid arthritis who had never been treated with antimalarials.

Although retinal changes seem to be rather improbable if the maximal daily dose according to ideal body weight is observed, ophthalmologic examinations were recommended (funduscopy, visual field testing, testing of color vision, and Amsler grid test) before the start of therapy and yearly; in patients older than 65 years, every 6 months (Maksymowych and Russell 1987, Ochsendorf et al. 1993, Rigaudiere et al. 2004). The baseline examination within 30 days before or after initiation of therapy could help to detect central red scotomata, which occur in up to 6% of the healthy population. Scotomata in patients with systemic LE (SLE) also can be caused by vasculitis, antiphospholipid syndrome, and glucocorticoid-induced diabetes mellitus; this investigation helps to detect those changes early, which are unrelated to chloroquine (Barthel et al. 1996). More intensive controls are necessary if kidney and liver functions are impaired, if the daily doses are higher than recommended, in patients older than 65 years, and in prolonged therapy (>5 years without interruption). The use of Amsler grids was advocated by some authors (Easterbrook 1985). This is a white grid superimposed on a black background, which can be used by the patient for regular testing at home. The development of wavy, gray, or indistinct lines during monocular fixation on the central white spot indicates incipient visual field defects. Recent case series of patients with hydroxychloroquine-induced retinopathy demonstrated the safety of the drug if renal function was normal (Bienfang et al. 2000, Mavrikakis et al. 2003). A Canadian consensus conference on hydroxychloroquine recommended the same controls as outlined for chloroquine (Canadian rheumatology association 2000).

Recently, a British group of ophthalmologists, dermatologists, and rheumatologists advocated that ophthalmologic baseline and follow-up examinations can be relinquished if maximal daily doses are observed and hydroxychloroquine is used. Only clinical controls at every visit and yearly controls of visual acuity were recommended. A special ophthalmologic examination was suggested only for special problems, such as weakness of vision, or in case of therapies longer than 5 years (Jones 1999). It is advisable to look for central visual field defects and to ask specifically for symptoms: flimmer scotoma, impaired vision by night, overlooking of words, or difficulties recognizing faces. If findings are conspicuous, an ophthalmologic examination should be initiated. Mackenzie recommended wearing sunglasses during chloroquine therapy for theoretical reasons (Mackenzie 1983).

Corneal deposits of chloroquine and the anterior stroma are common (30%–70%), but not dangerous. They are dose related and often asymptomatic. They are no reason to discontinue treatment. With hydroxychloroquine therapy, they are said to be rarer. Visual acuity is not impaired, but sometimes a "scattering" when looking into bright light was reported. The deposits may already be reversible during therapy, and they always disappear after discontinuation of the drug. A correlation to retinopathy was not observed according to the older literature. A recent consensus conference stated that corneal deposits should be recognized as evidence for possible overdose of hydroxychloroquine (Araiza-Casillas et al. 2004, Canadian rheumatology association 2000).

In cases of overdose, *difficulties in accommodating* occur (40% of patients with doses >500 mg/day). Mainly young patients notice blurred vision. A direct effect of chloroquine on the smooth muscles of the ciliary body is discussed as the cause. These difficulties in accommodating usually disappear spontaneously on continuation of therapy. There is no definite evidence that quinacrine is retinotoxic (Dubois 1976).

Skin

Chloroquine can induce hyperpigmentation, exanthema, exfoliative reactions, hypersensitivity to light, and pruritus.

Hyperpigmentation, that is, slate-gray to blue-black macules before the lower leg, in the face, the soft palate, or subungual are caused by hemosiderin and melanin. They disappear spontaneously within 11–20 months. In one case report, a depigmentation (such as vitiligo) was described that was reversible after discontinuation of chloroquine.

Exanthema can be maculopapular, lichenoid, or urticarial or can look like an erythema anulare centrifugum. Also, single cases with exfoliative reactions and toxic epidermal necrolyses were reported (Murphy and Carmichael 2001).

Chloroquine can induce *photoallergic and phototoxic reactions*. This has to be kept in mind if a light-sensitive dermatosis treated with chloroquine deteriorates (Metayer et al. 2001, Ochsendorf and Runne 1991).

Pruritus is mainly reported by black people during malaria prophylaxis and therapy (8%–74%). Within 11–48 h after intake of the drug, a generalized pruritus, especially on the palms, soles, and scalp, without visible skin changes starts. Antihistamines were of no benefit. Recently, the pruritus was attributed to opioidergic effects in a rat model. Promethazin and corticosteroids were of therapeutic benefit (Onigbogi 2000). Individuals with pruritus had an altered metabolism after therapeutic doses of chloroquine (Onyeji and Ogunbona 2001).

In prospective studies with large patient numbers, no exacerbation of psoriasis could be demonstrated statistically, and in some cases the psoriasis even got better. However, the psoriasis of individual patients may deteriorate under chloroquine.

Hair

A white discoloration is almost exclusively found in blond, ginger, or light-brown hair (about 60 case reports; see Ochsendorf and Runne 1991). These hair colors mainly are caused by pheomelanin, the syntheses of which is impaired by chloroquine. A toxic effect of chloroquine to the melanocyte was also reported (Ash et al. 1997). Daily dose seems to be the most relevant factor (mostly >400 mg/day), as a reduction in the daily dose to 250 mg/day was followed by recovery of the hair color despite continuation of therapy.

Nerve System and Muscles

A neuromyopathy during chloroquine therapy is rare (<1%). A slowly progressing weakness of the proximal arm and leg muscles was observed after treatment of at least 6 months with 250–500 mg chloroquine per day, after an overdose (1 g/day) already after 3 weeks (Ochsendorf and Runne 1991). The muscle reflexes are weakened or missing, the muscle enzyme levels rise, and the electromyogram shows neurogenic and myogenic changes. The same symptoms were reported after hydroxychloroquine therapy, especially in patients with renal insufficiency (Becerra-Cunat et al. 2003, Stein et al. 2000).

By light and electron microscopy, a granulovacuolar degeneration of muscle fibers as well as multiple osmophilic lamellar bodies at the neuromuscular junctions were demonstrated. Both clinical and histologic changes were reversible after discontinuation of the drug within a few weeks. In cases of clinical suspected cardiomyopathy, myocardial biopsy samples revealed the same morphologic changes in the heart muscle (Baguet et al. 1999). With normal doses, changes in the electrocardiogram, such as beveling of T waves, were observed. Hemodynamic changes, however, were not described. In long-term, high-dose treatment (>12 years, >250 mg/day), cases of complete heart blocks (Reuss-Borst et al. 1999) or cardiomyopathy were reported (Baguet et al. 1999, Nord et al. 2004).

Symptoms of the central nervous system include dizziness, vascular headache, hyperexcitability, seizures, and psychoses, which appear more likely in the case of excessive doses. In the case of predisposition, a seizure was described with normal doses in a young woman (Malcangi et al. 2000).

Ear

In adults, tinnitus and dizziness during chloroquine or hydroxychloroqine therapy are attributed to an ototoxic effect. This could be caused by an accumulation in the melanin of the stria vascularis or a destruction of sensory cells. Especially, parenteral application of chloroquine was associated with hearing loss, which was partially irreversible. After several years of hydroxychloroquine treatment of SLE/subacute cutaneous LE (SCLE), an irreversible hearing loss was reported in two patients (Johansen and Gran 1998). Chloroquine given during pregnancy can induce bilateral cochleovestibular paresis in the fetus.

Liver

Up to now, only two cases of liver toxicity have been reported after hydroxychloroquine use. No previous liver diseases were known in these patients, and the fulminant hepatic failures occurred within 2 weeks after starting the therapy (Makin et al. 1994). In patients with porphyria, excessive doses of chloroquine can induce a porphyria crisis.

Blood

Changes in the blood cell count, such as aplastic anemia, leukopenia, agranulocytosis, and hemolysis, were described rarely. The latter was observed almost exclusively in cases of glucose-6-phosphate dehydrogenase deficiency. The hemolytic effect of chloroquine, however, is so low grade that routine determination of the activity of this enzyme seems unnecessary. Some authors recommend doing this.

Other Symptoms

Recently, a hypersensitivity pneumonitis was described after chloroquine use (Mitja et al. 2000).

Pregnancy and Lactation

Therapy with chloroquine during pregnancy is discussed controversially. Chloroquine was associated with sensorineural hearing loss, blindness, malformations, abortion, and, in vitro, chromosomal damage. The frequency of these events was calculated with 1.2%–3.3% (control group <1%). On the other hand, there are several reports on healthy newborns after chloroquine therapy of the mother. It is agreed that malaria prophylaxis (2×500 mg/week) should be continued during pregnancy. In the case of a planned conception, however, it was recommended to discontinue chloroquine use in time. Here the potential risk of the treated disease, like activation of SLE (Wechsler et al. 1999), has to be weighed individually against the possible chloroquine side effects (Parke and West 1996). Recently, it was not recommended any longer to discontinue antimalarials in pregnant patients with SLE (Borden and Parke 2001). In a series of 21 newborns of mothers using chloroquine (daily dose, 332 mg) or hydroxychloroquine (daily dose, 317 mg) during pregnancy, no eye changes or other birth defects in the offspring were found (Klinger et al. 2001). This study suggests that when chloroquine or hydroxychloroquine are required to control symptoms of rheumatologic diseases in pregnant women, the risk-benefit ratio is favorable (Klinger et al. 2001). In a placebo-controlled study, hydroxychloroquine had beneficial effects with no side effects in the newborns (Costedoat-Chalumeau et al. 2003, Levy et al. 2001). No malformations were reported after hydroxychloroquine use (Barthel et al. 1996, Ostensen and Ramsey-Golderman 1998).

Chloroquine is excreted with the mother's milk. The chloroquine concentration is about the same as in saliva. Within 24 h, a breastfed baby takes up ca. 0.55% of the mother's dose. For hydroxychloroquine, the dose is 2% of the maternal dose per kilogram per day (Canadian rheumatology association 2000).

Quinacrine

Combining quinacrine with other 8-aminoquinolines increases their concentrations in plasma, and toxicity is enhanced.

Unspecific Symptoms

About half of the patients initially experience adverse reactions when taking 100 mg quinacrine, most of which are mild or reversible. About one-third experience headache, dizziness, or gastrointestinal symptoms (diarrhea, anorexia, nausea, or abdominal cramps). These reactions disappear spontaneously or after dose reduction, but approximately 20% of patients have to stop therapy. Some patients have persistent abdominal cramps or diarrhea; these symptoms can be ameliorated by bismuth-containing suspensions or spasmolytic agents.

Eye

Quinacrine has no retinal toxicity.

Skin

The skin may acquire a yellow stain from deposition of the drug in at least a third of the patients; according to others, it constantly discolors the skin (Leigh et al. 1979). The conjunctiva is also affected and resembles jaundice. However, plasma levels of bilirubin are normal. Also, hyperpigmentation and blue or black pigmentation the skin ("black and blue marks") and of the nails may occur. These marks consist of membrane-bound intracellular granules of quinacrine that contain large amounts of iron and some sulphur (Leigh et al. 1979). Discoloration was estimated to occur in about every second patient (Wallace 1989). The pigment may reduce its intensity or even disappear after a decrease in the daily dose of more than 50 mg. It resolves with drug withdrawal.

Rashes were reported in 1.6% of persons treated for malaria prophylaxis. Eighty percent were eczematous and 20% were lichenoid or exfoliative (Bauer 1981). The dermatitis resolved after discontinuation of the drug. In SLE, ca. 5% of patients developed a mild, reversible dermatitis with 25 to 100 mg/day of quinacrine. The incidence of lichenoid dermatitis was 1:2,000 with 100 mg/day and 1:500 with 200 mg/day. This dermatitis was followed by anhydrosis, cutaneous atrophy, alopecia, nail changes, altered pigmentation, and keratoderma (Bauer 1981). Even years later, lichenoid nodules, scaly red plaques, atrophic lesions on the soles, erosions, and leukoplakia of the tongue and fungating warty growths appeared. Progression to squamous cell carcinoma, especially on the palm, had occurred in several cases (Callaway 1979). Urticaria and exfoliative dermatitis, especially in patients with psoriasis, were reported in single cases.

Nerve System

Whereas in low doses psychic stimulation, alleviation of fatigue, and increased energy levels occurs, higher doses may be associated with restlessness, insomnia, nightmares, or psychosis, which quickly reverse within 2–4 weeks after discontinuation of the drug (Engel et al. 1947).

Liver

Reversible hepatitis was reported in single cases.

Blood

The most serious adverse reaction of quinacrine is aplastic anemia. The incidence increases with drug dose and duration of therapy. Only one case was reported with a daily dose of 100 mg (Wallace 1989). In every second patient, a premorbid lichen planus rash preceded the aplastic anemia. So, therapy has to be discontinued if a lichen planus rash occurs. The incidence of this aplasia with regular control of blood cell counts is estimated to be 1:500,000 (Wallace 1989).

Pregnancy and Lactation
The drug should not be given to pregnant women because it readily passes the placenta. However, successful pregnancies have been reported with concurrent quinacrine administration (Humphreys and Marks 1988).

Laboratory Surveillance

Up to now, published dermatologic expert opinions recommend all or some of the following tests before initiating therapy: complete blood cell counts, liver function tests, glucose-6-phosphate dehydrogenase levels, and urine porphyrin determinations, as well as blood cell count and liver function tests at follow-up every 3 to 4 months (Dutz and Ho 1998). However, this does not seem to be cost beneficial (Sontheimer 2000). In several studies, no significant hematologic or hepatic toxic effects were observed when using the previously mentioned dosing guidelines (Fox et al. 1996, Fries et al. 1993, Kuhn et al. 2000). It is questionable whether routine testing would have prevented the only three cases with severe side effects using the recommended doses: one report of a nonfatal case of serious hematologic toxic effects (McDuffie 1965) and two reports of idiosyncratic fatal hepatotoxic effects in the first 2 weeks of treatment (Makin and Wendon 1994).

Since 1996, the American College of Rheumatology guidelines for the use of hydroxychloroquine, although for rheumatoid arthritis, have stated explicitly that pretreatment and follow-up laboratory tests of any type are not necessary (American College of Rheumatology 1996). This recommendation is supported by the experience of Sontheimer and may hold true also for correctly dosed chloroquine (Sontheimer 2000). He estimates savings of approximately $1.1 million per year if routine laboratory tests for hydroxychloroquine would be abandoned by dermatologists and recommends cost-benefit analysis for laboratory analysis during the treatment of dermatologic diseases with antimalarials.

During quinacrine therapy, blood counts should be performed every 2–3 months. If significant decreases in hemoglobin levels and reticulocyte counts are observed, therapy has to be stopped.

Therapeutic Use

Discoid Lupus Erythematosus

Antimalarials should be considered in discoid LE (DLE) if no contraindications can be found, local therapy was ineffective, or relapses occurred soon after cessation of local therapy or the extent of the lesions is too large for local therapy.

Chloroquine and hydroxychloroquine especially improve the inflammatory manifestations of DLE. Spontaneous improvement of discoid lesions can be expected in approximately 15%, whereas antimalarials have a positive effect in more than 50% (up to 85%) of the plaques. If monotherapy is not satisfactory, the combination of chloroquine and hydroxychloroquine with quinacrine can improve efficacy (Feldmann et al. 1994, Wallace 2000).

Quinacrine (100 mg/day) has an onset of action of 3–4 weeks; its maximal effect occurs 6–8 weeks after initiation. With lower daily doses (50 mg), it takes longer to reach beneficial effects. Quinacrine monotherapy led to an excellent or improved response in approximately 73% (summary of 20 clinical trials in Wallace 1989). The application should be stopped or combined with other drugs, for example, chloroquine and hydroxychloroquine, if no effect is seen after 8 weeks.

In a recent Cochrane review, hydroxychloroquine was shown to improve or clear lesions of discoid LE in approximately 50% of patients, with fewer and less severe side effects than acitretine. There were not enough data, that is, randomized trials, to show reliable evidence for the effect of several other drugs (azathioprine, clofazimine, dapsone, gold, interferon alpha 1a, methotrexate, phenytoin, sulphasalazine, and thalidomide) (Jessop et al. 2001). However, several of those drugs are routinely and successfully used, also in combination with antimalarials. Smokers are less likely to respond to antimalarial therapy (Jewell and McCauliffe 2000).

Subacute Cutaneous/Systemic Lupus Erythematosus

In SLE, antimalarials can be used for early or mild cases without organ involvement or as a steroid-sparing agent. In cases of systemic involvement, antimalarial monotherapy is not indicated.

However, antimalarials can induce remissions and prevent exacerbations of chronic SLE ([No authors listed] 1995, Tsakonas et al. 1998). In a placebo-controlled randomized trial, chloroquine (250 mg) kept mild lupus in remission without serious side effects. The risk of an exacerbation of the disease was 4.6 times higher with placebo than with chloroquine (Meinao et al. 1996). Compared with nonsteroidal anti-inflammatory drugs, these compounds have the advantage of a lower risk for cutaneous, liver, and nephrotoxic reactions. In contrast to immunosuppressants, there is no risk of either bone marrow suppression or opportunistic infections. Therefore, chloroquine and hydroxychloroquine can be regarded as basic therapy for uncomplicated SLE (Barthel et al. 1996, D'Cruz 2001, Molad et al. 2002, Ruiz-Irastorza et al. 2000). In a recent survey, 70% of patients with SLE had received antimalarials (Wang et al. 1999). The average duration of therapy was 6.9 years per patient. Reasons for withdrawal of therapy were remission (42%), side effects (29%, see above), noncompliance (15%), and miscellaneous reasons, such as pregnancy (6%). Only in 8% was a lack of efficacy the reason for stopping therapy.

In SLE, the cutaneous symptoms, weariness, myalgias, and joint symptoms generally improve with antimalarial therapy (Williams et al. 1994). Also, mucosal lesions respond favorably (Orteu et al. 2001). If the heart, lungs, or kidneys are involved or if hematologic or vasculitic central nervous system manifestations occur, antimalarials should never be used alone (Barthel et al. 1996).

Whereas in SLE no exact data are available, a synergistic effect of the combination of methotrexate, sulfadiazine, and hydroxychloroquine was reported in rheumatoid arthritis. In addition, the hepatotoxicity of methotrexate was reduced (O'Dell et al.

1996, 2002). Exacerbations also were rare with continuation of hydroxychloroquine use (Clegg et al. 1997).

In SCLE, effectiveness of antimalarials of 50% to 80% was reported (Versapuech et al. 2000). Keep in mind that 90% of nonsmokers but only 40% of smokers with DLE/SCLE responded to antimalarials (Jewell and McCauliffe 2000). Therefore, smoking has to be regarded as a confounding factor impairing the therapeutic efficacy of antimalarials.

Quinacrine was also reported to add beneficial, steroid-sparing effects to a hydroxychloroquine therapy in SLE (Toubi et al. 2000) and SCLE (von Schmiedeberg et al. 2000). It can improve fever, adenopathy, sun sensitivity, mucous membrane lesions, alopecia, arthritis, headache, fatigue, and serositis. Quinacrine has no activity against nephritis, myocarditis, central nervous system involvement, or hematologic, hepatitis, or lung parenchymal involvement of lupus (Wallace 1989).

Other Lupus Variants

LE tumidus was treated effectively with antimalarials in 90% of patients (Kuhn et al. 2000). Therapeutic effects could mostly be seen after 4 to 6 weeks. Eight percent of the treated patients did not respond to chloroquine but could be successfully treated with hydroxychloroquine.

Lymphocytic infiltration of the skin recently was regarded as a photosensitive variant of LE (Weber et al. 2001). In 50% of cases, antimalarials were effective.

Lupus panniculitis was successfully treated with a combination of hydroxychloroquine and quinacrine (Chung and Hann 1997) and chloroquine and diltiazem (Morgan and Callen 2001). In the latter case, the lesions were calcified.

Prophylaxis of Thromboses, Antiphospholipid Syndrome

Chloroquine and hydroxychloroquine inhibit the aggregation of platelets. Given as thrombosis prophylaxis, hydroxychloroquine (600–800 mg/day for 1–2 weeks) reduced the rate of pulmonary emboli significantly in more than 10,000 patients with operative hip replacement (Loudon 1988). In another study, the rate of venous and arterial thromboembolic complications was significantly reduced in patients with SLE (Petri 1996). In a subgroup of SLE patients with phospholipid antibodies and a high risk of thrombotic events, thromboemboli occurred only in 4% (2/54) of the patients undergoing hydroxychloroquine therapy within 9 years, whereas in 20% of patients in the control group thromboemboli were observed within this time (Wallace et al. 1993). Therefore, chloroquine and hydroxychloroquine should be considered for the primary prophylaxis of thromboemboli in SLE. However, if thromboembolic complications have already occurred, anticoagulation is recommended.

Additional Effects

Antimalarials lowered the total cholesterol, low-density lipoprotein cholesterol, and triglyceride concentrations in patients with SLE, especially those who were concomitantly treated with corticosteroids (Borba and Bonfa 2001, Tam et al. 2000). Chloroquine lowered the blood glucose concentrations. These effects – reduction of the concentrations of lipids and blood sugar and the inhibition of platelet aggregation – could lower the risk of atherosclerosis (Barthel et al. 1996, Petri 1996, Rahmann et al. 1999, Wallace et al. 1993). Because SLE may be an additional risk factor for atherosclerosis, early therapy is discussed (Urowitz et al. 2000).

Conclusions

In the past, chloroquine and hydroxychloroquine became discredited because of possible severe side effects in the eye as a result of incorrect dosing. The rate of side effects, but not therapeutic efficacy, depends on plasma concentrations. Larger doses lead to accumulation of the drugs owing to their long half-lives. Therefore, maximal daily doses of 3.5 (to 4) mg/kg *ideal* body weight for chloroquine and 6 (to 6.5) mg/kg for hydroxychloroquine have to be observed. This is especially important for small people (women) and short corpulent persons. In case the of kidney or liver diseases, elimination may be impaired, and the dose has to be lowered. Control of the visual functions seems necessary. If these basic rules are observed, rather safe chloroquine and hydroxychloroquine therapy is possible for long periods. A combination of chloroquine and hydroxychloroquine with primaquine (or other substances) enhances the effectiveness. Because of their various effects (anti-inflammatory, corticosteroid sparing, lowering of corticosteroid side effects, antithrombotic), antimalarials are still essential drugs for the treatment of different variants of LE.

References

American College of Rheumatology Ad Hoc Committee on Clinical Guidelines (1996) Guidelines for monitoring drug therapy in rheumatoid arthritis. Arthritis Rheum 39:723–731

Araiza-Casillas R, Cardenas F, Morales Y, Cardiel MH (2004) Factors associated with chloroquine-induced retinopathy in rheumatic diseases. Lupus 13:119–124

Arnal C, Piette JC, Leone J, Taillan B, Hachulla E, Roudot-Thoraval F, Papo T, Schaeffer A, Bierling P, Godeau B (2002) Treatment of severe immune thrombocytopenia associated with systemic lupus erythematosus: 59 cases. J Rheumatol 29:75–83

Asch PH, Caussade P, Marquart-Elbaz C, Boehm N, Grosshans E (1997) Chloroquine-induced achromotrichia. An ultrastructural study. Ann Dermatol Venereol 124:552–556

Avina-Zubieta JA, Galindo-Rodriguez S, Newman S, Suarez-Almazor ME, Russell AS (1998) Long-term effectiveness of antimalarial drugs in rheumatic diseases. Ann Rheum Dis 57: 582–587

Baguet JP, Tremel F, Fabre M (1999) Chloroquine cardiomyopathy with conduction disorders. Heart 81:221–223

Barthel HR, Meier LG, Wallace DJ (1996) Antimalariamittel bei rheumatischen Erkrankungen. Dtsch med Wschr 121:1576–1582

Bauer F (1981) Quinacrine hydrochloride drug eruption (tropical lichenoid dermatitis). Its early and late sequelae and its malignant potential. A review. J Am Acad Dermatol 4:239–248

Becerra-Cunat JL, Coll-Canti J, Gelpi-Mantius E, Ferrer-Avelli X, Lozano-Sanchez M, Millan-Torne M, Ojanguren I, Ariza A, Olive A (2003) Chloroquine-induced myopathy and neuropathy: progressive tetraparesis with areflexia that simulates a polyradiculoneuropathy. Two case reports. Rev Neurol 36:523–526

Benagiano G (2001) Non-surgical female sterilization with quinacrine: an update. Contraception 63:239–245

Bienfang D, Coblyn JS, Liang MH, Corzillius M (2000) Hydroxychloroquine retinopathy despite regular ophthalmologic evaluation: a consecutive series. J Rheumatol 27:2703–2706

Boelaert JR, Piette J, Sperber K (2001) The potential place of chloroquine in the treatment of HIV-1-infected patients. J Clin Virol 20:137–140

Borba EF, Bonfa E (2001) Longterm beneficial effect of chloroquine diphosphate on lipoprotein profile in lupus patients with and without steroid therapy. J Rheumatol 28:780–785

Borden MB, Parke AL (2001) Antimalarial drugs in systemic lupus erythematosus: use in pregnancy. Drug Saf 24:1055–1063

Callaway JL (1979) Late sequelae of quinacrine dermatitis, a new premalignant entity. J Am Acad Dermatol 1:456–457

Canadian Hydroxychloroquine Study Group (1991) A randomized study of the effect of withdrawing hydroxychloroquine sulfate in systemic lupus erythematosus. New Engl J Med 324:150–154

Canadian rheumatology association (2000) Canadian Consensus Conference on hydroxychloroquine. J Rheumatol 27:2919–2921

Carmichael SJ, Charles B, Tett SE (2003) Population pharmacokinetics of hydroxychloroquine in patients with rheumatoid arthritis. Ther Drug Monit 25:671–681

Chung HS, Hann SK (1997) Lupus panniculitis treated by a combination therapy of hydroxychloroquine and quinacrine. J Dermatol 24:569–572

Clegg DO, Dietz F, Duffy J, Willkens RF, Hurd E, Germain BF, Wall B, Wallace DJ, Bell CL, Sleckman J (1997) Safety and efficacy of hydroxychloroquine as maintenance therapy for rheumatoid arthritis after combination therapy with methotrexate and hydroxychloroquine. J Rheumatol 24:1896–1902

Clemessy JL, Taboulet P, Hoffmann JF, Hantson P, Barriot P, Bismuth C, Baud J (1996) Treatment of acute chloroquine poisoning: a 5-year experience. Critical Care Med 24:1189–1195

Costedoat-Chalumeau N, Amoura Z, Duhaut P, Huong du LT, Sebbough D, Wechsler B, Vauthier D, Denjoy I, Lupoglazoff JM, Piette JC (2003) Safety of hydroxychloroquine in pregnant patients with connective tissue diseases: a study of one hundred thirty-three cases compared with a controll group. Arthritis Rheum 48:3207–3211

D'Cruz D (2001) Antimalarial therapy: a panacea for mild lupus? Lupus 10:148–151

Dereure O, Guilhou JJ (2002) Eosinophilic-like erythema: a clinical subset of Well's eosinophilic cellulitis responding to antimalarial drugs? Ann Dermatol Venereol 129:720–723

Dubois EL (1976) Lupus erythematosus, 2nd edn. University of Southern California Press, Los Angeles, pp 548, 588

Ducharme J, Farinotti R (1996) Clinical pharmacokinetics and metabolism of chloroquine. Focus on recent advancements. Clin Pharmacokin 31:257–274

Dutz JP, Ho VC (1998) Immunosuppressive agents in dermatology: an update. Dermatol Clin 16:235–251

Easterbrook M (1985) The sensitivity of Amsler grid testing in early chloroquine retinopathy. Trans Opthalmol Soc UK 104:204–207

Engel GL, Romano J, Ferris Eb (1947) Effect of quinacrine on the central nervous system. Arch Neurol 58:337–350

Erkan D, Yazici Y, Peterson MG, Sammaritano L, Lockshin MD (2002) A cross-sectional study of clinical thrombotic risk factors and preventive treatments in antiphospholipid syndrome. Rheumatology (Oxford) 41:924–929

Espinola RG, Pierangeli SS, Ghara AE, Harris EN (2002) Hydroxychloroquine reverses platelet activation induced by human IgG antiphospholipid antibodies. Thromb Haemost 87:518–522

Feldmann R, Salomon D, Saurat JH (1994) The association of the two antimalarials chloroquine and quinacrine for treatment-resistant chronic and subacute cutaneous lupus erythematosus. Dermatology 189:425–427

Ferrante A, Rowan-Kelly B, Seow WK, Thong YH (1986) Depression of human polymorphonuclear leucocyte function by anti-malarial drugs. Immunology 85:125–130

Fox RI, Dixon R, Guarrassi V, Krubel S (1996) Treatment of primary Sjogren's syndrome with hydroxychloroquine: a retrospective, open-label study. Lupus 5 (Suppl 6):S31–S36

Fries JF, Williams CA, Ramey DR, Block DA (1993) The relative toxicity of the disease-modifying antirheumatic drugs. Arthritis Rheum 36:297–306

Humphreys F, Mrks JM (1988) Mepacrine and pregnancy. Br J Dermatol 118:452

Jancinova V, Nosal R, Drabikova K, Danihelovaa E (2001) Cooperation of chloroquine and blood platelets in inhibition of polymorphonuclear leukocyte chemiluminescence. Biochem Pharmacol 62:1629–636

Jeong JY, Choi JW, Jeon KI, Jue DM (2002) Chloroquine decreases cell-surface expression of tumour necrosis factor receptors in human histiocytic U-937 cells. Immunology 105:83–91

Jessop S, Whitelaw D, Jordaan F (2004) Drugs for discoid lupus erythematosus (Cochrane Review). In: The Cochrane Library, Issue 2, Chichester, UK, Y. Wiley & Sons Ltd.

Jewell ML, McCauliffe DP (2000) Patients with cutaneous lupus erythematosus who smoke are less responsive to antimalarial treatment. J Am Acad Dermatol 42:983–987

Johansen PB, Gran JT (1998) Ototoxicity due to hydroxychloroquine: report of two cases. Clin Exp Rheumatol 16:472–474

Jones SK (1999) Ocular toxicity and hydroxychloroquine: guidelines for screening. Br J Dermatol 140:3–7

Jordan P, Brookes JG, Nikolic G, Le Couteur DG (1999) Hydroxychloroquine overdose: toxicokinetics and management. J Toxicol Clin Toxicol 37:861–864

Khoury H, Trinkaus K, Zhang MJ, Adkins D, Brown R, Vij R, Goodnough LT, Ma MK, McLeod HL, Shenoy S, Horowitz M, Dispersio JF (2003) Hydroxychloroquine for the prevention of acute graft-versus-host disease after unrelated donor transplantation. Biol Blood Marrow Transplant 9:714–721

Klinger G, Morad Y, Westall CA, Laskin C, Spitzer KA, Koren G, Ito S, Buncic RJ (2001) Ocular toxicity and antenatal exposure to chloroquine or hydroxychloroquine for rheumatic diseases. Lancet 358:813–814

Krishna S, White NJ (1996) Pharmacokinetics of quinine, chloroquine and amodiaquine. Clinical implications. Clin Pharmacokin 30:263–299

Kuhn A, Richter-Hintz D, Oslislo C, Ruzicka T, Megahed M, Lehmann P (2000) Lupus erythematosus tumidus – a neglected subset of cutaneous lupus erythematosus: report of 40 cases. Arch Dermatol 136:1033–1041

Laaksonen AL, Koskiahde V, Juva K (1974) Dosage of antimalarial drugs for children with juvenile rheumatoid arthritis and systemic lupus erythematosus. Scand J Rheumatol 3:103–109

Leigh JM, Kennedy CTC, Ramsey JD, Henderson WJ (1979) Mepacrine pigmentation in systemic lupus erythematosus. Br J Dermatol 101:147–153

Levy GD, Munz SJ, Paschal J (1997) Incidence of hydroxychloroquine retinopathy in 1207 patients in a large multicentre outpatient practice. Arthritis Rheum 40:1482–1486

Levy RA, Vilela VS, Cataldo MJ, Ramos RC, Duarte JL, Tura BR, Albuquerque EM, Jesus NR (2001) Hydroxychloroquine (HCQ) in lupus pregnancy: double-blind and placebo-controlled study. Lupus 10:401–404

Liu ST, Wang CR, Yin GD, Liu MF, Lee GL, Chen MY, Chuang CY, Chen CY (2001) Hydroxychloroquine sulphate inhibits in vitro apoptosis of circulating lymphocytes in patients with systemic lupus erythematosus. Asian Pac J Allergy Immunol 19:29–35

Loudon JR (1988) Hydroxychloroquine and postoperative thromboembolism after total hip replacement. Amer J Med 85(Suppl 4a):57–61

Mackenzie AH (1983) Dose refinements in long-term therapy of rheumatoid arthritis with antimalarials. Am J Med 75(Suppl):40–45

Makin AJ, Wendon J, Fitt S, Portmann BC, Williams R (1994) Fulminant hepatic failure secondary to hydroxychloroquine. Gut 35:569–570

Maksymowych W, Russell AS (1987) Antimalarials in rheumatology: efficacy and safety. Semin Arthritis Rheum 16:206–221

Malcangi G, Fraticelli P, Palmieri C, Cappelli M, Danieli MG (2000) Hydroxychloroquine-induced seizure in a patient with systemic lupus erythematosus. Rheumatol Int 20:31–33

Marquardt K, Albertson TE (2001) Treatment of hydroxychloroquine overdose. Am J Emerg Med 19:420–424

Mavrikakis I, Sfikakis PP, Mavrikakis E, Rougas K, Nikolaou A, Kostopoulos C, Mavrikakis M (2003) The incidence of irreversible retinal toxicity in patients treated with hydroxychloroquine: a reappraisal. Ophthalmology 110:1321–1326

McDuffie FC (1965) Bone marrow depression after drug therapy in patients with systemic lupus erythematosus. Ann Rheum Dis 24:289–292

Meinao IM, Sato EI, Andrade LE, Ferraz MB, Atra E (1996) Controlled trial with chloroquine diphosphate in systemic lupus erythematosus. Lupus 5:237–241

Metayer I, Balguerie X, Courville P, Lauret P, Joly P (2001) Photodermatosis induced by hydroxychloroquine: 4 cases. Ann Dermatol Venereol 128:729–731

Miller DR, Fiechtner JJ, Carpenter JR, Brown RR, Stroshane RM, Stecher VJ (1987) Plasma hydroxychloroquine concentrations and efficacy in rheumatoid arthritis. Arthritis Rheum 30:567–571

Minzi OM, Rais M, Svensson JO, Gustafsson LL, Ericsson O (2003) High-performance liquid chromatographic method for determination of amodiaquine, chloroquine and their monodesethyl metabolites in biological samples. J Chromatogr B Analyt Technol Biomed Life Sci 783:473–480

Mitja K, Izidor K, Music E (2000) Chloroquine-induced drug hypersensitivity alveolitis. Pneumologie 54:395–397

Molad Y, Gorshtein A, Wysenbeek AJ, Guedj D, Majadla R, Weinberger A, Amit-Vazina M (2002) Protective effect of hydroxychloroquine in systemic lupus erythematosus. Prospective long-term study of an Israeli cohort. Lupus 11:356–361

Morgan KW, Callen JP (2001) Calcifying lupus panniculitis in a patient with subacute cutaneous lupus erythematosus: response to diltiazem and chloroquine. J Rheumatol 28:2129–2132

Murphy M, Carmichael AJ (2001) Fatal toxic epidermal necrolysis associated with hydroxychloroquine. Clin Exp Dermatol 26:457–458

Nguyen K, Washenik K, Shupack J (2002) Necrobiosis lipoidica diabeticorum treated with chloroquine. J Am Acad Dermatol 45:S34–36

[No authors listed] (1995) A randomized trial of hydroxychloroquine in early rheumatoid arthritis: the HERA study. Amer J Med 98:156–168

Nord JE, Shah PK, Rinaldi RZ, Weisman MH (2004) Hydroxychloroquine cardiotoxicity in systemic lupus erythematosus: a report of 2 cases and review of the literature. Semin Arthritis Rheum 33:336–351

Ochsendorf FR, Runne U (1991) Chloroquin und Hydroxychloroquin: Nebenwirkungsprofil wichtiger Therapeutika. Hautarzt 42:140–146

Ochsendorf FR, Runne U (1991) Subakute Chloroquin-Überdosierung: Schwindel, körperliche Schwäche, bullöse Lichtreaktion, Sehstörungen und generalisierte Weißfärbung der Haare. Dtsch med Wschr 116:1513–1516

Ochsendorf FR, Runne U, Goerz G, Zrenner E (1993) Chloroquin-Retinopathie: durch individuelle Tagesdosis vermeidbar. Dtsch Med Wochenschr 118:1895–1898

Ochsendorf FR, Runne U (1997) Therapie des systemischen Lupus erythematodes. Dtsch Med Wochenschr 122:877

O'Dell JC, Haire C, Erikson N, Drymalski W, Palmer W, Eckhoff J, Garwood V, Maloley P, Klassen L, Wees S, Klein H, Moore G (1996) Treatment of rheumatoid arthritis with methotrexate alone, sulfasalazine and hydroxychloroquine or a combination of all three medications. New Engl J Med 344:1287–1291

O'Dell JR, Leff R, Paulsen G, Haire C, Mallek J, Eckhoff PJ, Fernandez A, Blakely K, Wees S, Stoner J, Hadley S, Felt J, Palmer W, Waytz P, Churchill M, Klassen L, Moore G (2002) Treatment of rheumatoid arthritis with methotrexate and hydroxychloroquine, methotrexate and sulfasalazine, or a combination of the three medications: results of a two-year, randomized, double-blind, placebo-controlled trial. Arthritis Rheum 46:1164–1170

Onigbogi O, Ajayi AA, Ukponmwan OE (2000) Mechanisms of chloroquine-induced body-scratching behavior in rats: evidence of involvement of endogenous opioid peptides. Pharmacol Biochem Behav 65:333–337

Onyeji CO, Ogunbona FA (2001) Pharmacokinetic aspects of chloroquine-induced pruritus: influence of dose and evidence for varied extent of metabolism of the drug. Eur J Pharm Sci 13:195–201

Orteu CH, Buchanan JA, Hutchison I, Leigh IM, Bull RH (2001) Systemic lupus erythematosus presenting with oral mucosal lesions: easily missed? Br J Dermatol 144:1219–1223

Ostensen M, Ramsey-Goldman R (1998) Treatment of inflammatory rheumatic disorders in pregnancy: what are the safest treatment options? Drug Saf 19:389–410

Parke AL, West B (1996) Hydroxychloroquine in pregnant patients with SLE. J Rheumatol 23:1715–1718

Petri M (1996) Hydroxychloroquine use in the Baltimore lupus cohort. Effects on lipids, glucose and thrombosis. Lupus 5(Suppl 1):S16–S22

Pinckers A, Broekhuyse RM (1983) The EOG in rheumatoid arthritis. Acta Ophthalmol 61:831–837

Rahman P, Gladman DD, Urowitz MB, Yuen K, Hallett D, Bruce IN (1999) The cholesterol lowering effect of antimalarial drugs is enhanced in patients with lupus taking corticosteroid drugs. J Rheumatol 26:325–330

Reeves GE, Boyle MJ, Bonfield J, Dobson P, Loewenthal M (2004) Impact of hydroxychloroquine therapy on chronic urticaria: chronic autoimmune urticaria study and evaluation. Intern Med J 34:182–186

Reuss-Borst M, Berner B, Wulf G, Muller GA (1999) Complete heart block as a rare complication of treatment with chloroquine. J Rheumatol 26:1394–1395

Rigaudiere F, Ingster-Moati I, Hache JC, Leid J, Verdet R, Haymann P, Rigolet MH, Zanlonghi X, Defoort S, Le Gargasson JF (2004) Up-dated ophthalmological screening and follow-up management for long-term antimalarial treatment. J Fr Ophthalmol 27:191–199

Ruiz-Irastorza G, Khamashta MA, Hughes GR (2000) Therapy of systemic lupus erythematosus: new agents and new evidence. Expert Opin Investig Drugs 9:1581–1593

Runne U, Ochsendorf FR, Schmid K, Raudonat HW (1992) Sequential concentration of chloroquine in human hair correlates with ingested dose and duration of therapy. Acta Derm Venereol (Stockh) 72:355–357

Savarino A, Gennero L, Sperber K, Boelaert JR (2001) The anti-HIV-1 activity of chloroquine. J Clin Virol 20:131–135

Scherbel AL, Mackenzie AH, Nousek JE, Adtjian M (1965) Ocular Lesions in Rheumatoid Arthritis and Related Disorders with Particular Reference to Retinopathy. N Engl J Med 273: 360–366

Sontheimer RD (2000) Questions answered and a $1 million question raised concerning lupus erythematosus tumidus: is routine laboratory surveillance testing during treatment with hydroxychloroquine for skin disease really necessary. Arch Dermatol 136:1044–1049

Stein M, Bell MJ, Ang LC (2000) Hydroxychloroquine neuromyotoxicity. J Rheumatol 27: 2927–2931

Tam LS, Gladman DD, Hallett DC, Rahman P, Urowitz MB (2000) Effect of antimalarial agents on the fasting lipid profile in systemic lupus erythematosus. J Rheumatol 27:2142–2145

Tett SE, McLachlan AJ, Cutler DJ, Day RO (1994) Pharmacokinetics and pharmacodynamis of hydroxychloroquine enantiomers in patients with rheumatoid arthritis receiving multiple doses of racemate. Chirality 6:355–359

Toubi E, Rosner I, Rozenbaum M, Kessel A, Golan TD (2000) The benefit of combining hydroxychloroquine with quinacrine in the treatment of SLE patients. Lupus 9:92–95

Tsakonas E, Joseph L, Esdaile JM, Choquette D, Senecal JL, Cidicino A, Danoff D, Osterland CK, Yeadon C, Smith CD (1998) A long-term study of hydroxychloroquine withdrawal on exacerbations in systemic lupus erythematosus. The Canadian hydroxychloroquine study group. Lupus 7:80–85

Urowitz M, Gladman D, Bruce I (2000) Atherosclerosis and systemic lupus erythematosus. Curr Rheumatol Rep 2:19–23

Versapuech J, Beylot-Barry M, Doutre MS, Beylot C (2000) Subacute cutaneous lupus. Evolutive and therapeutic features of a series of 24 cases. Presse Med 29:1596–1599

von Schmiedeberg S, Ronnau AC, Schuppe HC, Specker C, Ruzicka T, Lehmann P (2000) Combination of antimalarial drugs mepacrine and chloroquine in therapy refractory cutaneous lupus erythematosus. Hautarzt 51:82–85

Walker O, Ademowo OG (1996) A rapid, cost-effective liquid-chromatographic method for the determination for chloroquine and desethylchloroquine in biological fluids. Therap Drug Monitor 1:92–96

Wallace DJ (1989) The use of quinacrine (Atabrine) in rheumatic diseases: a reexamination. Semin Arthritis Rheum 18:282–296

Wallace DJ, Linker-Israeli M, Methger AL, Stecher VM (1993) The relevance of antimalarial therapy with regard to thrombosis, hypercholesterolemia and cytokines in SLE. Lupus 2(Suppl 1):S13–S15

Wallace DJ (1996) The use of chloroquine and hydroxychloroquine for non-infectious conditions other than rheumatoid arthritis or lupus: a critical review. Lupus 5(Suppl 1):S59–S64

Wallace DJ (2000) Is there a role for quinacrine (Atabrine) in the new millennium? Lupus 9:81–82

Weber F, Schmuth M, Fritsch P, Sepp N (2001) Lymphocytic infiltration of the skin is a photosensitive variant of lupus erythematosus: evidence by phototesting. Br J Dermatol 144:292–296

Wechsler B, Le Thi Huong D, Piette JC (1999) Pregnancy and systemic lupus erythematosus. Ann Med Interne (Paris) 150:408–418

Williams HJ, Egger MJ, Szinger JZ, Willkens RF, Kalunian KC, Clegg DO, Skosey JL, Brooks RH, Alarcon GS, Steen VD, Polisson RP, Ward JR (1994) Comparison of hydroxychloroquine and placebo in the treatment of the arthropathy of mild systemic lupus erythematosus. J Rheumatol 21:1457–1462

Wollheim FA, Hanson A, Laurell CB (1978) Chloroquine treatment in rheumatoid arthritis. Scand J Rheumatol 7:171–176

Zeidler GS (1995) Chloroquin (Resochin[R]) Synoptische Darstellung eines Pharmakons und seiner Indikation in der Medizin, speziell in der Dermatologie. In: Hautklinik. Düsseldorf: Heinrich-Heine University, Inaugural Dissertation

Ziering CL, Rabinowith LG, Esterly NB (1993) Antimalarials for children: indications, toxicities, and guidelines. J Am Acad Dermatol 28:764–770

CHAPTER 27

Dapsone and Retinoids 27

David Bacman, Annegret Kuhn, Thomas Ruzicka

Dapsone

Dapsone (4,4'-diaminodiphenylsulphone) has been in clinical use for more than 60 years. It is widely used in the treatment of a variety of infectious diseases, including leprosy and malaria, and it has some action against other parasites. In addition, it has been effective in the treatment of a diversity of cutaneous disorders, particularly those characterized by a neutrophilic infiltrate but also cutaneous manifestations of lupus erythematosus (LE), erythema nodosum, cutaneous vasculitides, pyoderma gangrenosum, bullous dermatoses, and dermatitis herpetiformis (Lang 1979, Mok et al. 1998).

Pharmacology

Chemistry
The chemical structure of dapsone is the simplest of the sulfones, all of which share a characteristic structure: a sulfur atom linking to two carbon atoms. Derivatives of dapsone, such as sulfoxone, are thought to be metabolized to the parent dapsone structure (Fig. 27.1) (Katz 1999, Zhu and Stiller 2001).

Pharmacokinetics
Absorption
After oral administration, dapsone is well absorbed from the gastrointestinal tract, with a bioavailibility of more than 86%. Peak serum levels are reached 2–6 h after a single dose is administered. After 8–10 days of therapy at a constant dosage level, the serum level stabilizes and remains at that point unless the dosage is changed. The elimination half-life ranges from 12–30 h, which may be due to the enterohepatic circulation of the drug and the extensive protein binding (Katz 1999, Lang 1979, Zhu and Stiller 2001, Zuidema et al. 1986).

Distribution
Dapsone is ca. 70%–90% bound to plasma protein, and its monoacetylated metabolite (monoacetyldapsone [MADDS]) is almost entirely (99%) protein bound. Dapsone seems to be distributed throughout the body, including the skin, liver, kidneys, and erythrocytes. Dapsone crosses the blood-brain barrier and the placenta and is excreted in breast milk. Nevertheless, there are no reports of harmful effects on the fetus in utero, and only a few cases of neonatal hemolysis have been described (Zhu and Stiller 2001, Zuidema et al. 1986).

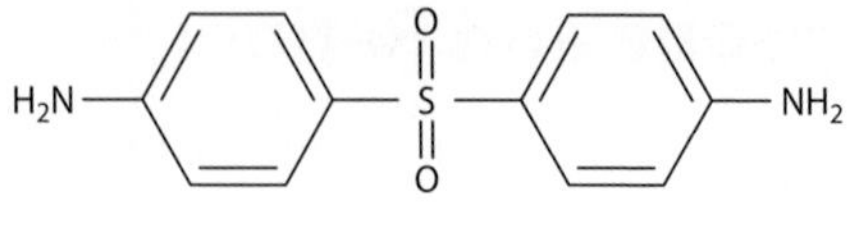

Fig. 27.1. Chemical structure of dapsone and its major metabolite

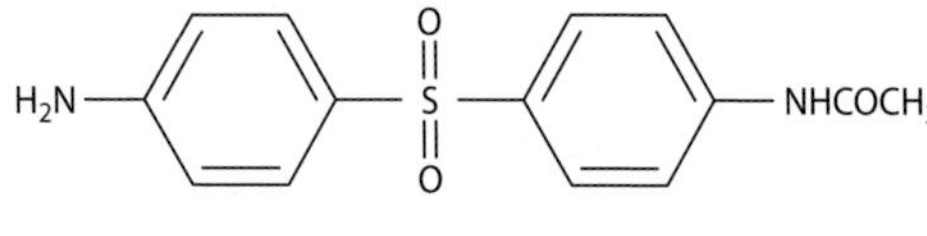

Dapsone

Monoacetyldapsone

Metabolism and Excretion

After absorption in the gastrointestinal tract, dapsone is transported to the liver, where it undergoes different metabolic transformations. The two major metabolic pathways involve N-acetylation and N-hydroxylation. Dapsone and its derivatives are acetylated by N-acetyltranferase to the nontoxic metabolites MADDS and diacetyl-dapsone. As with several other drugs, such as isoniazid and hydralazine, patients show genetic polymorphism in their ability to acetylate dapsone; some patients rapidly acetylate dapsone to MADDS ("rapid" acetylators), whereas in others this process occurs slowly ("slow" acetylators). Deacetylation occurs simultaneously, and a stable equilibrium between MADDS and dapsone is reached within a few hours of oral administration. However, it seems that the rate of acetylation does not relate to the half-life in the body and does not affect the efficacy of the drug. The other major metabolic pathway is hydroxylation, and it is responsible for hematologic side effects, such as methemoglobinemia, hemolysis, and Heinz-body formations. N-Hydroxylation is effected by a variety of cytochrome P-450 enzymes (CYP3A, CYP2E, and CYP2C) forming hydroxylamine, a potentially toxic metabolite, using hepatic microsomes. The levels of expression of these cytochrome P-450 enzymes may be crucial for individual vulnerability to dapsone side effects. Finally, dapsone, MADDS, and hydroxylamine are conjugated in the liver with glucuronic acid in preparation for excretion. Approximately 85%–90% of dapsone is excreted in the urine, primarily as glucuronide. Only 10% is excreted in the bile. Approximately 50% of a single dose of dapsone is excreted within the first 24 h. Probenecid decreases the renal clearance of dapsone, whereas rifampicin increases urinary excretion. Since dapsone is subject to enterohepatic circulation, administration of activated charcoal decreases its elimination half-life by 50% (Katz 1999, Lang 1979, Zhu and Stiller 2001, Zuidema et al. 1989).

Mode of Action

Antibacterial Action

Dapsone acts in leprosy and other infectious diseases in the same way as sulfonamides, inhibiting the synthesis of dihydrofolic acid through competition with para-aminobenzoate for the active site of dihydropteroate synthetase (Coleman 1993, Wozel and Barth 1988, Zhu and Stiller 2001).

Anti-inflammatory Action

The anti-inflammatory effect of dapsone is not related to its antibacterial effect. Dermatoses that respond to dapsone are in general associated with the accumulation of large numbers of polymorphonuclear leukocytes, mainly neutrophils. After stimulation, neutrophils release the heme-containing enzyme myeloperoxidase, which converts nicotinamide adenine dinucleotide phosphate-dependent oxygen to toxic oxygen intermediates, such as hydrogen peroxide, superoxide anion, hydroxyl radical, hydroxyl ion, and peroxide anion. These intermediates seem to allow microbial killing and to contribute to ongoing tissue injury during inflammation. Dapsone has been shown to protect cells from neutrophil-mediated auto-oxidative tissue injury by converting myeloperoxidase to an inactive compound (compound II), thus suppressing the formation of toxic oxygen intermediates. Dapsone has also been shown to suppress neutrophil chemotactic migration and to interfere with β2 integrin-mediated adherence of neutrophils. Furthermore, it has been suggested that dapsone inhibits the generation of 5-lipoxygenase products in polymorphonuclear leukocytes, lysosomal enzyme activity, and the alternative pathway of complement as well as leukotriene B_4 binding to neutrophils and the neutrophil chemotactic response to leukotriene B_4, thus reducing the inflammatory effect. In addition, it has been reported that dapsone may prevent the generation of prostaglandin D2 in mast cells (Coleman 1993, Lang 1979, Miyachi and Niwa 1982, Ruzicka et al. 1983, Wozel and Barth 1988, Zhu and Stiller 2001).

Indications

Used as an antibiotic, dapsone is effective in the treatment of leprosy and actinomycetoma and in the prophylaxis and treatment of *Pneumocystis carinii* pneumonia. Dapsone has been used in treating many diseases characterized by the abnormal infiltration of neutrophils or eosinophils (Table 27.1).

Dosage

Dapsone given in oral doses of 25–100 mg daily has been reported to be effective in the treatment of annular subacute cutaneous LE (SCLE); urticarial vasculitic lesions complicating systemic LE; the nonscarring form of chronic discoid LE (DLE), today designated as LE tumidus (Fig. 27.2) (Kuhn et al. 2000); bullous eruptions of systemic LE; and oral ulcerations (Coburn and Shuster 1982, Hall et al. 1982, McCormack et al. 1984, Ruzicka and Goerz 1981). In contrast, the response of chronic DLE to dapsone (100–150 mg/day) has been largely disappointing (<30% response rates), especially when lesions are widespread or disseminated (Lindskov and Reymann 1986, Ruzicka and Goerz 1981). Because exacerbation of cutaneous disease occurs when discontinuing therapy, a maintenance dose of 25–50 mg/day is almost always needed (Duna and Cash 1995). Dapsone might be an alternative to antimalarial agents when the latter cause adverse reactions (Lo et al. 1989).

Table 27.1. Indications for dapsone therapy in dermatology (Katz 1999, Lang 1979, Zhu and Stiller 2001)

Erythema elevatum diutinum
Dermatitis herpetiformis
Linear IgA dermatosis
Cicatricial pemphigoid
Bullous pemphigoid
Pemphigus vulgaris
Actinomycetoma
Sneddon-Wilkinson disease (subcorneal pustular dermatosis)
Pyoderma gangrenosum
Sweet syndrome
Eosinophilic cellulitis
Granuloma annulare
Erosive lichen planus
Relapsing polychondritis
Systemic lupus erythematosus
Subacute cutaneous lupus erythematosus
Discoid lupus erythematosus
Bullous lupus erythematosus

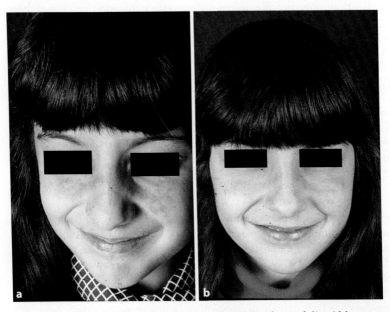

Fig. 27.2. a 10-year-old Turkish girl with non-scarring form of discoid lupus erythematosus before therapy. **b** Almost total clearing of skin lesions 3 weeks after therapy with dapsone

Monitoring and Prevention of Side Effects

Before therapy with dapsone is started, a complete blood cell count with differential white count should be obtained. Also, the glucose-6-phosphate dehydrogenase and methemoglobin levels should be tested, since hemolysis and methemoglobinemia are well-known dapsone-dependent side effects. Once therapy has been initiated, the complete blood cell count should be obtained weekly for the first month and then, if stable, every 2 weeks for another 2 months. Thereafter, the complete blood cell count should be done periodically. Serum creatinine and liver enzyme levels should also be measured before therapy starts and should be frequently monitored thereafter (Katz 1999, Lang 1979). To minimize the risk of side effects, the lowest effective dose of dapsone (generally 100 mg/day) should not be exceeded (Duna and Cash 1995, Lo et al. 1989). In addition, concomitant administration of drugs associated with hemolysis and blood dyscrasias, such as sulfonamides, isoniazid, aspirin, ibuprofen, and primaquine, should be avoided (Zhu and Stiller 2001).

Adverse Effects

Hemolysis
Hemolysis with Heinz-body formation is the second most important hematologic side effect of dapsone. Patients treated with 150 mg/day of dapsone will have a significant decrease in the hemoglobin level of almost 2 g/dl. Individuals with glucose-6-dehydrogenase deficiency have an even greater decrease in the hemoglobin level. In vivo and in vitro studies have demonstrated a direct involvement of hydroxylamines in hemolysis. Also, the presence of oxygen-free radicals seems to play a certain role. However, hemolysis does not correlate with the acetylator status of the patient.

Methemoglobinemia
Methemoglobinemia is the most common side effect of dapsone use. In healthy individuals, methemoglobin is constantly produced under physiologic conditions in very low amounts and is reduced by nicotinamide adenine dinucleotide-dependent methemoglobin reductase. After long-term administration of dapsone, more methemoglobin is formed by its hydroxylamine metabolite. Dapsone hydroxylamine reacts with oxyhemoglobin (Fe^{2+}) to form methemoglobin (Fe^{3+}). The methemoglobin level is more evident at the outset of treatment and is dose dependent. Usually, it is well tolerated if the dosage does not exceed 200 mg/day. Individuals with a deficiency of nicotinamide adenine dinucleotide-dependent methemoglobin reductase or with hemoglobinopathy are more susceptible to methemoglobinemia, whereas glucose-6-dehydrogenase-deficient patients are less subject to methemoglobinemia. Symptoms include cyanosis, weakness, tachycardia, dyspnea, dizziness, nausea, headache, and mild jaundice. Dapsone-induced methemoglobinemia can be reduced by coadministration of cimetidine, although this effect seems to vanish after about 3 months, possibly because of cytochrome P-450 enzyme induction (Coleman 1993, Katz 1999, Pfeiffer and Wozel 2003, Zhu and Stiller 2001, Zuidema et al. 1986).

Agranulocytosis

Most cases of agranulocytosis occur within the first 8 to 12 weeks of therapy in 0.2%–0.4% of patients. Although most patients recover, it may be fatal. Agranulocytosis is characterized by a neutrophil count of less than $0.5 \times 10^9/l$. The mechanism of dapsone-induced agranulocytosis is unclear. The hydroxylamine metabolite of dapsone is known to be toxic to human bone marrow and to human mononuclear cells in vitro. It is also produced by neutrophils in vitro during the respiratory burst. In addition, red blood cells seem to be involved. When exposed to hydroxylamine, erythrocytes liberate this metabolite and kill mononuclear leukocytes in vitro. Hydroxylamine binds strongly to red blood cells and reaches the bone marrow, where it can damage granulocyte precursors and lead to potentially fatal agranulocytosis (Coleman 1993, Katz 1999, Zhu and Stiller 2001).

Dapsone Hypersensitivity Syndrome

Another uncommon, but severe, adverse side effect is the dapsone or sulphone hypersensitivity syndrome (DHS). The syndrome was first noted by Lowe and colleagues in 1950 and was subsequently termed so by Allday and Barnes. This drug reaction was first noted in patients with lepromatous leprosy, and the incidence of the syndrome has increased in the leprosy population since the introduction of multidrug therapy during the past decades. However, DHS has also been seen in patients with various dermatologic diseases, including LE. It usually occurs during the first 3–5 weeks after the start of therapy and consists of fever, malaise, exfoliative dermatitis, hepatitis, lymphadenopathy, hemolytic anaemia, eosinophilia, leukocytosis, and atypical lymphocytosis. It is an infectious mononucleosis-like picture, although there is no serologic evidence of Epstein-Barr virus, cytomegalovirus, or toxoplasma infection. Age, sex, and initial dose of dapsone did not seem to predict the development of this life-threatening complication. The treatment strategy for DHS is unclear. It includes withdrawal of the drug and institution of systemic corticosteroids. A prolonged course of corticosteroids is needed as dapsone has a long half-life in tissues because of the enterohepatic circulation. The pathogenesis of DHS is unknown. Eosinophilia, corticosteroid response, improvement after drug withdrawal, and occurrence at a wide range of daily dosages from 50 to 300 mg suggest that DHS is an idiosyncratic hypersensitivity reaction to the drug (Mok and Lau 1996, 1998).

Other Side Effects

Neurologic and psychiatric side effects include peripheral neuropathy, depression, and psychosis. Cutaneous manifestations include, among others, erythema multiforme, erythema nodosum, and toxic epidermal necrolysis. Finally, dapsone may have renal (nephritic syndrome and renal papillary necrosis) and hepatic (cholestasis and toxic hepatitis) toxicity (Duna and Cash 1995, Lang 1979, Lo et al. 1989, Zhu and Stiller 2001).

Pregnancy and Lactation

Complications such as neonatal hemolytic disease, neonatal hyperbilirubinemia, and neonatal methemoglobinemia have been reported. However, treatment with dapsone during pregnancy is in general considered to be safe for both mother and fetus. Dapsone crosses the placenta and is excreted in breast milk (Zhu and Stiller 2001).

Retinoids

Retinoids (etretinate, acitretin, and isotretinoin) have revolutionized the treatment of acne, psoriasis, and other disorders of keratinization such as ichthyoses, Darier's disease, and pityriasis rubra pilaris. There is increasing evidence that oral retinoids can also exert effects on various other cutaneous diseases characterized histologically by dermal inflammation. Among these is CLE (Duken 1984, Lo et al. 1989, Windhorst 1982).

Pharmacology

Chemistry
Retinoids are naturally occurring compounds and synthetic derivatives of retinol (vitamin-A alcohol) that show vitamin A activity. There are three generations of synthetic retinoids today. Manipulation of the polar group and the polyene side chain of vitamin A forms the *first generation* of retinoids, which includes tretinoin (all-*trans*-retinoic acid), isotretinoin (13-*cis*-retinoic acid), and alitretinoin (9-*cis*-retinoic acid). The aromatic retinoids, etretinate and acitretin, are produced by replacing the cyclic end group of vitamin A with different substituted and nonsubstituted ring systems and are synthetic retinoids of the *second generation*. The *third-generation* retinoids, tazarotene and adapalene, known as polyaromatic compounds, are topical agents for the treatment of psoriasis and acne (Fig. 27.3). Bexarotene is also a third-generation retinoid and is approved for the systemic treatment of cutaneous T-cell lymphoma (Brecher and Orlow 2003, Orfanos et al. 1987).

Pharmacokinetics
Absorption
The bioavailability of isotretinoin (13-*cis*-retinoic acid) is approximately 25% after oral administration, and it can be increased by food 1.5- to 2-fold. After 30 min, the drug is detectable in the blood, and peak serum levels are reached 1–4 h after oral ingestion. As a result of enterohepatic circulation, secondary and tertiary blood concentration maxima may occur. About 6 h after oral administration, the main metabolite, 4-oxo-isotretinoin, is present in a 2- to 4-fold higher concentration. Isotretinoin and 4-oxo-isotretinoin reach steady-state concentrations within 10 days. The mean elimination half-life of isotretinoin is 19 h and of 4-oxo-isotretinoin is 29 h.

Similar to isotretinoin, the oral absorption of acitretin, the major metabolite of etretinate, is variable. Given with food, the bioavailibility is approximately 60% (range, 36%–95%). Peak serum levels are reached 2 h after a single dose is taken. Plasma concentrations of acitretin and its major metabolite, *cis*-acitretin, reach steady-state within 2–3 weeks. Mean peak concentrations of *cis*-acitretin are considerably higher at steady-state and result from the longer half-life and lower clearance of *cis*-acitretin compared with acitretin. The half-life after multiple doses of acitretin ranges from 3–96 h and of cis-acitretin from 35–148 h (Orfanos et al. 1987, 1997, Wiegand and Chou 1998b).

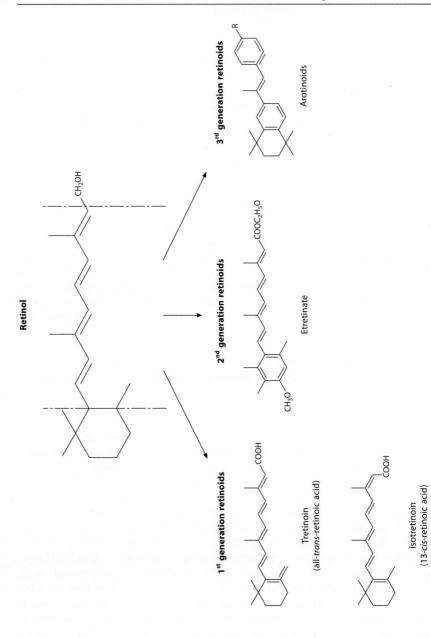

Fig. 27.3. Structural modification of the retinol molecule resulting in three generations of retinoids

Distribution

Isotretinoin is highly lipophilic and is therefore extensively (>99%) bound to plasma proteins, mainly albumin. It has been shown that isotretinoin is not stored in adipose tissue, and there is not specific retention in any organ.

As with isotretinoin, acitretin is to a great extent (98%) bound to plasma proteins, mostly to albumin, caused by its high lipophilicity. Acitretin is not stored in adipose tissue. Isotretinoin and acitretin seem to cross the placenta and to be excreted in breast milk (Orfanos et al. 1987, Wiegand and Chou 1998a).

Metabolism and Excretion

The major metabolites of isotretinoin in the blood following oral administration have been identified as 4-oxo-isotretinoin and 4-hydroxy-isotretinoin, and several glucuronide conjugates are measurable in the bile. In addition, tretinoin, its 4-oxo-metabolite, and 4-hydroxy-retinoic acid have also been detected. Approximately 20%–30% of isotretinoin isomerizes to tretinoin and is metabolized by this route. Excretion of isotretinoin occurs after conjugation with the feces or after metabolism with urine. Acitretin is metabolized into at least four compounds, the major metabolite being 13-*cis*-acitretin (Fig. 27.3). Because of their polar carboxylic acid group, both compounds are less lipophilic than etretinate and therefore do not accumulate in adipose tissue and are eliminated more rapidly in feces and urine. However, it is known that acitretin is in part converted into etretinate and that subsequently etretinate is stored in adipose tissue. It has been reported that the consumption of alcohol stimulates the formation of etretinate from acitretin, but it is not a necessary precondition for back-metabolization (Allen and Bloxham 1989, Lucek and Colburn 1985, Orfanos et al. 1997, Wiegand and Chou 1998b).

Mode of Action

The mode of action of the retinoids has not been completely elucidated, but they have profound effects on differentiation, cell growth, and immune response. Retinoids are capable of regulating epithelial differentiation in the skin, mucous membranes, and mesenchymal tissues. They promote cell proliferation in normal epidermis but inhibit epidermal keratinocytes in psoriatic lesions. Sebaceous glands are significantly reduced in size (up to 90%), and sebum excretion is reduced by isotretinoin. In general, retinoids are reported to stimulate humeral and cellular immunity, although immune-inhibitory effects have also been described. They can boost antibody production, increasing T-helper cells but not natural killer cells. Anti-inflammatory effects include inhibition of motility of neutrophils and eosinophils and their migration into the dermis. Isotretinoin seems to inhibit nitric oxide and tumor necrosis factor α production by keratinocytes and to reduce inducible nitric oxide synthase messenger RNA levels. The discovery of specific cellular binding proteins and nuclear receptors for retinoids has deeply advanced our understanding of the diverse biological processes of retinoids. These observations have also highlighted the complexity of interactions between retinoids and other hormonal signaling molecules. There are two groups of cellular binding proteins, the cellular retinol binding proteins (CRBP I and II) and the cellular retinoic acid binding proteins (CRABP I and II). CRABP II is the predominant form in human skin, although CRABP I is also present at low levels.

Expression of CRABP II is up-regulated by topical application of retinoic acid. CRABP II serves as an early marker for retinoic action in the skin and may regulate the bioavailability of retinoids by reducing the free levels available to reach the nucleus. Cellular retinoic acid binding proteins act as transporters across cell membranes and mediate transfer to the nucleus. In the nucleus of the target cell, retinoid molecules bind to their nuclear receptors. Two main classes of nuclear retinoid receptors have been identified, retinoic acid receptors (RARs) and retinoid X receptors (RXRs), each composed of α, β, and γ subtypes. In addition, there is more than one isoform of each receptor subtype. RARγ and RXRα are expressed predominantly in the skin. RARs can bind both all-*trans*-retinoic acid and 9-*cis*-retinoic acid, whereas RXRs interact with 9-*cis*-retinoic acid. In contrast, 13-*cis*-retinoic acid shows low affinity for RARs. The nuclear receptors combine, with the attached retinoid molecules, to form homodimers (RAR/RAR, RXR/RXR) or heterodimers (RAR/RXR) and then subsequently bind to stretches of DNA known as response elements. As a result, gene transcription of the target gene is stimulated and the production of proteins, which may directly mediate the effects of the retinoid, is activated (Allen and Bloxham 1989, Craven and Griffiths 1996, Orfanos et al. 1987, 1997).

Indications and Dosage

The efficacy of systemic retinoid therapy in a variety of dermatologic diseases, such as acne, psoriasis (pustular and erythrodermic types), and disorders of keratinization (ichthyoses, symmetric progressive erythrokeratoderma, Darier disease, pityriasis rubra pilaris, and palmoplantar hyperkeratosis), is well known. There are also reports of successful treatment of other dermatologic conditions, including disorders of epidermal differentiation (epidermodysplasia verruciformis, confluent and reticulated papillomatosis, and axillar granular parakeratosis) and inflammatory and immunodermatoses (atrophoderma vermiculatum, lichen planus, sarcoidosis, and granuloma annulare). Various synthetic retinoids have also been tried in the treatment of patients with different forms of cutaneous LE (CLE), and there are numerous reports of good responses to etretinate, acitretin, and isotretinoin (Duna and Cash 1995, Furner 1990b). Etretinate has been shown to be effective in the treatment of DLE, particularly the hyperkeratotic variant, and SCLE (Grupper and Berretti 1984, Lubach and Wagner 1984, Ruzicka et al. 1985). Subsequently, acitretin, the major metabolite of etretinate, given in oral doses of 50 mg/day initially, has also been reported to be effective in patients with DLE and SCLE (Fig. 27.4). The dose was individually adjusted according to clinical efficiency and side effects. The main advantage of using acitretin in the treatment of CLE compared with etretinate is the much shorter elimination half-life of the drug (although there is retroconversion to etretinate in some patients). The interesting observation that hydroxychloroquine leads to a decrease in serum triglyceride levels suggests that this effect may offset the acitretin-induced hypertriglyceridemia, a side effect frequently limiting the use of this drug. Therefore, the combination of low doses of acitretin with hydroxychloroquine should be considered (Ruzicka et al. 1988, 1992). Finally, there are also reports describing therapeutic responses of LE to isotretinoin. Isotretinoin given in doses from 0.5 to 1.0 mg/kg per day showed clinical improvement in patients with DLE and SCLE, particularly in those with erythematous, scaly lesions. The therapy was associ-

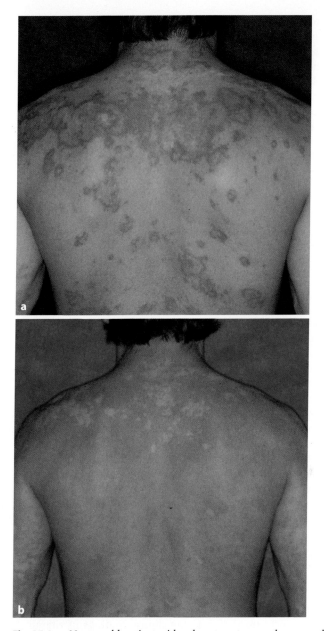

Fig. 27.4. a 29-year-old patient with subacute cutaneous lupus erythematosus before therapy. **b** Complete clearing of skin lesions with extensive depigmentation two weeks after therapy with acitretin

ated with the resolution of cutaneous histopathologic abnormalities, conversion of abnormal lesional direct immunofluorescence to normal, normalization of the epidermis on electron microscopy, and reduction in the number of T cells near the dermoepidermal junction without change in the ratio of T-helper (inducer) cells to T-suppressor (cytotoxic) cells. Retinoids may be useful in establishing rapid control of resistant lesions or in treating intermittent acute flare-ups, whether used as monotherapy or in combination with antimalarials or corticosteroids and in patients with CLE refractory to other drug regimens. Because of the recurrence of skin lesions after discontinuing medication use, long-term treatment may be needed to maintain control (Brecher and Orlow 2003, Duna and Cash 1995, Ellis and Krach 2001, Furner 1990a, Newton et al. 1986, Shornik et al. 1991).

Contraindications

Pregnancy, lactation, and severe hepatic and renal dysfunction (persistent elevated liver enzyme, urea, and creatinine levels) are absolute contraindications for oral retinoid treatment (Orfanos et al. 1987).

Monitoring and Prevention of Side Effects

Laboratory examinations of liver function (transaminases and γ-glutamyl transferase), alkaline phosphatase, serum lipids, and renal function tests (creatinine) should be performed before treatment is started, 3–4 weeks thereafter, and then at 3-month intervals. Patients with diabetes mellitus, obese patients, and alcoholic patients are at increased risk for hepatotoxicity and require more frequent liver function testing during therapy with retinoids. Concomitant use of other drugs (β-blockers, hormonal corticosteroid contraceptives, and thiazide diuretics) with an additive effect on lipid levels should be performed carefully. Other therapeutic agents that may interact with retinoids, such as antidiabetics (alterations in blood glucose), corticosteroids and tetracyclines (hyperlipidemia and pseudotumor cerebri), and methotrexate (hepatotoxicity), should be monitored cautiously or avoided. Supplementary therapy with vitamin A should be avoided while taking retinoids. To minimize skeletal toxicity, the lowest possible dosage in patients receiving long-term retinoid therapy should be used. Baseline radiography may be useful to document pretreatment bone status in addition to control x-rays once a year for individuals requiring prolonged treatment (Brecher and Orlow 2003, Katz et al. 1999, Orfanos et al. 1987).

Adverse Effects

The most common side effects are generally mucocutaneous and seem to be dose related. Many of these side effects are similar to the clinical findings in vitamin A intoxication but are less severe (Ellis and Krach 2001, Peck and DiGiovanna 1999).

Mucocutaneous
Acute mucocutaneous toxicity is a frequently observed side effect of retinoid use. Most of these symptoms are well tolerated, dose dependent, treatable, and reversible when treatment is discontinued or the dosage is reduced. Cheilitis and dry nasal

mucosa are the most common manifestations, and they occur in almost all patients receiving isotretinoin in sufficient dosage. Actually, the complete absence of these symptoms when associated with failure of drug response should raise the suspicion of noncompliance. Cheilitis generally responds to continual application of topical emollients during therapy. Lubrication to the anterior nares is also often required to alleviate dry nasal mucosa, which may cause nosebleeds in some patients. Xerosis cutis occurs in approximately 80% of patients and is often associated with pruritus. It has been suggested that tolerance of symptoms may develop during treatment. Photosensitivity affects approximately 10% of patients. Isotretinoin seems to stimulate granulation tissue, which can occasionally lead to pyogenic granuloma-like eruptions in sites of minor trauma and within acute lesions. Etretinate and acitretin show comparable mucocutaneous side effects. Although diffuse thinning of the hair and increased brittleness of the nails may occur during isotretinoin therapy, it is more common with administration of acitretin (Brecher and Orlow 2003, Ellis and Krach 2001, Peck and DiGiovanna 1999).

Ophthalmologic

Xerophthalmia occurs in one third of patients during isotretinoin therapy and is caused by decreased meibomian gland secrection, leading to an altered composition of the tear film and shortening of the tear film break-up time. This may lead to blepharoconjunctivitis, exposure keratitis, and corneal ulceration in extreme cases. Some patients may also develop a contact lens intolerance. Application of artificial tears several times a day can help alleviate these symptoms. Other ophthalmologic toxicities from retinoids include corneal opacities, decreased night vision (as a result of interference with steps in the rhodopsin cycle), transient acute myopia, papilledema, and cataracts. Rarely, dry eye syndrome and decreased night vision have been reported to persist after discontinuation of therapy. Etretinate and acitretin use have been shown to cause many of the same ocular side effects as isotretinoin therapy. However, isotretinoin seems to have a greater ability to suppress meibomian gland secretion (Brecher and Orlow 2003, Ellis and Krach 2001, Katz et al. 1999, Orfanos et al. 1987, Peck and DiGiovanna 1999).

Teratogenicity

Retinoids are known to be teratogenic and can lead to fetal abnormalities. The birth defects characteristically induced by retinoids, so-called retinoic acid embryopathy, include central nervous system abnormalities (hydrocephalus and microcephaly), external ear abnormalities (anotia and small or absent external auditory canals), cardiovascular abnormalities (septal wall and aortic defects), facial dysmorphia, eye abnormalities (microphthalmia), thymus gland and bone abnormalities. In addition, premature births, parathyroid hormone deficiency, and cases of low IQ in the absence of other central system abnormalities have been reported. Retinoid effects on neural crest cells during the fourth week after fertilization may be responsible for many of the observed malformations. Serum levels of the β subunit of human chorionic gonadotropin should be checked before therapy, and effective contraception is mandatory during and after treatment. Isotretinoin has a short half-life, and, therefore, contraceptive measures need to be taken for only 1 month after cessation of treatment. Etretinate and acitretin both have a long half-life. Although acitretin has a

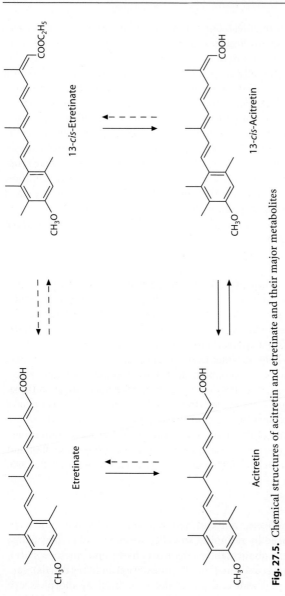

Fig. 27.5. Chemical structures of acitretin and etretinate and their major metabolites

much shorter half-life than etretinate, it is recommended that pregnancy should not occur for at least 3 years after the cessation of acitretin therapy, since some patients back-metabolize acitretin to etretinate (Fig. 27.5). Males can safely father children even when they are taking the drug (Brecher and Orlow 2003, Duna and Cash1995, Lo et al. 1989).

Skeletal Involvement
Administration of retinoids induces bone toxicities similar to those of chronic hypervitaminosis A (remodeling of long bones, cortical hyperostosis, decalcification, premature epiphyseal closure, periosteal thickening, and osteoporosis). In general, synthetic retinoids produce bony changes such as diffuse idiopathic skeletal hyperostosis, including anterior spinal ligament calcification, osteophytes, and bony bridges, but without narrowing of the disk space. Calcification of the anterior spinal ligament with bony bridging of vertebrae has been observed with long-term, high-dose (2 mg/kg per day) isotretinoin therapy, and minimal spinal hyperostosis has been reported in 10% of patients treated with short-term, low-dose isotretinoin. Ossification of the spinal posterior longitudinal ligament is rare. Extraspinal involvement (extraspinal tendon and ligament calcification) is significantly increased in patients receiving long-term etretinate therapy at an average dose of 0.8 mg/kg per day. Premature epiphyseal closure resulting in retardation of growth has been rarely described in children with oral retinoid treatment. The incidence of decreased bone mineral density is still under investigation. No changes in bone mineralization or in markers of bone turnover have been found after short-term therapy with isotretinoin. However, osteoporosis has been identified in patients who received long-term etretinate therapy (Brecher and Orlow 2003, Orfanos et al. 1987, Peck and DiGiovanna 1999).

Neuromuscular Involvement
Headache, fatigue, and lethargy may rarely occur during isotretinoin therapy. However, if headaches become persistent and are associated with nausea, vomiting, and visual changes, the drug should be discontinued immediately and pseudotumor cerebri should be excluded. Since tetracycline, doxycycline, and minocycline may increase the risk of intracranial hypertension, the concomitant use of these drugs and isotretinoin should be avoided. There is a single case report of pseudotumor cerebri in an adult patient receiving acitretin without concomitant antibiotic treatment. Myalgias, sometimes associated with elevated creatinine phosphokinase levels, occur in up to 15% of patients taking isotretinoin, particularly in physically active patients. It has been reported that the elevated creatinine phosphokinase levels return to normal within 2–4 weeks. In general, arthralgias are rarely seen in patients treated with retinoids, and they disappear after discontinuation of therapy. However, arthralgias and back pain in adolescents taking isotretinoin have been observed, although the cause of the back pain is unknown (Brecher and Orlow 2003, Ellis and Krach 2001, Peck and DiGiovanna 1999).

Gastrointestinal Involvement
Retinoids may alter liver function tests, most commonly the transaminases but also other tests (alkaline phosphatase, lactic dehydrogenase, and bilirubin). Elevations of transaminase levels occur in approximately 15% of patients, but they generally return

to normal within 2–4 weeks, even when therapy is continued. Severe hepatotoxic reactions resulting from retinoid use are rare and idiosyncratic. However, a correlation between long-term retinoid therapy and chronic liver toxicity has not been demonstrated. Nonspecific gastrointestinal side effects, such as nausea, diarrhea, and abdominal pain, have been reported with isotretinoin therapy but are infrequent. Although the oral administration of isotretinoin has been linked with inflammatory bowel disease flare-up, a causal relationship has not been established. In fact, isotretinoin has been given to patients with known Crohn's disease and ulcerative colitis without complications (Brecher and Orlow 2003, Ellis and Krach 2001, Katz et al. 1999, Peck and DiGiovanna 1999).

Lipid Involvement

Retinoid therapy may cause hyperlipidemia, probably due to both increased synthesis and decreased elimination of blood lipids. An elevation in serum triglyceride levels in excess of 800 mg/dl has been reported in approximately 25% of patients, a decrease in high-density lipoprotein levels has been shown in approximately 15% of patients, and an increase in cholesterol levels has been shown in approximately 7% of patients receiving isotretinoin therapy. Lipid levels normalize in most patients by reducing the daily retinoid dose, by introducing a diet low in fat and carbohydrates, or by administering lipid-lowering medication. Cessation of treatment should be considered only if abnormal lipid values persist for a long period. In cases of severe hypertriglyceridemia (triglyceride level >1000 mg/dl), patients are at risk for eruptive xanthomata and acute pancreatitis. Hypertriglyceridemia has also been observed during therapy with etretinate and acitretin. Increased serum lipid levels are of particular concern in patients with risk factors such as obesity, high alcohol intake, diabetes mellitus, and pretreatment hypertriglyceridemia (Brecher and Orlow 2003, Katz et al. 1999, Orfanos et al. 1987, Peck and DiGiovanna 1999).

Renal Involvement

Renal toxicity is not a characteristic effect of retinoid therapy. Isotretinoin can be safely administered to patients with end-stage kidney disease who undergo hemodialysis (Ellis and Krach 2001, Peck and DiGiovanna 1999).

Psychological Involvement

Psychiatric disorders such as depression, irritability, psychosis, attempted suicide, and actual suicide have been reported in individuals during and after isotretinoin therapy. However, there is no evidence that the use of isotretinoin is associated with an increased risk for depression or suicide. Psychiatric evaluation and treatment may still be needed (Brecher and Orlow 2003, Ellis and Krach 2001).

In conclusion, dapsone and retinoids may be useful alternatives in the treatment of resistant skin lesions and in patients with CLE refractory to other therapeutic regimens, given as monotherapy or in combination with antimalarials or corticosteroids, considering the indication and the possible side effects.

References

Allen JG, Bloxham DP (1989) The pharmacology and pharmacokinetics of the retinoids. Pharmacol Ther 40:1–27

Brecher AR, Orlow SJ (2003) Oral retinoid therapy for dermatologic conditions in children and adolescents. J Am Acad Dermatol. 49:171–182

Callen JP (1990) Treatment of cutaneous lesions in patients with lupus erythematosus. Dermatol Clin 8:355–365

Coburn PR, Shuster S (1982) Dapsone and discoid lupus erythematosus. Br J Dermatol 106:105–106

Coleman MD (1993) Dapsone: modes of action, toxicity and possible strategies for increasing patient tolerance. Br J Dermatol 129:507–513

Craven NM, Griffiths CE (1996) Topical retinoids and cutaneous biology. Clin Exp Dermatol 21:1–10

Duna GF, Cash JM (1995) Treatment of refractory cutaneous lupus erythematosus. Rheum Dis Clin North Am 21:99–115

Duken CM (1984) Retinoids: a review. J Am Acad Dermatol 11:541–552

Ellis CN, Krach KJ (2001) Uses and complications of isotretinoin therapy. J Am Acad Dermatol 45:S150–157

Furner BB (1990a) Treatment of subacute cutaneous lupus erythematosus. Int J Dermatol 29:542–547

Furner BB (1990b) Subacute cutaneous lupus erythematosus response to isotretinoin. Int J Dermatol 29:587–590

Grupper C, Berretti B (1984) Lupus erythematosus and etretinate. In: Cunliffe WJ, Miller AJ (eds) Retinoid therapy. MTP, Lancaster, pp 73–82

Hall RP, Lawley TJ, Smith HR, Katz SI (1982) Bullous eruption of systemic lupus erythematosus. Ann Intern Med 97:165–170

Katz SI (1999) Sulfones. In: Freeberg MI, Eisen ZA, Wolff K, Austen FK, Goldsmith AL, Katz IS, Fitzpatrick BT (eds) Dermatology in general medicine, 5th ed. McGraw-Hill, New York, pp 2790–2794

Katz HI, Waalen J, Leach EE (1999) Acitretin in psoriasis: an overview of adverse effects. J Am Acad Dermatol 41:S7–S12

Kuhn A, Richter-Hintz D, Oslislo C, Ruzicka T, Megahed M, Lehmann P (2000) Lupus erythematosus tumidus – a neglected subset of cutaneous lupus erythematosus: report of 40 cases. Arch Dermatol 136:1033–1041

Lang PG Jr (1979) Sulfones and sulfonamides in dermatology today. J Am Acad Dermatol 1:479–492

Lindskov R, Reymann F (1986) Dapsone in the treatment of cutaneous lupus erythematosus. Dermatologica 172:214–217

Lo JS, Berg RE, Tomecki KJ (1989) Treatment of discoid lupus erythematosus. Int J Dermatol 28:497–507

Lubach D, Wagner G (1984) Erfolgreiche Behandlung eines subakut kutanen Lupus erythematodes mit Etretinat. Aktuel Dermatol 10:142–144

Lucek RW, Colburn WA (1989) Clinical pharmacokinetics of the retinoids. Clin Pharmacokinet 10:38–62

McCormack LS, Elgart ML, Turner ML (1984) Annular subacute cutaneous lupus erythematosus responsive to dapsone. J Am Acad Dermatol 11:397–401

Miyachi Y, Niwa Y (1982) Effects of KI, colchicine and dapsone on the generation of PMNL-derived oxygen intermediates. Br J Dermatol 107:209–214

Mok CC, Lau CS (1996) Dapsone syndrome in cutaneous lupus erythematosus. J Rheumatol 23:766–768

Mok CC, Lau CS, Wong RW (1998) Toxicities of dapsone in the treatment of cutaneous manifestations of rheumatic diseases. J Rheumatol 25:1246–1247

Newton RC, Jorizzo JL, Solomon AR Jr, Sanchez RL, Daniels JC, Bell JD, Cavallo T (1986) Mechanism-oriented assessment of isotretinoin in chronic or subacute cutaneous lupus erythematosus. Arch Dermatol 122:170–176

Orfanos CE, Ehlert R, Gollnick H (1987) The retinoids. A review of their clinical pharmacology and therapeutic use. Drugs 34:459–503

Orfanos CE, Zouboulis CC, Almond-Roesler B, Geilen CC (1997) Current use and future potential role of retinoids in dermatology. Drugs 53:358–388

Peck GL, DiGiovanna JJ (1999) Retinoids. In: Freeberg MI, Eisen ZA, Wolff K, Austen FK, Goldsmith AL, Katz IS, Fitzpatrick BT (eds) Dermatology in general medicine. 5th ed. McGraw-Hill, New York, pp 2810–2821

Pfeiffer C, Wozel G (2003) Dapsone and sulfones in dermatology: overview and update. J Am Acad Dermatol 48:308–309

Ruzicka T, Goerz G (1981) Dapsone in the treatment of lupus erythematosus. Br J Dermatol 104:53–56

Ruzicka T, Wasserman SI, Soter NA, Printz MP (1983) Inhibition of rat mast cell arachidonic acid cyclooxygenase by dapsone. J Allergy Clin Immunol 72:365–370

Ruzicka T, Meurer M, Braun-Falco O (1985) Treatment of cutaneous lupus erythematosus with etretinate. Acta Derm Venereol 65:324–329

Ruzicka T, Meurer M, Bieber T (1988) Efficiency of acitretin in the treatment of cutaneous lupus erythematosus. Arch Dermatol 124:897–902

Ruzicka T, Sommerburg C, Goerz G, Kind P, Mensing H (1992) Treatment of cutaneous lupus erythematosus with acitretin and hydroxychloroquine. Br J Dermatol 127:513–518

Shornick JK, Formica N, Parke AL (1991) Isotretinoin for refractory lupus erythematosus. J Am Acad Dermatol 24:49–52

Wiegand UW, Chou RC (1998) Pharmacokinetics of oral isotretinoin. J Am Acad Dermatol 39:S8–12

Wiegand UW, Chou RC (1998) Pharmacokinetics of acitretin and etretinate. J Am Acad Dermatol 39:S25–33

Windhorst DB (1982) The use of isotretinoin in disorders of keratinisation. J Am Acad Dermatol 6:708–709

Wozel G, Barth J (1988) Current aspects of modes of action of dapsone. Int J Dermatol 27:547–552

Zhu YI, Stiller MJ (2001) Dapsone and sulfones in dermatology: overview and update. J Am Acad Dermatol 45:420–434

Zuidema J, Hilbers-Modderman ES, Merkus FW (1986) Clinical pharmacokinetics of dapsone. Clin Pharmacokinet 11:299–315

CHAPTER 28

Thalidomide in Cutaneous Lupus Erythematosus

Yousuf Karim, Maria J. Cuadrado

Thalidomide (α-N-phthalimidoglutarimide) was initially introduced into clinical practice in the mid-1950s; since that time, it has had a remarkable checkered history. It was used early on as an over-the-counter sedative (Mellin and Katzenstein 1962), and then in the treatment of morning sickness in pregnancy. However, in 1961, thalidomide was withdrawn from the market because of the discovery of its potential teratogenicity– it was associated with up to 12,000 cases of birth defects, particularly phocomelias (Mellin 1962, Randall 1990). Four years later, Sheskin serendipitously discovered that thalidomide had marked clinical efficacy in erythema nodosum leprosum (Sheskin 1965). Subsequently, a variety of conditions, including infectious, autoimmune, inflammatory, and malignant, have been shown to respond to thalidomide. Examples of these conditions include human immunodeficiency virus (HIV) infection (Reyes-Teran et al. 1996), rheumatoid arthritis (Gutiérrez-Rodriguez et al. 1989), Behcet's syndrome (Hamuryudan et al. 1998), graft-versus-host disease (Vogelsang et al. 1993), multiple myeloma (Singhal et al. 1999), and cutaneous features of lupus erythematosus (LE) (Knop et al. 1983). The latter include systemic LE (SLE) with cutaneous features, discoid LE (DLE), and subacute cutaneous LE (SCLE).

The common denominator of the previously mentioned differing conditions seems to be that they are all characterized by inflammation, immune dysregulation, or both. Thalidomide has been shown to have immunomodulatory, immunosuppressive, and anti-inflammatory actions, which may explain its therapeutic efficacy. Furthermore, thalidomide is often effective in conditions in which standard therapies have failed to make an impression, for example, severe ulceration in Behcet's syndrome or severe cutaneous lupus. Clinical use of thalidomide must, of course, be tightly regulated and supervised, not only because of the potential for teratogenicity, especially as many patients with lupus are young women, but also for the development of peripheral neuropathy. In this article, we discuss possible mechanisms of action and the clinical experience of thalidomide in the treatment of cutaneous features of LE.

Immunology and Possible Mechanisms of Action

Although substantial research has been undertaken into potential mechanisms of action of thalidomide, there are no definitive conclusions to explain its clinical efficacy. Indeed, as groups delve further into the effects of thalidomide, more and more putative mechanisms have been reported. Identifying which of these mechanisms are relevant, particularly with respect to its effects in different diseases, has proven difficult to dissect. Thalidomide has many metabolites, some of which may contribute to its biological activity. Here, we confine discussion to the actions of thalidomide itself. Thalidomide interferes with both innate and adaptive and cellular and molecular components of immunity.

Much work has focused on the effects of thalidomide on tumor necrosis factor (TNF)-α, a proinflammatory cytokine involved in host defense and identified as important in several infectious, inflammatory, and autoimmune diseases. In vitro studies show that thalidomide selectively and partially inhibits human monocyte synthesis of TNF-α, possibly via an increased rate of degradation of TNF-α messenger RNA (mRNA), with a reduction in half-life of TNF-α mRNA from 30 min to 17 min (Sampaio et al. 1991, Moreira et al. 1993, Corral and Kaplan 1999). Thalidomide may inhibit activation of NF-κB, a transcription factor that affects TNF-α and TNF-β genes (Keifer et al. 2001, Walchner et al. 1995).

This correlates with in vivo data from patients with erythema nodosum leprosum, a condition characterized by overproduction of TNF-α. Clinical improvement with thalidomide was accompanied by a corresponding decrease in serum TNF-α levels (Sampaio et al. 1991). In tuberculosis, regardless of whether there was associated HIV infection, plasma TNF-α and monocyte TNF-α mRNA levels fell on thalidomide treatment, in parallel with accelerated weight gain (Tramontana et al. 1995). In contrast, increased serum TNF-α levels were observed in thalidomide-treated HIV-associated oral ulceration (Jacobson et al. 1997) and in toxic epidermal necrolysis (Wolkenstein 1998).

It is clear, therefore, that in considering the relationship between thalidomide and TNF-α, attention must be paid to the difference between in vitro and in vivo scenarios, the pathophysiology of different diseases, and technical considerations of TNF-α measurement. Measurement of serum levels of TNF-α may not necessarily reflect TNF-α activity, as this may detect receptor-bound circulating homotrimer, which may be inactive. Technical difficulties, such as an undefined normal range, a short half-life, and phasic release of TNF-α, may also confound accurate measurement (Calabrese and Fleischer 2000).

TNF-α is elevated in active SLE, but the ratio of TNF-α to the soluble TNF-α receptor (TNF-sR) is lower in SLE than in rheumatoid arthritis. It has been suggested that the ratio of TNF-α to TNF-sR may be more critical than the absolute level of serum TNF-α. Indeed, there may be a relative deficiency of active TNF-α in SLE (Dean et al. 2000). Lee et al. reported an increased risk of nephritis in patients with low peripheral blood mononuclear cell TNF-α levels (Lee et al. 1997). TNF-α levels may relate to HLA haplotype. HLA-DR2, DQw1-positive patients with SLE have low levels of TNF-α inducibility and an increased incidence of lupus nephritis, whereas the DR4 haplotype, associated with high inducibility of TNF-α, has a negative relationship with lupus nephritis (Jacob et al. 1990). Although serum levels of TNF-α are important, local tissue expression of TNF-α may also be relevant to specific organ involvement. For example, Herrera-Esparza et al. reported glomerular and tubular deposition of TNF-α in 52% of renal biopsy samples from 19 patients with lupus nephritis (Herrera-Esparza et al. 1998).

In conclusion, the discovery of the in vitro effects of thalidomide on TNF-α in vitro does not allow direct extrapolation to clinical lupus, in which more complex interactions are likely to exist.

Thalidomide has multiple effects on T lymphocytes, which may have an important pathogenic role in lupus. Histopathologic examination in SLE and DLE typically reveals the presence of a lymphocytic infiltrate, predominantly T cell in nature, characterized by CD3 expression. These cells are typically activated, and the relative proportions of CD4 and CD8 may vary between SLE and DLE (Kohchiyama et al. 1985)

Thalidomide affected the ratio of peripheral blood T-helper (Th) to T-suppressor cells in healthy male volunteers, with a fall in Th cells and an apparent increase in T-suppressor cells (Gad et al. 1985). Thalidomide has been shown to affect Th1/Th2 cytokines in vitro. It inhibits production of the Th1 cytokine interferon (IFN)-γ and enhances production of the Th2 cytokines interleukin (IL)-4 and IL-5 in peripheral blood mononuclear cell cultures though effects vary with culture time (McHugh et al. 1995). It also inhibits monocyte production of the Th1 cytokine IL-12 in a dose-dependent manner.

Thalidomide has been shown in vitro to co-stimulate human T cells that have received signal 1 through the T-cell receptor complex, with resultant increased IL-2-mediated T-cell proliferation and IFN-γ production (Haslett et al. 1998). CD8[+] lymphocytes show a more marked co-stimulation than CD4[+] lymphocytes. In this setting, it is noteworthy that TNF-α production by anti-CD3-stimulated T cells was not inhibited by thalidomide, in contrast to its effects on monocytes. Thus, the effect of thalidomide may depend on the cell type and also on the nature of the stimulus. Despite its immunomodulatory effects, thalidomide does not seem to predispose to risk of significant infections, which may be related to its co-stimulatory effects on T cells.

Thalidomide also has effects on the humoral system, which of course is abnormal in SLE, characterized by hypergammaglobulinemia, and autoantibody production to multiple nuclear and cellular antigens. IgM levels fell in patients with erythema nodosum leprosum treated with thalidomide. Mice fed thalidomide for 5–7 days before immunization with sheep red blood cells exhibited lower IgM production (Shannon et al. 1981). In a series of patients with SLE and cutaneous features treated with thalidomide, the gammaglobulin level fell significantly in 10 of 13 patients (Atra and Sato 1993).

Innate immune mechanisms such as neutrophil and monocyte function are affected by thalidomide. For example, thalidomide inhibits neutrophil chemotaxis and phagocytosis and monocyte phagocytosis (Barnhill et al. 1984, Faure et al. 1980), which may be important in inflammatory diseases, including cutaneous forms of LE. Effects on phagocytes may relate to down-regulation of cell adhesion molecules. Vascular adhesion molecule expression has been noted in lesional, nonlesional, and non-sun-exposed skin in SLE (Belmont et al. 1994, Jones et al. 1996). Thalidomide may affect the density of TNF-α-induced intercellular adhesion molecule-1, vascular adhesion molecule-1, and E-selectin antigens in human endothelial cell cultures (Geitz et al. 1996, Settles et al. 2001).

Thalidomide has been shown to have antiangiogenic effects in vitro and in vivo. Endothelial cell proliferation in vitro has been shown to be inhibited by thalidomide (Moreira et al. 1999). Several growth factors are implicated in the development of human tumors, including basic fibroblast growth factor. The antiangiogenic properties of thalidomide may occur via inhibition of basic fibroblast growth factor-induced angiogenesis, as shown in vivo in a rabbit cornea micropocket assay (D'Amato et al.

1994). Thalidomide also has effects on other growth factors, for example, it is effective in inhibition of corneal angiogenesis induced by vascular endothelial growth factor (Kruse et al. 1998).

The antiangiogenic effects of thalidomide may correlate with its efficacy in malignant disease and with its teratogenicity, although not with TNF-α inhibition. It has been suggested that the effects of thalidomide on TNF-α and T cells may be more pertinent to its effect on immune and inflammatory disease, whereas antiangiogenic effects may have more impact on malignant disease; however, it seems likely that there is some degree of crossover in these effects.

Clinical Experience

Although thalidomide is well known to be an effective drug for the various manifestations of cutaneous lupus, it is not widely used to treat these disorders because of its serious side effects and because it is difficult to obtain. Probably for these reasons, there are no randomized, controlled trials proving its efficacy. The available data in the literature come from a few series of patients, which show agreement regarding the good response to treatment but major differences when optimal dose, safety, and relapse rate are analyzed. Table 28.1 shows the results of the main published series. Thalidomide was used to treat DLE in the first large series published almost 20 years ago (Knop et al. 1983). Further series published in the past decade (Atra and Sato 1993, Duong et al. 1999, Kyriakis et al. 2000, Ordi et al. 2000, Sato et al. 1998, Stevens et al. 1997) also included patients with SCLE and SLE with severe cutaneous features.

Response to Treatment

Complete or partial remission of the skin lesions has been reported in ca. 80% of patients treated, ranging from 73% (Ordi et al. 2000) to 100% (Sato et al. 1998). It is noteworthy that all studies included patients with severe skin involvement previously refractory to several treatments, such as topical and systemic steroids, antimalarials,

Table 28.1. Results of treatment with thalidomide in the main published series

Series and year	Patients (n)	Response (%)	Neuropathy (%)	Other side effects (%)	Recurrences (%)
Knop et al. 1983	60	90	25	42	75
Hasper MF, 1983	11	82	No data	64	36
Atra et al. 1993	23	87	13	52	35
Ochonisky et al. 1994	42	No data	21–50	No data	No data
Stevens et al. 1997	16	81	6	31	75
Sato et al. 1998	18	100	0	44	No data
Duong et al. 1999	7	86	0	57	No data
Ordi et al. 2000	22	73	5	45	50
Kyriakis et al. 2000	22	77	0	40	67
Walchner et al. 2000	10	100	40	20	80

and immunosuppressive agents, mainly azathioprine. In this context, this high rate of response is even more remarkable.

Factors influencing the response rate were analyzed in one study (Kyriakis et al. 2000). The only significant predictor of the final clinical outcome was the age of the patient, which was inversely correlated with the final remission rate. Cumulative dose of thalidomide, severity of the lesions, and disease duration did not have any effect on the final clinical outcome. The same study found that the remission rate after 1 month of treatment significantly correlated with the final remission rate. The authors suggested that the final clinical outcome is predictable since in their study a median 50% improvement in lesions during the first month was required to expect a final complete remission.

The starting dose of thalidomide varied between the different series. The earliest study used 400 mg daily (Knop et al. 1983), whereas more recent studies have used 50–100 mg/day (Stevens et al. 1997) to 200 mg/day (Kyriakis et al. 2000). The most common dose used was 100 mg/day (Duong et al. 1999, Ordi et al. 2000, Sato et al. 1998). In general, there were no differences in the response rate in relation to either dose used or severity of lesions treated. Most of the trials halved the starting dose after the first 4–8 weeks of treatment if marked improvement was achieved. Some authors reported exacerbation of the skin lesions when the dose was tapered (Kyriakis et al. 2000), whereas others described remission maintained with low-dose therapy (25–50 mg/day or alternate days) (Sato et al. 1998). Individual variability in the response to the drug might account for these different results since adjustment of the starting dose to lower or higher levels seems to be common in many patients in trials with thalidomide.

Thalidomide does not seem effective in the treatment of other manifestations of SLE, although some authors described improvement in joint pains (Sato et al. 1998). Thalidomide improved some immunologic parameters in patients with SLE (Walchner et al. 2000). Increased counts of peripheral blood lymphocytes and decreased anti-double-stranded DNA antibody titers were observed in 90% of the patients with SLE studied. These immunologic improvements lasted while treatment with thalidomide was maintained. No changes were observed in the anti-U1RNP, anti-Ro/SSA, and anti-La/SSB antibody titers or in C3, C4 complement factors.

Side Effects

Table 28.2 shows the frequency of the adverse reactions described in association with the use of thalidomide. Side effects are common during thalidomide treatment. Its original therapeutic use was as a sedative, and, accordingly, it is the cause of somnolence and drowsiness reported in a high percentage of patients. Although this adverse reaction improves with reduction in dose and is minimized if the drug is taken at night, sometimes it is severe enough to discontinue the treatment (Atra and Sato 1993, Kyriakis et al. 2000, Stevens et al. 1997).

The two most worrying side effects of thalidomide use are teratogenicity and neuropathy. The current availability of contraceptive methods has dramatically reduced the frequency of congenital malformation to almost zero. Nevertheless, a pregnancy test before treatment and the use of strict contraceptive measures during treatment for at least 3 months after taking the last dose are mandatory. Even the slightest doubt

Table 28.2. Side effects associated with thalidomide use

Side Effect	Percentage (%)	Series and year
Drowsiness	60	Knop et al. 1983
Dizziness	41	Kyriakis et al. 2000
Insomnia	8	Atra et al. 1993
Depression	13	Atra et al. 1993
Neuropathy	0	Sato et al. 1998
	25	Knop et al. 1983
	50	Ochonisky et al. 1994
Amenorrhea	24	Frances et al. 2002
	35.7	Ordi et al. 2000
Galactorrhea	4.3	Atra et al. 1993
Weight gain	18	Ordi et al. 2000
Constipation	31.6	Knop et al. 1983
Rash	11.6	Knop et al. 1983
Edema	6.6	Knop et al. 1983
Xerostomia	3.3	Knop et al. 1983

Up to 12,000 cases of teratogenicity have been reported (Mellin and Katzenstein 1962).
There is a series of four lupus patients who developed thrombosis (Flageul et al. 2000).
Mood alterations other than depression have been described in most series, but the percentage is not available.

about comprehension or compliance of safe contraception should be an absolute contraindication to treatment with thalidomide in women of fertile age.

Peripheral neuropathy is described in all trials with thalidomide, affecting a variable number of patients. Thalidomide mainly produces an axonal sensory neuropathy that typically manifests as painful, symmetrical paresthesia of the hands and feet, frequently accompanied by lower-limb sensory loss. Muscle weakness, muscle cramps, signs of pyramidal tract involvement, and carpal tunnel syndrome have been reported in many patients (Tseng et al. 1996).

The true incidence of thalidomide-induced neuropathy and its relationship to the cumulative dose is still controversial and varies between the conditions and the series. The incidence in prurigo nodularis is near 100%, whereas in Behcet's disease it is 25%–50%. In leprosy, despite neurologic involvement by the disease itself, the incidence seems to be quite low. In cutaneous LE, different series report peripheral neuropathy affecting 0% (Sato et al. 1998) to 25% (Knop et al. 1983). A study by Ochonisky et al. (Ochonisky et al. 1994) including 42 patients with different skin diseases found that 21% of patients had definite thalidomide-induced neuropathy and as many as 50% had clinical and/or electrophysiologic features of nerve damage. The discrepancies between the different studies might be due to the methods used to diagnose neuropathy, the frequency with which neurophysiologic studies were performed, and individual idiosyncrasy. Some reports have suggested that the development of neuropathy is related to the cumulative dose and the duration of the treatment (Clemmensen et al. 1984, De Iongh 1990), but most studies did not find any quantitative or qualitative correlation between neuropathy and total dose of thalidomide or duration of the therapy (Kyriakis et al. 2000, Ochonisky et al. 1994, Rovelli et al. 1998, Stevens et al. 1997). Patient-related factors such as female sex and older age seem to predispose to the development of neuropathy in the first few months of treatment (Fullerton and O'Sullivan 1968, Ochonisky et al. 1994). In the 1980s, a possible relationship between slow acetylation and the development of thalidomide-induced neuropathy was found (Hess et al. 1986), but a more recent study could not confirm this finding (Harland et al. 1995). The study included 16 patients with severe orogenital ulceration who were treated with thalidomide and 16 healthy controls. Forty percent of the patients and 35.7% of the controls were slow acetylators; 28.6% of the patients with neuropathy were slow acetylators compared with 50% without neuropathy.

Several electrophysiologic measures have been suggested for monitoring thalidomide toxicity. Use of the peripheral sensory nerve action potential (SNAP) index has been recommended based on a retrospective study of 59 patients treated with thalidomide (Gardner-Medwin et al. 1994). All patients were routinely assessed with three sensory potentials (medial, radial, and sural nerves). A baseline SNAP was calculated, giving each individual nerve an equal weighting of 100% and the three summated. A decrease of approximately 50% from this baseline total percentage SNAP was prospectively considered as an indication of subclinical neuropathy, and thalidomide therapy was discontinued. In the United Kingdom, the guidelines for the use of thalidomide (Powell and Gardner-Medwin, 1994) propose that electrophysiologic tests should be performed at baseline and should include at least three SNAPs and that thalidomide administration should be stopped immediately if either paresthesiae are developed or the SNAP index declines by more than 40%. They recommend electrophysiologic monitoring every 6 months. Recently, measures of F-wave chronodispersion have been proposed to monitor thalidomide-induced neuropathy (Rao et al. 2000). Further studies should be performed to establish the correlation of F-wave chronodispersion with the SNAP index.

The outcome of thalidomide-induced peripheral neuropathy is uncertain. Early reports of this side effect described 50% of cases with irreversible neuropathy after a long follow-up of 4–6 years (Fullerton et al. 1968). In all patients, recovery was very slow. Other studies have reported similar rates of poor recovery (Aronson et al. 1984, Mellin et al. 1962, Ochonisky et al. 1994). In some patients, recovery did not begin for years. Sural nerve biopsy samples showed severe degeneration of large axons with few signs of regeneration (Lagueny et al. 1986). Education of patients about the earliest symptoms of neuropathy and instructions to stop the drug and contact their physician may reduce the risk of permanent neuropathy. Careful examination for signs of neuropathy and electrophysiologic tests performed every 3 or 6 months should also help detect neuropathy early.

A poorly investigated side effect of thalidomide is amenorrhea. Although the first report was in 1989 in a small group of patients with rheumatoid arthritis treated with thalidomide (Gutierrez-Rodriguez et al. 1989), its importance has only recently been emphasized. Ordi-Ros et al. (Ordi-Ros et al. 1998) described 4 cases of amenorrhea in a series of 18 patients. Amenorrhea appeared 4–5 months after the drug was first administered and resolved 2–3 months after withdrawal. Reintroduction of the drug in two patients was again associated with amenorrhea. Ovarian biopsy performed in one patient showed severe ovarian atrophy. No patients had antiovarian antibodies. Three more cases more have been described in patients with aphthosis (Gompel et al.

1999) and in another two patients with DLE (Passeron et al. 2001). The most recent report (Frances et al. 2002) aimed to establish the prevalence of thalidomide-related amenorrhea retrospectively by studying a group of 21 patients treated with thalidomide. Five patients (24%) with cutaneous LE and one patient with aphthosis developed amenorrhea. All had high serum levels of pituitary gonadotropins (folliculestimulating hormone and luteinizing hormone). Amenorrhea as a side effect of thalidomide use might be underrecognized in diseases other than lupus since the combined oral contraceptive pill is a widely used contraceptive measure. Usually, patients with SLE use the progesterone-only pill, depot progestogens, or nonhormonal contraceptive measures. When the combined oral contraceptive pill is used, menstruation may continue even when endocrine abnormalities are present.

Thrombotic events have been described as occurring shortly after the onset of thalidomide treatment (Flageul et al. 2000). Four of five patients who developed thrombosis had SLE and were antiphospholipid antibody positive. Thrombosis has also been described in patients with multiple myeloma treated with thalidomide, dexamethasone, and chemotherapy (Osman et al. 2001). The possible underlying thrombogenic mechanism of thalidomide is still unknown and might only be exerted when other risk factors for thrombosis are present, such as antiphospholipid antibodies or malignancy. Although the role of thalidomide as a trigger factor to develop thrombosis has to be confirmed in larger series of patients, thalidomide should be used with caution in patients who are antiphospholipid antibody positive or who have other known risk factors for thrombosis.

Disease Relapses

Recurrences of the skin lesions are frequent when thalidomide is withdrawn. Most of the studies report that in approximately 70% of patients the skin lesions flare between 2 weeks and 3 months after discontinuing use of the drug (Knop et al. 1983, Kyriakis et al. 2000, Stevens et al. 1997). In other series (Atra and Sato 1993), the rate of recurrence is lower (35%), with milder symptoms than those before treatment (Kyriakis et al. 2000). Thalidomide probably exerts its immunomodulatory properties only while administered. The introduction of other drugs, such as antimalarials and low-dose steroids, at the time of thalidomide dose reduction might reduce the risk of relapses at complete withdrawal of thalidomide.

Thalidomide Analogues

Thalidomide analogues have been synthesized with the aim of developing drugs with better clinical efficacy and improved side effect profiles. These include thalidomide-template–based TNF-α inhibitors, which may be 50,000 times more effective in TNF-α inhibition. Two classes are described, according to inhibition of phosphodiesterase 4. Those without phosphodiesterase 4-inhibitory activity also co-stimulate T cells, although more potently than thalidomide (Corral and Kaplan 1999). However, there have been no reports to date of their clinical use in lupus, although they have been used in therapy of myeloma (M. Kazmi, personal communication). As the exact mechanisms for the efficacy of thalidomide in lupus are not known, it is difficult to know which properties would be important to retain in the analogue.

Conclusions

Thalidomide has shown excellent results in almost all cutaneous manifestations of lupus refractory to a variety of other drugs. Despite its serious side effects, with careful patient selection and monitoring, thalidomide may be very useful in the treatment of severe cutaneous lupus. Although it has immunosuppressive, immunomodulatory, and antiangiogenic actions, its precise mechanism of action in lupus has yet to be confirmed.

References

Aronson IK, Yu R, West DP, van den Broek H, Antel J (1984) Thalidomide induced peripheral neuropathy. Arch Dermatol 120:1466–1470

Atra E, Sato EI (1993) Treatment of the cutaneous lesions of systemic lupus erythematosus with thalidomide. Clin Exp Rheumatol 11:487–493

Barnhill RL, Doll NJ, Millikan LE, Hastings RC (1984) Studies on the anti-inflammatory properties of thalidomide: effects on polymorphonuclear leukocytes and monocytes. J Am Acad Dermatol 11:814–819

Belmont HM, Buyon J, Giorno R, Abramson S (1994) Up-regulation of endothelial cell adhesion molecules characterizes disease activity in systemic lupus erythematosus. The Shwartzman phenomenon revisited. Arthritis Rheum 37:376–383

Clemmensen OJ, Olsen PZ, Andersen KE (1984) Thalidomide neurotoxicity. Arch Dermatol 120:338–341

Corral LG, Kaplan G (1999) Immunomodulation by thalidomide and thalidomide analogues. Ann Rheum Dis 58(Suppl I):I 107–113

D'Amato RJ, Loughnan MS, Flynn E, Folkman J (1994) Thalidomide is an inhibitor of angiogenesis. Proc Natl Acad Sci USA 91:4082–4085

de Iongh RU (1990) A quantitative ultrastructural study of motor and sensory lumbosacral nerve roots in the thalidomide-treated rabbit fetus. J Neuropathol Exp Neurol 49:564–581

Dean GS, Tyrell-Price J, Crawley E, Isenberg DA (2000) Cytokines and systemic lupus erythematosus. Ann Rheum Dis 59:243–251

Duong DJ, Spigel GT, Moxley TR 3rd, Gaspari AA (1999) American experience with low-dose thalidomide therapy for severe cutaneous lupus erythematosus. Arch Dermatol 135:1079–1087

Faure M, Thivolet J, Gaucherand M (1980) Inhibition of PMN leukocytes chemotaxis by thalidomide. Arch Dermatol Res 269:275–280

Flageul B, Wallach D, Cavalier-Balloy B, Bachelez H, Carsuzaa F, Dubertret L (2000) Thalidomide and thrombosis. Ann Dermatol Venereol 127:171–174

Frances C, El Khoury S, Gompler A, Becherel PA, Chosidow O, Piette JC (2002) Transient secondary amenorrhea in women treated by thalidomide. Eur J Dermatol 12:63–65

Fullerton PM, O'Sullivan DJ (1968) Thalidomide neuropathy: a clinical, electrophysiological, and histological follow-up study. J Neurol Neurosurg Psychiatric 31:543–551

Gad SM, Shannon EJ, Krotoski WA, Hastings RC (1985) Thalidomide induces imbalances in T-lymphocyte sub-populations in the circulating blood of healthy males. Lepr Rev 56:35–39

Gardner-Medwin JM, Smith NJ, Powell RJ (1994) Clinical experience with thalidomide in the management of severe oral and genital ulceration in conditions such as Behcet's disease: use of neurophysiological studies to detect thalidomide neuropathy. Ann Rheum Dis 53:828–832

Geitz H, Handt S, Zwingenberger K (1996) Thalidomide selectively modulates the density of cell surface molecules involved in the adhesion cascade. Immunopharmacology 31:213–221

Gompel A, Frances C, Piette JC, Blanc AS, Cordoliani F, Piette AM (1999) Ovarian failure with thalidomide treatment in complex aphthosis: comment on the concise communication by Ordi et al. Arthritis Rheum 42:2259–2260

Gutiérrez-Rodriguez O, Starusta-Bacal P, Gutiérrez-Montes O (1989) Treatment of rheumatoid arthritis: the thalidomide experience. J Rheumatol 16:158–163

Hamuryudan V, Mat C, Saip S, Ozyazgan Y, Siva A, Yurdakul S, Zwingenberger K, Yazici H (1998) Thalidomide in the treatment of the mucocutaneous lesions of Behcet's syndrome. A randomised, double-blind, placebo controlled trial. Ann Intern Med 128:443–459

Haslett PA, Corral LG, Albert M, Kaplan G (1998) Thalidomide costimulates primary human T lymphocytes, preferentially inducing proliferation, cytokine production, and cytotoxic responses in the CD8+ subset. J Exp Med 187:1885–1892

Herrera-Esparza R, Barbosa-Cisneros O, Villalobos-Hurtando R, Avalos-Diaz E (1998) Renal expression of IL-6 and TNF alpha genes in lupus nephritis. Lupus 7:154–158

Jacob CO, Fronek Z, Lewis GD, Koo M, Hansen JA, McDevitt HO (1990) Heritable major histocompatibility complex class II-associated differences in production of tumor necrosis factor alpha: relevance to genetic predisposition to systemic lupus erythematosus. Proc Natl Acad Sci USA 87:1233–1237

Jones SM, Mathew CM, Dixey J, Lovell CR, McHugh NJ (1996) VCAM-1 expression on endothelium in lesions from cutaneous lupus erythematosus is increased compared with systemic and localized scleroderma. Br J Dermatol 135:678–686

Keifer JA, Guttridge DC, Ashburner BP, Baldwin AS Jr (2001) Inhibition of NF-kappa B activity by thalidomide through suppression of IkappaB kinase activity. J Biol Chem 276:22382–22387

Knop J, Bonsmann G, Happle R, Ludolph A, Matz DR, Mifsud EJ, Macher E (1983) Thalidomide in the treatment of sixty cases of chronic discoid lupus erythematosus. Br J Dermatol 108:461–466

Kohchiyama A, Oka D, Ueki H (1985) T-cell subsets in lesions of systemic and discoid lupus erythematosus. J Cutan Pathol 12:493–499

Kruse FE, Joussen AM, Rohrschneider K, Becker MD, Volcker HE (1998) Thalidomide inhibits corneal angiogenesis induced by vascular endothelial growth factor. Graefes Arch Clin Exp Ophthalmol 236:461–466

Kyriakis KP, Kontochristopoulos GJ, Panteleos DN (2000) Experience with low-dose thalidomide therapy in chronic discoid lupus erythematosus. Int J Dermatol 39:218–222

Lagueny A, Rommel A, Vignolly B, Taieb A, Vendeaud-Busquet M, Doutre MS, Julien J (1986) Thalidomide neuropathy: an electrophysiologic study. Muscle Nerve 9:837–844

Lee SH, Park SH, Min JK, Kim SI, Yoo WH, Hong YS, Park JH, Cho CS, Kim TG, Han H, Kim HY (1997) Decreased tumour necrosis factor-beta production in TNFB*2 homozygote: an important predisposing factor of lupus nephritis in Koreans. Lupus 6:603–609

McHugh SM, Rifkin IR, Deighton J Wilson AB, Lachmann PJ, Lockwood CM, Ewan PW (1995) The immunosuppressive drug thalidomide induces T helper type 2 (Th2) and concomitantly inhibits Th1 cytokine production in mitogen- and antigen-stimulated human peripheral blood mononuclear cell cultures. Clin Exp Immunol 99:160–167

Mellin GW, Katzenstein M (1962) The saga of thalidomide: neuropathy to embryopathy, with case reports and congenital abnormalities. N Engl J Med 23:1184–1190

Mellin GW (1962) The saga of thalidomide (concluded). N Engl J Med. 267:1238–1244

Moreira AL, Sampaio EP, Zmuidzinas A, Frindt P, Smith KA, Kaplan G (1993) Thalidomide exerts its inhibitory action on tumor necrosis factor α production by enhancing mRNA degradation. J Exp Med 177:1675–1680

Moreira AL, Friedlander DR, Shif B, Kaplan G, Zagzag D (1999) Thalidomide and a thalidomide analogue inhibit endothelial cell proliferation in vitro. J Neurooncol 43:109–114

Ochonisky S, Verroust J, Bastuji-Garin S, Gherardi R, Revuz J (1994) Thalidomide neuropathy incidence and clinicoelectrophysiologic findings in 42 patients. Arch Dermatol 130:66–69

Ordi-Ros J, Cortes F, Martinez N, Mauri M, de Torres I, Vilardell M (1998) Thalidomide induces amenorrhea in patients with lupus disease. Arthritis Rheum 41:2273–2275

Ordi-Ros J, Cortes F, Cucurull E, Mauri M, Bujan S, Vilardell M (2000) Thalidomide in the treatment of cutaneous lupus refractory to conventional therapy. J Rheumatol 27:1429–1433

Osman K, Comenzo R, Rajkumar SV (2001) Deep vein thrombosis and thalidomide therapy for multiple myeloma. N Engl J Med 344:1951–1952

Passeron T, Lacour JP, Murr D, Ortonne JP (2001) Thalidomide-induced amenorrhea: two cases. Br J Dermatol 144:1262–1295

Powell RJ, Gardner-Medwin JM (1994) Guideline for the clinical use and dispensing of thalidomide. Postgrad Med J 70:901–904

Randall T (1990) Thalidomide has 37-year history. JAMA 263:1474

Rao DG, Kane NM, Oware A (2000) Thalidomide neuropathy: role of F-wave monitoring. Muscle Nerve 23:1301–1302

Reyes-Teran G, Sierra-Madero JG, Martinez del Cerro V, Arroyo-Figueroa H, Pasquetti A, Calva JJ, Ruiz-Palacios GM (1996) Effects of thalidomide on HIV-associated wasting syndrome: a randomised, double-blind, placebo-controlled clinical trial. AIDS 10:1501–1507

Rovelli A, Amigo C, Nesi F, Balduzzi A, Nicolini B, Locasciulli A, Vassallo E, Miniero R, Uderzo C (1998) The role of thalidomide in the treatment of refractory chronic graft-versus-host disease following bone marrow transplantation. Bone Marrow Transplant 21:577–581

Sampaio EP, Sarno EN, Galilly R, Cohn ZA, Kaplan G (1991) Thalidomide selectively inhibits tumor necrosis factor α production by stimulated human monocytes. J Exp Med 173:699–703

Sato EI, Assis LS, Lorenzi VP, Andrade LE (1998) Long-term thalidomide use in refractory cutaneous lesions of systemic lupus erythematosus. Rev Assoc Med Bras 44:289–293

Settles B, Stevenson A, Wilson K, Mack C, Ezell T, Davis MF, Taylor LD (2001) Down-regulation of cell adhesion molecules LFA-1 and ICAM-1 after in vitro treatment with the anti-TNF-alpha agent thalidomide. Cell Mol Biol (Noisy-le-grand) 47:1105–1114

Shannon EJ, Miranda RO, Morales MJ, Hastings RC (1981) Inhibition of de novo IgM antibody synthesis by thalidomide as a relevant mechanism of action in leprosy. Scand J Immunol 13:553–562

Sheskin J (1965) Thalidomide in the treatment of lepra reactions. Clin Pharmacol Ther 6:303–306

Singhal S, Mehta J, Desikan R, Ayers D, Roberson P, Eddlemon P, Munshi N, Anaissie E, Wilson C, Dhodapkar M, Zeddis J, Barlogie B (1999) Antitumor activity of thalidomide in refractory multiple myeloma. N Engl J Med 341:1565–1571

Stevens RJ, Andujar C, Edwards CJ, Ames PRJ, Barwick AR, Khamashta MA, Hughes GRV (1997) Thalidomide in the treatment of the cutaneous manifestations of lupus erythematosus: experience in sixteen consecutive patients. Br J Rheumatol 36:353–359

Tseng S, Pak G, Washenik K, Pomeranz MK, Shupack JL (1996) Rediscovering thalidomide: a review of its mechanism of action, side effects, and potential uses. J Am Acad Dermatol 35:969–979

Vogelsang GB (1993) Acute and chronic graft-versus-host disease. Curr Opin Oncol 5:276–281

Walchner M, Messer G, Wierenga EA (1995) Reconstitution of transcription factor binding to the conserved lymphokine element-o and downregulation of NF-κB activity after thalidomide treatment of systemic lupus erythematosus. Arch Dermatol Res 287:347

Walchner M, Meurer M, Plewig G, Messer G (2000) Clinical and immunologic parameters during thalidomide treatment of lupus erythematosus. Int J Dermatol 39:383–388

Wolkenstein P, Latarjet J, Roujeau JC, Duguet C, Boudeau S, Vaillant L, Maignan M, Schuhmacher MH, Milpied B, Pilorget A, Bocquet H, Brun-Buisson C, Revuz J (1998) Randomised comparison of thalidomide versus placebo in toxic epidermal necrolysis. Lancet 352:1586–1589

CHAPTER 29

Immunosuppressive Drugs in Cutaneous Lupus Erythematosus

29

Michael Sticherling

In lupus erythematosus (LE), the skin organ is involved to a varying extent with gross intraindividual and interindividual differences. These differences have been referred to in detail in other chapters of this book. Dermatologic symptoms usually do not influence the survival of patients, but they do affect their quality of life and self-esteem to a great extent. In addition, cutaneous LE (CLE) mainly affects young and middle-aged patients and presents with a chronic course. Consequently, therapy has to be balanced for short- and long-term side effects and often may be restricted to safe yet effective local measures, including sun protection. Beyond these measures, antimalarials are the first-line treatment for cutaneous disease (Callen 2002, Duna and Cash 1995, Jessop et al. 2001, McCauliffe 2001, Patel and Werth 2002, Reid 2000, Werth 2001). However, physicians are often faced with the challenge of recalcitrant skin disease unresponsive to such conventional therapy and have to improve the patient's discomfort and cosmetic appearance as well as prevent development of further lesions. It is these cases that are referred to in this chapter. The order of agents herein does not reflect their priority and ranking. Critical evaluation of their use in CLE, namely, discoid LE (DLE) and subacute CLE (SCLE), which have been studied best, is given in each paragraph.

Optimal regimens still have to be defined regarding numerous uncontrolled, mostly retrospective treatment studies that are based on empirical knowledge or case reports and lack current prerequisites of evidence-based medicine. Comparison of many studies is further hampered by the fact that different disease manifestations have been included and dissection from systemic disease has only partly been performed or described. In many studies, CLE restricted to the skin and cutaneous manifestations among systemic disease have rather indiscriminately been included which, however, may differentially respond to the implemented therapy regimens.

Whereas in psoriasis our current rather detailed pathogenetic knowledge has led to novel and targeted therapeutic interventions, the immunologic background of LE seems heterogeneous, especially regarding skin involvement and its precise pathogenetic mechanisms, let alone precipitating factors. Despite the progress in our immunologic knowledge, treatment today is still symptomatic rather than curative.

Activation of self-reactive T and B cells by genetic and environmental factors seems to be centrally involved in LE, and, consequently, various immunomodulatory measures have been used in the past (Abu-Shakra and Buskila 2002, Callen 2002, Dequet and Wallace 2001, Duna and Cash 1995, Dutz 1998, Gescuk and Davis 2002, Jessop et al. 2001, McCauliffe 2001, Luger 2001, Patel and Werth 2002, Reid 2000, Robert and Kupper 1999, Solsky 2002, Sticherling 2001, Thoma-Uszynski and Hertl

2001, Wallace 2002, Werth 1993, 2001). Based on our current knowledge, these measures can influence both humoral and cellular responses of the immune system on cellular and functional levels and may consequently be divided into three subgroups: immunosuppressive agents (e.g., cylophosphamide), immunomodulatory agents with immunosuppressive activity (e.g., glucocorticosteroids and methotrexate), and immunomodulatory agents without immunosuppressive activity (e.g., macrolactame antibiotics and cyclosporine.

All regimens listed in this chapter are supposed to have immunomodulatory effects, which for some is based on experimental or clinical data and for others is based only on deduction from their empiric effectiveness in LE or other inflammatory disorders. Several recent reviews summarize therapeutic measures of CLE or cutaneous manifestation in the context of systemic LE (SLE) from various aspects (Abu-Shakra and Buskila 2002, Callen 2002, Dequet and Wallace 2001, Duna and Cash 1995, Gescuk and Davis 2002, Jessop et al. 2001, McCauliffe 2001, Patel and Werth 2002, Reid 2000, Robert and Kupper 1999, Solsky 2002, Sticherling 2001, Thoma-Uszynski and Hertl 2001, Wallace 2002, Werth 1993, 2001).

Often, a combination of different therapy regimens is needed either to increase clinical effectiveness or to reduce the extent of side effects of individual drugs. Still, the disease may relapse after tapering of daily doses or stopping the treatment, thus requiring persistent therapy for a long time. Positive clinical effects have to be balanced with short- and long-term side effects in each individual case. Infancy or old age, pregnancy, and comorbid conditions like arterial hypertension and diabetes mellitus have to be taken into account as well. After proper classification of cutaneous lesions and extensive evaluation of isolated skin vs systemic disease, effective and stage-adapted therapy has to be initiated. The therapeutic interventions summarized in this chapter comprise old, well-established drugs as well as novel ones and also include measures that have been described only anecdotally. The number of studies focusing on CLE is restricted and mainly comprises casuistic reports. In but a few studies on SLE, cutaneous symptoms are only generally referred to and mainly are referred to as rash.

Glucocorticosteroids

Glucocorticosteroids have been shown to influence various parameters involved in inflammatory processes, including migratory and resident cells like lymphocytes, mast cells, and endothelial cells. Thus, activation and extravasation of immune cells as well as subsequent edema is reduced or blocked. The advent of glucocorticosteroids in the 1960s has grossly improved the so far poor prognosis of SLE. Even with the availability of modern immunomodulatory substances, glucocorticosteroids are still needed for their rapid and distinct clinical effects. Yet, their long-term side effects have to be counterbalanced by combination with other drugs that will result in steroid-sparing effects (Callen 2002, Goldberg and Lidsky 1984, Wallace 2002, Werth 2002).

Some authors strongly discourage the use of oral glucocorticosteroids for CLE because of low efficacy on one hand and known toxicity on the other (McCauliffe 2001). Furthermore, several good alternatives are available before resorting to oral glucocorticosteroids. With rapid-onset disease or rapid progress, initial short courses of glucocorticosteroids can be effective before antimalarial therapy becomes effective. Whereas SCLE may respond to oral glucocorticosteroids, there is lack of efficacy especially in DLE. Doses well below 1 mg/kg body weight may suffice and should be tapered within 3–4 weeks. For CLE, the latter regimen seems efficient in most cases. Methylprednisolone, at doses of 1 g intravenously daily for 3 days, was shown to clear otherwise refractory SCLE within 1–2 weeks, with sustained improvement for 2–3 months (Werth 1993, Goldberg 1984). Such pulse regimens of glucocorticosteroids are preferred by some authors for their dose-sparing effects, whereas others suggest daily intake of low steroid doses.

For steroid-sparing effects, agents like azathioprine (see below) may be added that support clinical effects induced by glucocorticosteroids while tapering steroid doses. Cases in which steroid doses below 0.5 mg/kg body weight result in relapses of disease are sometimes referred to as steroid resistant and need other regimens to be initiated, as outlined later herein.

Cyclophosphamide

Although this drug is regarded as the gold standard for SLE, it is rarely needed for CLE (McCauliffe 2001, Wallace 2001). It may be applied at three dose levels (low, medium, and high, up to 50 mg/kg per day) and as pulse therapy. In a small study of low-dose cyclophosphamide (50–200 mg/d) comprising nine patients with DLE and SCLE, 50% showed an excellent response and another 30% a moderate response (Schulz and Menter 1971). Even with daily low doses of 100 mg, close monitoring of blood cell counts and liver enzymes has to be performed. Pulse therapy at 4-week intervals needs inward treatment and isolation to lower the risk of infection and is restricted to SLE manifestations. Apart from hematologic risks, both lung and urinary epithelia may be affected and may necessitate the prophylactic and timely application of mesna. Regarding the young age of most patients, the female preponderance, and the impact on reproduction, cyclophosphamide has to be critically evaluated, especially in the context of CLE.

Azathioprine

This antimetabolite of the purine synthesis represents the classic drug in autoimmune and rheumatologic disorders to be combined with glucocorticosteroids. Monotherapy may take 2–8 weeks to show clinical response (Abu-Shakra et al. 2001, Ashinoff et al. 1988, Callen et al. 1991, Tan et al. 1997, Tsokos et al. 1985). Before initiation of the therapy, activity of the metabolizing enzyme thiomethyltransferase should be evaluated to individually adapt the dosage of azathioprine and lower the incidence of side effects. With normal enzyme levels, doses of 2 mg/kg body weight and greater are recommended. Side effects include disturbances in blood cell counts and liver enzyme levels. Initially, these laboratory parameters should be checked at weeks 2, 4, and 8, and thereafter every 3 months. The incidence of infections seems to be only slightly increased in contrast to a distinct increase of tumors on long-term treatment. This, however, seems to apply to almost any immunosuppressive and most immunomodulatory drugs.

Methotrexate

Methotrexate was used extensively a couple of decades ago for various inflammatory processes (Jeffes et al. 1995, Cronstein 1996). Within dermatology, the drug has gone out of fashion by the misconception of dose restriction at a cumulative dose of 1.5–2 g because of possible liver damage and fibrosis. It is not clear if rheumatologic patients show different incidences of methotrexate-related liver disease than patients with psoriasis. Blood cell counts, liver enzyme levels, and fibrotic processes (procollagen III peptide at biannual intervals) should be monitored regularly.

Methotrexate was shown to be very effective in DLE and SCLE at doses as low as 15–20 mg once per week (Abe et al. 1994, Boehm et al. 1998, Bohm et al. 1997, Bottomley and Goodfield 1995a, b, Goldstein and Carey 1994, Kuhn et al. 2002). It may be used as a single agent or as adjunct therapy. In SLE, apart from synovitis, cutaneous disease may effectively be treated with distinct steroid-sparing effects (Abud-Mendoza et al. 1993, Rothenberg et al. 1988, Wilke et al. 1991). Methotrexate may be administered intravenously, thus circumventing individual variations of intestinal resorption, or orally in strictly compliant patients. Patients with LE might not tolerate oral methotrexate as well as other patients and may prefer the subcutaneous or intravenous application. To lower the incidence of side effects, tetrahydrofolate should be administered the following day. On induction of stable clinical effects, both dose and time intervals of application may be tapered. Immunologic effects at these low doses are probably induced by functional interaction with immunocompetent cells rather than by their physical eradication. Modulation of chemotaxis, migration and adhesion of polymorphonuclear leukocytes, and modulation of lymphocyte activity regarding interleukin (IL) 1ß, IL-6, and tumor necrosis factor (TNF)-α receptor expression seem to be the main effects (Boehm et al. 1998, Cronstein 1996, Jeffes et al. 1995).

Cyclosporine

This component is derived from the fungus streptomyces. Based on its effectiveness to suppress T-cell activity, it was introduced into transplantation medicine in the 1980s and is established within immunosuppressive regimens of transplanted solid organs. The drug interferes with the calmodulin-mediated intracellular signal transduction and thus inhibits the nuclear factor of activated T-cells (NFAT)-mediated transcription of several cytokines, mainly IL-2. Apart from T cells, various other cells are influenced, including mast cells, which are involved in different inflammatory processes.

Doses of 2.5–5 mg/kg body weight are usually applied to induce clinical effects and can often be tapered within 3–4 weeks. In CLE, however, prolonged treatment for several months may be needed to induce clinical improvement. Classic side effects include renal dysfunction and arterial hypertension. Thus, before initiation and during the first few months of therapy, these parameters should be monitored. Cyclosporine is approved for the treatment of rheumatoid arthritis and psoriasis. Beneficial effects were seen for thrombocytopenia, pancytopenia, and membranous nephritis associated with SLE, and steroid-sparing effects were suggested (Conti et al. 2000, Griffiths and Emery 2001). However, similar to arthralgia, myalgia, and fatigue, cutaneous disease is hardly improved (Conti et al. 2000, Lernia and Bisighini 1996, Obermoser et al. 2002, Saeki et al. 2000, Yell and Burge 1994). In a single patient, development of DLE was reported during treatment of psoriasis with cyclosporine (Lernia et al. 1996). Based on these results, the benign prognosis of CLE, and the possible side effects, cyclosporine should re regarded as second-line therapy in CLE.

Macrolactame Antibiotics

Another group of fungus-derived components, sometimes referred to as xenobiotics (Abu-Shakra and Busila 2002, Burkhardt and Kalden 1997, Luger 2001, Robert and Kupper 1999, Yokum 1996), is the macrolactams. Their antibiotic effects seem low compared with their immunologic potential. Similar to cyclosporine, tacrolimus and ascomycin can interfere with calmodulin by distinct binding proteins (Bergmann and Rico 2001, Burkhardt and Kalden 1997, Duddridge and Powell 1997, Furst 1999, Furukawa et al. 1995, Jayne 1999, Kilian et al. 1998, Kurtz et al. 1995, Singer and McCune 1998, Tran et al. 2001, Walker et al. 2002, Warner et al. 1995, Yokum 1996, Yoshimasu et al. 2002). Both drugs are well established within transplantation medicine. In off-label use outside this licensed application, data are so far mainly available on oral and topical tacrolimus and show positive effects on LE activity (Furukawa et al. 1995, Singer and McCune 1998, Tran 2001). However, no clinical data fulfilling the criteria of evidence-based medicine have been published except small studies and case reports (Bergmann and Rico 2001, Duddridge and Powell 1997, Kilian et al. 1998, Walker et al. 2002, Yoshimasu et al. 2002). This applies to many other drugs summarized in this chapter as well. Evidence-based trials are badly needed to compare their effectiveness to classical immunosuppressive regimens like glucocorticosteroids and azathioprine. Another component from this group, called "rapamycin" or "sirolimus", shows a distinctly different mechanism of action and is currently under clinical evaluation for different inflammatory disorders. Based on its promising effects, it may be used for various clinical forms of LE soon (Burkhardt et al. 1997, Singer and McCune 1998, Warner et al. 1995, Yocum 1996).

Inhibitors of Nucleic Acid Metabolism

Whereas the drugs described so far functionally or physically influence immune cells involved in the pathogenesis of LE, mycophenolate mofetil (MMF) and leflunomide were shown to decrease T- and B-cell proliferation by interfering with purine and pyrimidine metabolism, respectively. Whereas MMF is well established within transplantation medicine, leflunomide is licensed for use in rheumatoid arthritis. Both drugs have been used outside these indications in the context of LE (Furst 1999, Jayne 1999, Kurtz et al. 1995). MMF was shown to be effective for DLE and SCLE at doses of

2 g/d (Boehm and Bieber 2001, Goyal and Noussari 2001, Hanjani and Noussari 2002, Karim and Alba 2002, Schanz et al. 2002), whereas leflunomide was shown to positively influence accompanying cutaneous symptoms when applied for arthritic symptoms within SCLE as the main therapeutic target (10–20 mg/d) (Glant et al. 1998, Parnham 1995, Remer and Weisman 2001). However, gastrointestinal side effects, mainly diarrhea for MMF and hematologic and hepatic disturbances for leflunomide, may be limiting clinical application.

Clofazimine

The two classic antilepromatous drugs, dapsone and thalidomide, are referred to in other chapters of this book. Modulation of the inflammatory reaction and macrophage activity may in part explain their effects and may apply to another antilepromatous agent, clofazimine, as well. In fact, it has been successfully used in CLE (Arbisier and Moschella 1995, Krivanek and Paver 1980). Doses of 100 mg of Lamprene for 3 to 6 months improved skin symptoms in 60% of patients. The delayed effect is counteracted by only minimal side effects, mainly a pink-reddish discoloration of the skin and bodily secretions that is slowly reversible after discontinuation of the drug. This discoloration seems to be dose related, with deposits in the subcutaneous fat as well as in discoid plaques. Occasionally, gastrointestinal side effects like nausea and diarrhea may occur, as well as eosinophilic enteritis and splenic infarction.

Gold

Both parenteral (aurothioglucose) and oral gold (auranofin) have been successfully used for DLE, the latter at initial doses of 3 mg/day (Dalziel et al. 1986, Duna 1995, Steinkjer 1995, Werth 2001). An open trial showed improvement or complete remission in 19 of 23 patients (Steinkjer 1995). Infiltrated, but not hyperkeratotic, plaques were responsive. Diarrhea, nausea, and headache as well as renal and hematologic disturbances represent limiting side effects. Nonscarring forms of CLE seem to respond best. Possible lichenoid drug exanthema during the course of gold treatment should be dissected from LE-associated rash.

Miscellaneous

In a single study, 90% of 93 patients with chronic CLE showed very good results after oral phenytoin therapy at 300 mg/day for up to 6 months (Rodriquez-Castellanos et al. 1995). Prolonged remission of 6–12 months was observed in about one third of those patients in whom follow-up data were available. Minimal side effects seen in this study are counteracted by the potential risk of toxic epidermal necrolysis caused by phenytoin.

Sulfasalazine is well established in the treatment of inflammatory bowel diseases and various arthritides. Its effectiveness for CLE at a dose of 2 g/d has been suggested by a couple of case reports and small studies (Carmichael and Paul 1991, Delaporte et al. 1997, Ferda 1996). All patients that responded were rapid acetylators, whereas nonresponders were slow acetylators. However, severe side effects, especially hypersensitivity reactions, limit its use.

Another antibiotic with favorable effects was recently described in three cases of SCLE. The second-generation oral cephalosporin cefuroxime axetil cleared skin lesions within 6–8 weeks at a dose of 500 mg/d (Rudnicka 2000). The effect seems to be specific for this individual cephalosporin as others from this group did not work. Immunomodulatory effects beyond antibiotic activity may be involved.

Ambiguous results are found for vitamin E or tocopherol at doses of 800–2000 IU/d (Ayers and Mihan 1974, Duna 1995, Wallace 2001, 2002). Its mechanisms of action are unknown. Only fair responses have been found in open trials for DLE and SCLE at low doses, whereas adequate dosing resulted in marked improvement, especially in superficial disease of recent onset. These results, however, are discussed controversially, and vitamin E is not generally recommended.

Sex Hormone Treatment

Female preponderance and primary manifestation or exacerbation of preexisting LE during pregnancy is interpreted as involvement of sex hormones in the pathogenesis of LE (Piette et al. 1995, Wilder 1998). Consequently, therapeutic implementation of sex hormones has been controversially discussed in the past (Piette et al. 1995, Asherson and Lahita 1991). Nandrolone and danazol have been studied as weak androgens, but results have been ambiguous (Englert and Hughes 1988, Hazelton et al. 1983, Masse et al. 1980, Morley et al. 1982, Torrelo et al. 1990). Nandrolone did not show any effects in female patients but worsened symptoms in male patients. Whereas the beneficial role of danazol in the treatment of SLE-associated immune thrombocytopenia is appreciated, positive effects on CLE have been demonstrated in only a few patients. Hirsutism and weight gain as well as skin rash at higher doses further limit its therapeutic range. The adrenal steroid hormone dehydroepiandrosterone has been used in SLE for a decade, with controversial results regarding its effects (Gescuk and Davis 2002). Moreover, effects on skin symptoms have not been explicitly studied. Cyproterone acetate, a synthetic hydroxyprogesterone derivative, was shown to reduce the frequency of SLE flares as well as oral ulcerations (Jungers et al. 1985), whereas tamoxifen, an estrogen antagonist, was ineffective in a double-blind crossover study of SLE (Sturgess et al. 1984).

Intravenous Immunoglobulins

This biological agent based on polyclonal antibodies derived from human pool plasma has been used for a long time in diverse clinical conditions for antibody substitution as well as therapeutic intervention (Jolles et al. 1998, Rutter and Luger 2001, Sacher 2001). In the latter cases, divergent mechanisms on the humoral and cellular levels seem to be operative, including anticytokine effects, complement inactivation, and modulation of regulatory functions of different inflammatory cells. Autoimmune diseases are beyond the licensed applications yet are treated with partly beneficial results. No clinical studies are available on LE, but reports on a limited number of patients document beneficial effects in refractory CLE at high doses of 1–2 g/kg body weight every 4 weeks (De Vita et al. 1996, Genereau et al. 1999, Piette 1995). Minimal side effects are opposed to high costs. Therefore, intravenous immunoglobulins should only be used as an adjuvant in recalcitrant disease or initial treatment in combination with other immunosuppressive agents.

Biologicals

This novel group of therapeutics comprises proteins that are either purified from natural sources or produced as recombinant or synthetic proteins, and it reflects the recent progress of medical biotechnology and molecular biology. Monoclonal antibodies, fusion proteins, and cytokines can be allotted to this group (Gescuk and Davis 2002, Isenberg and Leckie 2002, Watts 2000). Many of these therapeutics are only just beginning to be introduced into the treatment of LE. The response of CLE to these agents has not been specifically addressed to date, apart from interferons, which have been extensively used in the past.

Cytokine Therapy

Local and systemic interferon α 2A and 2B have successfully been used for SCLE and DLE (Martinez et al. 1992, 1993, Nicolas and Thivolet 1989, Nicolas et al. 1990, Thivolet et al. 1990). Of four patients with SCLE, complete response was seen in two and partial response was seen in one, whereas the fourth showed progressive disease (Nicolas and Thivolet 1989). Aggravation/exacerbation of preexisting LE as well as induction/precipitation of hitherto unknown LE has to be taken into account as demonstrated by manifestation of SLE in patients treated with interferons for other chronic inflammatory or malignant disease (Garcia-Porrua et al. 1998, Graninger et al. 1991, Machlod and Smolen 1990, Morris et al. 1996, Noussari 1998, Ronnblom et al. 1991a, b, Schilling et al. 1991). Other side effects include fever and flulike symptoms.

Monoclonal Antibodies and Fusion Proteins

Various inflammatory parameters have been shown or suspected to be involved in the pathogenesis of LE, including humoral factors like cytokines or soluble cytokine receptors and cellular proteins like adhesion molecules, receptors, and the various participants of the T-cell receptor-mediated activation. A variety of monoclonal antibodies have become available within the past few years and are used in human disease, including phase I and II studies on SLE. They specifically target these proteins and may modulate inflammatory disease activity (Gelfand 2001, Isaacs 2001).

Blockage of co-stimulatory molecules has been accomplished by anti-CTLA4 immunoglobulin and anti-CD40 ligand. Their clinical effectiveness has been described within the context of systemic disease; effects on concomitant skin rash, however, have been reported. B-cell depletion parallel to improvement in rash, arthritis, and fatigue has been described for anti-CD20 antibody. Promising results have been found with anti-IL-8 antibodies as well as other anticytokine antibodies like anti-IL-10. Excellent reviews on treatment options with biologicals are given by Gescuk and Davis (Gescuk and Davis 2002), Isenberg and Leckie (Isenberg and Leckie 2002), and Watts (Watts 2000).

Refractory CLE has been successfully treated with chimeric monoclonal anti-CD4 antibody infusion in five patients with long-lasting remission and has regained responsiveness to conventional treatment (Prinz et al. 1996).

The therapeutic responses mediated by thalidomide are explained by modulation of TNF-α and suggest positive results by other strategies targeting this cytokine. Therefore, monoclonal anti-TNF-α antibody (infliximab) (Gescuk and Davis 2002, Pisetksky 2000) or soluble TNF-α receptor (etanercept) (DeBrandt et al. 2001), who, however, describe induction of SLE by this fusion proteins during treatment of rheumatoid arthritis) may play an important role in the treatment of LE in the future, including its cutaneous manifestations, and will have to be evaluated in future studies. However, propagation of infections as well as long-term side effects like induction of tumors or other autoimmune diseases will have to be evaluated (DeBrandt et al. 2001, Isenberg and Leckie 2002, Watts 2000).

In summary, in SLE, a variety of different biologicals have been applied with grossly diverging results. Targeting single, pathogenetically relevant parameters by monoclonal antibodies or receptor proteins is partly disappointing in clinical practice when moderate efficacy or unforeseen side effects are encountered. At this stage, any of these approaches are restricted to refractory or severely organ-threatening SLE and have not been specifically applied to CLE.

Ultraviolet (UV) Light

The issue of UV sensitivity in LE is well established and results in the recommendation of strict protection from sun and other UV-emitting sources (Gasparro 2000, McGrath et al. 1987, Millard and Hawk 2001). Based on these concepts, therapeutic use of UV light and its immunomodulatory activity seem contradictory. However, two approaches are feasible in this respect: extracorporeal photochemotherapy and UVA1 therapy. Modulation of DNA repair, cell-mediated immunity, and apoptotic phenomena have been discussed as possible explanations for the therapeutic effects observed.

Extracorporeal Photochemotherapy (Photopheresis)

In this therapy regimen, which is established for the treatment of T-cell lymphoma, UV exposure is restricted to circulating leukocytes. They are irradiated by low-energy UVA (312–400 nm) after oral ingestion of a photosensitizing drug (such as 8-methoxypsoralen). A variety of studies have shown beneficial effects on cutaneous manifestations restricted to the skin or among systemic disease that allowed tapering or discontinuation of glucocorticosteroids or cytotoxic medication (Knobler et al. 1992, Richter et al. 1998, Russell-Jones 2000, Wollina and Looks 1999). In an uncontrolled study of 10 patients with SLE, eight completed the treatment. Seven of these patients showed significant reduction of disease activity on photopheresis on 2 consecutive days each month for 6 months and following alternate months for another 6 months (Knobler et al. 1992). A case report on a patient with disseminated DLE refractory to classic drug therapy demonstrated beneficial results on photopheresis (Richter et al. 1998). The need for appropriate technical facilities and experience as well as the time lapse before clinical results appear restrict this therapy to recalcitrant cases in which the other, classic therapy regimens have failed.

UVA1 Therapy

The UV spectrum of electromagnetic radiation comprises UVB (280–315 nm) and UVA (315–400 nm) light. UVA constitutes the majority (90%–95%) of UV radiation on the earth's surface (Gasparro 2000, McGrath 1994). The biological, immunologic, and photochemical effects of both wavelengths seem divergent and partly opposing. LE-aggravating properties seem to be mainly attributable to UVB and the shorter part of UVA (UVA2, 315–340 nm). In contrast, UVA1 (340–400 nm) demonstrates the greatest efficacy in the treatment of LE. In this respect, LE may be attributed to other photodermatoses in which UV irradiation can be used for prophylaxis and treatment. Consequently, several studies have been published recently that document beneficial effects of UVA1 on both CLE and SLE (McGrath 1994, 1997, 1999, McGrath et al. 1996, Molina and McGrath 1997, Sonnichsen et al. 1993). Disease activity, therapeutic drug use, and anti-double-stranded DNA titers in SLE were shown to decrease after a 3-week course of UVA1 at 60 J/cm^2 per day for 5 days/week. Lower treatment frequencies of one or two irradiations per week for years seem to be effective as well (McGrath 1994, McGrath et al. 1996). In one case of SCLE, cutaneous symptoms improved after 9 weeks of treatment with UVA1 (Sonnichsen et al. 1993). In contrast to this, another case report described exacerbation in a patient with DLE on UVA1 treatment (McGrath 1999). As with other therapeutic regimens discussed in this chapter, UVA1 irradiation should only be implemented when other first-line therapies have failed, as, apart from possible LE aggravation, skin photocarcinogenesis and photoaging on long-term treatment have to be taken into account.

Stem Cell Transplantation

The progress in bone marrow and stem cell transplantation for malignant hematologic disorders has provided protocols that may be transferred to benign yet chronic or life-threatening immunologic disorders (Cohen and Nagler 2002, Moore et al. 2001, Traynor et al. 2002, Tyndall et al. 2000). Approximately 500 patients with severe autoimmune diseases have undergone autologous hematopoietic stem cell transplantation in the past 5 years (Cohen and Nagler 2002, Furst 2002, Gratwohl et al. 2001, Moore et al. 2001, Openshaw et al. 2002, Traynor et al. 2002, Tyndall and Koike 2002, Tyndall et al. 2000). Data have been compiled by Tyndall and Koike (Tyndall and Koike 2002), including patients with severe, organ-threatening SLE. For isolated CLE, this therapy certainly does not represent a feasible option. Even for SLE, this approach is controversially discussed, as data suggest no major improvement compared with high-dose cyclophosphamide immunoablative therapy without stem cell rescue (Traynor et al. 2002, Tyndall and Koike 2002). Therefore, this concept of "immunologic resetting" needs further evaluation with longer follow-up and multi-center randomized studies.

Summary and Perspectives

CLE may be regarded as its own disease entity or as a manifestation within multiorgan disease. Irrespective of this view, any patient with CLE has to be examined carefully to exclude systemic disease, which in turn will influence the timeliness and the extent of therapy. CLE may often be successfully and satisfactorily treated by local measures, including UV protection and antimalarial drugs. In cases of recalcitrant disease, other measures, including the systemic immunomodulatory regimens summarized in this chapter, have to be introduced. Many of these approaches lack sufficient scientific and clinical data to prove their general effectiveness. On the other hand, heterogeneity of skin disease and its low impact on the general prognosis of the afflicted patient limit clinical and scientific interest in solid clinical studies, which are, however, badly needed. CLE should be regarded as a severe, if only distressing, disease that needs ample drug treatment and intensive patient care. Consequently, modern immunomodulatory approaches have to be evaluated that may be more effective yet less toxic than established treatment regarding both short- and, even more important, long-term treatment.

References

Abe Y, Seno A, Tada J, Arata J (1994) Discoid lupus erythematosus: successful treatment with oral methotrexate. Arch Dermatol 130:938–939

Abud-Mendoza C, Sturbaum AK, Vazquez-Compean R, Gonzalez-Amaro R (1993) Methotrexate therapy in childhood systemic lupus erythematosus. J Rheumatol 20:731–733

Abu-Shakra M, Buskila D (2002) Update on the treatment of systemic lupus erythematosus: therapeutic highlights from the Sixth International Lupus Conference. Isr Med Assoc J 4:71–73

Abu-Shakra M. Shoenfeld Y (2001) Azathioprine therapy for patients with systemic lupus erythematosus. Lupus 10:152–153

Arbisier JL, Moschella SL (1995) Clofazimine. A review of its medical uses and mechanisms of action. J Am Acad Dermatol 32:241–247

Asherson RA, Lahita RG (1991) Sex hormone modulation in systemic lupus erythematosus. Still a therapeutic option? Ann Rheum Dis 50:897–898

Ashinoff R, Werth VP, Frank AG Jr (1988) Resistant discoid lupus erythematosus of palms and soles: successful treatment with azathioprine. J Am Acad Dermatol 19:961–965

Ayers S Jr, Mihan R (1974) Lupus erythematosus and vitamin E: an effective and non-toxic therapy. Cutis 23:49–52

Bergman J, Rico MJ (2001) Tacrolimus clinical studies for atopic dermatitis and other conditions. Semin Cutan Med Surg 20:250–259

Boehm I, Bieber T (2001) Chilblain lupus erythematosus Hutchinson: successful treatment with mycophenolate mofetil. Arch Dermatol 137:235–236

Boehm IB, Boehm GA, Bauer R (1998) Management of cutaneous lupus erythematosus with low-dose methotrexate: indication for modulation of inflammatory mechanisms. Rheumatol Int 18:59–62

Bohm L, Uerlich M, Bauer R (1997) Rapid improvement of subacute lupus erythematosus with low-dose methotrexate. Dermatology 194:307–308

Bottomley WW, Goodfield MJ (1995a) Methotrexate for the treatment of discoid lupus erythematosus. Br J Dermatol 133:655–656

Bottomley WW, Goodfield MJ (1995b) Methotrexate for the treatment of severe mucocutaneous lupus erythematosus. Br J Dermatol 133:311–314

Burkhardt H, Kalden JR (1997) Xenobiotic immunosuppressive agents: therapeutic effects in animal models of autoimmune diseases. Rheumatol Int 17:85–90

Callen JP (2002) Management of skin disease in patients with lupus erythematosus. Best Pract Res Clin Rheumatol 16:245–264

Callen JP, Spencer LV, Burruss JB, Holtman J (1991) Azathioprine: an effective, corticosteroid-sparing therapy for patients with recalcitrant cutaneous lupus erythematosus or with recalcitrant cutaneous leukocytoclastic vasculitis. Arch Dermatol 127:515–522

Carmichael AJ, Paul CJ (1991) Discoid lupus erythematosus responsive to sulphasalazine. Br J Dermatol 125:291–294

Cohen Y, Nagler A (2002) Treatment of refractory autoimmune diseases with lymphoablation and hematopoietic stem cell support. Isr Med Assoc J 4:865–867

Conti F, Priori R, Alessandri C, Spinelli FR, Medda E, Valesini G (2000) Safety profile and causes of withdrawal due to adverse events in systemic lupus erythematosus patients treated long-term with cyclosporine A. Lupus 9:676–680

Cronstein BN (1996) Molecular therapeutics. Methotrexate and its mechanism of action. Arthritis Rheum 39:1951–1960

Dalziel K, Going G, Cartwright PH, Marks R, Beveridge GW, Rowell NR (1986) Treatment of chronic discoid lupus erythematosus with an oral gold component (auranofin). Br J Dermatol 115:211–216

De Vita S, Ferraccioli GF, Di Poi E, Bartoli E, Bombardieri S (1996) High dose intravenous immunoglobulin therapy for rheumatic diseases: clinical relevance and personal experience. Clin Exp Rheumatol 14:S85–92

DeBandt M, Descamps V, Meyer O (2001) Etanercept-induced systemic lupus erythematosus: two cases on patients with rheumatoid arthritis. Lupus 10:S118

Delaporte E, Catteau B, Sabbagh N, Gosselin P, Breuillard F, Doutre M-S, Broly F, Piette F, Bergoend H (1997) Traitement du lupus erythemateux chronique par la sulfasalazine: 11 observations. Ann Dermatol Venereol 124:151–156

Dequet CR, Wallace DJ (2001) Novel therapies in the treatment of systemic lupus erythematosus. Curr Opin Investig Drugs 2:1045–1053

Duddridge M, Powell RJ (1997) Treatment of severe and difficult cases of systemic lupus erythematosus with tacrolimus. A report of three cases. Ann Rheum Dis 56:690–692

Duna GF, Cash JM (1995) Treatment of refractory cutaneous lupus erythematosus. Rheum Dis Clin North Am 21:99–115

Dutz JP, Ho VC (1998) Immunosuppressive agents in dermatology. An update. Dermatol Clin 16:235–251

Englert HJ, Hughes GVR (1988) Danazol and discoid lupus. Br J Dermatol 119:407–409

Ferda A (1996) Efficacy of sulfasalazine in discoid lupus erythematosus. Int J Dermatol 10:746–748

Furst DE (1999) Leflunomide, mycophenolic acid and matrix metalloproteinase inhibitors. Rheumatology (Oxford) 38:14–18

Furst DE (2002) Stem cell transplantation for autoimmune disease: progress and problems. Curr Opin Rheumatol 14:220–224

Furukawa F, Imamura S, Takigawa M (1995) FK506: therapeutic effects on lupus dermatosis in autoimmune-prone MRL/Mp-lpr/lpr mice. Arch Dermatol Res 287:558–563

Garcia-Porrua C, Gonzales Gay MA, Fernandez-Lamelo F, Paz-Carreira JM, Lavilla E, Gonzales-Lopez MA (1998) Simultaneous development of SLE-like syndrome and autoimmune thyroiditis following alpha-interferon treatment. Clin Exp Rheumatol 16:107–108

Gasparro FP (2000) Photodermatology: progress, problems and prospects. Eur J Dermatol 10:250–254

Gelfand EW (2001) Antibody-directed therapy: Past, present and future. J Allergy Clin Immunol 108:111–116

Genereau T, Chosidow O, Danel C, Cherin P, Herson S (1999) High-dose intravenous immunoglobulin in cutaneous lupus erythematosus. Arch Dermatol 135:1124–1125

Gescuk BD, Davis JC Jr (2002) Novel therapeutic agents for systemic lupus erythematosus. Curr Opin Rheumatol 14:515–521

Glant TT, Mikecz K, Brennan F, Negroiu G, Bartlett R (1998) Suppression of autoimmune responses and inflammatory events by leflunomide in an animal model for rheumatoid arthritis. J Rheumatol 25:20–26

Goldberg JW, Lidsky MD (1984) Pulse methylprednisolone therapy for persistent subacute cutaneous lupus. Arthritis Rheum 27:837–838

Goldstein E, Carey W (1994) Discoid lupus erythematosus: successful treatment with oral methotrexate. Arch Dermatol 130:938–939

Goyal S, Noussari HC (2001) Treatment of resistant discoid lupus erythematosus of the palms and soles with mycophenolate mofetil. J Am Acad Dermatol 45:142–144

Graninger WB, Hassfeld W, Pesau BB, Machold KP, Zielinski CC, Smolen JS (1991) Induction of systemic lupus erythematosus by interferon-gamma in a patient with rheumatoid arthritis. J Reumatol 18:1621–1622

Gratwohl A, Passweg J, Gerber I, Tyndall A (2001) International Stem Cell Project for Autoimmune Diseases. Stem cell transplantation for autoimmune diseases. Best Pract Res Clin Haematol 14:755–776

Griffiths B, Emery P (2001) The treatment of lupus with cyclosporine A. Lupus 10:165–170

Hanjani NM, Noussari CH (2002) Mycophenolate mofetil for the treatment of cutaneous lupus erythematosus with smoldering systemic involvement. Arch Dermatol 138:1616–1618

Hazelton RA, McCruden AB, Sturrock RD, Stimson WH (1983) Hormonal manipulation of the immune response in systemic lupus erythematosus: a drug trial of an anabolic steroid, 19-nortestosterone. Ann Rheum Dis 42:155–157

Isaacs JD (2001) From bench to bedside: discovering rules for antibody design, and improving serotherapy with monclonal antibodies. Rheumatol 40:724–738

Isenberg D, Leckie MJ (2002) Biological treatments for systemic lupus erythematosus. Scand J Rheumatol 31:187–191

Jansen GT, Dillaha CJ, Honeycutt WM (2001) Discoid lupus erythematosus. Is systemic treatment necessary? Arch Dermatol 92:283–285

Jayne D (1999) Non-transplant uses of mycophenolate mofetil. Curr Opin Nephrol Hypertens 8:563–567

Jeffes EW 3rd, McCullough JL, Pittelkow MR, McCormick A, Almanzor J, Liu G (1995) Methotrexate therapy of psoriasis: differential sensitivity of proliferating lymphoid and epithelial cells to the cytotoxic and growth – inhibitory effects of methotrexate. J Invest Dermatol 104: 183–188

Jessop S, Whitelaw D, Jordaan F (2001) Drugs for discoid lupus erythematosus. Cochrane Database Syst Rev CD002954

Jolles S, Hughes J, Whittaker S (1998) Dermatological uses of high-dose intravenous immunoglobulin. Arch Dermatol 134:80–86

Jungers P, Kuttenn F, Liote F, Pelissier C, Athea N, Laurent MC, Viriot J, Dougados M, Bach JF (1985) Hormonal modulation in systemic lupus erythematosus. Preliminary clinical and hormonal results with cyproterone acetate. Arthritis Rheum 28:1243–1250

Karim MY, Alba P, Cuadrado MJ, Abbs IC, D'Cruz DP, Khamashta MA, Hughes GR (2002) Mycophenolate mofetil for systemic lupus erythematosus refractory to other immunosuppressive agents. Rheumatology (Oxford) 41:876–882

Kilian K, Banyai A, Karadi A, Miklos K, Patranyi GG, Paloczi K (1998) FK-506 (tacrolimus) therapy for an unusual SLE-like disease. Transplant Proc 30:4130–4131

Knobler RM, Graninger W, Lindmaier A, Trautinger F, Smolen JS (1992) Extracorporeal photochemotherapy for the treatment of systemic lupus erythematosus. A pilot study. Arthrit Rheum 32:319–324

Krivanek JFC, Paver WKA (1980) Further studies on the use of clofazimine in discoid lupus erythematosus. Australas J Dermatol 21:169–171

Kuhn A, Specker C, Ruzicka T, Lehmann P (2002) Methotrexate treatment for refractory sub-acute cutaneous lupus erythematosus. J Am Acad Dermatol 46:600–603

Kurtz ES, Bayley SC, Arshad F, Lee AA, Przekop PA (1995) Leflunomide: an active antiin-flammatory and antiproliferative agent in models of dermatologic disease. Inflamm Res 44:187–188

Lernia VD, Bisighini G (1996) Discoid lupus erythematosus during treatment with cyclosporine. Acta Derm Venereol 76:87–88

Luger T (2001) Treatment of immune-mediated skin diseases: future perspectives. Eur J Derma-tol 11:343–347

Machlod KP, Smolen JS (1990) Interferon-gamma induced exacerbation of systemic lupus ery-thematosus. J Rheumatol 17:831–832

Martinez J, de Misa RF, Torrelo A, Ledo A (1992) Low-dose intralesional interferon alfa for dis-coid lupus erythematosus. J Am Acad Dermatol 26:494–496

Martinez J, de Misa RF, Boixeda P, Arrazola JM, Ledo A (1993) Long-term results of intralesional interferon alpha-2B in discoid lupus erythematosus. J Dermatol 20:444–446

Masse R, Youinou P, Dorval JC, Cledes J (1980) Reversal of lupus-erythematosus-like disease with danazol. Lancet 20:651

McCauliffe DP (2001) Cutaneous lupus erythematosus. Semin Cutan Med Surg 20:14–26

McGrath HJ (1994) Ultraviolet A1 irradiation decreases clinical disease activity and autoanti-bodies in patients with systemic lupus erythematosus. Clin Exp Rheumatol 12:129–135

McGrath H Jr (1997) Prospects for UV-A1 therapy as a treatment modality in cutaneous and sys-temic LE: Lupus 6:209–217

McGrath HJ (1999) Ultraviolet A1 (340–400 nm) irradiation and systemic lupus erythematosus. J Invest Dermatol 4:79–84

McGrath HJ, Bak E, Michalski JP (1987) Ultraviolet-A light prolongs survival and improves immune function (New Zealand black × New Zealand white) F_1 hybrid mice. Arthritis Rheum 30:557–561

McGrath HJ, Martinez-Osuna P, Lee FA (1996) Ultraviolet A1 (340–400 nm) irradiation therapy in systemic lupus erythematosus. Lupus 5:269–274

Millard TP, Hawk JLM (2001) Ultraviolet therapy in lupus. Lupus 10:185–187

Molina N, McGrath HJr. Longterm ultraviolet A1 irradiation therapy in systemic lupus erythe-matosus. J Rheumatol 24:1072–1074

Moore J, Tyndall A, Brooks P (2001) Stem cells in the aetiopathogenesis and therapy of rheu-matic disease. Best Pract Res Clin Rheumatol 15:711–726

Morley KD, Parke A, Hughes GRV (1982) Systemic lupus erythematosus: two patients treated with danazol. Br Med J 284:1431–1432

Morris LF, Lemak NA, Arnett FC Jr, Jordon RE, Duvic M (1996) Systemic lupus erythematosus diagnosed during interferon alfa therapy. South Med J 89:810–814

Nicolas JF, Thivolet J (1989) Interferon alpha therapy in severe unresponsive subacute cutaneous lupus erythematosus. N Engl J Med 321:1550–1551

Nicolas JF, Thivolet J, Kanitakis J, Lyonnet S (1990) Response of discoid and subacute cutaneous lupus erythematosus to recombinant interferon alpha 2a. J Invest Dermatol 95:142S-145S

Nousari HC, Kimyai-Asadi A, Tausk FA (1998) Subacute cutaneous lupus erythematosus asso-ciated with interferon beta-1a. Lancet 352:1925–1825

Obermoser G, Weber F, Sepp N (2001) Discoid lupus erythematosus in a patient receiving cyclosporin for liver transplantation. Acta Derm Venereol 81:319

Openshaw H, Nash RA, McSweeney PA (2002) High-dose immunosuppression and hematopoi-etic stem cell transplantation in autoimmune disease: clinical review. Biol Blood Marrow Transplant 8:233–248

Parnham MJ (1995) Leflunomide: a potential new disease modifying anti-rheumatic drug. Exp Opin Invest Drugs 4:777–779

Patel PP, Werth V (2002) Cutaneous lupus erythematosus: a review. Dermatol Clin 20:373–385

Piette JC (1995) High-dose immunoglobulins in the treatment of refractory cutaneous lupus erythematosus. Open trial in 5 cases. Arthritis Rheum 38:S304

Piette JC, Du LT, Papo T (1995) Postmenopausal hormone therapy and systemic lupus erythematosus. Ann Intern Med 122:961–962

Pisetksky DS (2000) Tumor necrosis α blockers and the induction of anti-DNA autoantibodies. Arthritis Rheum 43:2381–2382

Prinz JC, Meurer M, Reiter C, Rieber EP, Plewig G, Riethmuller G (1996) Treatment of severe cutaneous lupus erythematosus with a chimeric CD4 monoclonal antibody, cM-T412. J Am Acad Dermatol 34:244–252

Reid C (2000) Drug treatment of cutaneous lupus. Am J Clin Dermatol 1:375–379

Remer CF, Weisman MH, Wallace DJ (2001) Benefits of leflunomide in systemic lupus erythematosus: a pilot observational study. Lupus 10:480–483

Richter HI, Krutmann J, Goerz G (1998) Extrakorporale Photopherese bei therapie-refraktärem disseminiertem diskoiden Lupus erythematodes. Hautarzt 49:487–491

Robert C, Kupper TS (1999) Inflammatory skin diseases, T cells and immune surveillance. N Engl J Med 341:1817–1828

Rodriquez-Castellanos MA, Rubio JB, Gomez JFB, Mendoza AG (1995) Phenytoin in the treatment of discoid lupus erythematosus. Arch Dermatol 131:620–621

Ronnblom LE, Alm GV, Oberg KE (1991a) Autoimmunity after alpha-interferon therapy for malignant carcinoid tumors. Ann Intern Med 115:178–183

Ronnblom LE, Alm GV, Oberg KE (1991b) Autoimmune phenomena in patients with malignant carcinoid tumors during interferon-alpha treatment. Acta Oncol 30:537–540

Rothenberg RJ, Graziano FM, Grandone JT, Goldberg JW, Bjarnason DF, Finesilver AG (1988) The use of methotrexate in steroid-resistant systemic lupus erythematosus. Arthritis Rheum 31:612–615

Rudnicka L, Szymanska E, Walecka I, Slowinska M (2000) Long-term cefuroxime axetil in subacute cutaneous lupus erythematosus. Dermatology 200:129–131

Russell-Jones R (2000) Extracorporeal photopheresis in cutaneous T-cell lymphoma. Inconsistent data underline the need for randomized studies. Br J Dermatol 142:16–21

Rutter A, Luger T (2001) High-dose intravenous immunoglobulins: an approach to treat severe immune-mediated and autoimmune diseases of the skin. J Am Acad Dermatol 44:1010–1024

Sacher RA (2001) Intravenous immunoglobulin consensus statement. J Allergy Clin Immunol 108:139–146

Saeki Y, Oshima S, Kurimoto I, Miura H, Suemura M (2000) Maintaining remission of lupus erythematosus profundus (LEP) with cyclosprin A. Lupus 9:390–392

Schanz S, Ulmer A, Rassner G, Fierlbeck G (2002) Successful treatment of subacute lupus erythematosus with mycophenolate mofetil. Br J Dermatol 147:174–178

Schilling PJ, Kurzrock R, Kantarjian H, Gutterman JU, Talpaz M (1991) Development of systemic lupus erythematosus after interferon therapy for chronic myelogenous leukemia. Cancer 68:1536–1537

Schulz EJ, Menter MA (1971) Treatment of discoid and subacute cutaneous lupus erythematosus with cyclophosphamide. Br J Dermatol 85:60–65

Singer NG, McCune WJ (1998) Update on immunosuppressive therapy. Curr Opin Rheumatol 10:169–173

Solsky M, Wallace DJ (2002) New therapies in systemic lupus erythematosus. Best Pract Res Clin Rheumatol 16:293–312

Sonnichsen N, Meffert H, Kunzelmann V, Audring H (1993) UV-A-1 therapy of subacute cutaneous lupus erythematosus. Hautarzt 44:723–725

Steinkjer B (1995) Auranofin in the treatment of discoid lupus erythematosus. J Dermatol Treat 2:27–29

Sticherling M (2001) Chronic cutaneous lupus erythematosus. In: Hertl M (ed) Autoimmune disease of the skin – pathogenesis, diagnosis, management. Springer, Vienna Berlin Heidelberg New York, pp 337–364

Sturgess AD, Evans DT, Mackay IR, Riglar A (1984) Effects of the oestrogen antagonist tamoxifen on disease indices in systemic lupus erythematosus. J Clin Lab Immunol 13:11–14

Tan BB, Lear TJ, Gawkrodger DJ, English JS (1997) Azathioprine in dermatology: a survey of current practice in the UK. Br J Dermatol 136:351–355

Thivolet J, Nicolas JF, Kanitakis J, Lyonnet S, Chouvet B (1990) Recombinant interferon alpha 2a is effective in the treatment of discoid and subacute cutaneous lupus erythematosus. Br J Dermatol 122:405–409

Thoma-Uszynski S, Hertl M (2001) Novel therapeutic approaches in autoimmune skin disorders. In: Hertl M (ed) Autoimmune disease of the skin – pathogenesis, diagnosis, management. Springer, Vienna Berlin Heidelberg New York, pp 337–364

Torrelo A, Espana A, Medina S, Ledo A (1990) Danazol and discoid lupus erythematosus. Dermatologica 181:239

Tran QHD, Guay E, Chartier S, Tousignant J (2001) Tacrolimus in dermatology. J Cutan Med Surg 5:329–335

Traynor AE, Barr WG, Rosa RM, Rodriguez J, Oyama Y, Baker S, Brush M, Burt RK (2002) Hematopoietic stem cell transplantation for severe and refractory lupus. Analysis after five years and fifteen patients. Arthritis Rheum 46:2917–2923

Tsokos GC, Caughman SW, Klippel JH (1985) Successful treatment of generalized discoid lesions with azathioprine. Its use in a patient s with systemic lupus erythematosus. Arch Dermatol 121:1323–1325

Tyndall A, Koike T (2002) High-dose immunoablative therapy with hematopoietic stem cell support in the treatment of severe autoimmune disease: current status and future direction. Intern Med 41:608–612

Tyndall A, Passweg J, Grathwohl A (2000) Haemopoietic stem cell transplantation in the treatment of severe autoimmune diseases. Ann Rheum Dis 60:702–707

Walker SL, Kirby B, Chalmers RJ (2002) The effect of topical tacrolimus on severe recalcitrant chronic discoid lupus erythematosus. Br J Dermatol 147:405–406

Wallace D (2001) Current and emerging lupus treatments. Am J Manag Care 7:S490–495

Wallace DJ (2002) Management of lupus erythematosus: recent insights. Curr Opin Rheumatol 14:212–219

Warner LM, Cummons T, Nolan L, Sehgal SN (1995) Sub-therapeutic doses of sirolimus and cyclosporin A in combination reduce SLE pathologies in the MRL mouse. Inflamm Res 44:S205–206

Watts RA (2000) Musculoskeletal and systemic reactions to biological therapeutic agents. Curr Opin Rheumatol 12:49–54

Werth V (2001) Current treatment of cutaneous lupus erythematosus. Dermatol Online J 7:2–12

Werth VP (1993) Management and treatment with systemic glucocorticoids. Adv Dermatol 8:81–101

Wilder RL (1998) Hormones, pregnancy, and autoimmune diseases. Ann NY Acad Sci. 840:45–50

Wilke WS, Krall PL, Scheetz RJ, Babiak T, Danao T, Mazanec DJ, Segal AM, Clough JD (1991) Methotrexate for systemic lupus erythematosus: a retrospective analysis of 17 unselected cases. Clin Exp Rheumatol 9:581–587

Wollina U, Looks A (1999) Extracorporeal photochemotherapy in cutaneous lupus erythematosus. J Eur Acad Dermatol Venereol 13:127–130

Yell JA, Burge SM (1994) Cyclosporine and discoid lupus erythematosus. Br J Dermatol 131:132–133

Yocum DE (1996) Cyclosporine, FK-506, rapamycin, and other immunomodulators. Rheum Dis Clin North Am 22:133–154

Yoshimasu T, Ohtani T, Sakamoto T, Oshima A, Furukawa F (2002) Topical FK506 (tacrolimus) therapy for facial erythematous lesions of cutaneous lupus erythematosus and dermatomyositis. Eur J Dermatol 12:50–52

CHAPTER 30

Experimental Therapies in Cutaneous Lupus Erythematosus

STEFAN W. SCHNEIDER, THOMAS A. LUGER

Experimental therapy of cutaneous lesions in patients with lupus erythematosus (LE) involves an empirical as well as a scientific approach. Unfortunately, to evaluate the efficacy of different therapeutic strategies for the treatment of cutaneous LE (CLE), the data of few double-blind, placebo-controlled trials are available. Most of the clinical studies using novel therapies were performed in patients with systemic LE (SLE) to monitor improvement of specific organ function such as nephritis, proteinuria, and nerve system or using the Systemic Lupus Activity Measure (SLAM) and Systemic Lupus Erythematosus Disease Activity Index (SLEDAI) scales (Dequet et al. 2001). However, skin involvement is one of the most frequent clinical complaints and can be found in 70% of patients during the course of disease.

The major goals in the management of the cutaneous lesions are to improve skin inflammation and thus to prevent the development of deforming scars, atrophy, or dyspigmentation. The present chapter summarizes the clinical experience with novel, not-yet-established therapeutic strategies in the treatment of LE, with a focus on their efficacy in improving skin lesions (see Table 30.1).

Immunomodulating Drugs

Methotrexate

Methotrexate (MTX) is a folate antagonist that has profound anti-inflammatory activities. Accordingly, MTX inhibits the activity of the proinflammatory cytokine interleukin (IL)-1β by blocking its binding to the IL-1 receptor (Sauder et al. 1993). On the other hand, the synthesis and release of IL-1β is not affected by MTX (Boehm et al. 1998). Moreover, there is evidence that patients with LE have a defective IL-1 receptor antagonist synthesis, which results in impaired down-regulation of this proinflammatory mediator (Hsieh et al. 1995). In addition to IL-1, MTX also inhibits other proinflammatory cytokines, such as IL-6 and tumor necrosis factor (TNF)-α, which, via activating B cells, are involved in the regulation of immunoglobulin production in patients with SLE (Linker-Israeli et al. 1991).

Most studies using MTX for the treatment of LE have been performed in patients with SLE. Apparently, MTX is helpful in treating synovitis and mild forms of SLE but seems not to be very effective for organ-threatening disease (Carneiro and Sato 1999). However, promising studies on MTX for the treatment of refractory CLE have been published. Twelve patients with CLE refractory to antimalarials or low-dose oral glu-

Table 30.1. New therapeutic modalities for lupus erythematosus

Immunomodulating drugs	Biological agents	Dehydroepiandrosterone
Methotrexate	INF-α	**Intravenous Immunoglobulin**
Calcineurin inhibitors	Anti-CD4	
Mycophenolate Mofetil	Rituximab	**Plasmapheresis and**
Leflunomide	CTLA-4Ig	**immunoadsorption**
	Anti-B7	
	Anti-IL-10	
	Anti-TNF-α	**Stem cell transplantation**
	LJP-994	
	Anti-C5	
Antibiotics	**Tazarotene**	**Other experimental therapies**
Cefuroxime Axetil		
Sulfasalazine	**Phenytoin**	

Anti-IL-10, anti-interleukin-10; INF-α, interferon-α; anti-TNF-α, anti-tumor necrosis factor-α.

cocorticosteroids were switched to MTX therapy (Boehm et al. 1998). On weekly administration of 10–25 mg MTX, marked improvement was observed in 10 of 12 patients. In 2 patients, the skin lesions cleared within 4 weeks, whereas most patients improved after an average of 6 weeks. Concomitant permanent or temporary treatment with systemic corticosteroids was necessary in six patients. Five patients showed long-term remissions of 5–24 months and a decrease in elevated circulating autoantibodies. All patients tolerated low-dose MTX treatment very well, and no withdrawal due to side effects was necessary. In two patients, MTX administration was discontinued because of lack of efficacy. Another recently published study showed complete clearing of skin lesions in one patient with severe SCLE refractory to therapy with antimalarials and corticosteroids (Kuhn et al. 2002).

Calcineurin Inhibitors

Cyclosporine (CsA) and tacrolimus (FK-506) both down-regulate T-cell activation by inhibiting calcineurin, a phosphatase required for the activation of nuclear factor of activated T cells (NFAT), a transcription factor that is required for the generation of many immunomodulating and proinflammatory cytokines. Subsequently, the synthesis of cytokines such as interferon (IFN)-γ, IL-2, IL-3, IL-4, granulocyte colony-stimulating factor, and TNF-α is inhibited. CsA and tacrolimus have different cytoplasmatic binding sites. CsA binds to cyclophylin, whereas tacrolimus connects with high affinity to FK-binding protein, which is also termed "macrophilin-12". Compared with CsA, tacrolimus exhibits a stronger immunosuppression activity.

Among other indications, CsA is approved for the treatment of rheumatoid arthritis, psoriasis, and atopic dermatitis, and its efficacy in the treatment of SLE has been reported in several studies (Caccavo et al. 1997, Manger et al. 1996). Accordingly, 10 patients with biopsy-proven membranous lupus nephropathy were treated with CsA (3.8 mg/kg for at least 12 months) and a decrease in proteinuria and an improvement in serum albumin levels over more than 1 year was observed. However, one major problem of CsA treatment is nephrotoxicity, which was responsive to a dose reduction or the addition of antihypertensive drugs (Hallegua et al. 2000). Two other studies reported on 56 and 18 patients with LE being treated with CsA either as an adjunctive steroid-sparing agent or because other treatments had failed. In the study including 56 patients, only in 5.3% was renal toxicity detectable (Conti et al. 2000, Dammacco et al. 2000). According to a National Institutes of Health trial of the treatment of membranous lupus nephritis, cyclophosphamide is more effective than CsA. However, the efficacy of steroids and CsA was found to be superior compared with that of steroids alone (Austin et al. 2000). Furthermore, a study of 43 patients with lupus given CsA, 4 mg/kg daily, for 4 years revealed a good response regarding thrombocytopenia but minor improvements in arthralgia, myalgia, and fatigue (Morton and Powell 2000). Unfortunately, 83% of the patients had to stop treatment because of adverse events.

Evidence from animal studies suggests that tacrolimus may have a protective effect against lupus nephritis (Entani et al. 1993). However, no data are available on the efficacy of tacrolimus in the treatment of patients with renal SLE. The efficacy of tacrolimus therapy in three patients with severe SLE whose disease had been poorly controlled by cyclophosphamide and CsA treatment has been reported (Duddrige and Powell 1997). In two of these patients, the treatment was successful; however, the third patient with cutaneous vasculitis did not experience improvement after 2 months of therapy, and administration of tacrolimus was discontinued because of nephrotoxity.

In several studies, topical tacrolimus has been shown to be an effective alternative for the treatment of atopic dermatitis as well as other inflammatory skin diseases. Systemic absorption usually is minimal, and, unlike topical corticosteroids, tacrolimus ointment does not cause skin atrophy (Paller et al. 2001). Therefore, it was tempting to evaluate the efficacy of topical tacrolimus for the treatment of CLE. In one study, 11 patients with facial skin lesions were treated with tacrolimus ointment twice daily (Yoshimasu et al. 2002). Six patients (three with SLE, one with discoid LE [DLE], and two with dermatomyositis) experienced marked regression of their skin lesion, whereas four patients (three with DLE and one with dermatomyositis) were resistant to topical therapy with tacrolimus. Therefore, the facial rash in SLE seems to improve well on local therapy with tacrolimus ointment, whereas DLE lesions seem to be more resistant. In a recent study, topical tacrolimus plus topical corticosteroids was used to treat two women with DLE resistant to antimalarials, thalidomide, and potent topical corticosteroids (Walker et al. 2002). Facial skin lesions were treated twice daily with a combination of 0.03% tacrolimus and 0.05% clobetasol propionate, and control lesions were treated with clobetasol monotherapy. The combined application of tacrolimus and a steroid resulted in a significant improvement within 10 days. In contrast, lesions treated with a topical steroid only did not significantly improve. Tapering off topical tacrolimus administration resulted in recurrence of the skin lesion, but on subsequent resumption of local tacrolimus therapy twice daily, DLE lesions improved again. Moreover, one of these patients discontinued concomitant hydroxychloroquine therapy and reduced the prednisolone dosage from 12.5 to 5.0 mg daily without relapse.

The macrolactam ascomycin derivate pimecrolimus, like tacrolimus, binds to some cytoplasmic proteins and also functions as a calcineurin inhibitor. One of the striking features of pimecrolimus is its preferential distribution to the skin and other epithelial tissues. Pimecrolimus has been introduced for the topical treatment of atopic dermatitis, and, according to preliminary data, this compound also seems to be suited for the treatment of inflammatory skin diseases such a psoriasis, hand eczema, seborrhoic eczema, and rosacea. Currently, there is only limited experience on the efficacy of pimecrolimus cream in CLE. Pimecrolimus also has been developed as an oral drug, and a first clinical trial with this compound has shown high efficacy in the treatment of psoriasis (Tomi and Luger 2002). In this 4-week dose-finding study, patients receiving 40 or 60 mg of pimecrolimus by mouth daily experienced a 60% or 75% improvement in the Psoriasis Area and Severity Index score, respectively, and, in contrast to tacrolimus or CsA therapy, no severe side effects such as nephrotoxicity were observed (Rappersberger et al. 2000). Further clinical trials are currently being performed to prove the efficacy and safety of oral pimecrolimus in the treatment of inflammatory skin diseases. Because of its high affinity to the skin and its low toxicity, this drug in the future may turn out to be very well suited for the treatment of LE.

Mycophenolate Mofetil

Mycophenolate mofetil (MMF) (CellCept) is a purine synthesis inhibitor that is hydrolysed to mycophenolic acid, a potent inhibitor of inosine monophosphate dehydrogenase required for purine synthesis in B and T lymphocytes as well as the inhibition of adhesion molecule glycosylation and the activation of monocytes (Frieling and Luger 2002, Kitchin et al. 1997). MMF therapy has been proved to be effective for the prevention of organ transplant rejection and for the therapy of rheumatoid arthritis and Crohn's disease. In addition, skin diseases such as bullous pemphigoid, pemphigus, psoriasis, and atopic dermatitis have been shown to significantly improve with MMF treatment (Beissert and Luger 1999, Geilen et al. 2000). In some case reports, MMF also was found to improve SLE, particularly lupus nephritis (Chan et al. 2000, Gaubitz et al. 1999). Moreover, treatment of diffuse proliferative lupus nephritis with MMF and prednisolone compared with cyclophosphamide and prednisolone was equally effective but remarkably less toxic (Chan et al. 2000). MMF also seems to be a successful approach to treat therapy-resistant skin lesions of SCLE (Schanz et al. 2002). Accordingly, two patients with extended SCLE that did not respond to administration of azathioprine and antimalarials or high-dose corticosteroids were treated with MMF, 2 g daily. Within a few weeks, the skin lesion improved and finally disappeared. There is evidence that a daily dose of 1 g may be sufficient to maintain remission, whereas 500 mg daily in one case was followed by the recurrence of the skin lesions. One patient received MMF for more than 24 months without reporting significant side effects. Furthermore, two cases of refractory DLE involving the palms and soles have been reported to be successfully treated with MMF (Goyal and Nousari 2001). Patients received 45 mg or 35 mg/kg daily, and within 4 months marked improvement of the skin lesion was documented. No side effects were reported, and the results of routine laboratory investigations remained within normal limits. These data indicate that MMF seems to be an effective and safe treatment for SLE as well as CLE. However, further controlled clinical trials are required to ultimately establish the role of MMF in LE therapy.

Leflunomide

The isoxazole derivate leflunomide (Arava) is a pyrimidine synthesis inhibitor that is rapidly converted to its active form malononitrilamide (A-771726). The active metabolite functions as an inhibitor of pyrimidine synthesis and thereby suppresses T-lymphocyte proliferation and the production of autoantibodies by B lymphocytes. Preliminary reports suggest that leflunomide may also be effective in the management of LE (Petera et al. 2000, Remer et al. 2001). According to two studies on treatment with leflunomide, the lupus activity scores (European Consensus Lupus Activity Measurement [ECLAM] or SLE Disease Activity Index [SLEDAI]) decreased, and in some patients the concomitant use of steroids could be reduced. Leflunomide was well tolerated, and no severe side effects have been observed. Currently leflunomide may be considered as a valuable additive therapy for severe (organ-threatening) cases of SLE (Petri 2001). However, the ultimate role of leflunomide in the treatment of the different forms of LE remains to be evaluated in further studies.

Antibiotics

Cefuroxime Axetil

Cefuroxime axetil is a β-lactamase–stable, second-generation, oral cephalosporine, which in vivo is rapidly hydrolysed to the active compound cefuroxime. It has a broad spectrum of antibacterial activities that encompasses methicillin-sensitive staphylococci, *Streptococcus pneumoniae, Haemophilus influenzae, Moraxella (Branhamella) catarrhalis,* group A β-hemolytic streptococci, and several other bacteria. Major indications for cefuroxime are lower and upper respiratory tract infections and bacterial skin diseases. Moreover, this drug also seems to exert some immunomodulating activities. In one study, cefuroxime axetil was used to treat three patients with SCLE (Rudnicka et al. 2000). With a dose of 500 mg daily, skin lesions cleared almost completely within 30–40 days. Moreover, in one patient, leukopenia, the erythrocyte sedimentation rate, and arthralgia improved. None of the patients experienced severe side effects. A not yet fully understood immunomodulating mechanism seems to be responsible for the improvement in SCLE. This activity seems to be specific for cefuroxime axetil, since other related antibiotics were not effective (Rudnicka et al. 2000).

Sulfasalazine

The anti-inflammatory drug sulfasalazine is an established and effective treatment for inflammatory bowel disease and various forms of arthritis. The successful use of sulfasalazine (2 mg/d) in 8 of 11 patients with LE has been reported (Delaporte et al. 1997). Drug metabolism could be one possible explanation for this discrepancy, since responders belonged to the group of rapid acetylators and nonresponders were slow acetylators. Moreover, no serious toxicity was noted in this small open-label clinical trial. In contrast, another study reported drug eruptions in five of six patients being treated with sulfasalazine, and in only two patients was a beneficial effect observed (Lagrange et al. 1998).

Biological Agents

IFN-α

Recombinant IFN-α has antiviral as well as immunomodulating properties and is considered to be associated in many aspects with the pathogenesis of autoimmune diseases. High amounts of IFN have been detected in the serum of patients with LE (Shou-Nee et al. 1987), and it has been speculated that increased IFN levels could result from a homeostatic attempt to control aberrant immune reactions in LE (Huddlestone et al. 1979). However, IFN-α and IFN-γ were found to accelerate the course of the autoimmune diseases in mice and to induce, even in normal mice, the development of an autoimmune nephropathy (Schattner 1988). Moreover, in many conditions, systemic application of IFN-α was associated with the development of autoantibodies (Fleischmann et al. 1996). However, there is also evidence from two clinical studies that IFN-α may improve the clinical course of certain autoimmune diseases (Nicolas et al. 1990, Tebbe et al. 1992). One study reports on IFN-α treatment of 10 patients with DLE or SCLE. Some of the patients were pretreated with hydroxy-chloroquine, systemic or topical corticosteroids, or thalidomide with or without clinical improvement. Before initiating IFN-α treatment, patients were not allowed to receive specific treatment for at least 1 month. After an average treatment duration of 6 weeks at a mean dose of 35×10^6 units of IFN-α per week, five of six patients with DLE experienced an improvement in their skin lesions. Similar results were obtained in three of four patients with SCLE, but time until remission was longer (~10 weeks), and a mean weekly dose of 80×10^6 units of IFN-α was required. In one patient with SCLE receiving IFN-α, an exacerbation of skin lesions was observed, and one patient did not respond to IFN-α treatment. Although, IFN-α therapy may lead to the improvement of CLE, in particular DLE, its mode of action in diseases with an autoimmune pathogenesis is still obscure. Currently, one has to evaluate very carefully the initiation of IFN therapy in patients with LE because the induction of autoantibodies on application of IFN has to be considered. Moreover, there is evidence for the induction of an LE-like disease in patients being treated with IFN-α for other reasons (Ronnblom et al. 1990).

Anti-CD4

The CD4 molecule is expressed on T lymphocytes and acts as a co-receptor for the T-cell receptor (TCR) by direct interaction with the major histocompatibility complex class II molecule on antigen-presenting cells. TCR-independent engagement of the CD4 molecule by monoclonal antibodies leads to T-cell inactivation. Moreover, T-helper cells may contribute directly to cutaneous tissue damage in LE by stimulating both macrophages and cytotoxic T cells. Therefore, specific inhibition of T-helper cells using anti-CD4 was considered as a suitable approach to suppress disease activity (Prinz et al. 1996). Accordingly, in vitro, a recombinant chimeric CD4 monoclonal antibody (cM-T412) was found to block T-helper cell functions such as proliferative response to recall antigens, IL-2 challenge, or allogeneic blood mononuclear cells (Riethmuller et al. 1992). Because of the low toxicity and the lack of immunogenicity, this antibody was chosen for first clinical trials (Riethmuller et al. 1992). Five patients with DLE, including two with systemic involvement, were treated with anti-CD4. The antibody was given in two cycles of seven and four infusions, separated by an interval of 4–7 weeks with a total dose of 275 mg (two patients with DLE) or 400 or 475 mg (one patient with SCLE and two with SLE). After antibody treatment, an immediate improvement in lesional inflammatory activity and healing of cutaneous lesions was observed. Long-lasting improvement with a restoration of responsiveness to conventional anti-inflammatory agents also was noticed. Moreover, proteinuria as an index of lupus nephropathy was fully resolved. The antibody was well tolerated, and side effects such as nausea and diarrhea were controlled by application of metoclopramide and loperamide. Further controlled clinical trials are required to prove these very promising but preliminary results.

Rituximab

Rituximab, is a chimeric mouse/human monoclonal antibody (Rituxan) specific for the B-cell surface molecule CD20 that has been approved for the treatment of CD20$^+$ low-grade or follicular non-Hodgkin's lymphoma. Since B lymphocytes play a crucial role in the pathogenesis of LE, anti-CD20 was considered to be valuable for the treatment of SLE. Therefore, a single-center, open-label, dose-escalation phase I/II trial was performed in 18 patients with active, but not organ-threatening, disease(Anolik et al. 2000). The treatment was well tolerated, and symptoms such as rash, arthritis, and fatigue markedly improved. Moreover, even low-dose rituximab therapy resulted in B-lymphocyte depletion. Further studies will reveal whether this promising approach ultimately will be a useful therapy for LE (Anolik et al. 2000).

CTLA-4Ig

CTLA-4 is expressed on the surface of a subpopulation of activated T lymphocytes and binds with high affinity to molecules of the B7 family that are present on B cells and antigen-presenting cells. CTLA-4Ig is a fusion protein of the extracellular domain of CTLA-4 with the Fc portion of IgG1, which serves as a soluble receptor. Therefore, this molecule prevents CTLA-4/B7 interaction by blocking T-cell activation and T-cell-dependent B-cell functions in vivo. In animal studies, treatment of New Zealand Black/New Zealand White (NZB/NZW) mice resulted in an improved survival rate as well as regression of nephritis (Finck et al. 1994). Moreover, there is evidence that the combination of CTLA-4Ig with an ICOS-Ig fusion protein that blocks the binding of ICOS expressed on activated T cells to its ligand potentiates the beneficial effects of CTLA-4Ig in a murine model of SLE (Ramanujam et al. 2002). Clinical studies with CTLA-4Ig in patients with lupus nephritis are being initiated, and one compound (BMS-188667) currently is being investigated in clinical trials for patients with rheumatoid arthritis and psoriasis.

Anti-B7

Targeting directly molecules of the B7 family which are crucial for providing costimulatory signals required for T-cell activation may be another effective strategy for the treatment of autoimmune diseases (Diamond et al. 2001, Theofilopoulos et al. 2001).

Accordingly, studies in NZB/NZW mice have shown that the combined application of monoclonal antibodies directed against both B7-1 and B7-2 decreases anti-double-stranded (ds) DNA antibodies and prolongs survival. Treatment with either mAb alone did not have a similar strong efficacy. The results of first clinical trials using anti-B7 (IDEC-114) for the treatment of patients with psoriasis (Schopf 2001) and clinical studies based on these strategies in patients with lupus nephritis are forth-coming (Diamond et al. 2001).

Anti-IL-10

According to several reports IL-10 seems to play a pivotal role in the pathogenesis of SLE, although its exact function in vivo is not fully understood (Llorente et al. 2000). Among many immunomodulating activities, IL-10 is known to inhibit the production of several proinflammatory cytokines and to promote a Th2 immune response. Accordingly, IL-10 promotes B-cell differentiation and hyperactivity, but at high doses also seems to have an inhibitory effect on B-cell functions. Moreover, IL-10 upregulates Fas ligand-expression in vitro which may result in augmented T-cell death in vivo (Solsky and Wallace 2002). In mice IL-10 inhibits antigen presentation and Th1-lymphocyte activation (Yin et al. 2000). In patients with SLE an increased production of IL-10 by peripheral blood mononuclear cells was found to be associ-ated with overproduction of pathogenic auto-antibodies. Therefore, it seemed rea-sonable to investigate whether blocking IL-10 may provide an useful approach to treat autoimmune diseases such as LE. Accordingly, six steroid-dependent patients with SLE were treated for 21 consecutive days with intravenous infusion of anti-IL-10 (20 mg/d). Patients experienced a significant decrease in disease activity and were able to reduce concomitant steroid medication. In addition, a significant improve-ment of vasculitis and skin lesions was observed. Clinical scores remained stable through a follow-up of 6 months and no significant adverse events have been reported (Llorente et al. 2000).

Anti-TNF-α

TNF-α blockers such as humanized antibodies (infliximab) or fully human anti-bodies (adalizumab) and a fusion protein between the TNF-αR and Ig (etanercept) recently have been used successfully for the treatment autoimmune diseases such as rheumatoid arthritis, Crohn's disease as well as psoriasis (Luger 2001). The experi-ence using this compounds to treat LE is limited and one has carefully to consider their potential to induce autoantibodies which may cause exacerbation of the disease (Charles et al. 2000, Pisetsky 2000). However, one patient with rheumatoid arthritis and with SCLE was reported to be treated with etanercept which resulted in a signifi-cant improvement of the previously therapy-resistant skin lesions within 15 days (Fautrel et al. 2002). After 6 months, the rheumatoid arthritis remained improved, there were no signs of active lupus, ANA were stable and no anti-ds-DNA antibodies were present. Further controlled clinical trials ultimately will reveal the role of anti TNF-α strategies in the treatment of LE.

LJP-394

LJP-394 (abetimus) is an anti-anti-ds-DNA B-cell toleragen consisting of four synthetic double-stranded oligodeoxyribonucleotides. Toleragens have been shown to suppress antibody synthesis by targeted B cells. They cross-link B-cell surface antibodies without providing the second T-cell activating signal, thereby making the B cells unresponsive. The consequence is a down-regulation of anti-ds-DNA antibody, an autoantibody presumed to be a causative factor in lupus nephritis. Therefore, a double-blind placebo-controlled study including 230 SLE patients with a history of renal disease has been performed (Alacron-Segovia et al. 2000, Furie et al. 2001, McNeely et al. 2001). Although the initial evaluation of the results indicated no efficacy in the improvement of renal disease, upon a second analysis it appeared that LJP-394 provided clinical benefit only in those patients with high levels of anti-ds-DNA antibodies. Moreover, the compound was well tolerated with a low risk for serious side effects (Wallace 2001b).

Anti-C5

Decreased levels of complement components, including C3, C4, and CH50, is one of the characteristic laboratory parameters of SLE that also correlates with disease activity. C3b, derived from C3 by either the classic or alternative pathway of complement activation, provides a binding site for C5, making it susceptible to the action of C5 convertase. This activity triggers the terminal sequence of complement activation that leads to membrane damage (Moxley and Ruddy 1997). A monoclonal antibody designed to interfere with C5 activity decreased proteinuria and improved survival in treated NZB/NZW mice (Matis and Rollins 1995, Strand 2000). Moreover, in a single-site, dose-finding, phase I trial, 24 patients with SLE have been treated with a humanized anti-C5 monoclonal antibody (5G1.1), and a phase II trial is under way. However, the results of these trials are not yet available.

Tazarotene

The topical retinoid tazarotene is a member of a novel, conformationally rigid non-isomerizable class of retinoids, the acetylenic retinoids. It is hypothesized that the ability to adopt different shapes enables these retinoids to interact indiscriminately with many of the retinoid acid receptors and to activate multiple retinoid pathways. This receptor-selective topical retinoid decreases inflammation as well as abnormal differentiation and hyperproliferation of keratinocytes. Therefore, tazarotene successfully was introduced for the treatment of psoriasis (Chandraratna 1997). In one patient resistant to conventional therapies, topical tazarotene was used to treat hyperkeratotic lesions of DLE (Edwards and Burke 1999). A daily dose of 0.05% tazarotene gel was applied, and within several weeks facial lesions cleared, and the patient remained disease free for several months without experiencing any therapy-related side effects.

Phenytoin

Phenytoin is an anticonvulsive drug that plays a pivotal role in the management of convulsive diseases. Because there is evidence for immunomodulating and anti-inflammatory activity of phenytoin, it was also considered a valuable alternative to treat LE. Accordingly, in one study, patients with DLE were treated with phenytoin for an average of 5 months, and cutaneous lesions were evaluated every 4 weeks (Rodriguez-Castellanos et al. 1995). Patients received 100 mg of sodium diphenyl-hydantoin by mouth three times daily. In 9 of 10 patients with disseminated DLE, the response was reported to be excellent, and in 1 patient the response was considered to be very good (Callen 1982). Similar results were reported in another study demonstrating that 90% of patients (35 of 39 patients) with DLE significantly improved on treatment with phenytoin. Moreover, the remaining 4 patients (10%) also noted very good resolution of skin lesions. Toxicity was minimal in prevalence and severity. Within a follow-up period of 6–12 months, approximately 33% of patients remained without relapse, whereas approximately 16% relapsed. Follow-up data were not available in the remaining approximately 51% of the patients. Although, the exact mechanism of action of phenytoin in improving DLE is unclear, the promising clinical results may encourage further controlled clinical trials.

Dehydroepiandrosterone

The androgen dehydroepiandrosterone (DHEA) belongs to the group of steroid hormones that are produced by the adrenal cortex. In vitro, T lymphocytes, on exposure with DHEA, have been shown to produce increased amounts of Th1 cytokines such as IFN-γ and IL-2, whereas the production of Th2 cytokines such as IL-4 was decreased (Daynes et al. 1990). Moreover, DHEA and DHEA-sulphate serum levels were found to be decreased in patients with SLE unrelated to disease activity or treatment (Jungers et al. 1982). In an animal model of lupus (female NZB/NZW mice), treatment with androgens resulted in an improvement in disease activity. The ability of androgens to promote an immunodeviation toward Th1 as well as their efficacy in lupus mice prompted studies in humans (Melez et al. 1980). Accordingly, patients with lupus nephritis or severe cytopenias were treated with DHEA, 200 mg/d. As a result of this treatment, no difference in SLE disease indices compared with placebo was noted. Only the loss of bone mineral density was lower in DHEA-treated patients (Solsky and Wallace 2002). Three pivotal trials involving nearly 500 patients with mild to moderate disease activity suggest that DHEA (200 mg/day) has favorable effects in SLE, including steroid-sparing properties, improvement of bone mineralization, increase in patient visual assessment scores, and a decrease in SLEDAI and SLAM indices (Chang et al. 2000, Mease et al. 2000). Therefore, DHEA is currently being proposed as an adjunct to antimalarials that may be particularly effective in improving cognitive function and fatigue (Ferrario et al. 2000, Hallegua et al. 2000). However, in women, virilization has to be considered as a possible side effect of DHEA therapy.

Intravenous Immunoglobulin

The exact mechanisms of action of intravenous immunoglobulin (IVIg) are unknown, but there is evidence for the solubilization of immune complexes or anti-idiotypic down-regulation of autoantibody production as well as induction of immunomodulating cytokines such as transforming growth factor β and IL-10 (Ballow 1997, McMurray 2001, Rutter and Luger 2002). Considering the role of autoantibodies such as anti-ds-DNA antibodies in the pathogenesis of SLE, treatments such as IVIg designed to remove or neutralize these antibodies seemed to be promising. IVIg is currently approved for the treatment of Kawasaki disease, immune thrombocytopenic purpura, and Guillain-Barre syndrome. In addition, skin diseases such as autoimmune blistering diseases, scleroderma, and dermatomyositis have been successfully treated with IVIg. Some studies using IVIg for the management of LE indicate improvement in nephritis, SLAM scores, myocardial dysfunction, cerebritis, and autoantibodies titers (Levy et al. 2000, Traynor et al. 2000). Moreover, IVIg was effectively used in two patients with SLE and acquired factor VII inhibition who failed to respond to corticosteroids or other immunosuppressive agents (Lafferty et al. 1997). In another study, 10 patients with refractory skin lesions were treated with 1 g/kg per day for 2 days monthly. Although an excellent response was reported in 4 of the 10 patients, the improvement was short lived (Callen 2002). One patient with antimalarial-resistant DLE (Genereau et al. 1999) that could not receive thalidomide because of cutaneous adverse drug reaction was treated with high-dose IVIg (2 g/kg per month) in combination with hydroxychloroquine sulphate and topical betamethasone dipropionate. The skin lesions improved within 3 months and almost completely disappeared after 6 months. In none of the reported studies were severe adverse events observed. Controlled clinical trials are required to further evaluate the efficacy of IVIg in the treatment of LE. Furthermore, for economical reasons, the long-term application of IVIg may be limited.

Plasmapheresis and Immunoadsorption

Impaired clearance of immune complexes and the production of autoantibodies are characteristic features of LE. Therefore, it was conceivable that the extracorporal removal of these proteins may help improve LE lesions or support current treatments. Plasmapheresis is a procedure that separates plasma/proteins from whole blood by cell centrifugation techniques or membrane technology. Subsequently, the plasma is replaced by albumin and saline. Usually plasmapheresis is combined with an immunosuppressive therapy to prevent antibody rebound or rapid resynthesis of immunoglobulins. This modality was first considered for therapy of lupus patients with hyperviscosity, cryoglobulinemia, pulmonary hemorrhage, or thrombotic thrombocytopenic purpura (Wallace 2001a). It also has been used successfully in the management of acute central nervous system involvement of lupus when other therapies have failed (Neuwelt et al. 1995). However, in a large international prospective controlled trial in patients with SLE, plasmapheresis did not reveal any additional benefit compared with conventional treatment (Leweis et al. 1992). Therefore, plasmapheresis currently is not recommended for the treatment of SLE, unless the disease is complicated by hyperviscosity, cryoglobulinemia, pulmonary hemorrhage, or thrombotic thrombocytopenic purpura.

A promising alternative to plasmapheresis is immunoadsorption (Terman et al. 1979), which via the use of different technologies, such as sepharose columns coupled with polyclonal sheep antibodies binding human IgG heavy and light chains (Ig-Therasorb), allows for a more specific approach to eliminate antibodies as well as immune complexes. Accordingly, selective immunoadsorption of immunoglobulin, anti-ds-DNA antibodies, immune complexes, antiphospholipid antibodies, and anti-C1q antibodies was applied successfully in single cases or uncontrolled trials of SLE. In addition, patients with SLE suffering from nephritis, pneumonitis, hemolytic anemia, central nervous system involvement, and skin lesions refractory to immunosuppression were treated with immunoadsorption and subsequently substituted with normal human immunoglobulins to avoid the rebound of autoantibody production (Gaubitz et al. 1998, Graninger et al. 2002, Viertel et al. 2000). All patients showed an improvement in clinical and laboratory signs of disease activity. The therapy was well tolerated without significant side effects. During follow-up (up to 1 year), organ function remained stable, requiring only low-dose prednisolone (5–7.5 mg daily per os).

C1q is believed to contribute to the defective clearance of apoptotic cells (Walport et al. 1998), and high titers of C1q autoantibodies correlate with the relapse of lupus nephritis (Haseley et al. 1997, Walport et al. 1998). Therefore, clearance of C1q by a specific immunoadsorption seemed to be a promising approach for the treatment of SLE. Eight patients with non–life-threatening disease flares were treated with C1q immunoadsorption (Pfuller et al. 1998). Five patients experienced improvement of organ involvement, and no severe side effects have been reported (Hiepe et al. 1999). In a recent case report, a 25-year-old women with SLE, relapsing malar, and discoid rash, which extended to almost the whole integument, was treated by C1q immunoadsorption (MIRO adsorbers) (Berner et al. 2001). The cutaneous lesions have been refractory to previous treatment with chloroquine or MTX in combination with prednisone (up to >60 mg daily). During C1q immunoadsorption, a rapid and complete resolution of skin involvement was observed, as was a decrease of ds-DNA and C1q autoantibodies. However, the persisting proteinuria indicated that lupus nephritis did not improve. During follow-up of 12 months after stopping C1q immunoadsorption and therapy with MTX (15 mg/wk) as well as low-dose prednisone (5 mg/d), no relapse of CLE lesions or increase in clinical disease activity has been reported. Finally, the therapy was well tolerated, without any evidence of severe side effects after 12 therapy courses.

Stem Cell Transplantation

Autologous stem cell transplantation recently has been introduced for the treatment of autoimmune diseases. Accordingly, in nine patients with life-threatening SLE who failed to respond to intravenous cyclophosphamide therapy, autologous hematopoietic stem cell transplantation in combination with high-dose chemotherapy (intravenous cyclophosphamide, 50 mg/kg) has been performed. One patient died of disseminated mucormycosis, and one patient developed cytomegalovirus viremia before transplantation. The remaining seven patients showed an improvement and remained free of active lupus during 25 months of follow-up (Traynor et al. 2000).

However, because of the severe side effects and the sometimes insufficient response rate, this treatment may be considered only for patients with life-threatening disease that cannot be controlled by conventional immunosuppressive measures.

Other Experimental Therapies

The development of cladarabine, a purine nucleoside analogue that preferentially targets resting and proliferating T and B lymphocytes while sparing neutrophils, monocytes, red blood cells, and platelets for the treatment of LE, was discontinued because of an unacceptable risk-benefit ratio. A similar compound, fludarabine, is currently undergoing a National Institutes of Health-sponsored trial (Strand 2000).

Bindarit is a propioic acid inhibitor that modulates cytokine and chemokine production in animal models of inflammation (Zoja et al. 1998). In an open-label pilot study using bindarit in 10 patients with lupus nephritis, a decrease in proteinuria was observed (Vigano et al. 1995). However, a follow-up placebo-controlled trial was never initiated.

Tamoxifen is an antiestrogen used for the treatment and prevention of breast cancer. In an SLE mice model (MRL-Ipr/Ipr), tamoxifen decreased proteinuria and increased murine survival (Wu et al. 2000). However, a double-blind crossover study in 11 patients with SLE did not reveal any significant clinical improvement, and most of the patients experienced severe side effects (Sturgess et al. 1984).

Many biologicals have been developed, and, according to preclinical data, some of them seemed to be promising candidates for the treatment of LE. Among several antibodies and fusion proteins that have been effective in first trials, many failed to be of significant clinical benefit and are not being further developed for LE therapy. This includes, for example, anti-CD154, the ligand for CD40 (Dumont 2002), anti-CD4, anti-CD5, ricin, an immunoconjugate, 3E10 monoclonal antibody vaccine, anti-CD40L hu5 c9, and human recombinant DNAse.

Conclusion

The enormous progress in biotechnology and in the understanding of the underlying pathomechanisms of autoimmune diseases such as LE has allowed for a more specific and hopefully efficient strategy to target disease-relevant mechanisms. However, until the mechanisms responsible for autoimmunity are not completely resolved, which ultimately may allow the cure of these diseases, the search for effective, safe, and not impairing life quality strategies is mandatory. Accordingly, the number of drugs currently being evaluated for their efficacy and safety in the treatment of the various forms of LE is rapidly increasing. However, many compounds that, according to laboratory data and animal studies, seemed to be promising finally had to be withdrawn. Whether in the future chemotherapeuticals or biologicals will end up as the most efficient therapy with a minimal profile of adverse events is not clear and also may vary depending on the course, activity, and organ involvement of the disease. In addition, the combination of newly developed drugs and other immunomodulating strategies may allow the increase of efficacy and the minimization of adverse events.

References

Alarcon-Segovia D, Tumlin J, Furie R, McKay J, Cardiel M, Linnik M, Hepburn B (2000) SLE trial shows fewer renal flares in LJP 394 treated patients with high-affinity antibodies to LJP 394: 90-05 trial results. Arthritis Rheum 43:S272

Anolik J, Campbell D, Ritchlin C, Holyst M, Rosenfeld S, Sanz I, Young F, Felgar R, Kunkel L, Benyunes M, Grillo-Lopez A, Rosenblatt J, Looney RJ (2000) PhaseI/II open-label, dose-escalation trial of rituximab (Rituxan) in patients with SLE. Arthritis Rheum 43:2860

Austin HA, Vaughan EM, Balow JE (2000) Lupus membranous nephropathy: randomized, controlled trial of prednisone, cyclosporine and cyclophosphamide. J Am Soc Nephrol 11:81A

Ballow M (1997) Mechanisms of action of intravenous immune serum globulin in autoimmune and inflammatory diseases. J Allergy Clin Immunol 100:151–157

Beissert S, Luger TA (1999) Future developments of antipsoriatic therapy. Dermatol Therapy 11:104–117

Berner B, Scheel AK, Schettler V, Hummel KM, Reuss-Borst MA, Muller GA, Oestmann E, Leinenbach HP, Hepper M (2001) Rapid improvement of SLE-specific cutaneous lesions by C1q immunoadsorption. Ann Rheum Dis 60:898–899

Boehm IB, Boehm GA, Bauer R (1998) Management of cutaneous lupus erythematosus with low-dose methotrexate: indication for modulation of inflammatory mechanisms. Rheumatol Int 18:59–62

Caccavo D, Lagana B, Mitterhofer AP, Ferri GM, Afeltra A, Amoroso A, Bonomo L (1997) Long-term treatment of systemic lupus erythematosus with cyclosporin A. Arthritis Rheum 40:27–35

Callen JP (1982) Chronic cutaneous lupus erythematosus. Clinical, laboratory, therapeutic, and prognostic examination of 62 patients. Arch Dermatol 118:412–416

Callen JP (2002) Management of skin disease in patients with lupus erythematosus. Best Pract Res Clin Rheumatol 16:245–264

Carneiro JR, Sato EI (1999) Double blind, randomized, placebo controlled clinical trial of methotrexate in systemic lupus erythematosus. J Rheumatol 26:1275–1279

Chan TM, Li FK, Tang CS, Wong RW, Fang GX, Ji YL, Lau CS, Wong AK, Tong MK, Chan KW, Lai KN (2000) Efficacy of mycophenolate mofetil in patients with diffuse proliferative lupus nephritis. Hong Kong-Guangzhou Nephrology Study Group. N Engl J Med 343:1156–1162

Chandraratna RA (1997) Tazarotene: the first receptor-selective topical retinoid for the treatment of psoriasis. J Am Acad Dermatol 37:S12-S17

Chang DM, Lan JL, Lin HY, Taipei LSF, Taiwan T (2000) GL 701 (prasterone, dehydroepiandrosterone) significantly reduces flares in female patients with mild to moderate systemic lupus erythematosus (SLE). Arthritis Rheum 43:S241

Charles PJ, Smeenk RJT, de Jong J, Feldmann M, Maini RN (2000) Assessment of antibodies to double-stranded DNA induced in rheumatoid arthritis patients following treatment with infliximab, a monoclonal antibody to tumor necrosis factor alpha: Findings in open-label and randomized placebo-controlled trials. Arthritis Rheum 43:2283–2390

Conti F, Priori R, Alessandri C, Spinelli FR, Medda E, Valesini G (2000) Safety profile and causes of withdrawal due to adverse events in systemic lupus erythematosus patients treated long-term with cyclosporine A. Lupus 9:676–680

Dammacco F, Della Casa AO, Ferraccioli G, Racanelli V, Casatta L, Bartoli E (2000) Cyclosporine-A plus steroids versus steroids alone in the 12-month treatment of systemic lupus erythematosus. Int J Clin Lab Res 30:67–73

Daynes RA, Dudley DJ, Areano BA (1990) Regulation of murine lymphokine production in vivo. Dehydroepiandrosterone is a natural enhancer of interleukin 2 synthesis by helper T cells. Eur J Immunol 20:793–802

Delaporte E, Catteau B, Sabbagh N, Gosselin P, Breuillard F, Doutre MS, Broly F, Piette F, Bergoend H (1997) Treatment of discoid lupus erythematosus with sulfasalazine: 11 cases. Ann Dermatol Venereol 124:151–156

Dequet CR, Wallace, DJ (2001) Novel therapies in the treatment of systemic lupus erythematosus. Curr Opin Investig Drugs 2:1045–1053

Diamond B, Bluestone J, Wofsy D (2001) The immune tolerance network and rheumatic disease: immune tolerance comes to the clinic. Arthritis Rheum 44:1730–1735

Duddridge M, Powell RJ (1997) Treatment of severe and difficult cases of systemic lupus erythematosus with tacrolimus. A report of three cases. Ann Rheum Dis 56:690–692

Dumont FJ (2002) IDEC-131. IDEC/Eisai. Curr Opin Investig Drugs 3:725–734

Edwards KR, Burke WA (1999) Treatment of localized discoid lupus erythematosus with tazarotene. J Am Acad Dermatol 41:1049–1050

Entani C, Izumino K, Iida H, Fujita M, Asaka M, Takata M, Sasayama S (1993) Effect of a novel immunosuppressant, FK506, on spontaneous lupus nephritis in MRL/MpJ-lpr/lpr mice. Nephron 64:471–475

Fautrel B, Foltz V, Frances C, Bourgeois P, Rozenberg S (2002) Regression of subacute cutaneous lupus erythematosus in a patient with rheumatoid arthritis treated with a biologic tumor necrosis factor alpha-blocking agent: comment on the article by Pisetsky and the letter from Aringer et al. Arthritis Rheum 46:1408–1409

Ferrario L, Bellone M, Bozzolo E, Baldissera E, Sabbadini MG (2000) Remission from lupus nephritis resistant to cyclophosphamide after additional treatment with cyclosporin A. Rheumatology (Oxford) 39:218–220

Finck BK, Linsley PS, Wofsy D (1994) Treatment of murine lupus with CTLA4Ig. Science 265:1225–1227

Fleischmann M, Celerier P, Bernard P, Litoux P, Dreno B (1996) Long-term interferon-alpha therapy induces autoantibodies against epidermis. Dermatology 192:50–55

Frieling U, Luger TA (2002) Mycophenolate mofetile and leflunomide: promising compounds for the treatment of skin diseases. Clin Exp Dermatol 27:562–570

Furie RA, Cash JM, Cronin ME, Katz RS, Weisman MH, Aranow C, Liebling MR, Hudson NP, Berner CM, Coutts S, de Haan HA (2001) Treatment of systemic lupus erythematosus with LJP 394. J Rheumatol 28:257–265

Gaubitz M, Schorat A, Schotte H, Kern P, Domschke W (1999) Mycophenolate mofetil for the treatment of systemic lupus erythematosus: an open pilot trial. Lupus 8:731–736

Gaubitz M, Seidel M, Kummer S, Schotte H, Perniok A, Domschke W, Schneider, M (1998) Prospective randomized trial of two different immunoadsorbers in severe systemic lupus erythematosus. J Autoimmun 11:495–501

Geilen CC, Orfanos-Boeckel H, Offermann G, Orfanos CE (2000) Mycophenolate mofetil: a new immunosuppressive drug in dermatology and its possible uses. Hautarzt 51:63–69

Genereau T, Chosidow O, Danel C, Cherin P, Herson S (1999) High-dose intravenous immunoglobulin in cutaneous lupus erythematosus. Arch Dermatol 135:1124–1125

Goyal S, Nousari HC (2001) Treatment of resistant discoid lupus erythematosus of the palms and soles with mycophenolate mofetil. J Am Acad Dermatol 45:142–144

Graninger M, Schmaldienst S, Derfler K, Graninger WB (2002) Immunoadsorption therapy (therasorb) in patients with severe lupus erythematosus. Acta Med Austriaca 29:26–29

Hallegua D, Wallace DJ, Metzger AL, Rinaldi RZ, Klinenberg JR (2000) Cyclosporine for lupus membranous nephritis: experience with ten patients and review of the literature. Lupus 9:241–251

Haseley L, Wisnieski J, Denburg M, Michael-Grossman, AR, Ginzler EM, Gourley MF, Hoffman JH, Kimberly RP, Salmon JE (1997) Antibodies to C1q in systemic lupus erythematosus: Characteristics and relation to Fc-gamma RIIA alleles. Kidney Int 52:1375–1380

Hiepe F, Pfuller B, Wolbart K, Bruns A, Leinenbach HP, Hepper M, Schossler W, Otto V, (1999) C1q: a multifunctional ligand for a new immunoadsorption treatment. Ther Apher 3:246–251

Hsieh SC, Tsai CY, Sun KH, Tsai YY, Tsai ST, Han SH, Yu HS, Yu CL (1995) Defective spontaneous and bacterial lipopolysaccharide-stimulated production of interleukin-1 receptor antagonist by polymorphonuclear neutrophils of patients with active systemic lupus erythematosus. Br J Rheumatol 34:107–112

Huddlestone JR, Merigan TC Jr, Oldstone MB (1979) Induction and kinetics of natural killer cells in humans following interferon therapy. Nature 282:417–419

Jungers P, Nahoul K, Pelissier C, Dougados M, Tron F, Bach JF (1982) Low plasma androgens in women with active or quiescent systemic lupus erythematosus. Arthritis Rheum 25:454–457

Kitchin JE, Pomeranz MK, Pak G, Washenik K, Shupack JL (1997) Rediscovering mycophenolic acid: a review of its mechanism, side effects, and potential uses. J Am Acad Dermatol 37:445–449

Kuhn A, Specker C, Ruzicka T, Lehmann P (2002) Methotrexate treatment for refractory subacute cutaneous lupus erythematosus. J Am Acad Dermatol 46:600–603

Lafferty TE, Smith JB, Schuster SJ, DeHoratius RJ (1997) Treatment of acquired factor VIII inhibitor using intravenous immunoglobulin in two patients with systemic lupus erythematosus. Arthritis Rheum 40:775–778

Lagrange S, Piette JC, Becherel PA, Cacoub P, Frances C (1998) Sulfasalazine in the treatment of cutaneous lupus erythematosus: open trial in six cases. Lupus 7:21

Levy Y, Sherer Y, George J, Rovensky J, Lukac J, Rauova L, Poprac P, Langevitz P, Fabbrizzi F, Shoenfeld Y (2000) Intravenous immunoglobulin treatment of lupus nephritis. Semin Arthritis Rheum 29:321–327

Lewis EJ, Hunsicker LG, Lan SP, Rohde RD, Lachin JM (1992) A controlled trial of plasmapheresis therapy in severe lupus nephritis. The Lupus Nephritis Collaborative Study Group. N Engl J Med 326:1373–1379

Linker-Israeli M, Deans RJ, Wallace DJ, Prehn J, Ozeri-Chen T, Klinenberg JR (1991) Elevated levels of endogenous IL-6 in systemic lupus erythematosus. A putative role in pathogenesis. J Immunol 147:117–123

Llorente L, Richaud-Patin Y, Garcia-Padilla C, Claret E, Jakez-Ocampo J, Cardiel MH, Alcocer-Varela J, Grangeot-Keros L, Alarcon-Segovia D, Wijdenes J, Galanaud P, Emilie D (2000) Clinical and biologic effects of anti-interleukin-10 monoclonal antibody administration in systemic lupus erythematosus. Arthritis Rheum 43:1790–1800

Luger T (2001) Treatment of immune-mediated skin diseases: future perspectives. Eur J Dermatol 11:343–347

Manger K, Kalden JR, Manger B (1996) Cyclosporin A in the treatment of systemic lupus erythematosus: results of an open clinical study. Br J Rheumatol 35:669–675

Matis LA, Rollins SA (1995) Complement-specific antibodies: designing novel anti-inflammatories. Nat Med 1:839–842

McMurray RW (2001) Nonstandard and adjunctive medical therapies for systemic lupus erythematosus. Arthritis Rheum 45:86–100

McNeely PA, Iverson GM, Furie RA, Cash JM, Cronin ME, Katz RS, Weisman MH, Aranow C, Linnik MD (2001) Pre-treatment affinity for LIP 394 influences pharmacodynamic response in lupus patients. Lupus 10:526–532

Mease PJ, Ginzler EM, Gluck OS, Schiff MH, Schmeer P, Gurwith M, Schwarz KE (2000) Improvement in bone mineral density in steroid-treated patients during treatment with GL 701 (prasterone, DHEA). Arthritis Rheum 43 (Suppl):206

Melez KA, Boegel WA, Steinberg AD (1980) Therapeutic studies in New Zealand mice. VII. Successful androgen treatment of NZB/NZW F1 females of different ages. Arthritis Rheum 23:41–47

Morton SJ, Powell RJ (2000) An audit of cyclosporin for systemic lupus erythematosus and related overlap syndromes: limitations of its use. Ann Rheum Dis 59:487–489

Moxley G, Ruddy S (1997) Immune complexes and complement. In: Kelley WN, Harris ED, Ruddy S, Sledge CB (eds) Textbook of rheumatology, 5th edn. Saunders, Philadelphia, pp 232–235

Neuwelt CM, Al-Baude HA, Webb RL (1995) Role of intravenous cyclophosphamide in the treatment of severe neuropsychiatric systemic lupus. Am J Med 98:32–41

Nicolas JF, Thivolet J, Kanitakis J, Lyonnet S (1990) Response of discoid and subacute cutaneous lupus erythematosus to recombinant interferon alpha 2a. J Invest Dermatol 95:142S-145S

Paller A, Eichenfield LF, Leung DY, Stewart D, Appell M (2001) A 12-week study of tacrolimus ointment for the treatment of atopic dermatitis in pediatric patients. J Am Acad Dermatol 44:S47-S57

Petera P, Manger B, Manger K, Rosenburg R, Smolen JS, Kalden JR (2000) A pilot study of leflunomide in systemic lupus erythematosus (SLE). Arthritis Rheum 43:S241

Petri M (2001) High dose Arava in lupus (HAIL). Arthritis Rheum 44:S280

Pfuller B, Wolbart K, Claunitzer A et al. (1998) Successful treatment of systemic lupus erythematosus by C1q-immunoadsorption. Arthritis Rheum 41:S110

Pisetsky DS (2000) Tumor necrosis factor alpha blockers and the induction of anti-DNA autoantibodies. Arthritis Rheum 43:2381–2382

Prinz JC, Meurer M, Reiter C, Rieber EP, Plewig G, Riethmuller G (1996) Treatment of severe cutaneous lupus erythematosus with a chimeric CD4 monoclonal antibody, cM-T412. J Am Acad Dermatol 34:244–252

Ramanujam M, Wang X, Ghosh SS, Huang W, Akkerman A, Roy-Chowdhury I, Davidson A (2002) Treatment of murine SLE using a double expressing CTLA4-Ig/ICOS-Ig adenovirus. Arthritis Rheum 46:S226

Rappersberger LE, Komar M, Ebelin ME, Scott G, Bueche M, Burtin P, Wolff K (2000) Oral SDZ ASM981: Safety, pharmacokinetics and efficacy in patients with moderate to severe chronic plaque psoriasis. J Invest Dermatol 114:776

Remer CF, Weisman MH, Wallace DJ (2001) Benefits of leflunomide in systemic lupus erythematosus: a pilot observational study. Lupus 10:480–483

Riethmuller G, Rieber EP, Kiefersauer S, Prinz J, van der LP Meiser B, Breedveld F, Eisenburg J, Kruger K, Deusch K (1992) From antilymphocyte serum to therapeutic monoclonal antibodies: first experiences with a chimeric CD4 antibody in the treatment of autoimmune disease. Immunol Rev 129:81–104

Rodriguez-Castellanos MA, Rubio JB, Gómez JFB, Mendoza AG (1995) Phenytoin in the Treatment of Discoid Lupus Erythematosus. Arch Dermatol 131:620–621

Ronnblom LE, Alm G, Vberg KE (1990) Possible induction of systemic lupus erythematosus by interferon-alpha treatment in a patient with a malignant carcinoid tumour. J Intern Med 227:207–210

Rudnicka L, Szymanska E, Walecka I, Slowinska M (2000) Long-term cefuroxime axetil in subacute cutaneous lupus erythematosus. A report of three cases. Dermatology 200:29–131

Rutter A, Luger TA (2002) Intravenous immunoglobulin: An emerging treatment for immune-mediated skin diseases. Curr Opin Investig Drugs 3:713–719

Sauder DN, Wong D, Laskin C (1993) Epidermal cytokines in murine lupus. J Invest Dermatol 100:42S–46S

Schanz S, Ulmer A, Rassner G, Fierlbeck G (2002) Successful treatment of subacute cutaneous lupus erythematosus with mycophenolate mofetil. Br J Dermatol 147:174–178

Schattner A (1988) Interferons and autoimmunity. Am J Med Sci 295:532–544

Schopf RE (2001) IDEC-114 (IDEC). Curr Opin Ivestig Drugs 2:635–638

Shou-Nee S, Fang FS, Yumei W (1987) Serum interferon in systemic lupus erythematosus. Br J Dermatol 117:155–159

Solsky MA, Wallace DJ (2002) New therapies in systemic lupus erythematosus. Best Pract Res Clin Rheumatol 16:293–312

Strand V (2000) New therapies for systemic lupus erythematosus. Rheum Dis Clin North Am 26:389–405

Sturgess AD, Evans DT, Mackay IR, Riglar A (1984) Effects of the oestrogen antagonist tamoxifen on disease indices in systemic lupus erythematosus. J Clin Lab Immunol 13:11–14

Tebbe B, Lauy M, Gollnick H (1992) Therapy of cutaneous lupus erythematosus with recombinant interferon alpha-2a. Eur J Dermatol 2:253–255

Terman DS, Buffaloe G, Mattioli C, Cook G, Tillquist R, Sullivan M, Ayus JC (1979) Extracorporeal immunoadsorption: initial experience in human systemic lupus erythematosus. Lancet 2:824–827

Theofilopoulos AN, Drummer W, Kono DH (2001) T cell homeostasis and systemic autoimmunity. J Clin Invest 108:335–340

Tomi NS, Luger TA (2003) The treatment of atopic dermatitis with topical immunomodulators. Clinics Dermatol 21:215–224

Traynor AE, Schroeder J, Rosa RM, Cheng D, Stefka J, Mujais S, Baker S, Burt RK (2000) Treatment of severe systemic lupus erythematosus with high-dose chemotherapy and haemopoietic stem-cell transplantation: a phase I study. Lancet 356:701–707

Viertel A, Weidmann E, Wigand R, Geiger H, Mondorf UF (2000) Treatment of severe systemic lupus erythematosus with immunoadsorption and intravenous immunoglobulins. Intensive Care Med 26:823–824

Vigano G, Gotti E, Casiraghi F, Noris M, Taddei I, Dionisio P, Remuzzi G (1995) Bindarit reduces urinary albumin excretion (UAB) and urinary interleukin 6 (IL-6) in patients with proliferative lupus nephritis. J Am Soc Nephrol 6:434

Walker SL, Kirby B, Chalmers RJ (2002) The effect of topical tacrolimus on severe recalcitrant chronic discoid lupus erythematosus. Br J Dermatol 147:405

Wallace DJ (2001a) Apheresis for lupus erythematosus: state of the art. Lupus 10:193–196

Wallace DJ (2001b) Clinical and pharmacological experience with LJP-394. Expert Opin Investig Drugs 10:111–117

Walport MJ, Davies KA, Botto M (1998) C1q and systemic lupus erythematosus. Immunobiology 199:265–285

Wu WM, Suen JL, Lin BF, Chiang BL (2000) Tamoxifen alleviates disease severity and decreases double negative T cells in autoimmune MRL-lpr/lpr mice. Immunology 100:110–118

Yin Z, Bahtiyar G, Lanzhen L (2000) IL-10 down-modulates murine lupus. Arthritis Rheum 43:S438

Yoshimasu T, Ohtani T, Sakamoto T, Oshima A, Furukawa F (2002) Topical FK506 (tacrolimus) therapy for facial erythematous lesions of cutaneous lupus erythematosus and dermatomyositis. Eur J Dermatol 12:50–52

Zoja C, Corna D, Benedetti G, Morigi M, Donadelli R, Guglielmotti A, Pinza M, Bertani T, Remuzzi G (1998) Bindarit retards renal disease and prolongs survival in murine lupus autoimmune disease. Kidney Int 53:726–734

CHAPTER 31

Management of Cutaneous Lupus Erythematosus

Jeffrey P. Callen

The treatment of cutaneous lesions of lupus erythematosus (LE) involves both an empiric and a scientific approach (Callen 2001). Unfortunately, there are few double-blind, placebo-controlled trials of drugs used to treat cutaneous LE (CLE). I generally approach patients with "specific" cutaneous lesions of LE (e. g., subacute CLE [SCLE], discoid LE [DLE], or lupus profundus/panniculitis) in a similar manner (Table 31.1). Several other chapters in this text deal with individual therapies and their risks and potential uses in depth; this chapter includes an overview of my approach that encompasses most of the therapies mentioned elsewhere in this volume.

The goals of management of the patient with DLE or SCLE are to improve the patient's appearance and to prevent the development of deforming scars, atrophy, or dyspigmentation. In addition, most patients with chronic CLE or SCLE have disease that primarily affects their skin, and they may be reassured that their prognosis is relatively benign.

A complete list of the patient's medications will assist in the exclusion of drug-induced CLE (Bleumink et al. 2001, Bonsmann et al. 2001, Callen et al. 2001, Crowson and Magro 1997, Reed et al. 1985). Also, patients who smoke may have more severe clinical disease than nonsmokers (Gallego et al. 1999).

Cosmetic problems are often of major importance to the patient with CLE. Dyspigmentation may follow both DLE and SCLE and may be effectively hidden by agents such as Covermark or Dermablend. Scarred lesions may be excised if they are inactive, but the possibility of reactivation resulting from manipulation exists because the Koebner phenomenon has been reported to occur in some patients with LE.

Photosensitivity is generally prevalent in patients with CLE (Lehmann et al. 1990, Millard et al. 2000). Of patients with systemic LE, 57%–73% have a history of photosensitivity, whereas 70%–90% of those with SCLE and 50% of those with DLE report photosensitivity. An issue in the patient with LE is whether they may also have another photosensitive eruption – polymorphous light eruption (PLE). Scandinavian investigators (Nyberg et al. 1997) suggested that 49% of patients with LE also have PLE, whereas Millard et al. (Millard et al. 2000) reported that 50% of their patients with DLE and 60%–70% of their patients with SCLE have PLE. The PLE often precedes the diagnosis of CLE, but it may continue to manifest after the diagnosis. Furthermore, these investigators noted that CLE is a rare consequence of PLE. I observed PLE in patients who were later identified as having SCLE, but it has been my contention that these patients actually had SCLE from the onset of their photosensitivity. Regardless of whether this issue is merely a matter of terminology usage, it is evident

Table 31.1. Therapy for cutaneous lupus erythematosus

Standard therapy:
Thorough evaluation
Is the patient taking any drugs that might exacerbate the disease?
Is the patient a smoker?
Reassurance and education
Sunscreens, sun-protective clothing, and lifestyle alterations
Topical agents – corticosteroids, retinoids
Intralesional corticosteroids
Antimalarial agents – hydroxychloroquine, chloroquine, quinacrine

When standard therapy fails:
Is the patient using the therapy appropriately?
Dapsone
Auranofin
Thalidomide
Retinoids – isotretinoin, acitretin
Immunosuppressive/cytotoxic agents – azathioprine, methotrexate, mycophenolate mofetil, cyclosporine, other
Intravenous immune globulin
Cytokines – interferon α, chimeric CD4 monoclonal antibody
Systemic corticosteroids

that many patients with CLE are photosensitive. The action spectrum has been defined by photoprovocation testing and includes UVA, UVB, and, occasionally, visible light. Phototesting does not reproduce lesions in all or even most patients, and it should be reserved for investigations or for individual circumstances in which it is necessary for worker's compensation or other medicolegal circumstances.

Sunscreens are a cornerstone of therapy, but their importance is often forgotten as the physician manipulates the topical or systemic therapies that the patient is using. The ideal sunscreen would have a broad spectrum and be water resistant. Unfortunately, no sunscreen can block all UV radiation that might exacerbate CLE; therefore, patients should also be encouraged to alter their sun-related behavior and to use sun-protective measures, including sun-protective clothing. A recent study (Stege et al. 2000) examined the capacity of three sunscreens to prevent the development of skin lesions by provocative phototesting. Although each of the three sunscreens tested prevented lesions, the extent to which they did so varied greatly. The sunscreen that was most effective contained octocrylene as the UVB protectant; Mexoryl SX, Mexoryl XL, and Parsol 1789 as UVA protectants; and titanium oxide. This sunscreen's sun protective factor (SPF) was 60. Their study was of only 11 patients (9 men and 2 women), of whom 8 had SCLE and 3 had DLE. This preparation is not available in the United States at the present time. Therefore, it is my recommendation that the patient apply a high SPF, broad-spectrum sunscreen daily.

Topical corticosteroids are usually prescribed for patients with CLE. An appropriate topical corticosteroid is selected for the area of the body being treated as well as the type of lesions that are present. Facial lesions should be treated with low- to mid-potency agents such as 2.5% hydrocortisone, desonide, aclomethasone, or hydrocortisone valerate. Lesions on the trunk and arms may be treated with mid-potency agents such as triamcinolone acetonide or betamethasone valerate. Lesions on the palms or soles and hypertrophic lesions often require superpotent corticosteroids such as clobetasol or halobetasol. Patients prefer creams over ointments; however, ointments may be more potent and are possibly more effective. For lesions on hairy areas, most patients prefer a lotion or foam. Although topical corticosteroids are effective in study settings, in the office setting they do not seem to be as effective, probably because of their expense and messiness. Last, the prescribing physician should consider the total amount of corticosteroid that the patient applies, as it is possible to cause hypothalamic-pituitary-adrenal axis suppression with use of even as little as 2 oz/day of the superpotent corticosteroids.

Several other topical agents might be of use in individual patients with CLE. However, none of these agents have been tested in any systematic manner. Retinoids, specifically, tretinoin, might be effective and have primarily been used in patients with DLE and hypertrophic LE. Tazarotene (Tazorac, a topical retinoid) might also be used. Topical application of calcipotriene (Dovonex, a topical vitamin D derivative) has been reported to be effective in patients with localized scleroderma, but it might also be tried in patients with CLE. Another nonsteroidal agent that might be considered in the future is tacrolimus or pimicrolimus. Finally, because it is known that systemically administered interferon is effective for CLE, it might be helpful to apply imiquimod to individual lesions.

Intralesional injections of corticosteroids are often effective in patients with lesions that are refractory to topical corticosteroids. Small amounts of triamcinolone acetonide may be injected with a 30-gauge needle into multiple areas. These injections are often very effective in the control of lesions, but they do not prevent the development of new lesions. The potential for cutaneous atrophy or dyspigmentation similar to that seen with the disease should be discussed with the patient; however, in most cases, an experienced dermatologist is able to inject without great risk. Also, as noted with topical corticosteroids, the total dose of intralesional corticosteroids should be noted. Alternative agents for intralesional injection have not been well tested. Interferon has been successfully used when given subcutaneously, and it would be interesting to see if lower doses injected into individual lesions would be effective, without systemic ill effects.

When existing lesions are not controlled with topical agents or intralesional corticosteroids, systemic therapy is often indicated. First-line therapy is the use of an antimalarial drug. Antimalarials seem to work less well in patients who smoke (Jewell and McCauliffe 2000, Rahman et al. 1998). The antimalarial agent that I prefer is hydroxychloroquine sulfate (Plaquenil). This drug is used in doses of 200 mg orally once or twice per day or in a dose of less than 6.5 mg/kg per day. The onset of action of the antimalarial agents is roughly 4–8 weeks, and for this reason some physicians have advocated higher initial loading doses. Hydroxychloroquine is also of benefit to the joint symptoms and malaise that may accompany CLE. Hydroxychloroquine is less toxic but also less effective than chloroquine phosphate (Aralen), which is used in doses of 250–500 mg/day. Thus, patients who fail to fully respond to hydroxychloroquine may be switched to chloroquine; however, I believe that these two agents should not be used together because of concern that ophthalmologic toxicity may be enhanced. Another antimalarial, quinacrine hydrochloride (Atabrine), may add benefit to either hydroxychloroquine or chloroquine and is not associated with ophthalmologic toxicity (Feldmann et al. 1994). This agent is not readily available, but several compounding pharmacies in the United States offer it.

Antimalarial drugs may cause nausea, diarrhea, myopathy, cardiomyopathy, or psychosis. Cutaneous eruptions have also been reported with antimalarial drug therapy, as have hyperpigmentation, generalized or localized pruritus, lichenoid drug eruption, or hypopigmentation of the hair, nails, and mucous membranes. Hematologic toxicity may occur and may be manifest late in the course of therapy. Hematologic toxicity seems to be more common with quinacrine therapy than with use of other antimalarials. Fortunately, the frequency of these side effects with antimalarials is relatively uncommon, with the exception of the gastrointestinal tract side effects.

Ocular toxicity, including irreversible retinopathy, has been reported with chloroquine and hydroxychloroquine therapy but not with quinacrine use. The risk of ocular changes is greater with chloroquine therapy. Ophthalmologic toxicity is probably related to the dose and duration of therapy. If detected early, these changes often do not progress if use of the drug is stopped. However, there are patients in whom the drug therapy is discontinued but the retinopathy continues. Although other ocular changes, including blurring of vision and corneal deposition of the antimalarial, occur, these are reversible on cessation of drug therapy. Ophthalmologic evaluation, preferably by a physician familiar with these agents, should be performed at baseline or shortly after initiation of therapy and then periodically (e. g., every 6–12 months).

In difficult cases, multiple other approaches have been advocated for the treatment of CLE. In general, low-dose systemic corticosteroids (< 1 mg/day of prednisone or its equivalent) are rarely effective for DLE and only partially effective for SCLE lesions. Corticosteroids are effective for the acute lesions of photosensitivity, malar rash, or vasculitic lesions that may complicate LE. The long-term use of oral or intramuscular corticosteroids for patients with cutaneous disease should be avoided.

Dapsone, given in doses of 25–200 mg daily, has been useful for patients with vasculitic lesions that may accompany LE, SCLE lesions, bullous LE, and oral ulcerations (Neri et al. 1999). In open-label clinical trials, dapsone treatment resulted in improvement in some patients with DLE or SCLE; however, the level of benefit has been judged as "excellent" in only approximately 25% of patients. In contradistinction, clofazimine failed to demonstrate efficacy in all but one report (Krivanek and Paver 1980). There are several special circumstances in which dapsone may be useful. The first is bullous LE. In addition, patients with urticarial vasculitis along with SCLE lesions may benefit from the use of dapsone. In my practice, I have observed only one patient who seemed to benefit from dapsone therapy; therefore, it is the first line of therapy for only a few patients.

A variety of other antibiotics have been used for the treatment of CLE. Recently, Rudnicka et al. (Rudnicka et al. 2000) reported that use of the antibiotic cefuroxime axetil resulted in the clearing of skin lesions in three patients with SCLE at a dose of 500 mg daily. Cefuroxime axetil is a second-generation β-lactamase oral cephalosporin. Others must replicate this observation before it can be recommended for widespread use; however, it is a relatively benign form of treatment. Another group has reported the successful use of sulfasalazine in 8 of 11 patients (Delaporte et al. 1997). Sulfasalazine is used for inflammatory bowel disease and various arthritides.

These authors administered 2 g daily, but they noted that the minimal effective daily dose was 1.5 g. The eight patients who responded were all rapid acetylators, whereas the three who failed to respond were all slow acetylators. No serious toxicity was noted in this small open-label case series. In contrast, Lagrange et al. noted a drug eruption in five of six patients they treated with sulfasalazine, and in only two patients did they believe that there was a beneficial effect (Lagrange et al. 1998).

Auranofin (Ridura), an oral form of gold, has been used for CLE (Dalziel et al. 1986). Complete remission occurs in a few patients, approximately 15%, whereas a partial response has been noted in about two thirds of those treated. My personal experience has been encouraging in a few patients. Auranofin is begun at a dose of 3 mg/day, and after 1 week the dose may be raised to twice daily if the patient experiences no problem with nausea, diarrhea, or headache. I have treated patients with as high as 3 mg three times daily without difficulty. Monitoring with regular complete blood cell counts and urinalysis is suggested. Responsiveness may be best in patients with non-scarring forms of CLE. I have seen one patient with a lichenoid drug eruption presumed to be due to auranofin use. She had been treated with auranofin for "anti-malarial-resistant" SCLE, and the dose had been raised when the eruption occurred. Cessation of the drug led to resolution of the eruption, and control of her SCLE was achieved with aggressive sun-protection measures and chloroquine therapy.

Thalidomide has recently become more available and is being used for patients with CLE with some regularity (Atra and Sato 1993, Duong et al. 1999, Ordi-Ros et al. 2000). Its mechanism of action is believed to involve a decrease in inflammatory mediators, particularly tumor necrosis factor (TNF)-α and Fas-ligand. Open-label trials suggest that it is highly effective and may result in an increase in the lymphocyte count and a decrease in the C-reactive protein level. Induction with 100–300 mg daily at bedtime results in improvement in 90% of the patients who can tolerate the drug. Toxicity commonly associated with thalidomide use includes drowsiness, headache, weight gain, amenorrhea, and dizziness. Drowsiness and dizziness may persist during the following day. Neuropathy, usually sensory, may limit the ability of patients to continue thalidomide therapy on a long-term basis. Neuropathy may be reversible, but there are patients whose neuropathy has progressed despite discontinuing the drug therapy. Whether nerve conduction studies should be performed at the onset of therapy and periodically is not known. Thalidomide is a potent teratogen and, accordingly, the company has developed a program to prevent the chance of pregnancy in patients exposed to the drug. The program requires that the prescribing physician and the pharmacy be registered with the company and that the patient take extra precautions in taking the drug. No more than a 1-month supply may be written for at any one time. Unfortunately, the response to thalidomide therapy is not durable in most patients; therefore, long-term, low-dose maintenance therapy may be necessary.

Rodriquez-Castellanos and coworkers (Rodriquez-Castellanos et al. 1995) treated 93 patients with CLE with oral phenytoin (up to 300 mg/day) and observed excellent results in 90%. Relapse occurred in at least one third of the patients in whom follow-up data were available, but prolonged remission of 6–12 months was noted in 33 patients. Toxicity was minimal in prevalence and severity.

Oral retinoids are effective in many patients who have failed previous less toxic therapies. Isotretinoin (Accutane) and acitretin (Soriatane) have both been used in doses similar to those used for acne vulgaris and psoriasis, respectively (Newton et al. 1986, Ruzicka et al. 1985). The response is not durable, and after short courses the patient will still need further suppressive therapy. These agents are particularly helpful in patients with hypertrophic lesions or those with lesions on the palms or soles. These patients are monitored for lipid abnormalities, liver enzyme elevations, and cytopenias. In addition, these agents are teratogenic and should not be used in potentially pregnant women. If the clinician decides to use these agents in women of childbearing age, pregnancy prevention counseling should take place at each visit and pregnancy prevention methods should be provided to the patient.

Several cytotoxic agents have been reported to be beneficial for the control of CLE lesions. Azathioprine has perhaps had the greatest number of reports (Callen et al. 1991), but methotrexate (Boehm et al. 1998) and mycophenolate mofetil (Pashinian et al. 1998, Goyal and Nousari 2001) have also been reported to benefit patients with "recalcitrant" disease. We treated six patients with refractory disease, and most improved within 4–8 weeks. Continued therapy is required to maintain the remission. Small case series or individual reports have suggested that cytarabine, cyclophosphamide, and cyclosporine may be effective.

High-dose intravenous immune globulin was used by Lagrange et al. (Lagrange et al. 2004) in nine patients and by Genereau et al. (Genereau et al. 1999) in one patient. One gram per kilogram per day for 2 consecutive days monthly was administered to patients who had failed multiple previous therapies. There was an excellent result in 4 of the 10 patients, but the response is short-lived. Toxicity is minimal, but this therapy is extremely expensive.

The use of cytokine therapy has been reported. I predict that there will be additional reports of newer agents that are available and are just beginning to be tested for some dermatologic indications, as well as others that are not currently on the market. Because thalidomide may be effective through its effects on TNF-α, it might be possible that infliximab or etanercept therapy might also prove to be of benefit to patients with CLE. However, at least one patient developed SCLE while taking etanercept (Bleumink et al. 2001). Interferon-α has been used successfully (Nicolas et al. 1990, Tebbe et al. 1992); however, all patients taking this regimen develop toxicity, and long-term remission is rarely achieved. In contrast, Prinz and colleagues (Prinz et al. 1996) used chimeric CD4 monoclonal antibody infusions in five patients with severe, refractory CLE. Long-lasting improvement was noted, with restoration of responsiveness to conventional treatments. If other cytokines can be administered and result in the restoration of response with less toxic therapy, then perhaps we will be able to induce remission with one agent and maintain it with another.

Conclusion

In summary, patients with LE may manifest a variety of skin lesions. A thorough evaluation of any given patient is needed before therapy. Patients may have factors that exacerbate their disease, such as light from the sun or from artificial sources, drugs, or smoking. If possible, therapy should begin with the removal of any identified exacerbating factors and include sunscreens, protective clothing, behavioral alteration, and topical corticosteroids. Calcipotriene or retinoids may be effective in some patients. Intralesional injection of corticosteroids and oral antimalarials are the other parts of a standard therapy program. The choice of alternative therapy is personal, and discussions of the risks and benefits should be carefully documented. Successful therapy for CLE is possible in almost all well-motivated, cooperative patients.

References

Atra E, Sato EI (1993) Treatment of cutaneous lesions of systemic lupus erythematosus with thalidomide. Clin Exp Rheumatol 11:487–493

Bleumink GS, ter Borg EJ, Ramselaar CG, Ch Stricker BH (2001) Etanercept-induced subacute cutaneous lupus erythematosus. Rheuamtology (Oxford) 40:1317–1319

Boehm IB, Boehm GA, Bauer R (1998) Management of cutaneous lupus erythematosus with low-dose methotrexate: indication for modulation of inflammatory mechanisms. Rheumatol Int 18:59–62

Bonsmann G, Schiller M, Luger TA, Stander S (2001) Terbinafine-induced subacute cutaneous lupus erythematosus. J Am Acad Dermatol 44:925–931

Callen JP, Kulp-Shorten CL, Hughes AP (2001) Subacute cutaneous lupus erythematosus associated with terbinafine therapy. Arch Dermatol 137:1196–1198

Callen JP, Spencer LV, Burruss JB, Holtman J (1991) Azathioprine: an effective, corticosteroids-sparing therapy for patients with recalcitrant cutaneous lupus erythematosus or with recalcitrant cutaneous leukocytoclastic vasculitis. Arch Dermatol 127:515–522

Callen JP (2001) Therapy of cutaneous lupus erythematosus. Dermatologic Therapy 14:61–69

Crowson AN, Magro CM (1997) Subacute cutaneous lupus erythematosus arising in the setting of calcium channel blocker therapy. Hum Pathol 28:67–73

Dalziel K, Going G, Cartwright PH, Marks R, Beveridge GW, Rowell NR (1986) Treatment of chronic discoid lupus erythematosus with an oral gold compound (Auranofin) Br J Dermatol 115:211–216

Delaporte E, Catteau B, Sabbagh N, Gosselin P, Breuillard F, Doutre MS, Broly F, Piette F, Bergoend H (1997) Traitment du lupus erythemateux chronique par la sulfasalazine: 11 observations. Ann Dermatol Venereol 124:151–156

Duong JD, Spigel T, Moxley RT III, Gaspari AA (1999) American experience with low-dose thalidomide therapy for severe cutaneous lupus erythematosus. Arch Dermatol 135:1079–1087

Feldmann R, Salomon D, Saurat JH (1994) The association of the two antimalarials chloroquine and quinacrine for treatment-resistant chronic and subacute cutaneous lupus erythematosus. Dermatology 189:425–427

Gallego H, Crutchfield CE III, Lewis EJ, Gallego HJ (1999) Report of an association between discoid lupus erythematosus and smoking. Cutis 63:231–234

Genereau T, Chosidow O, Danel C, Cherin P, Herson S (1999) High-dose intravenous immunoglobulin in cutaneous lupus erythematosus. Arch Dermatol 135:1124–1125

Goyal S, Nousari HC (2001) Treatment of resistant discoid lupus erythematosus of the palms and soles with mycophenolate mofetil. J Am Acad Dermatol 45:142–144

Jewell ML, McCauliffe DP (2000) Patients with cutaneous lupus erythematosus who smoke are less responsive to antimalarial treatment. J Am Acad Dermatol 42:983–987

Krivanek JFC, Paver WKA (1980) Further study of the use of clofazimine in discoid lupus erythematosus. Australasian J Dermatol 21:169–171

Lagrange S, Piette JC, Becherel PA, Cacoub P, Frances C (1998) Sulfasalazine in the treatment of cutaneous lupus erythematosus: open trial in six cases. Lupus 7:21

Lagrange S, Frances C, Roy S, Papo T, Piette JC (2004) High dose intravenous immune globulin in the treatment of refractory severe discoid lupus erythematosus. J Am Acad Dermatol, in press

Lehmann P, Holzle E, Kind P, Goerz G, Plewig G (1990) Experimental reproduction of skin lesions in lupus erythematosus by UVA and UVB radiation. J Am Acad Dermatol 22:181–187

Millard TP, Hawk JLM, McGregor JM (2000) Photosensitivity in lupus. Lupus 9:3–10

Neri R, Mosca M, Bernacchi E, Bombardieri S (1999) A case of SLE with acute, subacute and chronic cutaneous lesions successfully treated with dapsone. Lupus 8:240–243

Newton RC, Jorizzo JL, Solomon AR, Sanchez R, Bell JD, Cavallo T (1986) Mechanism-oriented assessment of isotretinoin in chronic of Subacute cutaneous lupus erythematosus. Arch Dermatol 122:180–186

Nicolas JF, Thivolet J, Kanitkis J, Lyonnet S (1990) Response of discoid and Subacute cutaneous lupus erythematosus to recombinant interferon alpha 2a. J Invest Dermatol 95:142S–145S

Nyberg F, Hassan T, Puska P, Stephansson E, Hakkinen M, Ranki A, Ros AM (1997) Occurrence of polymorphous light eruption in lupus erythematosus. Br J Dermatol 136:217–221

Ordi-Ros J, Cortes F, Cucurull E, Mauri M, Bujan S, Vilardell M (2000) Thalidomide in the treatment of cutaneous lupus erythematosus refractory to conventional therapy. J Rheumatol 27:1429–1433

Pashinian N, Wallace DJ, Klinenberg JR (1998) Mycophenolate mofetil for systemic lupus erythematosus. Arthritis Rheum 41:S110

Prinz JC, Meurer M, Reiter C, Rieber EP, Plewig G, Riethmuller G (1996) Treatment of severe cutaneous lupus erythematosus with a chimeric CD4 monoclonal antibody, cM-T412. J Am Acad Dermatol 34:244–252

Rahman P, Gladman DD, Urowitz MB (1998) Smoking interferes with efficacy of antimalarial therapy in cutaneous lupus. J Rheumatol 25:1716–1719

Reed BR, Huff JC, Jones SK, Orton PW, Lee LA, Norris DA (1985) Subacute cutaneous lupus erythematosus associated with hydrochlorothiazide therapy. Ann Intern Med 103:49–51

Rodriquez-Castellanos MA, Rubio JB, Gomez JFB, Mendoza AG (1995) Phenytoin in the treatment of discoid lupus erythematosus. Arch Dermatol 131:620–621

Rudnicka L, Szymanska E, Walecka I, Stowinska M (2000) Long-term cefuroxime axetil in subacute cutaneous lupus erythematosus. A report of three cases. Dermatology 200:129–131

Ruzicka T, Meurer M, Brown-Falco O (1985) Treatment of cutaneous lupus erythematosus with etretinate. Acta Derm Venereol 65:324–329

Stege H, Budde MA, Grether S, Krutmann J (2000) Evaluation of the capacity of sunscreens to photoprotect lupus erythematosus patients by employing the photoprovocation test. Photodermatol Photoimmunol Photomed 16:256–259

Tebbe B, Lauy M, Gollnick H (1992) Therapy of cutaneous lupus erythematosus with recombinant interferon alpha-2a. Eur J Dermatol 2:253–255

Acknowledgements

The editors thank Lisa Cluver, Editorial Today, Sunrise Beach, Missouri, USA; Sigrid Petermann and Assem Dittmann, Department of Dermatology, University of Düsseldorf, Germany, for copy editing the manuscripts; and Essex Pharma GmbH, München, Germany, for financial support which made possible the use of color illustrations. Furthermore, this work was supported by a Heisenberg professorship from the German Research Association (DFG) to A. Kuhn.

Subject Index